The C...
Coun...

FOR

DUMMIES

by Rosanne Rust, MS, RD, LDN
with Meri Raffetto, RD, LDN

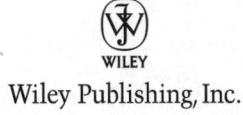

WILEY

Wiley Publishing, Inc.

The Calorie Counter For Dummies®

Published by
Wiley Publishing, Inc.
111 River St.
Hoboken, NJ 07030-5774
www.wiley.com

For general information on our other products and services, please contact our Customer Care Department within the U.S. at 877-762-2974, outside the U.S. at 317-572-3993, or fax 317-572-4002.

For technical support, please visit www.wiley.com/techsupport.

Wiley also publishes its books in a variety of electronic formats. Some content that appears in print may not be available in electronic books.

Library of Congress Control Number: 2009939353

ISBN: 978-0-470-56834-7

Manufactured in the United States of America

10 9 8 7 6 5 4 3 2 1

WILEY

Contents at a Glance

Introduction

According to recent data from the National Center for Health Statistics, about two-thirds of adults in the United States are overweight, and almost one-third are obese. Consumers must come to terms with the fact that eating *behavior and choices* are what drive their struggles with excessive weight. Changing your eating behaviors is a multifaceted process that involves commitment and support, but one thing remains true: You must consume fewer calories.

A major influence on today's high calorie intake is restaurant dining. On a typical day in the United States in 2009, more than 130 million individuals patronized a food-service establishment, and there's no sign that this trend will change. But just because more people are dining out doesn't mean they're any less concerned about making healthy food choices. What they may not realize, though, is that diet plays a role in disease risk and management.

Getting the right amount of calories from a variety of foods and with a focus on whole grains, fruits, and vegetables creates the healthiest diet. The foods you eat should provide key nutrients, such as vitamins A, C, and E; B-vitamins, vitamin D; fiber; and omega-3 fatty acids. A healthy diet should also be low in saturated fat and sodium.

Whether you're eating at home or dining out, considering calorie intake and proper nutrition is a good idea. *The Calorie Counter For Dummies* is the perfect companion to eating on the go because it includes nutritional information for everyday foods as well as many popular restaurants foods and beverages. With it, you have the information you need to balance your diet for better health.

About This Book

The Calorie Counter For Dummies is your handy nutritional reference guide for common foods and popular restaurants. You can keep it in your car, your purse, or at your desk at work.

Why count calories? Well, we don't recommend obsessing over every calorie you eat all day, but having an idea of how many calories are in different foods is useful knowledge. Think of it as "calorie awareness."

This book will help you understand how different foods compare to each other so you can make an informed choice about what you eat. You'll gain a better understanding of how you can balance your diet throughout the week and discover how to decipher nutrient profiles so you can determine what's important to your health.

The Calorie Counter For Dummies is for anyone interested in good health. Although we're casting a wide net with that statement, we think it rings true. If one or more of these descriptions hits home, you've come to the right place:

✔ You only use fast food in situations where you're on the road or away from home, and you want to make the best choices.

✔ You frequent restaurants on a daily basis, and you feel now is the time to take control of your dietary decisions.

✔ You're watching your total calorie and/or sodium intake.

✔ You're concerned about weight control, heart health, diabetes, or high blood pressure.

If you're a parent, here's a special note for you: As the guardian of your child's health, it's up to you to pass along good habits for your children to model. By showing your child that you're aware of the types of foods you choose to eat and are making healthier choices in order to manage your own health, you'll be setting a good example.

Conventions Used in This Book

This guide provides you with nutritional data for common foods and nearly 140 popular restaurants. We've chosen to highlight a few key nutrients that have the greatest impact on health and disease risk: calories (Cal), fat, saturated fat (Sfat), sodium (Sod), carbohydrates (Carb), fiber, sugar, and protein (Prot).

Following is a quick primer on how these different nutritional values are measured (we skip over calories because that one's pretty self explanatory):

Nutritional Value	Measured in
Fat	Grams
Saturated fat	Grams
Sodium	Milligrams
Carbohydrates	Grams
Fiber	Grams
Sugar	Grams
Protein	Grams

Here's a cheat sheet to some other abbreviations we use within the nutritional data:

Abbreviation	Meaning
&	and
amt	amount
approx.	approximately
avg	average
diam	diameter
ea	each
equiv	equivalent
g	grams
indv	individual
lrg	large
med	medium
mg	milligrams
NP	not provided
oz	ounce
pc	piece
reg	regular

Abbreviation	*Meaning*
sml	small
std	standard
tbsp	tablespoon
tsp	teaspoon
vit A/C	vitamin A or C
w/	with
w/o	without

We also want to mention that we didn't really have room to include trademark symbols for all the various nuggets, nibblers, uperchinos, and other brand-name items offered by the fine restaurants in this book. So we reiterate what's on the copyright page: All trademarks listed in this book are the property of their respective owners. Wiley Publishing, Inc., is not associated with any product or vendor mentioned in *The Calorie Counter For Dummies.*

How This Book Is Organized

The three parts in this book are designed to provide you with guidance in making better food choices whether you're dining out or eating in.

Part 1: Healthy Eating 101

Here we've outlined some basic guidelines for healthier eating and included tips based on a few common health concerns: weight control, high cholesterol, diabetes, and high blood pressure. Take note of the specific guidelines that apply to your needs to make the best choices for your situation.

Part II: Restaurant Guide

In a perfect world, you'd have the time and energy to cook a fresh, healthy meal every night, but that's just not how most folks live these days. Because we don't expect you to be perfect, we're giving you the nutrition facts for 150 popular restaurants so you can make informed choices when dining out. You can even impress your friends with these handy facts too! (Beware the fallout of reporting the calories in that three-cheese, triple-patty burger with bacon that your friend just ate for lunch though.)

Part III: Common Food Guide

We by no means want to discourage you from preparing meals at home because that's the best way to control calories and provide your body with adequate nutrients. So we've included a part that provides the nutrient data for common foods. If you do a quick comparison between the two types of products, you can see why eating at home is usually a better option. (And if this part inspires you to cook more at home, consider picking up a copy of *Lowfat Cooking For Dummies* or *30-Minute Meals For Dummies,* both published by Wiley.)

Where to Go from Here

If you need to brush up on some healthy eating guidelines, take a look at the chapters in Part I. If you're curious about the nutritional content of food items at your favorite restaurants, dive in to Part II. You're likely to find some shocking information.

Part I
Healthy Eating 101

The 5th Wave
By Rich Tennant

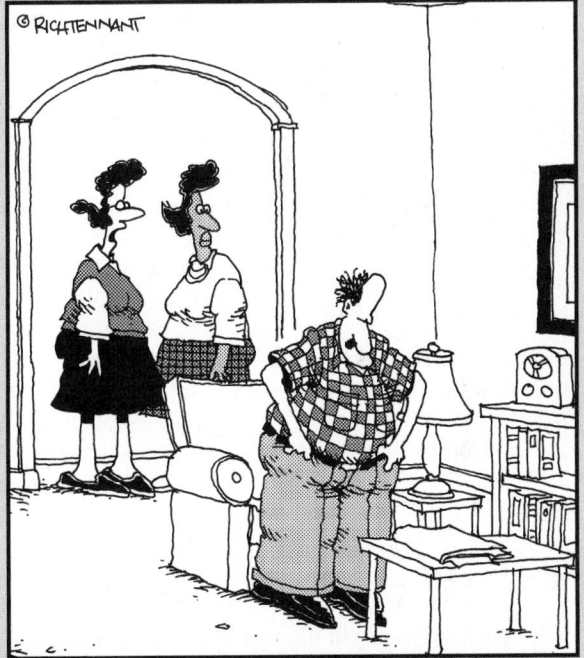

"Phillip's doctor told him diet, exercise, and genes can effect your cholesterol levels, so he cut out fatty foods, walks everyday, and switched to chinos."

In this part . . .

*N*o matter what your personal situation may be, eating healthfully is easy to do when you have a few basic guidelines in mind. That's why this part introduces you to the concept of balanced eating and explains the basics of how to go about it — whether you're enjoying a nice meal at home or dining at your favorite restaurant.

If you want to lose weight, or if you have high blood pressure, high cholesterol, or diabetes, this part is also your resource for specific healthy-eating information geared toward your needs.

Chapter 1

Keep Your Balance

● ●

In This Chapter

▶ Developing a balanced lifestyle

▶ Making healthier decisions when dining out

● ●

*B*alance is what a healthy body is all about. Every system within your body constantly strives for balance, and it's this balance that keeps your health stable and your systems functioning.

We bet you're no stranger to the phrase *balanced diet*. However, do you have any idea what that phrase really means? This chapter takes a stab at defining it for you. It also features tips for healthy eating when dining out so you can find balance even at your favorite restaurant.

Balancing Act

So what exactly is a balanced diet? There's no one perfect diet, but a balanced diet is one that includes a variety of foods from each basic food group every day. Eating different foods from each food group guarantees you're getting adequate carbohydrates, proteins, fats, vitamins, and minerals. A balanced diet also infers that energy needs are balanced with physical activity; that is, you take in the exact amount of calories your body needs to function and maintain a healthy weight.

Of course, most people can't eat perfectly at every meal of every day. To really succeed in achieving a balanced diet, consider your diet through the week, not necessarily at only one meal.

Strive for a little variety

Nobody likes to eat the same thing all the time. One of the ways you can help yourself eat a balanced diet on a daily basis is to really make an effort to choose a variety of foods. By *variety* we mean you should pick different types of foods within each food group. So even if you love bananas, you should try to mix things up and eat an apple, a plum, some melon, or berries every week. Hey, go crazy: Try a kiwifruit or mango once in a while too!

Eat fruits and vegetables

Fruits and vegetables are nutritional powerhouses, and they play a vital role in a balanced diet. When you're on the go, bring fruit to work or school with you, or grab an apple on your way out the door. This behavior strategy helps round out your diet by providing important vitamins and minerals, thereby balancing out the higher-fat, higher-calorie choices you may make at other times. It also adds fiber to your diet, and fiber helps control hunger, aiding in weight control.

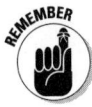

Eat at least two servings of fruit daily, gradually increasing this amount to three or four.

And what about those pesky vegetables? Well, they're very low in calories and rich in vitamins and fiber, plus they add color and healthy *phytochemicals* (nonnutritive plant chemicals that have protective or disease-preventive properties). And despite what you may recall from childhood, vegetables can be delicious if prepared properly.

Grilling is a really quick and easy way to prepare vegetables as a side dish or pasta topping. Vegetables such as bell peppers, eggplant, zucchini, onions, potatoes, and portobello mushrooms all do well on the grill.

Adding more fruits and vegetables to your diet when you eat at home is important because choices are slim and sometimes nonexistent in many restaurants, especially the fast-food variety. If you can choose a fruit or vegetable when dining out, do so, but in some restaurants, your best bet is simply to make lower-calorie, lower-sodium choices. Doing so gives you a better shot at balancing out nutrients to meet your body's needs overall.

Embrace exercise and sleep

The diets of people who are overweight are usually unbalanced. Being overweight is a risk factor for

Type 2 diabetes and heart disease. If you need to lose weight, check with your physician and do the following:

- ✔ **Exercise regularly.** Including physical activity (also known as exercise) with a balanced diet is a great way to stimulate weight loss.

- ✔ **Get more sleep.** Research has shown that getting adequate sleep helps with weight control. When you're well rested, you're able to make reasonable decisions, thereby passing up that 460-calorie sweet potato casserole in favor of the 60-calorie steamed vegetables.

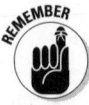

Losing weight is all about finding balance. (There's that word again.) Make exercise a habit, but also make sure you get enough rest.

Perhaps you're on a high-protein diet in an effort to lose weight. Although this type of diet can lead to successful weight loss, fast-food restaurants aren't the place to stick to it because most of the high-protein foods offered there are also high in fat. So, please, no "double bacon cheeseburger without the bun" orders.

Basic Tips When Dining Out

Dining out can be an enjoyable experience, but it can also be a high-calorie one. However, with a bit of planning ahead, you can manage to enjoy your dining experience without the worry of eating too many calories or sacrificing health. Consider these tips to save calories the next time you dine out:

✔ Ask for dressings or sauces on the side, or skip the mayo.

✔ Consider an appetizer or side dish as an entrée, or choose the regular, small, or kid-sized portion. (Skip anything that's extra-large or supersized.)

✔ Choose nonfat or lowfat milk and coffee drinks (pick the small or "tall" size for the latter).

✔ Select grilled or oven-roasted items and skip the deep-fried foods.

✔ Drink more water with your meals.

✔ Review beverage sizes and calories. You can rack up several hundred calories a day in liquid if you don't monitor your intake.

✔ Watch out for salads; they aren't always the low-calorie choice.

✔ Include as many vegetable toppings as possible on your sandwich, in your omelet, or on your pizza.

✔ Skip the butter on breakfast items such as waffles or pancakes and use smaller amounts of syrup.

✔ Enjoy your eggs with toast, but skip the extra meat item.

✔ Skip the extra cheese on anything whatsoever.

✔ Choose pastas with marinara or olive oil–based sauces rather than cream or Alfredo-type ones.

✔ Consider splitting an item with a friend and ordering a side salad to round out your meal (unless of course you're splitting dessert).

✔ Bring this guide with you and choose wisely!

If you currently eat out daily, consider cutting back to eating no more than three meals per week away from home (not counting packed lunches). Ideally, you should limit dining out to two or fewer times a week.

Chapter 2

Dietary Guidelines for Optimal Health

* *

In This Chapter

▶ Watching calories to lose weight

▶ Limiting fats to prevent high cholesterol

▶ Cutting back on sodium to regulate blood pressure

▶ Spreading out your carbs to control diabetes

* *

*I*f you're like most people, you're concerned about your overall health. Maybe you just want to lose weight. Perhaps you're trying to prevent conditions such as heart disease, high cholesterol, and high blood pressure. You may even be trying to eat better in order to treat an existing condition, such as diabetes.

This chapter provides some dietary guidelines based on these five common health concerns and offers recommendations on healthy restaurant menu options for each one.

Weight Loss

Excess body weight is associated with risk factors for several diseases, namely heart disease and diabetes. Being overweight or obese may also aggravate your joint health and either hasten or worsen arthritis. It can also affect high blood pressure.

The current standard for determining healthy body weights is the Body Mass Index (BMI). BMI measures your overall "fatness" and is a better indicator of health than simply body weight for one's height. You should strive for a normal BMI, valued between 19 and 24. A BMI of 25 to 29 indicates you're overweight, and a BMI of 30 or higher indicates you're obese. Check with your doctor or registered dietitian to determine what a healthy weight is for you.

General dietary considerations for weight loss:

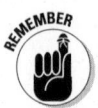

✔ To lose weight, you must reduce your total calorie intake. Eating 500 calories less a day will promote the loss of 1 pound per week.

✔ Check out the calories in common foods that you eat each week to determine where you can make a change or reduce portion sizes.

✔ Include fiber in your diet. Fiber (found in fruits, vegetables, beans, lentils, and foods made with whole grains) provides denseness without the calories, meaning you can actually eat a bit more without upping your calorie intake. Shoot for 3 grams of fiber or more per serving.

✔ Add one to two vegetable servings to your diet daily. Have carrots available to snack on, slice an apple, or eat a banana. You'll be surprised how easy this is to do if you plan on it.

✔ Drink at least six to eight 8-ounce glasses of water every day.

✔ Analyze your eating behaviors to see whether any of them are possibly sabotaging your weight-loss efforts. Skipping meals, avoiding food groups, and eating when you're stressed or bored can all hinder weight loss.

✔ Get support. If you need to lose weight, find a professional to help you do it. Talk to your doctor about consulting a registered dietitian (RD) or certified personal trainer (CPT).

Quick tips for eating fast food if you're trying to lose weight:

✔ Try to limit a meal's calories to between 400 and 600 for women and between 500 and 700 for men.

✔ Choose an appetizer for a main entrée and order a side salad to go with it.

✔ Select lowfat salad dressings when available, or just use less of the full-fat ones.

✔ Share a side dish or dessert with someone.

✔ Drink your whole glass of water (or more!) but limit other beverages to just one glass.

✔ Take home half the meal for a delicious lunch the next day. You may even want to physically split the meal in half when it arrives at your table and ask for the to-go box right away so as to avoid the uncomfortable stomach pain that follows from eating the whole thing.

✔ Fit exercise into your day whenever possible. If you dine out for lunch for business, arrange to walk to your destinations. Every little bit helps.

Menu options for weight loss:

✔ Add fiber to your salad bar selection with beans and other fresh vegetables. For example, you can top leafy greens with garbanzo beans and three-bean salad. Whatever you do, avoid the creamy premade salads or sweet salad toppings.

✔ When it comes to prepared entrée salads, look for ones that have less than 300 calories.

✔ Choose the small or "junior" burger or roast beef sandwich with lettuce, tomato, ketchup, mustard, pickle, and onion. Hold the cheese and mayo.

✔ Be mindful of sodium. Sodium, found in salt, can cause your body to retain fluid (which leads to excess water weight). Ideally, you should aim for less than 240 milligrams of sodium per serving.

✔ Choose whole-wheat bread over white bread whenever possible to up your fiber intake. (***Remember:*** Fiber makes you feel fuller longer.)

✔ Order a side salad rather than French fries, or share a small order of fries with someone.

✔ Choose low-calorie grilled items.

✔ Order baked or grilled fish if it's available.

Heart Disease or High Cholesterol

Diet is an important part of treatment for high cholesterol (which can increase your risk for heart disease if left unchecked). If you have this condition, perhaps your doctor told you to follow a lowfat diet. Just what does that mean? In general, it means you should pay close attention to the amount of fats in foods, particularly saturated fat (less than 7 percent of your daily calories should be from saturated fat). The amount of fat you need daily depends on your height, weight, and activity; most men only need about 65 to 75 grams of fat per day, and most women only need about 50 to 60 grams per day.

You should work to limit dietary cholesterol (which by the way is found only in animal products; so eat more plants!), but your focus should be on reducing fat. Trans fats have been linked to heart disease, so we encourage you to limit them as much as possible. Talk with your doctor about consulting a registered dietitian for help changing your diet to lower your blood cholesterol.

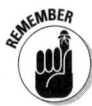

A lowfat diet should also contain adequate amounts of fiber (about 20 to 30 grams per day). So try to eat a lowfat, high-fiber diet.

General dietary considerations for heart disease or high cholesterol:

- ✔ Limit your intake of saturated fat found in high-fat meats (such as prime rib, beef or pork ribs, salami, pepperoni, sausage, and chicken skin) and whole-milk products (such as sour cream, half and half, butter, and cheese).

- ✔ Include more fish in your heart-healthy diet — just make sure it's not fried. Choose grilled fish or seafood when it's available.

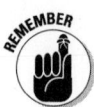

✔ Keep your portion sizes under control. Portion size is of utmost importance when you're trying to maintain a lowfat diet or cut calories to promote weight loss. Even the healthiest roasted chicken, for example, can provide too much fat if you eat the whole chicken in one sitting.

✔ Consider choosing smaller portions of foods you love. If you have a craving for French fries, choose the smallest order and "count" that fat as part of your overall fat intake for the day.

✔ Use food labels to help you make lowfat choices. U.S. food label guidelines require a food to have less than 3 grams of fat per serving to qualify as lowfat and less than 1 gram of saturated fat to be considered low in saturated fat. When it comes to fast food, you may loosen that guideline for one meal, but then make lower-fat choices at other meals that day.

✔ Be aware that there may be some "hidden fat" in your diet because not all foods come with complete nutritional information.

Quick tips for eating fast food if you have heart disease or high cholesterol:

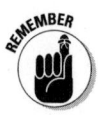

✔ Check both the fat and the saturated fat. Total fat per 500-calorie meal should be about 15 grams or less. Saturated fat per meal should be less than 4 grams per 500-calorie meal (or less than 1 gram per 100 calories).

✔ To keep fat in check when eating out, the best choices include grilled, oven-roasted, and baked items rather than deep-fried ones. Check the nutrition information before making this assumption, however, because sometimes seemingly healthy entrées, such as a chicken salad, may have quite a bit of fat and calories compared to a sandwich.

✔ Look for foods that also add some fiber to your meal, such as a green salad, vegetable toppings for your sandwich, or a fruit choice. This simple effort will increase your overall daily fiber intake and add important vitamins and minerals to your diet.

✔ Skip the cheese on your sandwich and save about 10 grams of fat (7 grams of which are saturated) and 80 to 120 calories.

Menu options for heart disease or high cholesterol:

✔ Oven-baked or oven-roasted chicken or turkey

✔ Grilled fish

✔ Baked potatoes with nonfat topping

✔ Side salads

✔ Lowfat fruit and yogurt parfaits

✔ Applesauce, an apple, or fruit slices

High Blood Pressure

Hypertension, or high blood pressure, is an important disorder to monitor. It increases your risk of heart disease or stroke. If your doctor has informed you that you have high blood pressure, be sure to follow his or her advice. You may need medication to reduce it, but diet also plays a role. For most people, lowering the sodium in their diet helps regulate blood pressure. (***Note:*** Making sure you're getting adequate amounts of calcium, vitamins, and minerals is important too.)

General dietary considerations for high blood pressure:

- ✔ Eat a diet rich in fruits and vegetables, whole grains, and nonfat or lowfat dairy, fish, poultry, and nuts.

- ✔ Limit your sodium intake. Your total sodium for the day should be around 1,500 to 2,000 milligrams. However, if you can keep it to 3,000 milligrams, that's a good place to start.

- ✔ Remember that a low-sodium food is one that contains less than 140 milligrams per serving. Limit foods that exceed this amount.

- ✔ Add calcium to your diet. Calcium is found in lowfat dairy products and some vegetables such as broccoli, bok choy, spinach, kale, and collard greens.

- ✔ Limit added salt and processed foods that are high in sodium.

- ✔ Lose weight if you're overweight. Even losing 10 pounds can make a difference in your blood pressure readings.

Quick tips for eating fast food if you have high blood pressure:

- ✔ Investigate sodium levels. Try to pick items that have less than 500 milligrams per serving. (*Note:* Many restaurant foods contain much more than that. See for yourself in Part II.)

- ✔ Skip the soup. Soup is often low in calories, but processed soups are loaded with sodium. Save your soup craving for a home-cooked soup that you can prepare with much less salt.

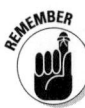

✔ Pass over processed meats such as bacon, sausage, and ham. They tend to have lots of sodium.

✔ Skip the salt shaker. Don't add any additional salt to your foods.

✔ Choose smaller portions and lower-calorie options. (**Remember:** The smaller the portion, the less sodium there is.)

✔ Pick lowfat items. Even though fat itself doesn't directly affect blood pressure, it does affect your overall calorie intake and waistline.

✔ Get your low-calorie calcium by ordering a glass of lowfat or nonfat milk when dining out.

Menu options for high blood pressure:

✔ Small and regular-sized burgers generally have more sodium than a home-cooked burger, but ordering the smallest size saves you sodium.

✔ Most beverages are fine sodium-wise; just remember to still watch out for consuming too many calories.

✔ Chicken salads or garden salads can be safe options; be sure to check the sodium from various vendors.

✔ Choose vinegar- and oil-based dressings or dressings that contain less than 300 milligrams of sodium. Always check the sodium content on various types of dressing because it varies greatly.

✔ Choose fresh toppings, such as onion, tomato, and lettuce, over pickled items, such as jarred pepper strips or pickles.

✔ Say "no cheese" and save about 100 calories and up to 500 milligrams of sodium.

✔ Opt for one egg with toast, a pancake, or a bowl of oatmeal for breakfast over combination meals that include high-fat, high-sodium meats (think sausage, ham, and bacon). Also, consider trying an egg white or "egg substitute" omelet or scramble.

✔ Order baked fish.

✔ Try a fruit cup or piece of fresh fruit as a side dish.

Diabetes

Diet plays a huge role in the management of diabetes, so if you have this disease, you want to pay close attention to how much, and when, you eat. Because having diabetes increases your risk for heart disease, you should maintain a low fat intake in addition to watching your blood sugar.

General dietary considerations for diabetes:

✔ Don't skip meals. For most people, eating three small meals a day plus one or two snacks is a good strategy.

✔ Distribute your carbohydrate intake throughout the day with a fairly equal amount at each meal. Most people need about 45 to 60 grams of carbohydrates per meal, but this amount can vary depending on individual needs.

✔ Don't go overboard on protein and fat. They have calories too and will raise your blood sugar or widen your waistline.

✔ Include fiber in your diet. Fiber slows down the absorption of your meal, thereby reducing how quickly your blood sugar rises and sustaining you for a longer period of time.

✔ Include regular physical activity every week, with your doctor's approval. Exercise helps keep blood sugar in good control.

✔ Maintain a reasonable weight as well as a diet that's low in total fat and saturated fat.

✔ Meet with a registered dietitian or certified diabetes educator (CDE) to help you set up an appropriate meal plan that fits your lifestyle.

Quick tips for eating fast food if you have diabetes:

✔ Look for special healthy menu items. More and more restaurants are adding such items to their menus.

✔ Ask for dressings or sauces on the side.

✔ Assess portion sizes. Use this guide to determine calories, carbohydrates, and fat per serving and modify your serving appropriately by either sharing an entrée or getting a to-go box. Always skip the jumbo or super-sized portions.

✔ Choose a lowfat appetizer as a meal and order a side salad to go with it.

✔ If a fast-food meal is overboard on fat or sodium, make up for it by consuming lower-fat, lower-sodium foods at other meals and snacks.

✔ Look for foods that are high in fiber.

✔ Skip the cheese, or extra cheese, because it racks up 100 calories or more per ounce.

✔ Watch out for what sounds like a better choice. Items such as fat-free muffins may indeed contain no fat, but they may also contain plenty of sugar and calories.

Menu options for diabetes:

✔ A salad or steamed vegetable as a side dish and a fruit for dessert

✔ Thin-crust pizza

✔ Small or "junior" burger

✔ Grilled chicken sandwich

✔ Seafood salad

✔ Scrambled egg whites or egg substitute

✔ Turkey sausage, one patty

✔ Baked salmon

✔ Half of a baked potato (restaurant potatoes are usually so large that they may have 50 grams of carbohydrates each)

Part II
Restaurant Guide

The 5th Wave   By Rich Tennant

"Oh, I have a very healthy relationship with food. It's the relationship I have with my scale that's not so good."

In this part . . .

*E*ver wonder what the calorie content is for that delicious-looking salad from Panera? Not sure whether you should order the chicken or the fish at McDonald's if you're trying to watch your fat intake? All the mysteries are revealed in this part, which presents nutrition information for nearly 140 popular restaurants. Use this data to make informed decisions about what you're eating so you can continue to create balance in your diet even when you're not wearing that "Kiss the Cook" apron.

Description & Serving	Cal	Fat	Sfat	Sod	Carb	Fiber	Sugar	Prot

Arby's

Breakfast

Description & Serving	Cal	Fat	Sfat	Sod	Carb	Fiber	Sugar	Prot
Bacon, Egg, & Cheese Wrap	515	29	8	1367	50	2	2	16
Ham, Egg, & Cheese Wrap	575	31	10	2005	51	2	3	25
Sausage, Egg, & Cheese Wrap	689	45	15	1849	50	2	2	21
Biscuit, plain	273	15	4	786	28	1	3	5
Bacon Biscuit	340	21	6	1028	29	1	3	9
Bacon, Egg, & Cheese Biscuit	461	30	10	1446	30	1	4	17
Chicken Biscuit	417	23	5	1240	39	1	3	15
Ham Biscuit	323	17	4	1315	29	1	4	14
Ham, Egg, & Cheese Biscuit	444	26	8	1734	31	1	4	21
Sausage Biscuit	436	31	9	1160	28	1	3	10
Sausage Gravy Biscuit	1040	60	22	4700	107	1	4	7
Sausage, Egg, & Cheese Biscuit	557	40	13	1579	30	1	3	18
Croissant	190	10	6	190	21	1	2	3
Bacon & Egg Croissant	337	22	10	651	23	1	3	11
Bacon, Egg, & Cheese Croissant	378	25	12	850	23	1	3	14
Ham & Cheese Croissant	281	15	9	918	22	1	3	14
Ham, Egg, & Cheese Croissant	361	21	10	1138	23	1	4	19
Sausage & Egg Croissant	433	32	13	784	23	1	3	12
Sausage, Egg, & Cheese Croissant	475	35	15	982	23	1	3	15
Egg & Cheese Sourdough	392	17	7	1058	40	2	5	17
Bacon, Egg, & Cheese Sourdough	437	21	8	1220	40	2	5	20
Ham, Egg, & Cheese Sourdough	442	19	7	1586	41	2	6	26
Sausage, Egg, & Cheese Sourdough	556	33	12	1431	40	2	5	22
Blueberry Muffin	320	12	2	490	49	1	26	4
French Toastix	312	13	2	492	44	1	11	6
Sausage Patty	210	20	7	480	0	0	0	6
Breakfast Syrup	78	0	0	25	20	0	11	0

Sandwich

Description & Serving	Cal	Fat	Sfat	Sod	Carb	Fiber	Sugar	Prot
Arby's Melt	298	12	4	922	36	2	5	16
Beef 'n Cheddar, reg	440	21	6	1275	43	2	8	22
Beef 'n Cheddar, med	536	27	9	1701	44	2	8	32
Beef 'n Cheddar, lrg	657	36	12	2309	46	3	8	42
Bacon Cheddar Roastburger	443	18	8	1448	44	2	7	23
Bacon Cheddar Roastburger w/ Double Meat	562	27	12	1980	44	2	7	36
All American Roastburger	412	18	7	1305	45	2	9	19
All American Roastburger w/ Double Meat	531	27	11	1837	45	2	9	32
Bacon & Bleu Roastburger	466	23	9	1397	44	2	8	21
Bacon & Bleu Roastburger w/ Double Meat	585	32	12	1929	44	2	8	34
Super Roast Beef	399	19	6	1061	40	2	10	21
Roast Beef Sandwich, lrg	547	28	12	1869	41	3	6	42
Roast Beef Sandwich, med	415	21	9	1379	34	2	5	31
Roast Beef Sandwich, reg	320	14	5	953	34	2	5	21
Ham & Swiss Melt Sandwich	268	8	3	1042	35	1	6	17
Arby-Q	340	11	4	1089	48	2	18	17
Chicken Bacon & Swiss - Crispy	544	25	7	1632	50	2	9	32
Chicken Cordon Bleu Sandwich - Crispy	577	28	7	1936	47	2	7	37

Description & Serving	Cal	Fat	Sfat	Sod	Carb	Fiber	Sugar	Prot
Chicken Fillet Sandwich - Crispy	488	23	4	1210	47	2	6	26
Chicken Bacon & Swiss - Roast	439	18	6	1343	40	2	10	30
Chicken Cordon Bleu Sandwich - Roast	472	20	6	1646	37	2	8	34
Chicken Fillet Sandwich - Roast	383	16	3	921	37	2	7	23
Roast Chicken Club Sandwich	498	20	7	1540	46	2	9	30
Roast Turkey Ranch & Bacon Sandwich	818	38	11	2146	75	5	17	46
Pecan Chicken Salad Sandwich	769	39	10	1240	79	9	17	30
Corned Beef Reuben Sandwich	590	32	9	1685	55	3	6	32
Roast Ham & Swiss Sandwich	691	31	8	1952	75	5	19	33
Roast Turkey & Swiss Sandwich	708	30	8	1677	74	5	17	41
Ultimate BLT Sandwich	779	45	11	1571	75	6	18	23
BBQ Bacon Cheddar Roastburger	581	25	10	2128	61	3	17	25
Fajita Flatbread Melt - Roast Beef	514	35	13	1716	28	2	3	26
Fajita Flatbread Melt - Roast Chicken	470	26	8	1608	30	2	4	28
Subs								
French Dip & Swiss Toasted Sub	533	19	8	2169	67	3	3	29
Classic Italian Toasted Sub	596	27	7	1831	65	3	4	25
Philly Beef Toasted Sub	610	30	9	1549	62	3	3	29
Turkey Bacon Club Toasted Sub	605	24	6	1701	65	3	3	35
Chicken								
Popcorn Chicken, reg	363	16	3	930	27	2	0	24
Popcorn Chicken, lrg	529	24	4	1354	39	3	0	35
Salad								
Chopped Italian Salad	386	28	12	1420	11	3	5	21
Chopped Turkey Club Salad	230	11	6	801	9	3	5	22
Chopped Farmhouse Chicken Salad - Crispy	395	19	7	857	25	4	5	25
Chopped Farmhouse Chicken Salad - Grilled	229	11	6	579	9	3	6	20
Side								
Cheddar Fries, med	546	33	5	1525	62	6	0	7
Curly Fries, sml	338	20	4	791	39	4	0	4
Curly Fries, med	496	29	5	1160	58	6	0	7
Curly Fries, lrg	604	36	7	1413	70	7	0	8
Jalapeno Bites, reg, 5 pc	305	21	9	526	29	2	3	5
Loaded Potato Bites, reg, 5 pc	353	22	7	800	27	2	0	11
Mozzarella Sticks, reg, 4	426	28	13	1370	38	2	5	18
Onion Petals, reg	248	17	3	249	26	2	5	3
Onion Petals, lrg	480	33	5	482	51	3	10	6
Potato Cakes, 2	246	18	4	391	26	2	0	2
Topping/Dressing/Condiment								
Bacon, 4 pc	77	6	2	301	1	0	1	5
Arby's Sauce	15	0	0	177	4	0	1	0
Horsey Sauce	62	5	1	173	3	0	1	0
Mayonnaise Packet	105	11	2	74	0	0	0	0
Arby-Q Spicy Three Pepper Sauce	22	1	0	140	3	0	3	0
Balsamic Vinaigrette Dressing	130	12	2	460	5	0	4	0
Buttermilk Ranch Dressing	230	24	4	390	2	0	2	1
Dijon Honey Mustard Dressing	180	17	3	240	8	0	7	1

Description & Serving	Cal	Fat	Sfat	Sod	Carb	Fiber	Sugar	Prot
Buffalo Dipping Sauce	11	1	0	782	2	0	0	0
Honey Mustard Dipping Sauce	129	12	2	151	6	0	5	0
Ranch Dipping Sauce	158	16	4	277	2	0	1	1
BBQ Dipping Sauce	44	0	0	343	11	0	8	0
Tangy Southwest Sauce	249	26	4	278	3	0	3	0
Bronco Berry Dipping Sauce	92	0	0	27	23	0	21	0
Marinara Sauce	30	2	0	0	4	1	3	1
Cheddar Cheese Sauce - side	25	2	0	182	2	0	0	0
Ketchup Packet	13	0	0	158	3	0	3	0
Kids								
Junior Roast Beef Sandwich	272	10	4	740	34	2	5	16
Curly Fries	234	14	3	548	27	3	0	3
Popcorn Chicken	272	12	2	698	20	1	0	18
Applesauce	90	0	0	10	22	2	19	0
Dessert								
Apple Turnover w/ Icing	380	14	7	287	58	3	37	4
Cherry Turnover w/ Icing	364	13	7	269	58	1	35	4
Gourmet Chocolate Chunk Cookies, 2	209	10	5	163	27	0	17	2
Chocolate Swirl Shake	620	17	10	449	101	1	98	16
Jamocha Swirl Shake	611	17	10	485	99	1	95	16
Chocolate Malt Swirl Shake	620	17	10	454	101	1	97	16
Vanilla Shake	572	18	11	458	86	0	85	17
Beverage								
Mandarin Peach Iced FruiTea	90	0	0	0	23	0	23	0
Diet Blackberry Iced FruiTea	0	0	0	0	4	0	0	0
Diet Peach Iced FruiTea	0	0	0	0	4	0	0	0
Passion Fruit Iced FruiTea	100	0	0	0	25	0	25	0

Au Bon Pain

Breakfast

Description & Serving	Cal	Fat	Sfat	Sod	Carb	Fiber	Sugar	Prot
Asiago Cheese Bagel	340	6	4	620	56	2	5	15
Cinnamon Crisp Bagel	410	7	4	400	77	4	25	11
Cinnamon Raisin Bagel	320	1	0	450	68	3	13	11
Everything Bagel	340	5	0	990	61	3	4	13
Honey 9 Grain Bagel	350	4	0	490	69	6	7	12
Jalapeno Double Cheddar Bagel	340	10	6	640	53	2	5	17
Onion Dill Bagel	280	1	0	430	57	3	4	11
Plain Bagel	280	1	0	430	56	2	4	11
Poppy Bagel	320	4	1	430	58	4	4	12
Sesame Seed Bagel	330	5	1	440	59	3	4	12
White Chocolate Toffee Bagel Braid	350	6	3	500	63	2	15	11
Almond Croissant	600	38	14	300	55	4	15	13
Apple Croissant	280	11	6	160	44	3	19	5
Chocolate Croissant	440	22	13	210	58	3	27	7
Ham & Cheese Croissant	400	20	11	660	38	2	5	15
Plain Croissant	310	17	9	220	31	1	3	7

Description & Serving	Cal	Fat	Sfat	Sod	Carb	Fiber	Sugar	Prot
Raspberry Cheese Croissant	370	17	9	280	46	2	17	8
Spinach & Cheese Croissant	290	16	9	300	28	2	3	10
Sweet Cheese Croissant	400	19	11	320	49	1	21	9
Cherry Danish	420	20	10	340	54	1	23	7
Lemon Danish	440	20	10	360	57	1	24	7
Sweet Cheese Danish	470	24	13	390	54	1	23	9
Blueberry Muffin	490	17	2	510	74	2	31	9
Carrot Walnut Muffin	560	27	6	820	72	4	40	9
Chocolate Chip Muffin	580	23	6	480	83	3	47	9
Corn Muffin	490	17	3	600	75	3	31	10
Cranberry Walnut Muffin	540	25	3	500	66	4	28	10
Double Chocolate Chunk Muffin	620	25	8	540	86	4	47	11
Low-Fat Triple Berry Muffin	300	3	0	720	65	2	33	4
Raisin Bran Muffin	480	11	2	600	85	10	43	12
Southwest Jalapeno Muffin	560	30	5	720	64	2	32	8
Chocolate Orange Pecan Scone	580	28	13	360	74	3	36	10
Cinnamon Scone	530	27	16	400	60	2	22	9
Orange Scone	470	23	13	420	57	1	17	10
Apple Strudel	440	24	14	270	50	1	21	5
Cherry Strudel	460	26	16	270	50	1	26	5
Bacon & Bagel	340	6	2	650	58	2	4	16
Bacon & Egg Melt on Ciabatta	510	26	14	1270	41	2	2	26
Egg & Broccoli Baked Sandwich	350	10	5	910	42	3	2	23
Egg on a Bagel	360	4	1	790	60	3	5	21
Egg on a Bagel w/ Bacon	420	8	3	1000	60	3	5	25
Egg on a Bagel w/ Bacon & Cheese	510	15	6	1140	61	3	5	31
Egg on a Bagel w/ Cheese	450	10	5	930	61	3	5	26
Portobello, Egg and Cheddar	500	26	14	1160	42	3	2	22
Prosciutto & Egg on Asiago Bagel	520	16	7	1690	60	1	5	34
Sausage, Egg & Cheddar on Asiago Bagel	810	47	23	1540	58	1	5	38
Smoked Salmon & Wasabi on Onion Dill Bagel	430	11	5	1090	64	1	7	23
Apple Croissants Tart, 1 oz	80	4	2	55	12	1	4	1
Cinnamon Walnut Quinoa, 1 oz	45	3	0	0	4	1	1	2
French Pecan Toast, 1 oz	70	4	2	45	8	0	4	2
Pineapple Blueberry Cobbler, 1 oz	45	2	0	35	8	1	4	1
Roasted Potatoes, 1 oz	35	1	0	110	6	1	0	1
Sausage w/ Peppers & Onions, 1 oz	50	5	2	90	1	0.	1	2
Scrambled Eggs, 1 oz	35	3	1	90	1	0	1	3
Southwest Corn Casserole, 1 oz	60	4	2	85	4	0	2	3
Oatmeal, sml (8.75 oz)	150	3	0	10	28	4	1	6
Blueberry Yogurt w/ Blueberries, sml (8.5 oz)	250	3	2	135	50	0	43	8
Granola Topping, 2 oz	230	8	1	75	37	3	11	5
Strawberry Yogurt w/ Blueberries, sml (8.5 oz)	250	2	2	135	50	0	43	7
Vanilla Yogurt w/ Blueberries, sml (8.5 oz)	220	3	2	180	41	0	32	9

Sandwich/Wrap

Description & Serving	Cal	Fat	Sfat	Sod	Carb	Fiber	Sugar	Prot
Arizona Chicken Sandwich	690	28	11	1600	60	4	6	47
Baja Turkey Sandwich	700	27	10	1680	71	5	4	46
BBQ Brisket Sandwich	660	21	6	1660	81	5	18	36
BBQ Chicken Sandwich	560	13	3	1500	83	6	18	29

Description & Serving	Cal	Fat	Sfat	Sod	Carb	Fiber	Sugar	Prot
Caprese Sandwich	680	32	15	1200	65	4	2	30
Chicken Pesto Sandwich	660	24	5	1560	66	4	5	43
Eggplant & Mozzarella Sandwich	670	30	12	1550	73	6	7	27
Mozzarella Chicken Sandwich	680	24	8	1460	67	4	6	48
Portobello & Goat Cheese Sandwich	550	25	9	1340	62	6	5	19
Prosciutto Mozzarella Sandwich	810	41	16	2290	71	4	5	41
Roast Beef Caesar Sandwich	680	27	9	1560	68	3	5	40
Spicy Tuna Sandwich	470	16	3	1180	60	11	8	29
Steakhouse on Ciabatta	720	30	11	1850	76	4	8	44
Tuna Melt	690	30	10	1160	71	5	5	42
Turkey Club Sandwich	700	31	13	1970	59	2	2	45
Turkey Melt	810	32	13	2040	79	3	16	47
Demi Chicken Sandwich on Baguette	370	9	2	850	49	3	3	22
Demi Chicken Sandwich w/ Cheddar Cheese on Baguette	440	15	5	980	50	3	3	27
Demi Ham Sandwich on Baguette	330	5	2	1190	56	3	10	17
Demi Ham Sandwich w/ Swiss Cheese on Baguette	400	10	5	1230	56	3	9	23
Demi Roast Beef Sandwich on Baguette	360	8	2	830	49	3	3	19
Demi Roast Beef Sandwich w/ Brie Cheese on Baguette	460	18	8	1040	49	3	2	24
Demi Tuna Sandwich on Baguette	320	7	2	770	49	3	3	17
Demi Tuna Sandwich w/ Cheddar Cheese on Baguette	400	14	5	900	50	3	3	22
Demi Turkey Sandwich on Baguette	320	6	2	1000	49	2	3	18
Demi Turkey Sandwich w/ Swiss Cheese on Baguette	400	12	5	1040	49	2	3	24
Half Sandwich Ham & Swiss on Farmhouse Roll	320	13	5	950	34	2	2	21
Half Sandwich Roast Beef & Brie on Farmhouse Roll	350	14	6	630	34	2	2	20
Half Sandwich Tuna & Cheddar on Farmhouse Roll	360	16	5	660	35	2	3	19
Half Sandwich Turkey & Swiss on Farmhouse Roll	320	11	5	700	34	2	2	22
Whole Sandwich Ham & Swiss on Country White	530	17	9	1930	60	2	2	39
Whole Sandwich Roast Beef & Brie on Country Style Bread	600	21	11	1290	59	3	2	39
Whole Sandwich Tuna & Cheddar on Country White Bread	610	25	9	1330	63	3	4	37
Whole Sandwich Turkey & Swiss on Country White Bread	530	14	8	1410	60	2	2	42
BBQ Brisket Wrap	690	28	10	1730	82	8	16	32
BBQ Chicken Wrap	640	24	8	1650	83	9	16	29
Chicken Caesar Asiago Wrap	610	28	9	1440	61	5	9	34
Mayan Chicken Hot Wrap	580	13	3	1300	93	6	6	24
Mediterranean Wrap	610	29	7	1770	73	8	9	18
Southwest Tuna Wrap	750	40	13	1470	66	7	11	39
Thai Peanut Chicken Wrap	530	15	2	1340	79	6	16	30

Salad

BBQ Chicken Salad	300	11	5	690	25	6	7	24
Caesar Asiago Salad	220	12	6	480	18	3	4	11
Chef's Salad	250	15	7	1030	7	3	4	24

Description & Serving	Cal	Fat	Sfat	Sod	Carb	Fiber	Sugar	Prot
Chickpea & Tomato Cucumber Salad	230	12	5	810	23	7	3	11
Garden Salad	70	2	0	85	13	3	3	3
Grilled Chicken Caesar Asiago Salad	300	13	6	740	18	3	4	28
Mandarin Sesame Chicken Salad	310	17	1	410	29	3	10	20
Mediterranean Chicken Salad	290	16	6	1230	12	3	2	23
Thai Peanut Chicken Salad	240	8	0	280	19	4	5	22
Tuna Garden Salad	240	12	2	480	15	4	5	20
Turkey & Strawberry Salad	110	4	0	280	10	4	5	11
Turkey Cobb Salad	330	19	8	930	14	4	4	27

Soup

Description & Serving	Cal	Fat	Sfat	Sod	Carb	Fiber	Sugar	Prot
Baked Stuffed Potato Soup, sml (8 oz)	230	13	7	660	20	1	4	6
Beef & Vegetable Soup, sml (8 oz)	210	10	2	720	17	2	3	12
Black Bean Soup, sml (8 oz)	170	1	0	740	30	17	2	10
Broccoli Cheddar Soup, sml (8 oz)	200	14	6	660	13	1	5	7
Carrot Ginger Soup, sml (8 oz)	90	3	0	640	15	2	6	1
Chicken & Dumpling Soup, sml (8 oz)	140	5	2	850	19	1	4	7
Chicken Florentine Soup, sml (8 oz)	170	8	4	700	17	1	3	5
Chicken Gumbo Soup, sml (8 oz)	120	5	1	590	14	1	1	4
Chicken Noodle Soup, sml (8 oz)	90	2	1	700	12	1	2	6
Clam Chowder, sml (8 oz)	210	12	5	680	18	1	5	6
Corn & Green Chili Bisque, sml (8 oz)	170	10	5	1030	18	2	4	4
Corn Chowder, sml (8 oz)	230	12	6	750	27	2	7	6
Cream of Chicken & Wild Rice Soup, sml (8 oz)	160	9	4	650	15	1	2	4
Curried Rice & Lentil Soup, sml (8 oz)	110	2	0	840	20	5	3	5
French Moroccan Tomato Lentil Soup, sml (8 oz)	120	2	0	710	21	7	4	7
French Onion Soup, sml (8 oz)	80	3	2	870	13	1	4	2
Garden Vegetable Soup, sml (8 oz)	50	1	0	720	9	2	3	2
Gazpacho, sml (8 oz)	60	3	0	1020	8	2	4	1
Hearty Cabbage Soup, sml (8 oz)	80	3	1	690	10	2	3	3
Italian Wedding Soup, sml (8 oz)	110	5	2	870	13	2	3	5
Jamaican Black Bean Soup, sml (8 oz)	160	1	0	290	29	16	4	10
Mediterranean Pepper Soup, sml (8 oz)	110	3	0	400	17	5	2	5
Old Fashioned Tomato Soup, sml (8 oz)	130	5	2	770	18	2	10	4
Pasta E Fagioli Soup, sml (8 oz)	170	5	2	670	23	6	2	8
Portuguese Kale Soup, sml (8 oz)	80	4	1	820	10	2	1	4
Potato Cheese Soup, sml (8 oz)	170	9	6	840	16	1	3	4
Potato Leek Soup, sml (8 oz)	200	13	7	670	18	1	2	3
Red Beans, Italian Sausage and Rice Soup, sml (8 oz)	180	4	1	720	27	11	2	9
Southern Black-Eyed Pea Soup, sml (8 oz)	120	1	0	650	19	6	2	7
Southwest Tortilla Soup, sml (8 oz)	130	7	2	770	15	3	2	3
Southwest Vegetable Soup, sml (8 oz)	120	3	0	260	18	4	2	4
Split Pea w/ Ham Soup, sml (8 oz)	170	1	0	810	28	10	2	12
Thai Coconut Curry Soup, sml (8 oz)	110	5	1	700	14	1	4	3
Tomato Basil Bisque, sml (8 oz)	140	6	4	330	18	2	10	4
Tomato Cheddar Soup, sml (8 oz)	160	11	4	710	12	1	4	6
Tomato Florentine Soup, sml (8 oz)	80	2	1	680	12	2	4	4
Tomato Rice Soup, sml (8 oz)	80	1	0	190	16	1	4	2

Description & Serving	Cal	Fat	Sfat	Sod	Carb	Fiber	Sugar	Prot
Tuscan Vegetable Soup, sml (8 oz)	110	4	2	790	15	2	2	5
Vegetable Beef Barley Soup, sml (8 oz)	90	2	1	670	14	3	2	6
Vegetarian Chili, sml (8 oz)	150	2	0	650	26	13	3	8
Vegetarian Lentil Soup, sml (8 oz)	120	1	0	800	20	7	3	6
Vegetarian Minestrone Soup, sml (8 oz)	80	1	0	750	14	3	4	3
Wild Mushroom Bisque, sml (8 oz)	120	6	2	680	15	2	4	3
BBQ Chicken & Beef Stew, sml (8 oz)	200	7	3	760	24	2	11	13
Baked Stuffed Potato, sml (8 oz)	230	13	7	660	20	1	4	6
Chicken & Vegetable Stew, sml (8 oz)	190	11	3	630	17	2	3	7

Pasta/Rice

Description & Serving	Cal	Fat	Sfat	Sod	Carb	Fiber	Sugar	Prot
Chicken Broccoli Alfredo Penne, 12 oz	680	43	18	1100	38	2	4	28
Meat Lasagna, 10.7 oz	470	24	11	1080	41	5	7	22
Macaroni & Cheese, sml (8 oz)	330	19	12	920	24	1	3	13
BBQ Brisket Harvest Rice Bowl	790	19	6	1560	118	10	22	37
BBQ Brisket Harvest Rice Bowl w/ Brown Rice	740	21	6	1530	103	12	23	37
BBQ Chicken Harvest Rice Bowl	690	11	2	1400	120	12	22	31
BBQ Chicken Harvest Rice Bowl w/ Brown Rice	650	12	2	1370	105	13	23	31
Mayan Chicken Harvest Rice Bowl	560	12	3	1100	87	5	6	27
Mayan Chicken Harvest Rice Bowl w/ Brown Rice	510	13	3	1070	72	7	6	27

Side/Snack

Description & Serving	Cal	Fat	Sfat	Sod	Carb	Fiber	Sugar	Prot
Apples, Blue Cheese & Cranberries, 5 oz	200	10	4	270	27	3	21	4
Baked Potato, 1 oz	25	0	0	20	5	1	0	1
BBQ Beef Salad, 1 oz	35	1	0	90	4	0	1	2
Beef Stroganoff Penne, 1 oz	40	2	1	75	4	0	0	2
Black Bean & Corn Salad, 6 oz	130	0	0	310	25	5	2	5
Brie, Fruit & Crackers, 3.5 oz	200	11	6	280	18	0	9	6
Brown Rice, 1 oz	30	0	0	20	6	0	0	1
Brown Rice & Hazelnut Waldorf Salad, 4.5 oz	180	9	2	160	22	2	8	2
Brown Rice & Mushrooms, 5 oz	200	13	2	280	18	2	1	3
Brown Rice Waldorf Salad, 1 oz	45	3	0	40	5	0	2	0
Cheddar, Fruit & Crackers, 3.5 oz	200	12	6	280	18	0	9	8
Chicken Broccoli Alfredo Penne, 1 oz	60	4	2	90	3	0	0	2
Chicken Marsala Penne, 1 oz	35	1	0	75	4	0	1	2
Chicken Penne Pesto, 1 oz	60	3	1	90	4	0	0	3
Chicken Pesto Salad, 4.1 oz	160	8	3	420	1	1	1	20
Chicken Provencal, 1 oz	25	0	0	90	4	0	1	2
Chickpea & Tomato Salad, 6 oz	100	1	0	200	19	6	2	5
Chocolate Covered Almonds	230	15	5	10	20	2	17	4
Creamed Spinach, 1 oz	30	2	2	125	2	1	1	1
Egg & Cucumber Salad, 1 oz	40	3	1	90	1	0	1	2
Eggplant Parmesan, 1 oz	50	3	1	150	4	1	1	2
Fire Roasted Exotic Grains & Vegetables, 1 oz	40	1	0	85	7	1	0	1
Fresh Grapes, 8 oz	160	0	0	0	41	2	35	2
Fresh Pineapple, 8 oz	110	0	0	0	30	3	22	1
Fresh Watermelon, 8 oz	70	0	0	0	17	1	14	1
Fruit Cup, sml (6 oz)	70	0	0	15	18	1	15	1
Fruit Romanoff w/ Almonds, 5.3 oz	200	7	2	15	34	3	25	3

Description & Serving	Cal	Fat	Sfat	Sod	Carb	Fiber	Sugar	Prot
Herb Cheese, Fruit & Crackers, 4 oz	190	11	6	450	20	1	12	4
Hummus & Cucumber, 4.3 oz	130	8	0	460	10	3	1	3
Italian Sausage, Peppers & Onions, 1 oz	25	1	0	80	1	0	0	2
Jambalaya, 1 oz	25	1	0	85	2	0	1	1
Macaroni & Cheese, 1 oz	40	3	2	115	3	0	0	2
Meat Lasagna, 1 oz	45	2	1	100	4	0	1	2
Meatballs & Marinara Sauce, 1 oz	50	4	2	125	2	1	1	2
Meatloaf w/ Wine Sauce, 1 oz	50	3	1	75	2	0	1	2
Mediterranean Tuna Salad, 4.4 oz	120	8	1	280	4	1	3	9
Mixed Nuts, 1.1 oz	180	16	3	60	7	1	2	5
Mozzarella & Tomato, 4.7 oz	180	14	7	280	5	1	4	10
Muesli, 8 oz	390	8	2	50	76	7	39	11
Orzo Toscana Salad, 1 oz	35	1	0	90	6	1	1	1
Penne Marinara, 1 oz	30	1	0	55	5	0	1	1
Polenta Marinara, 1 oz	25	1	0	90	3	0	1	1
Potato Bacon Salad, 1 oz	40	2	0	125	5	1	1	1
Quinoa, 1 oz	25	0	0	50	4	1	0	1
Roasted Apple Cranberry Orzo, 1 oz	45	1	0	25	9	1	3	1
Roasted Carrots, 1 oz	15	0	0	60	3	1	1	0
Roasted Green Beans w/ Almonds, 1 oz	20	1	0	60	2	1	0	1
Roasted Zucchini & Summer Squash, 1 oz	5	0	0	15	1	0	1	0
Sesame Brown Rice & Orange Salad, 1 oz	45	3	0	50	6	0	1	1
Side Caesar Asiago Salad	130	6	3	270	12	2	2	6
Side Garden Salad	50	1	0	65	8	2	1	2
Smoked Salmon, Egg & Guacamole, 5.1 oz	140	10	2	270	6	3	2	8
Southwest Fusilli Pasta Salad, 1 oz	45	3	0	65	4	0	1	1
Southwest Panzanella Salad, 1 oz	50	3	0	55	7	0	3	1
Stuffed Peppers w/ Beef, 1 oz	20	1	0	40	2	0	1	1
Stuffed Peppers w/ Lentils, 1 oz	20	0	0	35	3	1	1	1
Thai Beef & Peanut, 3.7 oz	120	5	1	290	5	1	4	12
Tomato Cucumber Salad, 1 oz	10	0	0	40	2	0	1	0
Tomato, Green Bean & Almond Salad, 1 oz	20	2	0	50	2	0	1	0
Tuna Salad, 1 oz	40	3	0	100	1	0	1	4
Turkey, Asparagus, Cranberry Chutney & Gorgonzola, 4.8 oz	140	5	3	550	10	1	7	15
Turkish Apricots, 1.4 oz	120	0	0	10	29	4	15	1
Vegetarian Lasagna, 1 oz	20	0	0	55	4	1	1	1
Watermelon, Feta & Almonds, 3.9 oz	70	3	1	55	11	1	9	2
Watermelon & Feta Salad, 1 oz	15	1	0	25	3	0	2	0
White Rice, 1 oz	35	0	0	20	8	0	0	1

Kids

Kid's Cheese Sandwich on Farmhouse Roll	360	22	12	550	32	1	1	11
Kid's Grilled Chicken Sandwich on Multigrain Bread	230	6	1	640	28	5	3	19
Kid's Roasted Turkey Sandwich on Farmhouse Roll	270	7	2	800	33	1	2	17
Kid's Macaroni & Cheese, 6 oz	250	14	9	690	18	0	2	10

Dessert

Banana Nut Pound Cake	480	26	5	430	56	1	31	7
Blondie	460	33	5	580	59	2	38	5

Description & Serving	Cal	Fat	Sfat	Sod	Carb	Fiber	Sugar	Prot
Chocolate Cheesecake Brownie	460	19	6	400	74	1	50	5
Chocolate Cherry Tulip	410	21	5	370	54	2	33	5
Chocolate Chip Brownie	510	19	6	380	74	1	51	6
Chocolate Chip Cookie	280	13	7	210	40	2	24	3
Chocolate Covered Strawberry	35	2	2	5	5	1	4	0
Chocolate Dipped Cranberry Almond Macaroon	300	15	11	190	36	4	29	4
Chocolate Dipped Shortbread	380	22	12	310	42	1	15	4
Chocolate Duo, 2.1 oz	160	9	5	40	18	0	14	3
Confetti Cookie w/ M&M's	280	13	6	210	39	0	24	3
Crème de Fleur	500	25	14	410	57	2	28	11
Crumb Cake	750	40	17	980	97	1	53	8
English Toffee Cookie	250	14	6	170	27	1	17	2
Gelatin Dessert, Lemon, 8 oz	120	0	0	210	29	0	29	2
Gelatin Dessert, Lime, 8 oz	120	0	0	190	29	0	30	2
Gelatin Dessert, Orange, 8 oz	130	0	0	160	30	0	30	2
Hazelnut Mocha Brownie	490	22	5	350	74	3	47	6
Iced Cinnamon Roll	410	15	8	270	60	2	22	8
Lemon Drop Tulip	410	19	5	330	55	1	31	5
Lemon Pound Cake	520	25	5	490	67	1	43	6
Mango Coconut Mousse, 2.1 oz	170	10	6	45	18	0	11	3
Marble Pound Cake	490	26	5	520	59	1	35	6
Mini Chocolate Chip Cookie	70	3	2	55	10	0	6	1
Mini Oatmeal Raisin Cookie	60	3	1	50	10	1	6	1
Mint Chocolate Pound Cake	530	29	6	580	64	3	42	7
Oatmeal Raisin Cookie	230	8	4	190	36	2	23	3
Palmier	440	23	15	330	53	1	19	1
Pecan Roll	810	41	14	430	99	3	47	12
Raspberry Mousse, 2.5 oz	150	6	4	45	20	0	13	3
Rocky Road Brownie	490	22	6	370	74	2	48	6
Shortbread Cookie	340	20	10	300	37	1	11	4
Tiramisu, 2.1 oz	170	11	6	45	15	0	11	3
White Chocolate Chunk Macadamia Nut Cookie	300	16	8	240	36	1	21	3

Bread

Artisan Baguette, sandwich size	310	3	1	760	61	2	1	10
Artisan Baguette, salad size	230	2	1	570	46	2	1	8
Artisan Honey Multigrain Baguette, sandwich size	340	5	0	670	66	6	1	11
Artisan Honey Multigrain Baguette, salad size	250	3	0	500	49	4	1	8
Artisan Sundried Tomato Bread, 4 oz	270	1	0	750	57	2	2	10
Asiago Breadstick	190	4	3	350	28	1	3	9
Bread Bowl	620	3	1	1720	123	6	3	26
Cheddar Jalapeno Breadstick	130	2	1	260	26	1	2	6
Ciabatta, sml	180	1	0	480	38	2	1	6
Ciabatta, lrg	310	1	0	820	64	3	2	11
Cinnamon Raisin Breadstick	190	1	0	230	41	2	13	6
Country White Bread, 4 oz	270	1	0	670	56	2	1	9
Everything Breadstick	170	3	0	500	31	1	2	7
Farm House Rolls, 4.5 oz	360	7	1	670	63	3	2	12
Focaccia, 4.6 oz	360	7	1	700	62	3	3	12
Lahvash, 4 oz	280	4	1	660	56	4	5	9

Description & Serving	Cal	Fat	Sfat	Sod	Carb	Fiber	Sugar	Prot
Rosemary Garlic Breadstick	190	5	1	720	31	2	3	6
Sesame Breadstick	180	4	1	220	30	2	2	7
Whole Wheat Multigrain Bread, 4 oz	260	3	0	630	53	9	4	11

Dressing/Condiment

Description & Serving	Cal	Fat	Sfat	Sod	Carb	Fiber	Sugar	Prot
Balsamic Vinaigrette Dressing, 2 oz	120	9	2	360	8	0	8	0
Blue Cheese Dressing, 2 oz	310	33	6	460	2	0	2	2
Caesar Dressing, 2 oz	270	28	5	370	4	0	2	1
Fat Free Raspberry Vinaigrette, 2 oz	50	0	0	190	12	0	12	0
Hazelnut Vinaigrette Dressing, 2 oz	270	25	4	300	11	0	10	1
Light Ranch Dressing, 2 oz	120	11	2	410	3	0	2	2
Lite Honey Mustard Dressing, 2 oz	170	9	2	380	20	0	12	1
Lite Olive Oil Vinaigrette, 2 oz	110	10	2	420	6	0	5	0
Pomegranate Vinaigrette Dressing, 2 oz	250	22	4	160	12	0	11	0
Sesame Ginger Dressing, 2 oz	230	20	3	680	12	0	11	1
Thai Peanut Dressing, 2 oz	160	8	1	740	20	0	17	2
Artichoke Aioli Spread, 1 oz	70	6	1	230	2	0	1	1
Basil Pesto, 1 oz	120	12	2	220	1	0	0	2
Chili Dijon, 1 oz	120	12	2	130	3	1	2	1
Guacamole, 1 oz	50	5	1	115	2	2	0	0
Herb Bagel Spread, 2 oz	140	12	8	340	4	0	3	5
Herb Mayonnaise, 1 oz	110	11	2	160	1	0	1	0
Honey Mustard Sauce, 2.5 oz	200	3	0	240	41	1	39	2
Honey Pecan Cream Cheese, 2 oz	200	16	10	135	10	0	9	2
Jalapeno Mayonnaise, 1 oz	50	5	1	310	1	0	1	2
Lite Cream Cheese Spread, 2 oz	120	9	6	280	5	0	3	4
Mayonnaise, 1 oz	70	7	1	220	2	0	2	0
Mediterranean Spread, 1 oz	120	11	3	430	2	1	1	2
Mustard, 1 tsp	0	0	0	70	0	0	0	0
Sun-Dried Tomato Spread, 0.5 oz	45	4	0	70	1	0	1	0
Sundried Tomato Cream Cheese, 2 oz	140	11	7	170	5	1	4	4
Tsaziki, 1 oz	15	0	0	40	2	0	2	1
Vegetable Cream Cheese, 2 oz	170	16	10	270	3	0	2	3

Topping

Description & Serving	Cal	Fat	Sfat	Sod	Carb	Fiber	Sugar	Prot
All Natural Chicken Breast, 1 portion	120	2	0	420	0	0	0	26
Bacon, 1 portion	60	5	2	210	0	0	0	5
Brie Cheese, 1.5 oz	170	15	9	320	1	1	0	7
Cheddar Cheese, 2 slices	160	13	7	270	1	0	0	10
Feta Cheese, 1 oz	80	6	4	320	1	0	0	5
Goat Cheese, 1 oz	45	4	2	110	1	0	1	3
Gorgonzola Cheese, 1 oz	200	16	12	770	2	0	0	12
Ham, 1 portion	100	4	2	1190	0	0	0	18
Mozzarella Cheese, 2 oz	120	9	6	105	0	0	0	9
Prosciutto, 1.5 oz	110	6	3	940	2	0	0	14
Roast Beef, 1 portion	150	6	2	300	0	0	0	23
Roasted Red Pepper Hummus, 1 portion	80	5	0	250	6	2	0	2
Roasted Red Peppers, 2 oz	10	0	0	105	2	0	1	0
Sausage Patty, 2 oz	210	20	7	360	0	0	0	8
Swiss Cheese, 1 portion	150	12	8	90	2	0	0	12

Description & Serving	Cal	Fat	Sfat	Sod	Carb	Fiber	Sugar	Prot
Tuna Salad Mix, 1 portion	160	10	2	400	3	1	2	17
Turkey Breast, 1 portion	90	1	0	650	1	0	0	20

Beverage

Description & Serving	Cal	Fat	Sfat	Sod	Carb	Fiber	Sugar	Prot
Caffe Americano, sml (12 oz)	5	0	0	15	1	0	1	0
Caffe Latte, sml (12 oz)	200	11	7	170	17	0	17	11
Cappuccino, sml (12 oz)	120	7	4	85	10	0	10	0
Caramel Macchiato, sml (12 oz)	350	10	6	160	53	0	50	10
Chai Latte, sml (12 oz)	290	11	7	130	38	0	26	11
Frozen Watermelon Lemonade, 16 oz	260	0	0	15	64	5	52	2
Hot Chocolate, sml (12 oz)	350	11	7	125	58	3	54	12
Iced Caffe Latte, sml (12 oz)	110	6	4	80	19	0	10	6
Iced Caramel Macchiato, sml (12 oz)	290	7	5	125	49	0	46	7
Iced Chai Latte, sml (12 oz)	190	5	4	65	31	0	18	5
Iced Mocha Latte, sml (12 oz)	210	11	7	70	27	1	26	6
Iced Vanilla Latte, sml (12 oz)	240	5	3	65	44	0	44	5
Iced White Chocolate Latte, sml (12 oz)	250	11	7	135	35	0	32	5
Mocha Latte, sml (12 oz)	300	16	10	160	35	1	33	11
Orange Juice, sml (8 oz)	110	0	0	0	26	0	26	2
Vanilla Latte, sml (12 oz)	320	9	6	120	50	0	50	9
White Chocolate Latte, sml (12 oz)	310	14	9	180	41	0	38	9

Auntie Anne's

Pretzel

Description & Serving	Cal	Fat	Sfat	Sod	Carb	Fiber	Sugar	Prot
Garlic Pretzel	350	5	3	990	65	2	10	8
Garlic Pretzel w/o Butter	310	1	0	990	65	2	10	8
Garlic Pretzel w/o Butter or Salt	310	1	0	400	65	2	10	8
Garlic Pretzel w/o Salt	350	5	3	400	65	2	10	8
Jalapeño Pretzel	330	5	3	1060	63	2	9	8
Jalapeño Pretzel w/o Butter	300	1	0	1060	63	2	9	8
Jalapeño Pretzel w/o Butter or Salt	300	1	0	480	63	2	9	8
Jalapeño Pretzel w/o Salt	330	5	3	480	63	2	9	8
Jumbo Pretzel Dog	610	29	13	1150	67	2	10	19
Jumbo Pretzel Dog w/o Butter	580	25	10	1150	67	2	10	19
Original Pretzel	340	5	3	1060	63	2	9	8
Original Pretzel w/o Butter	310	1	0	990	65	2	10	8
Original Pretzel w/o Butter or Salt	310	1	0	400	65	2	10	8
Original Pretzel w/o Salt	340	5	3	400	65	2	10	8
Party Pretzels, 12 pc	2140	32	18	6150	405	12	61	49
Pepperoni Pretzel	480	16	8	860	65	2	10	15
Pepperoni Pretzel w/o Butter	440	12	5	860	65	2	10	15
Pretzel Dog	360	20	9	740	33	1	5	11
Pretzel Dog w/o Butter	320	16	6	740	33	1	5	11
Pretzel Pocket - Bacon, Egg, & Cheese	580	23	10	790	71	2	12	23
Pretzel Pocket - Bacon, Egg, & Cheese w/o Butter	550	20	8	790	71	2	12	23
Pretzel Pocket - Pepperoni	650	27	12	1120	75	2	11	25
Pretzel Pocket - Pepperoni w/o Butter	620	24	10	1120	75	2	11	25
Pretzel Pocket - Turkey & Cheddar	470	10	5	1050	73	2	14	20

Description & Serving	Cal	Fat	Sfat	Sod	Carb	Fiber	Sugar	Prot
Pretzel Pocket - Turkey & Cheddar w/o Butter	440	6	2.5	1050	73	2	14	20
Raisin Pretzel	360	5	3	390	69	2	16	8
Raisin Pretzel w/o Butter	330	1	0	390	69	2	16	8
Sesame Pretzel	400	10	3.5	990	67	3	10	10
Sesame Pretzel w/o Butter	360	6	1	990	67	3	10	10
Sesame Pretzel w/o Butter or Salt	360	6	1	400	67	3	10	10
Sesame Pretzel w/o Salt	400	10	3.5	400	67	3	10	10
Sour Cream & Onion Pretzel	360	5	3	1180	68	2	12	9
Sour Cream & Onion Pretzel w/o Butter	330	1.5	0	1180	68	2	12	9
Sour Cream & Onion Pretzel w/o Butter or Salt	330	1.5	0	590	68	2	12	9
Sour Cream & Onion Pretzel w/o Salt	360	5	3	590	68	2	12	9

Dessert

Almond Pretzel	390	6	3.5	400	74	2	17	8
Almond Pretzel w/o Butter	350	2	1	400	74	2	17	8
Cinnamon Sugar Party Pretzels, 12 pc	2940	72	455	2460	519	12	177	49
Cinnamon Sugar Pretzel	470	12	7	400	84	2	29	8
Cinnamon Sugar Pretzel w/o Butter	380	1	0	400	84	2	29	8
Cinnamon Sugar Stix, 6 pc	470	12	7	400	84	2	29	8
Cinnamon Sugar Stix w/o Butter, 6 pc	380	1	0	400	84	2	29	8
Original Stix, 6 pc	340	5	3	990	65	2	10	8
Original Stix w/o Butter, 6 pc	310	1	0	990	65	2	10	8

A&W

Burger/Sandwich/Hot Dog

Papa Burger	690	39	14	1350	44	4	8	40
Papa Single Burger	470	25	8	1000	38	4	7	23
Original Bacon Double Cheeseburger	760	45	17	1570	45	4	8	44
Original Double Baconburger	680	38	14	1330	44	4	7	40
Original Bacon Cheeseburger	530	30	10	1160	39	4	7	26
Hamburger	380	19	6	860	33	3	6	21
Cheeseburger	420	21	7	1040	37	4	6	23
Grilled Chicken Sandwich	400	15	3	820	31	4	7	35
Crispy Chicken Sandwich	550	25	4.5	1130	52	5	6	30
Hot Dog, plain	310	19	8	740	23	1	4	11
Coney (Chili) Dog	340	20	9	900	26	2	5	14
Coney (Chili) Cheese Dog	380	23	9	1100	28	2	5	14
Chicken Strips, 3 pc	500	29	5	1050	32	2	2	28

Side

French Fries, kids/sml	200	8	2	290	28	3	0	2
French Fries, reg	310	12	3	460	45	4	0	3
French Fries, lrg	430	17	4	640	61	6	1	5
Corn Dog Nuggets, kids/sml, 5 pc	180	8	2	520	20	1	6	5
Corn Dog Nuggets, reg, 8 pc	280	13	3	830	32	2	9	9
Chili Cheese Fries	410	17	5	990	52	5	2	8
Cheese Fries	390	18	4.5	870	50	4	0	4
Breaded Onion Rings, reg	350	16	3.5	710	45	2	3	5

Description & Serving	Cal	Fat	Sfat	Sod	Carb	Fiber	Sugar	Prot
Breaded Onion Rings, lrg	480	27	7	990	62	3	4	7
Cheese Curds	570	40	21	1220	27	2	3	27
Extra Burger Patty (1)	170	12	5	170	2	0	0	15

Condiment

Ranch Dipping Sauce	160	17	2.5	240	2	0	1	0
BBQ Dipping Sauce	40	0	0	230	10	0	6	0
Honey Mustard Dipping Sauce	100	6	1.5	170	12	0	6	0

Dessert

Polar Swirl, M&Ms, 12 oz	710	25	16	290	107	2	93	15
Polar Swirl, Oreo, 12 oz	690	24	11	570	107	3	79	14
Polar Swirl, Reese's, 12 oz	740	31	14	380	97	3	85	18
Milkshake, Strawberry, sml (16 oz)	670	29	18	180	90	0	52	11
Milkshake, Strawberry, med (20 oz)	840	36	23	230	113	0	65	14
Milkshake, Vanilla, sml (16 oz)	720	31	19	210	97	0	57	12
Milkshake, Vanilla, med (20 oz)	900	39	24	260	121	0	71	15
Milkshake, Chocolate, sml (16 oz)	700	29	18	200	100	2	60	11
Milkshake, Chocolate, med (20 oz)	880	36	23	250	125	3	75	14
Vanilla Cone	260	7	4	145	41	0	29	7
A&W Root Beer Freeze, sml (16oz)	430	9	5	200	79	0	37	9
A&W Root Beer Freeze, med (20 oz)	530	11	7	260	99	0	47	11
A&W Root Beer Freeze, lrg (32 oz)	850	18	11	410	158	0	75	18
Sundae, Strawberry	300	8	4	140	47	0	12	7
Sundae, Chocolate	320	8	4	180	53	0	15	8
Sundae, Hot Fudge	350	11	6	140	54	1	15	8
Sundae, Caramel	340	9	4	250	57	0	13	8
A&W Root Beer Float, sml (16 oz)	330	5	3	100	70	0	57	2
A&W Root Beer Float, med (20 oz)	350	5	3	105	77	0	64	2
A&W Root Beer Float, lrg (32 oz)	640	10	6	200	136	0	110	4
A&W Diet Root Beer Float, sml (16 oz)	170	5	3	100	30	0	17	2
A&W Diet Root Beer Float, med (20 oz)	170	5	3	105	30	0	17	2
A&W Diet Root Beer Float, lrg (32 oz)	350	10	6	200	60	0	34	4

Beverage

A&W Regular Root Beer, sml (11 oz)	220	0	0	40	57	0	29	0
A&W Regular Root Beer, med (14 oz)	290	0	0	50	76	0	76	0
A&W Regular Root Beer, lrg (22 oz)	460	0	0	85	121	0	121	0
A&W Diet Root Beer, sml (11 oz)	0	0	0	40	0	0	0	0
A&W Diet Root Beer, med (14 oz)	0	0	0	50	0	0	0	0
A&W Diet Root Beer, lrg (22 oz)	0	0	0	85	0	0	0	0

Back Yard Burgers

Salad

BYB Blackened Chicken Salad	330	15	3	1360	25	5	7	27
BYB Fried Chicken Salad	410	19	3.5	1000	41	5	6	21
BYB Garden Fresh Salad	100	2	0	160	20	4	5	4
BYB Grilled Chicken Salad	220	4	0	950	23	4	7	27
BYB Side Salad	30	0	0	25	6	2	3	1

Description & Serving	Cal	Fat	Sfat	Sod	Carb	Fiber	Sugar	Prot
Burger								
BYB Back Yard American Cheeseburger, 1/3 lb	780	48	19	1560	47	3	6	41
BYB Back Yard American Cheeseburger, 2/3 lb	1270	88	36	2160	47	3	6	74
BYB Back Yard American Cheeseburger, Jr.	630	36	14	1520	47	3	6	31
BYB Back Yard Bleu Cheeseburger, 1/3 lb	780	47	19	1430	47	3	6	42
BYB Back Yard Bleu Cheeseburger, 2/3 lb	1270	86	36	1900	47	3	6	76
BYB Back Yard Bleu Cheeseburger, Jr.	630	35	14	1390	47	3	6	32
BYB Back Yard Burger, 1/3 lb	680	39	14	1040	47	3	6	36
BYB Back Yard Burger, 2/3 lb	1070	70	26	1130	47	3	6	64
BYB Back Yard Burger, Jr.	530	27	9	1010	47	3	6	26
BYB Back Yard Cheddar Cheeseburger, 1/3 lb	790	48	20	1220	47	3	6	43
BYB Back Yard Cheddar Cheeseburger, 2/3 lb	1290	88	38	1490	47	3	6	78
BYB Back Yard Cheddar Cheeseburger, Jr.	640	36	15	1190	47	3	6	33
BYB Back Yard Pepper Jack Cheeseburger, 1/3 lb	740	45	17	1370	47	3	6	39
BYB Back Yard Pepper Jack Cheeseburger, 2/3 lb	1190	82	32	1790	47	3	6	70
BYB Back Yard Pepper Jack Cheeseburger, Jr.	590	33	12	1340	47	3	6	29
BYB Back Yard Swiss Cheeseburger, 1/3 lb	790	48	19	1170	47	3	6	44
BYB Back Yard Swiss Cheeseburger, 2/3 lb	1290	88	36	1390	47	3	6	80
BYB Back Yard Swiss Cheeseburger, Jr.	640	36	14	1140	47	3	6	34
BYB Bacon Cheddar Burger	850	54	22	1420	48	3	6	46
BYB Black Jack Burger	780	49	17	1340	48	4	4	40
BYB Mushroom Swiss Burger	790	49	19	820	45	3	4	45
BYB Garden Veggie Burger	400	8	1.5	1560	57	7	8	27
Sandwich								
BYB Blackened Chicken Sandwich	540	24	4	1810	53	4	9	32
BYB Crispy Chicken Sandwich	590	26	5	1360	65	4	5	25
BYB Grilled Chicken Sandwich	350	4.5	0.5	1280	47	3	6	31
BYB Hawaiian Chicken Sandwich	450	11	1.5	1610	59	3	18	32
Chicken Tender/Hot Dog								
BYB Chicken Tender Meal	1260	79	14	2830	102	8	2	39
BYB Bak-Pak Chicken Tender Meal	1110	71	12	2410	91	7	1	31
BYB Back Yard Big Dog	500	33	13	1480	32	1	9	16
BYB Bak-Pak Dog	320	18	6	950	29	1	7	10
BYB Chili Cheese Big Dog	630	44	20	1770	34	1	9	25
Side								
BYB Chili	150	9	3	690	8	1	3	8
BYB Seasoned Fries, lrg	960	68	11	1740	87	8	0	8
BYB Seasoned Fries, reg	640	45	7	1160	58	6	0	6
Dressing/Condiment								
Honey Mustard Dressing	240	23	3.5	160	7	0	7	0
Balsamic Vinaigrette	170	17	2.5	330	3	0	3	0
Bleu Cheese Dressing	220	24	4.5	440	1	0	1	2
Ranch Dressing	150	15	2.5	380	2	0	1	1
Lite Ranch Dressing	150	15	2.5	390	2	0	1	1
Margarine Cup	50	6	1	65	0	0	0	0
Light Mayonnaise, packet	40	4	0.5	85	1	0	0	0
Real Mayonnaise, packet	90	10	1.5	65	0	0	0	0

Description & Serving	Cal	Fat	Sfat	Sod	Carb	Fiber	Sugar	Prot
Beverage								
BYB Lemonade, 20 oz	490	0	0	0	130	0	125	0
BYB Tea, Sweetened, 20 oz	180	0	0	15	47	0	47	0
BYB Tea, Unsweetened, 20 oz	0	0	0	15	0	0	0	0
Dessert								
BYB Apple Cobbler	360	14	6	330	59	1	35	3
BYB Apple Cobbler A La Mode	510	21	11	390	78	1	53	5
BYB Blackberry Cobbler	290	8	3	170	51	5	30	3
BYB Blackberry Cobbler A La Mode	440	15	8	220	71	5	49	5
BYB Cherry Cobbler	350	12	5	270	59	1	35	3
BYB Cherry Cobbler A La Mode	500	20	10	330	78	1	53	5
BYB Ice Cream, A La Carte	150	8	5	55	20	0	19	2
BYB Peach Cobbler	330	11	5	240	56	1	35	3
BYB Peach Cobbler A La Mode	480	18	9	300	75	1	53	5
BYB Pecan Cobbler	740	26	6	270	119	2	60	9
BYB Pecan Cobbler A La Mode	890	33	11	330	139	2	79	11
BYB Chocolate Shake	640	30	18	280	83	3	77	11
BYB Strawberry Shake	620	28	18	230	83	0	77	11
BYB Vanilla Shake	620	28	18	230	83	0	77	11

Baja Fresh

Description & Serving	Cal	Fat	Sfat	Sod	Carb	Fiber	Sugar	Prot
Entrée								
Chicken								
Chicken Burrito Ultimo	880	36	18	2190	84	9	NP	54
Chicken Baja Burrito	790	38	15	2140	65	8	NP	52
Chicken Burrito Mexicano	790	13	3.5	2270	117	20	NP	50
Cabo Style Salad Burrito	980	52	20	1770	81	11	NP	50
Caesar Style Salad Burrito	940	50	19	1930	75	8	NP	48
Chicken Bean & Cheese Burrito	970	35	18	2230	96	21	NP	67
Chicken Bare Burrito (served in bowl)	640	7	1	2330	97	20	NP	45
Chicken Baja Taco	210	5	1	230	28	2	NP	12
Chicken Americano Soft Taco	230	10	4.5	590	20	2	NP	16
Charbroiled Chicken Quesadilla	1330	80	37	2590	84	9	NP	75
Charbroiled Chicken Nachos	2020	110	41	2980	164	32	NP	91
Mexican Torta w/ Chips	880	35	9	1580	96	9	NP	54
Mexican Torta w/o Chips	620	23	6	1330	64	6	NP	45
Chicken w/ Flour Tortillas	1140	33	10	3240	147	27	NP	69
Chicken w/ Corn Tortillas	860	24	7	2400	105	24	NP	61
Chicken w/ Mixed Tortillas	1070	30	9	2960	137	26	NP	67
Pork								
Carnitas Burrito Ultimo	920	44	21	2330	86	9	NP	46
Carnitas Baja Burrito	830	45	18	2280	67	8	NP	45
Carnitas Burrito Mexicano	830	20	6	2420	119	19	NP	42
Carnitas Bean & Cheese Burrito	1010	42	20	2370	98	21	NP	59
Carnitas Bare Burrito (served in bowl)	680	14	4	2480	99	20	NP	37
Carnitas Baja Taco	220	7	2	280	29	2	NP	10

Description & Serving	Cal	Fat	Sfat	Sod	Carb	Fiber	Sugar	Prot
Carnitas Americano Soft Taco	250	12	5	640	21	2	NP	13
Savory Pork Carnitas Quesadilla	1370	87	40	2730	86	9	NP	67
Savory Pork Carnitas Nachos	2060	117	43	3120	166	32	NP	83
Carnitas w/ Flour Tortillas	1190	43	14	3450	150	26	NP	58
Carnitas w/ Corn Tortillas	920	34	11	2610	108	23	NP	50
Carnitas w/ Mixed Tortillas	1120	40	13	3170	140	26	NP	55
Seafood								
Shrimp Burrito Ultimo	860	36	18	2280	85	8	NP	48
Breaded Fish Burrito Ultimo	940	42	19	1950	96	8	NP	41
Mahi Mahi Burrito Ultimo	880	36	18	1890	84	8	NP	52
Shrimp Baja Burrito	760	37	15	2230	66	7	NP	47
Breaded Fish Baja Burrito	850	44	16	1900	78	7	NP	40
Mahi Mahi Baja Burrito	780	38	15	1840	66	7	NP	51
Shrimp Burrito Mexicano	770	13	3.5	2370	117	18	NP	44
Breaded Fish Burrito Mexicano	850	19	4	2040	129	18	NP	37
Mahi Mahi Burrito Mexicano	790	13	3.5	1970	117	18	NP	49
Shrimp Bean & Cheese Burrito	950	34	17	2320	96	20	NP	61
Breaded Fish Bean & Cheese Burrito	1030	41	18	1990	108	20	NP	54
Mahi Mahi Bean & Cheese Burrito	960	35	18	1930	96	20	NP	65
Shrimp Baja Taco	200	5	1	280	28	2	NP	11
Shrimp Americano Soft Taco	230	10	4.5	640	21	2	NP	15
Breaded Fish Americano Soft Taco	240	11	4.5	490	23	2	NP	10
Mahi Mahi Americano Soft Taco	240	10	4.5	490	20	2	NP	17
Fried Baja Fish Taco	250	13	2	420	27	2	NP	8
Grilled Mahi Mahi Taco	230	9	1.5	300	26	4	NP	12
Charbroiled Shrimp Quesadilla	1310	79	37	2680	84	8	NP	69
Breaded Fish Quesadilla	1400	86	38	2350	96	8	NP	62
Charbroiled Mahi Mahi Quesadilla	1330	79	37	2290	84	8	NP	73
Charbroiled Shrimp Nachos	2000	110	41	3060	164	31	NP	85
Breaded Fish Nachos	2090	116	41	2740	176	31	NP	78
Charbroiled Mahi Mahi Nachos	2020	110	41	2680	164	31	NP	90
Shrimp w/ Flour Tortillas	1120	32	10	3410	148	25	NP	62
Shrimp w/ Corn Tortillas	840	23	7	2570	106	22	NP	55
Shrimp w/ Mixed Tortillas	1045	29	9	3130	138	24	NP	60
Mahi Mahi w/ Flour Tortillas	1120	32	10	2800	147	25	NP	64
Mahi Mahi w/ Corn Tortillas	840	23	7	1960	105	22	NP	57
Mahi Mahi w/ Mixed Tortillas	1050	29	9	2520	138	24	NP	62
Breaded Fish w/ Flour Tortillas	1340	46	12	3020	172	25	NP	59
Breaded Fish w/ Corn Tortillas	1060	37	9	2180	130	22	NP	51
Breaded Fish w/ Mixed Tortillas	1260	43	11	2740	162	24	NP	57
Steak								
Steak Burrito Ultimo	950	44	21	2310	85	8	NP	50
Steak Baja Burrito	850	46	18	2260	67	7	NP	49
Steak Burrito Mexicano	860	21	7	2400	118	18	NP	47
Steak Bean & Cheese Burrito	1030	43	21	2350	97	20	NP	64
Steak Bare Burrito (served in bowl)	700	15	4.5	2450	99	19	NP	41
Steak Baja Taco	230	8	2	260	28	2	NP	11
Steak Americano Soft Taco	260	13	6	640	21	2	NP	15

Description & Serving	Cal	Fat	Sfat	Sod	Carb	Fiber	Sugar	Prot
Charbroiled Steak Quesadilla	1430	87	41	2600	84	8	NP	80
Charbroiled Steak Nachos	2120	118	44	2990	163	31	NP	96
Steak w/ Flour Tortillas	1240	45	15	3440	149	25	NP	65
Steak w/ Corn Tortillas	960	36	12	2600	107	22	NP	58
Steak w/ Mixed Tortillas	1170	42	14	3160	139	24	NP	63
Vegetarian								
Bean & Cheese Burrito	840	33	17	1790	96	20	NP	39
Grilled Veggie Burrito	800	33	17	1880	94	16	NP	32
Veggie & Cheese Bare Burrito (served in bowl)	580	10	4	1950	101	20	NP	19
Cheese Quesadilla	1200	78	37	2140	84	8	NP	47
Veggie Quesadilla	1260	78	37	2310	96	11	NP	48
Kids								
Chicken Taquitos	630	33	7	990	60	4	NP	18
Chicken Taquitos w/ Beans	780	40	12	1810	68	17	NP	39
Chicken Taquitos w/ Rice	740	40	11	1770	66	8	NP	30
Mini Bean & Cheese Burrito	540	14	7	1050	84	11	NP	18
Mini Bean & Cheese Burrito w/ Chicken	590	15	7	1200	84	12	NP	28
Mini Cheese Quesadilla	610	26	13	940	72	5	NP	19
Mini Cheese Quesadilla w/ Chicken	650	27	13	1090	72	5	NP	28
Side								
Cheese Nachos	1890	108	40	2530	163	31	NP	63
Side Salad	130	6	1.5	430	16	4	NP	5
Chips and Guacamole	1340	83	8	950	141	20	NP	21
Pronto Guacamole	560	34	3	370	60	8	NP	9
Chips and Salsa Baja	810	37	4	1140	98	14	NP	13
Rice & Beans Plate	420	5	1.5	1320	72	18	NP	18
Rice	280	4	0.5	980	55	4	NP	5
Black Beans	360	2.5	1	1120	61	26	NP	23
Pinto Beans	320	1	0	840	56	21	NP	19
Veggie Mix	110	0	0	330	24	6	NP	3
Steak	330	14	6	670	0	0	NP	48
Chicken	230	3.5	0.5	760	0	2	NP	48
Carnitas	300	16	6	1010	4	2	NP	35
Shrimp	150	2	0.5	740	1	0	NP	31
Breaded Fish	390	16	2.5	410	25	0	NP	30
Mahi Mahi	210	3	1	240	1	0	NP	44
Tostada Shell	490	28	3.5	600	44	4	NP	7
Corn Tortilla Chips, 1.5 oz	210	9	1	55	29	3	NP	3
Corn Tortilla Chips, 5 oz	740	34	3.5	170	90	9	NP	10
Soup								
Chicken Tortilla Soup w/o Charbroiled Chicken	270	14	4	2600	29	4	NP	8
Chicken Tortilla Soup w/ Charbroiled Chicken	320	14	4	2760	29	4	NP	17
Salad								
Charbroiled Chicken Baja Ensalada	310	7	2	1210	18	7	NP	46
Charbroiled Steak Baja Ensalada	450	18	7	1240	18	6	NP	54
Savory Pork Carnitas Baja Ensalada	370	18	6	1410	20	7	NP	35

Description & Serving	Cal	Fat	Sfat	Sod	Carb	Fiber	Sugar	Prot
Charbroiled Shrimp Baja Ensalada	230	6	2	1110	18	6	NP	28
No Meat Tostada Salad	1010	53	13	1930	98	25	NP	32
Charbroiled Chicken Tostada Salad	1140	55	14	2370	98	27	NP	60
Charbroiled Steak Tostada Salad	1230	63	17	2380	98	25	NP	65
Savory Pork Carnitas Tostada Salad	1180	62	17	2520	100	26	NP	52
Charbroiled Shrimp Tostada Salad	1120	55	14	2460	99	25	NP	55
Breaded Fish Tostada Salad	1200	61	15	2140	111	25	NP	47
Charbroiled Fish Tostada Salad	1130	55	14	2070	99	25	NP	59
Dressing/Condiment								
"Enchilado" Style Addition (for burritos)	630	40	19	1450	45	7	NP	23
Olive Oil Vinaigrette, 71 g	290	31	4.5	290	2	0	NP	0
Ranch Dressing, 71 g	260	26	6	470	4	0	NP	2
Fat Free Salsa Verde, 71 g	15	0	0	370	3	1	NP	0
Guacamole, 8 oz	310	35	5	710	14	6	NP	6
Salsa Baja, 8 oz	70	2.5	0	970	7	4	NP	2
Salsa Verde, 8 oz	50	0	0	1170	11	3	NP	2
Salsa Roja, 8 oz	70	1	0	1080	13	4	NP	3
Pico de Gallo, 8 oz	50	0.5	0	890	12	3	NP	2

Blimpie

Breakfast

Description & Serving	Cal	Fat	Sfat	Sod	Carb	Fiber	Sugar	Prot
Plain Bluffin	129	1	0	242	25	2	2	5
Bacon, Egg & Cheese Biscuit	432	24	17	1579	37	1	3	17
Egg & Cheese Biscuit	385	21	15	1377	37	1	3	14
Plain Biscuit	263	11	10	830	34	1	3	6
Ham, Egg & Cheese Biscuit	420	21	16	1655	39	1	5	19
Sausage, Egg & Cheese Biscuit	535	35	20	1687	37	1	3	20
Bacon, Egg & Cheese Bluffin	293	14	7	973	27	2	2	16
Egg & Cheese Bluffin	245	10	5	771	27	2	2	13
Ham, Egg, & Cheese Bluffin	280	11	6	1049	29	2	4	18
Sausage, Egg & Cheese Bluffin	395	24	10	1081	27	2	2	19
Bacon, Egg & Cheese Burrito	553	24	12	2095	56	5	3	31
Egg & Cheese Burrito	506	20	11	1892	56	5	3	28
Ham, Egg & Cheese Burrito	559	21	11	2310	58	5	5	36
Sausage, Egg & Cheese Burrito	656	34	16	2202	56	5	3	34
Bacon, Egg & Cheese Croissant	396	115	12	1026	30	1	4	16
Egg & Cheese Croissant	349	111	11	823	30	1	4	12
Ham, Egg & Cheese Croissant	384	112	11	1102	31	1	6	17
Plain Croissant	233	102	6	295	28	1	4	5
Sausage, Egg & Cheese Croissant	499	125	16	1133	30	1	4	18
Cinnamon Roll	449	20	9	729	60	2	17	9
Panini Breakfast, 4"	494	14	5	1408	67	2	7	26

Sandwich

Description & Serving	Cal	Fat	Sfat	Sod	Carb	Fiber	Sugar	Prot
Blimpie Best Sub, 4"	268	8	4	910	33	2	6	16
Blimpie Best Sub, Super Stacked, 6"	523	19	8	2128	52	3	12	37
Blimpie Trio Sub, Super Stacked, 6"	488	12	5	1773	52	3	11	41
BLT Sub, Regular, 6"	447	22	5	933	46	3	7	15

Description & Serving	Cal	Fat	Sfat	Sod	Carb	Fiber	Sugar	Prot
BLT Sub, Super Stacked, 6"	639	41	9	1438	43	2	6	22
Chicken Cheddar Bacon Ranch Sub, Regular, 6"	642	34	10	1648	48	3	8	36
Chicken Teriyaki Sub, Regular, 6"	428	9	4	1315	50	1	12	35
Chicken Teriyaki, Wheat, 6"	416	10	5	1255	47	5	12	36
Club, 4"	254	6	3	743	33	2	6	16
Club, Wheat, 6"	363	11	5	1003	43	6	8	26
Cuban, Regular, 6"	413	11	5	1628	43	1	6	29
French Dip Sub, 6"	413	11	5	1652	46	1	3	30
Ham & Swiss Sub, 4"	257	6	3	724	33	2	7	16
Ham & Swiss Sub, Wheat, 6"	368	11	5	965	44	6	9	26
Ham, Salami & Cheese Sub, Regular, 6"	443	16	7	1306	49	3	9	25
Meatball Sub, Regular, 6"	607	32	14	2072	51	4	6	28
Hot Pastrami Sub, 6"	435	16	7	1354	42	1	5	30
Hot Pastrami Sub, Super Stacked, 6"	571	23	10	2113	43	1	7	46
Philly Steak & Onion Sub, Regular, 6"	499	24	10	1233	45	1	6	26
Reuben, Regular, 6"	571	24	7	1221	54	3	8	34
Roast Beef & Provolone Sub, 4"	262	7	3	676	31	2	5	20
Roast Beef & Provolone Sub, Wheat, 6"	385	12	5	990	40	6	6	32
Roast Beef, Turkey & Cheddar Sub, Regular, 6"	571	30	9	1769	48	3	8	27
Seafood Sub, Regular, 6"	333	7	1	840	56	4	9	13
Special Vegetarian Sub, 6"	593	30	10	1766	66	4	10	17
Tuna Sub, 4"	282	11	2	458	31	2	5	14
Turkey & Avocado Sub, 6"	381	9	1	1406	52	4	8	21
Turkey & Cranberry Sub, 6"	350	4	1	1219	58	3	14	20
Turkey & Bacon Sub, Super Stacked, 6"	582	24	11	2622	48	2	8	40
Turkey & Provolone Sub, 4"	247	6	2	858	33	2	5	16
Turkey & Provolone Sub, Wheat, 6"	370	10	5	1344	43	6	7	27
Veggie Supreme Sub, 6"	553	28	16	1415	48	3	7	29
VegiMax Sub, 6"	522	20	6	1272	56	5	8	28
VegiMax Sub, Wheat, 6"	499	21	6	1212	50	8	7	30

Specialty Sandwich/Wrap

Ciabatta, Buffalo Chicken	583	27	7	2050	50	3	5	32
Ciabatta, Grilled Chicken Caesar	617	24	6	1584	63	3	4	34
Ciabatta, Mediterranean	447	8	2	1719	65	3	6	26
Ciabatta, Roast Beef, Turkey & Cheddar	588	30	9	1941	51	3	6	28
Ciabatta, Sicilian	637	25	7	2520	68	3	10	33
Ciabatta, Tuscan	600	23	7	2150	65	3	6	29
Ciabatta, Turkey Italiano	502	11	4	2164	64	3	5	30
Ciabatta, Ultimate Club	480	21	6	1538	47	2	5	27
Chicken Caesar Wrap, Regular	607	29	9	1586	56	4	5	30
Roast Beef & Cheddar Wrap, Regular	684	36	12	1928	59	6	5	32
Southwestern Wrap, Regular	530	22	6	1771	61	4	10	23
Steak & Onion Wrap, Regular	774	47	15	1795	62	6	7	28
Zesty Wrap, Regular	569	26	10	1979	59	6	6	28

Salad

Antipasto Salad	245	14	6	1627	12	4	6	20
Buffalo Chicken Salad	222	9	5	842	10	4	5	25
Chef Salad, Regular	176	7	4	805	10	2	5	18

Description & Serving	Cal	Fat	Sfat	Sod	Carb	Fiber	Sugar	Prot
Chicken Caesar Salad	192	8	4	463	6	3	3	25
Garden Salad	29	0	0	16	6	3	3	2
Seafood Salad, Regular	122	4	1	582	17	3	5	6
Tuna Salad, Regular	272	18	3	517	7	2	3	18
Ultimate Club Salad	287	16	9	1196	10	3	6	25

Soup

Bean w/ Ham Soup	140	1	0	1070	23	11	2	8
Beef Steak & Noodle Soup	120	3	2	780	14	0	4	8
Beef Stew	170	4	2	890	18	2	2	17
Captain's Corn Chowder	210	7	3	890	29	4	7	6
Chicken & Dumping Soup	170	5	3	970	19	3	4	11
Chicken Gumbo	90	2	0	1280	13	2	4	6
Chicken Noodle Soup	130	4	1	1040	18	2	5	7
Chicken w/ White & Wild Rice Soup	150	10	3	1030	15	4	4	14
Cream of Broccoli w/ Cheese Soup	190	8	5	940	15	3	5	6
Cream of Potato Soup	190	9	3	860	24	3	3	5
French Onion Soup	0	4	1	1020	11	1	6	2
Grande Chili w/ Bean & Beef	250	9	5	1230	30	18	7	18
Harvest Vegetable Soup	100	1	0	920	19	3	4	4
Italian Style Wedding Soup	130	4	2	900	17	0	0	7
Minestrone Soup	90	3	0	1150	14	4	4	4
New England Clam Chowder	170	3	2	1060	28	2	5	7
Pasta Fagioli w/ Sausage Soup	150	5	2	910	22	4	2	7
Pilgrim Turkey Vegetables w/ Rice Soup	110	2	1	800	19	2	2	4
Seafood Gumbo	100	2	1	850	16	2	3	4
Split Pea w/ Ham Soup	130	2	0	1090	21	6	1	8
Tomato Basil w/ Raviolini Soup	110	1	0	720	22	0	5	4
Yankee Pot Roast Soup	80	2	1	750	12	2	2	5

Side

Cole Slaw	160	9	2	240	20	2	17	1
Macaroni Salad	330	22	5	790	28	2	8	5
North West Potato Salad	260	17	4	390	22	3	3	3
Potato Salad	230	12	3	490	28	3	8	3

Kids

3" Ham & American Cheese Kids Meal	262	9	5	901	32	2	6	15
3" Tuna Kids Meal	277	11	2	457	30	2	4	14
3" Turkey Kids Meal	187	2	0	598	31	2	5	10

Dessert

Brownie	182	7	3	115	28	1	19	2
Chocolate Chunk Cookie	196	10	4	153	25	0	16	2
Oatmeal Raisin Cookie	170	7	3	142	26	1	15	2
Peanut Butter Cookie	198	12	5	161	20	1	12	3
Sugar Cookie	327	17	6	286	41	1	22	3
White Chocolate Macadamia Nut Cookie	198	12	5	161	20	1	12	3
Apple Turnover	340	21	10	190	35	1	11	4
Cherry Turnover	350	21	10	190	35	1	14	4

Description & Serving	Cal	Fat	Sfat	Sod	Carb	Fiber	Sugar	Prot
Bread								
Cheddar Jalapeno Bread, 6"	213	4	2	434	36	1	3	8
Ciabatta Bread	230	3	0	590	43	2	2	8
Honey Oat Bread, 6"	259	8	1	405	41	5	5	10
Marble Rye, 6"	242	2	1	NP	46	2	2	9
Wheat Bread, 6"	190	4	1	357	34	4	2	9
White Bread, 6"	213	3	1	418	40	1	3	7
Zesty Parmesan Bread, 6"	236	4	2	488	39	2	4	9
Spinach Herb Wrap	310	8	3	840	52	3	3	9
Traditional Wrap	310	8	3	670	52	5	1	9
Topping								
Bacon	105	8	3	447	0	0	0	7
Cappacola	18	1	0	164	0	NP	0	3
Chicken Strips	93	3	1	253	0	0	0	16
Corned Beef	106	2	1	759	2	0	2	18
Egg	45	3	1	188	2	0	0	4
Ham	35	1	0	278	2	NP	2	5
Meatballs	292	21	8	1342	11	3	3	15
Pastrami	114	6	3	633	1	0	1	14
Pepperoni	66	6	3	233	1	NP	NP	3
Philly Steak & Onion	210	15	6	630	5	NP	3	13
Prosciuttini	13	0	0	177	1	0	1	2
Roast Beef	46	1	0	220	0	0	0	8
Salami	36	3	1	137	0	0	0	2
Seafood Salad	92	4	1	415	10	1	2	4
Tuna	241	18	2	350	0	0	0	16
Turkey	30	0	0	316	1	NP	1	5
American Cheese	104	9	6	507	1	NP	NP	6
Cheddar Cheese	75	6	4	382	1	NP	0	4
Shredded Parmesan Cheese	52	4	2	145	1	0	0	4
Shredded Mild Cheddar Cheese	114	9	6	176	0	0	0	7
Pepper Jack Cheese	77	7	4	135	0	0	0	6
Provolone Cheese	76	6	4	190	0	NP	NP	5
Swiss Cheese	79	6	4	44	0	0	0	6
Guacamole, 1 oz	45	4	1	135	2	1	0	0
Lettuce, 1.5 oz	6	0	0	4	1	0	1	0
Olives, 0.5 oz	16	2	0	124	1	0	0	0
Onion, 3 pc	11	0	0	1	3	0	1	0
Hot Ring Peppers, 12 pc	0	0	0	450	1	0	0	0
Jalapeno Peppers, 18 pc	10	0	0	486	1	0	0	0
Red Roasted Peppers, 1.7 oz	11	0	0	112	2	0	1	0
Sweet Pepper Strips, 6 pc	20	0	0	116	5	0	5	0
Tomato, 2 pc	7	0	0	2	2	0	1	0
Dressing/Condiment								
Blue Cheese Dressing	230	24	5	440	2	NP	2	2
Buttermilk Ranch Dressing	230	24	4	380	2	NP	1	1
Creamy Caesar Dressing	210	21	4	520	2	NP	1	1

Description & Serving	Cal	Fat	Sfat	Sod	Carb	Fiber	Sugar	Prot
Creamy Italian Dressing	180	18	3	420	4	0	3	0
Dijon Honey Mustard Dressing	180	17	3	240	8	NP	7	1
Fat-Free Italian Dressing	25	0	NP	390	5	0	3	0
Light Buttermilk Ranch Dressing	70	4	1	310	8	NP	3	1
Light Italian Dressing	20	1	0	770	2	NP	2	0
Peppercorn Dressing	240	26	4	453	1	0	1	1
Special Dressing	70	7	1	0	0	NP	NP	0
Thousand Island Dressing	210	20	3	350	6	0	6	0
Mayonnaise	202	22	3	202	0	0	0	0
Mustard, Deli Style	5	0	0	60	0	0	0	0
Mustard, Honey	43	1	0	168	7	1	5	1
Mustard, Spicy Brown	5	0	0	60	0	NP	0	0
Oil, Blend	130	14	2	0	0	0	0	0
Red Wine Vinegar	5	0	0	0	1	0	0	0
Original Red Hot Sauce	10	0	0	760	2	0	0	0

Bob Evans

Breakfast

Crepe/Parfait

	Cal	Fat	Sfat	Sod	Carb	Fiber	Sugar	Prot
Blueberry Banana & Yogurt Crepe, 1	366	11	4	291	59	5	39	8
Blueberry Crepe, 1	396	25	9	296	37	2	24	5
Plain Crepe, 1	345	25	9	289	25	1	12	5
Strawberry Banana Crepe, 1	448	25	9	290	51	4	34	6
Strawberry Banana Fruit & Yogurt Crepe, 1	345	11	4	287	53	5	34	8
Strawberry Blueberry Fruit & Yogurt Crepe, 1	327	12	4	292	48	5	31	8
Blueberry & Banana Yogurt Parfait	177	1	0	61	39	3	34	4
Strawberry Banana Mini Fruit & Yogurt Parfait	151	1	0	55	33	3	28	4
Strawberry Blueberry Mini Fruit & Yogurt Parfait	158	1	0	62	34	3	30	4

Eggs

	Cal	Fat	Sfat	Sod	Carb	Fiber	Sugar	Prot
Bob Evans Egg Lites Omelet Shell	85	0	0	357	1	0	2	17
Border Scramble Omelet	621	44	18	1569	16	3	9	40
Border Scramble Omelet, Bob Evans Egg Lites	441	25	13	1248	15	3	9	38
Border Scramble Omelet, Egg White	431	25	13	1159	15	3	8	38
Egg White Omelet Shell	75	0	0	269	2	0	0	17
Egg, 1	131	11	3	68	1	0	1	7
Farmer's Market Omelet	621	43	21	2209	14	1	6	38
Farmer's Market Omelet, Bob Evans Egg Lites	440	25	16	1888	13	1	6	36
Farmer's Market Omelet, Egg White	427	25	16	1791	13	1	4	36
Garden Harvest Omelet	503	34	17	1726	14	2	6	29
Garden Harvest Omelet, Bob Evans Egg Lites	323	16	12	1405	13	2	6	28
Garden Harvest Omelet, Egg White	313	16	12	1317	13	2	4	27
Ham & Cheddar Benedict	836	53	20	3166	44	0	8	43
Ham & Cheddar Omelet	477	33	13	1773	4	0	2	39
Ham & Cheddar Omelet, Bob Evans Egg Lites	296	14	8	1451	3	0	2	37
Ham & Cheddar Omelet, Egg White	286	14	8	1363	3	0	0	37
Hardcooked Egg, 1	57	4	1	52	1	0	0	6
Omelet Shell, 4 oz	185	13	4	452	2	0	1	13

Description & Serving	Cal	Fat	Sfat	Sod	Carb	Fiber	Sugar	Prot
Omelet Shell, 6 oz	265	19	5	678	3	0	2	19
Sausage & Cheddar Omelet	640	49	19	1538	4	0	2	42
Sausage & Cheddar Omelet, Bob Evans Egg Lites	459	31	14	1217	3	0	2	40
Sausage & Cheddar Omelet, Egg White	449	31	14	1128	3	0	0	40
Scrambled Egg Lites, 1 egg equiv	28	0	0	119	1	0	1	6
Scrambled Egg Whites, 1 egg equiv	25	0	0	90	1	0	0	6
Scrambled Eggs, 1 egg equiv	80	5	2	226	1	0	1	6
Spinach, Bacon & Tomato Country Benedict	760	51	17	1972	43	1	8	31
Three Cheese Omelet	490	37	17	1415	4	0	2	31
Three Cheese Omelet, Bob Evans Egg Lites	309	18	12	1094	3	0	2	29
Three Cheese Omelet, Egg White	299	18	12	1005	3	0	0	29
Turkey & Spinach Omelet	580	37	16	2386	7	1	5	48
Turkey & Spinach Omelet, Bob Evans Egg Lites	400	18	11	2065	6	1	5	46
Turkey & Spinach Omelet, Egg White	389	18	11	1976	6	1	3	46
Western Omelet	487	32	13	1744	7	1	4	39
Western Omelet, Bob Evans Egg Lites	310	14	8	1453	6	1	4	38
Western Omelet, Egg White	300	14	8	1364	6	1	2	37

Hotcakes

Description & Serving	Cal	Fat	Sfat	Sod	Carb	Fiber	Sugar	Prot
Blueberry Hotcake w/o topping, 1	343	10	2	792	58	2	18	7
Buttermilk Hotcake w/o topping, 1	337	10	2	792	56	2	16	7
Cinnamon Hotcake w/o topping, 1	382	12	4	792	62	2	22	7
Multigrain Hotcake w/o topping, 1	374	11	4	897	61	4	18	8
Stacked & Stuffed Blueberry Cream Hotcakes	1047	36	16	1852	165	6	80	18
Stacked & Stuffed Caramel Banana Pecan Hotcakes	1493	70	21	2265	204	9	110	20
Stacked & Stuffed Cinnamon Cream Hotcakes	1070	43	20	1911	155	4	72	17
Stacked & Stuffed Strawberry Banana Cream Hotcakes	1168	36	16	1837	197	12	103	19

Specialty Breakfast

Description & Serving	Cal	Fat	Sfat	Sod	Carb	Fiber	Sugar	Prot
Border Scramble Burrito w/ Egg	812	46	17	1989	57	9	9	43
Border Scramble Burrito w/ Egg Lites	683	33	13	1775	56	9	10	42
Border Scramble Burrito w/ Egg Whites	677	33	13	1716	56	9	8	42
Country Biscuit Breakfast	666	46	16	1697	39	0	6	25
Fit from the Farm Breakfast w/ Parfait	306	4	1	703	41	3	36	25
Fit from the Farm Breakfast w/ Oatmeal	347	6	2	813	46	3	29	26
Fit from the Farm Breakfast w/ Yogurt Crepe	495	15	5	933	61	6	41	29
French Toast, ea	164	3	1	283	18	1	9	4
Fruit & Yogurt Plate	347	2	0	74	82	9	69	7
Meat Lover's BoBurrito	799	49	19	2427	41	3	7	47
Meat Lover's BoBurrito, Egg Lites	670	36	16	2212	41	3	7	46
Meat Lover's BoBurrito, Egg Whites	663	36	16	2154	41	3	6	46
Pot Roast Hash	701	45	14	1210	34	4	19	37
Stuffed French Toast w/o topping	627	19	9	977	65	3	37	14
Sunshine Skillet	638	41	14	1905	36	4	17	30
Sweet Cream Waffles w/o topping	394	8	4	849	66	2	20	10
Turkey Sausage Breakfast	362	7	2	1009	48	5	18	27
Western BoBurrito	677	37	14	2392	42	3	7	44
Western BoBurrito, Egg Lites	548	24	10	2178	42	3	7	43
Western BoBurrito, Egg Whites	542	24	10	2119	42	3	6	43

Description & Serving	Cal	Fat	Sfat	Sod	Carb	Fiber	Sugar	Prot
Breakfast Side/Condiment								
Apple Butter, 0.5 oz	34	0	0	2	8	0	7	0
Bacon, 1 pc	36	4	2	54	0	0	0	1
Banana Nut Bread	215	8	1	125	34	2	21	4
Beef Gravy, 2.2 oz	25	1	0	419	3	0	0	1
Biscuit	274	14	4	885	32	0	3	5
Blueberry Bread	261	12	2	338	36	1	20	3
Bowl of Grits	265	10	4	257	40	2	1	4
Bowl of Oatmeal	167	3	0	259	31	4	1	6
Bowl of Sausage Gravy	313	20	13	1480	26	0	2	8
Chicken-Roasted Gravy, 2 oz	54	4	1	262	3	0	0	1
Cinnamon Swirl, frosted	532	28	0	602	67	0	21	10
Cinnamon Swirl, unfrosted	616	30	1	623	82	0	35	11
Country Gravy, 3 oz	56	4	1	303	6	0	2	0
Cup of Grits	148	6	2	143	22	1	0	2
Cup of Oatmeal	91	2	0	140	17	2	0	3
Cup of Sausage Gravy	182	12	8	860	15	0	1	5
Diet Blackberry Jam, 0.4 oz	5	0	0	5	2	1	1	0
Grape Jelly, 0.5 oz	36	0	0	2	9	0	9	0
Mush	171	7	1	1012	25	5	10	2
Orange Marmalade, 0.5 oz	36	0	0	0	9	0	8	0
Pancake Syrup, 3 oz	213	0	0	101	55	0	44	0
Sausage Breakfast Patty, 1	140	11	4	313	0	0	0	8
Sausage Link, 1	133	12	3	184	0	0	0	5
Smoked Ham, 1 pc	99	3	1	1293	3	0	1	16
Strawberry Jam, 0.5 oz	36	0	0	1	9	0	9	0
Sugar Free Pancake Syrup, 3 oz	39	0	0	79	10	0	0	0
Turkey Sausage, 1 pc	72	4	1	404	1	0	0	9
Appetizer								
Blue Ribbon Apple Pie	503	12	2	712	96	4	57	3
Country Fair Cheese Bites	942	66	33	1757	47	5	4	41
Itsy Bitsy Trio	1134	55	15	1898	111	5	12	50
Itsy Bitsy Trio, Mini Pot Roast Sandwich	243	11	4	582	23	1	5	12
Itsy Bitsy Trio, Mini Pulled Pork Sandwich	281	14	3	502	22	1	3	20
Itsy Bitsy Trio, Mini Sausage Sandwich	298	17	6	767	20	1	3	13
Loaded Potato Bites	1008	63	16	2180	93	6	7	16
Wildfire Chicken Quesadilla	766	34	17	1581	55	6	19	62
Salad								
Chili & Cheese Taco Salad, Savor size	616	44	14	1104	43	8	7	20
Chili & Cheese Taco Salad	855	64	18	1565	52	11	10	26
Cobb Salad, Savor size	413	28	12	1146	7	2	3	36
Cobb Salad	568	37	18	1673	10	3	4	51
Country Caesar Salad, Savor size	547	38	10	1355	19	1	4	32
Country Caesar Salad	746	53	12	1712	20	1	4	44
Country Spinach Salad, Savor size	435	30	8	1082	10	4	4	35
Country Spinach Salad	479	31	8	1297	12	5	4	44
Cranberry Pecan Chicken Salad, Savor size	673	45	15	1658	38	4	28	32
Cranberry Pecan Chicken Salad	894	60	17	2338	45	5	34	46

Description & Serving	Cal	Fat	Sfat	Sod	Carb	Fiber	Sugar	Prot
Garden Salad	58	1	0	132	9	1	2	2
Heritage Chef Salad, Savor size	294	18	9	923	7	2	4	26
Heritage Chef Salad	398	25	12	1320	10	3	6	35
Specialty Garden Salad	124	7	3	334	10	1	2	6
Wildfire Fried Chicken Salad, Savor size	543	27	8	995	54	5	13	23
Wildfire Fried Chicken Salad	711	34	9	1332	70	7	18	32
Wildfire Grilled Chicken Salad, Savor size	391	18	6	769	35	5	13	24
Wildfire Grilled Chicken Salad	440	19	6	963	37	6	14	32

Soup/Chili

	Cal	Fat	Sfat	Sod	Carb	Fiber	Sugar	Prot
Bean Soup, cup	110	2	1	549	15	4	0	8
Bean Soup, bowl	204	4	1	1016	28	8	1	14
Cheddar Baked Potato Soup, cup	172	9	6	744	15	0	2	8
Cheddar Baked Potato Soup, bowl	242	13	8	1046	22	1	3	12
Vegetable Beef Soup, cup	90	2	1	503	13	2	6	6
Vegetable Beef Soup, bowl	135	3	1	759	20	3	8	8
Sausage Chili, cup	215	14	5	550	15	6	1	13
Sausage Chili, bowl	351	22.	8	898	24	9	2	21

Sandwich

	Cal	Fat	Sfat	Sod	Carb	Fiber	Sugar	Prot
Bob's BLT & E	639	41	15	1021	26	3	7	19
Bob-B-Q Pulled Pork Sandwich	599	25	4	741	67	4	26	34
Chicken Salad Sandwich, half	319	19	3	646	27	3	6	11
Fried Chicken Club Sandwich	637	31	11	1567	47	3	4	40
Fried Chicken Sandwich	489	18	4	1109	47	3	4	35
Fried Haddock Sandwich	732	33	10	1596	71	4	6	38
Grilled Cheese Sandwich	350	15	6	729	22	2	4	9
Grilled Chicken Club Sandwich	583	31	11	1420	34	2	4	40
Grilled Chicken Sandwich	441	19	4	971	33	2	4	35
Knife & Fork Bob-B-Q Chicken Sandwich	670	20	9	1438	60	5	31	35
Knife & Fork Bob-B-Q Pulled Pork Sandwich	859	32	9	1176	91	7	53	33
Knife & Fork Meatloaf Sandwich	820	37	17	3182	51	3	13	24
Knife & Fork Turkey Sandwich	718	37	12	2784	46	2	7	27
Pot Roast Sandwich, half	371	18	7	829	30	2	8	22
Turkey Bacon Melt, half	292	14	6	1035	23	1	3	17

Burger

	Cal	Fat	Sfat	Sod	Carb	Fiber	Sugar	Prot
Bacon Cheeseburger	719	38	17	1355	35	2	5	25
Cheeseburger	648	31	13	1247	35	2	5	24
Hamburger	542	22	8	776	34	2	4	18
Hamburger Patty, 1	336	17	7	186	0	0	0	12

Entrée

Beef

	Cal	Fat	Sfat	Sod	Carb	Fiber	Sugar	Prot
Country Fried Steak	496	33	11	1217	31	0	0	18
Country Fried Steak w/ Gravy	550	37	12	1510	37	0	2	19
Italian Sausage & Pepper Pasta	696	40	12	2001	54	5	13	23
Italian Sausage Link, 1 pc	363	28	10	1021	1	0	1	20
Meatloaf	435	22	8	1958	22	1	11	17
Open-Faced Roast Beef	476	24	8	1041	22	1	9	32
Pot Roast Beef Stew Deep-Dish	727	34	14	2900	67	3	10	24

Description & Serving	Cal	Fat	Sfat	Sod	Carb	Fiber	Sugar	Prot
Sirloin Steak	421	29	9	638	3	0	0	33
Steak Tip Stir-Fry	1008	43	11	3687	87	6	28	70
Steak Tips & Noodles	947	54	13	3558	50	3	5	67
Steak Tips	266	15	4	828	3	0	0	29
Chicken/Turkey								
Bob-B-Q Roasted Chicken	326	14	4	1151	15	1	15	35
Chicken Fried Chicken Deep-Dish Dinner	1087	60	19	3106	90	2	7	34
Chicken Parmesan	691	28	9	2365	65	5	13	39
Chicken Salad Plate	712	43	6	974	70	12	56	20
Chicken Stir-Fry	636	20	4	2635	78	6	27	38
Fried Chicken Breast	285	12	3	758	13	1	0	29
Fried Chicken Strips, 1 pc	137	8	1	301	10	0	0	7
Garden Vegetable & Chicken Alfredo	851	46	18	2224	60	6	10	46
Garlic Butter Grilled Chicken Breast	242	14	3	691	1	0	0	29
Grilled Chicken Breast	242	14	3	635	0	0	0	29
Grilled Chicken Tenders, 1 pc	87	6	1	188	0	0	0	8
Slow-Roasted Chicken-N-Noodles	289	16	3	695	23	1	3	13
Slow-Roasted Chicken Pot Pie	886	60	22	2710	66	5	13	31
Wildfire Grilled Chicken Breast	299	14	3	719	15	1	14	29
Slow-Roasted Turkey	136	5	1	972	1	0	2	20
Turkey & Dressing	622	31	9	3059	36	2	8	45
Pork								
Pork Bob-B-Q Ribs Dinner	759	26	10	1889	77	5	54	52
Pork Bob-B-Q Ribs	377	13	5	937	38	2	27	26
Seafood								
Fried Haddock	363	18	4	608	27	2	2	24
Garden Vegetable & Salmon Alfredo	975	54	20	1715	60	6	10	58
Garlic Butter Salmon	300	15	3	172	1	0	0	40
Potato-Crusted Flounder	218	12	3	531	9	0	1	19
Salmon Stir-Fry	760	28	5	2126	78	6	27	50
Salmon	294	14	3	101	0	0	0	40
Wildfire Salmon	357	14	3	200	15	1	14	40
Vegetarian								
Chicken-N-Noodles Deep-Dish, dinner size	785	38	13	2312	66	2	6	30
Garden Vegetable Alfredo	809	48	20	1860	72	10	14	21
Green Pepper & Onion Pasta	468	21	4	1498	59	6	16	8
Vegetable Stir-Fry	507	14	2	2050	87	9	31	13
Side								
Applesauce	69	0	0	11	18	2	13	0
Baked Potato	220	3	0	525	51	6	6	8
Broccoli Florets	44	1	0	41	8	5	3	5
Coleslaw	208	14	2	243	19	1	17	1
Corn	166	11	4	258	17	2	2	2
Corn & Pepper Relish	16	0	0	2	4	1	1	0
Cottage Cheese	92	4	2	310	4	1	3	11
Cranberry Relish	68	0	0	7	16	1	15	0
Dinner Roll	201	5	1	268	34	1	6	5

Description & Serving	Cal	Fat	Sfat	Sod	Carb	Fiber	Sugar	Prot
French Fries	319	13	3	92	46	1	0	4
Fruit Cup	148	1	0	8	38	4	32	1
Fruit Dish	58	0	0	7	14	1	13	1
Garden Vegetables	160	11	4	307	15	5	6	3
Glazed Carrots	75	3	1	85	13	3	6	1
Green Beans	47	2	1	515	6	2	1	3
Grilled Mushrooms	87	5	1	865	10	5	0	4
Home Fries	183	6	1	685	28	3	14	3
Loaded Baked Potato	388	16	8	983	53	6	7	18
Mashed Potatoes	192	7	4	428	16	1	1	2
Onion Petals	301	18	2	464	35	2	3	3
Parmesan Crusted Garlic Bread, 1 pc	195	9	3	430	23	1	0	6
Rice Pilaf	133	5	1	620	21	1	1	2
Strawberry Yogurt	93	1	0	54	18	0	17	4

Kids

Description & Serving	Cal	Fat	Sfat	Sod	Carb	Fiber	Sugar	Prot
Fresh Garden Salad	49	4	2	74	1	1	0	3
Fried Chicken Strips, 1 pc	137	8	1	301	10	0	0	7
Fruit & Yogurt Dippers	222	1	0	62	51	5	44	5
Fudge Blast Sundae	216	9	6	83	31	0	22	3
Grilled Cheese Triangles	313	15	7	851	32	1	3	10
Grilled Chicken Tenders, 1 pc	87	6	1	188	0	0	0	8
Hot Cocoa, 8.2 oz	253	10	9	233	39	1	36	3
Kids Pasta	139	3	1	404	23	2	4	2
Macaroni & Cheese	318	11	3	774	44	2	11	11
Mini Cheeseburgers	284	15	6	507	22	1	4	12
Plenty-O-Pancakes	337	12	5	685	52	1	18	6
Reese I'm Smiling Sundae	274	13	7	117	35	1	27	5
Smiley Faced Potatoes	271	16	3	334	29	2	1	3
Strawberry Sundae, 4.4 oz	177	8	6	41	24	1	19	3
Turkey Lurkey	163	7	2	1102	2	0	1	20

Seniors

Description & Serving	Cal	Fat	Sfat	Sod	Carb	Fiber	Sugar	Prot
Chicken Parmesan	552	25	9	1961	41	4	8	37
Chicken Stir-Fry	365	12	2	1359	45	5	16	21
Garden Vegetable Alfredo	415	25	10	972	36	5	7	11
Garden Vegetable & Chicken Alfredo	501	28	11	1277	36	5	7	25
Green Pepper & Onion Pasta	329	18	4	1094	36	5	11	6
Italian Sausage & Pepper Pasta	557	36	11	1597	31	3	9	21
Steak Tip Stir-Fry	546	24	5	1882	48	5	16	37
Steak Tips & Noodles	486	27	7	1989	27	1	3	34
Turkey & Dressing	486	26	8	2087	35	2	6*	26
Vegetable Stir-Fry	279	9	1	1054	45	5	16	7

Dressing/Condiment

Description & Serving	Cal	Fat	Sfat	Sod	Carb	Fiber	Sugar	Prot
Avocado Ranch Dressing, 1.6 oz	219	23	4	383	2	0	1	1
Blue Cheese Dressing, 1.6 oz	235	25	5	360	3	0	2	2
Bread & Celery Dressing	148	8	2	427	16	1	2	3
Buttermilk Ranch Dressing, 1.6 oz	166	17	3	333	2	0	2	2
Caesar Dressing, 1.6 oz	247	27	4	375	1	0	0	1

Description & Serving	Cal	Fat	Sfat	Sod	Carb	Fiber	Sugar	Prot
Citrus Stir-Fry Sauce, 2 oz	51	0	0	335	12	0	10	1
Cocktail Sauce, 1 oz	25	0	0	334	6	0	4	0
Colonial Dressing, 1.6 oz	247	22	3	206	12	0	12	0
French Dressing, 1.6 oz	234	22	4	263	10	0	9	0
Hollandaise Sauce, 1 oz	25	1	1	155	3	0	1	0
Honey Mustard Dressing, 1.6 oz	205	18	3	263	9	0	7	0
Hot Bacon Dressing, 1.6 oz	113	3	1	202	19	0	18	0
Lite Ranch Dressing, 1.6 oz	110	11	2	402	2	0	1	1
Marinara Sauce, 3 oz	35	1	0	374	5	1	3	1
Pork-Roasted Gravy, 2 oz	64	5	3	304	3	0	0	1
Queso Sauce, 4 oz	159	9	5	923	8	0	4	13
Ranchero Picante, 1.3 oz	37	0	0	92	0	0	0	9
Sour Cream, 0.6 oz	34	3	2	14	1	0	1	1
Sweet Italian Dressing, 1.6 oz	184	17	3	539	9	0	7	0
Swiss Bacon Dressing, 1.6 oz	242	27	5	423	2	0	2	2
Tartar Sauce, 0.7 oz	116	12	2	123	1	0	1	0
Thousand Island Dressing, 1.6 oz	227	21	3	378	8	0	6	0
Vinegar & Oil Dressing, 1.5 oz	27	3	0	0	0	0	0	0
Wildfire BBQ Sauce, 1 oz	62	0	0	99	15	1	14	0
Wildfire Ranch Dressing, 1.6 oz	129	10	2	328	9	0	2	1

Topping

American Cheese, 1 pc	53	4	3	235	1	0	0	3
Bacon Bits	145	11	5	553	1	0	1	10
Blue Cheese	97	8	5	381	0	0	0	6
Captain Wafers Crackers	28	1	0	43	4	0	0	0
Cranberries	68	0	0	0	17	1	13	0
Dill Pickle Slices	2	0	0	239	0	0	0	0
Honey Roasted Pecans	132	13	1	67	5	2	3	2
Lettuce & Tomato	9	0	0	4	2	1	1	1
Lettuce, Tomato & Pickle	12	0	0	244	2	1	1	1
Monterey Jack Cheese, 1 pc	71	6	4	340	0	0	0	4
Raisins	84	0	0	3	20	1	15	1
Shredded Cheddar Cheese	112	9	6	179	1	1	0	7
Tomato Slices, 2 pc	11	0	0	5	2	1	1	0

Dessert

Coconut Cream Pie	528	28	19	423	64	4	41	8
French Silk Pie	662	44	26	320	60	2	44	6
NSA Apple Pie	499	30	5	426	56	4	19	4
NSA Apple Pie a la mode	610	36	9	461	69	4	30	6
Oreo Ice Cream Pie	883	42	19	692	121	3	44	9
Red, White & Blue Supreme Pie	693	50	24	336	63	3	44	5
Strawberry Shortcake	569	22	11	924	86	4	49	9
Strawberry Sundae	419	20	14	113	56	2	44	8
Strawberry Supreme Pie	651	47	22	333	58	3	40	5
Vanilla Ice Cream	111	6	4	36	13	0	10	2

Dessert Topping

Blueberry Topping, 3 oz	103	0	0	14	25	2	23	1
Brown Sugar	95	0	0	2	24	0	24	0

Description & Serving	Cal	Fat	Sfat	Sod	Carb	Fiber	Sugar	Prot
Caramel Topping, 1 oz	74	0	0	79	18	0	14	1
Chocolate Fudge Topping, 1 oz	86	2	1	46	16	0	11	1
Strawberry Topping, 3 oz	55	0	0	0	14	2	12	1
Whipped Topping, 0.4 oz	37	3	2	2	3	0	3	0
Beverage								
Arnold Palmer	47	0	0	7	11	0	11	0
Caramel Mocha	268	9	8	149	45	1	41	2

Bojangles' Famous Chicken 'n Biscuits

Breakfast

Biscuit (plain)	243	12	3	663	29	2	NP	4
Bacon Biscuit Sandwich	290	17	5	810	26	1	NP	8
Bacon, Egg & Cheese Biscuit Sandwich	550	42	14	1250	27	1	NP	17
Cajun Filet Biscuit Sandwich	454	21	6	949	46	1	NP	20
Country Ham Biscuit Sandwich	270	15	4	1010	26	1	NP	9
Egg Biscuit Sandwich	400	30	6	630	26	1	NP	8
Sausage Biscuit Sandwich	350	23	7	810	26	1	NP	9
Smoked Sausage Biscuit Sandwich	380	26	9	940	27	1	NP	10
Steak Biscuit Sandwich	649	49	13	1126	37	1	NP	49

Chicken

Cajun Spiced Chicken Breast	278	17	NP	565	12	<1	NP	33
Cajun Spiced Chicken Leg	122	16	NP	530	11	<1	NP	10
Cajun Spiced Chicken Thigh	310	23	NP	465	11	<1	NP	16
Cajun Spiced Chicken Wing	160	25	NP	630	11	<1	NP	9

Sandwich

Cajun Filet Sandwich	337	11	5	401	41	3	NP	22
Grilled Filet Sandwich	235	5	3	540	25	2	NP	23
Cajun Filet Sandwich w/ mayo	437	22	7	506	41	3	NP	22
Grilled Filet Sandwich w/ mayo	335	16	5	645	25	2	NP	23

Side

Botato Rounds	235	11	4	328	31	3	NP	3
Cajun Pintos	110	0	0	480	18	6	NP	6
Marinated Cole Slaw	136	3	0	454	26	3	NP	1
Dirty Rice	166	6	2	762	24	1	NP	5
Green Beans	25	0	0	710	5	2	NP	0
Macaroni & Cheese	198	14	5	418	12	<1	NP	7
Potatoes w/o gravy	80	1	0	380	16	1	NP	2
Seasoned Fries	344	19	5	480	39	4	NP	5
Chicken Supremes	337	16	6	629	26	1	NP	21
Buffalo Bites	180	5	2	720	5	0	NP	27

Dessert

Bo Berry Sweet Biscuit	220	10	3	410	29	1	NP	3
Cinnamon Sweet Biscuit	320	18	4	560	37	1	NP	4

Description & Serving	Cal	Fat	Sfat	Sod	Carb	Fiber	Sugar	Prot
Boston Market								
Individual Meal								
Award Winning Sirloin	290	15	6	440	0	0	0	39
Beef Brisket	280	20	1.5	260	1	0	0	26
BBQ Brisket	400	20	1.5	760	28	1	18	26
Meatloaf	520	36	16	1030	21	0	4	29
1/4 White BBQ Chicken	430	13	4	1400	28	1	18	52
3 Piece BBQ Dark Chicken	430	13	4	1400	28	1	18	52
Half BBQ Chicken	730	30	9	2360	28	1	19	90
3 Piece Dark Individual Meal	390	22	6	1270	1	0	1	51
3 Piece Dark (2 Thighs & Drumstick)	490	29	8	1600	0	0	1	60
3 Piece Dark Skinless (Thigh & 2 Drumsticks)	290	11	3.5	1010	0	0	1	45
3 Piece Dark Skinless (2 Thighs & Drumstick)	350	15	4.5	1210	0	0	1	52
1/4 White Rotisserie Chicken	320	12	4	900	0	0	0	52
1/4 White Rotisserie Chicken, No Skin	240	4	1	890	1	0	0	50
Half Rotisserie Chicken	610	29	9	1860	1	0	1	89
1 Thigh & 1 Drumstick	290	17	5	950	0	0	1	37
Crispy Country Chicken w/ Country Gravy	480	23	4.5	1150	36	1	2	33
Pastry Top Chicken Pot Pie	800	48	18	1090	59	4	4	32
Roasted Turkey	150	2.5	1	500	0	0	0	31
Family Meal, per serving								
Beef Brisket	280	20	1.5	260	1	0	0	26
Meatloaf	480	36	16	1030	21	0	4	29
Rotisserie Chicken	310	15	4.5	930	0	0	0	44
Roasted Turkey	180	3	1	635	0	0	0	38
Soup/Side								
Baked Beans	270	1.5	0	1000	53	11	13	11
Caesar Side Salad w/o Dressing	40	2	1.5	75	3	1	1	3
Caesar Side Salad	180	17	3.5	410	4	1	2	4
Caesar Salad Dressing	360	38	6	910	4	1	2	2
Chicken Noodle Soup	250	8	2.5	1420	23	2	2	22
Chicken Tortilla Soup w/ Toppings	410	26	7	2100	30	2	3	17
Chicken Tortilla Soup w/o Toppings	160	8	1.5	1690	13	2	3	10
Cinnamon Apples	210	3	0	15	47	3	42	0
Coleslaw	300	20	4.5	280	27	4	22	2
Creamed Spinach	280	23	15	580	12	4	1	9
Fresh Steamed Vegetables LF	60	2	0	40	8	3	3	2
Fresh Vegetable Stuffing	190	8	1	580	25	2	4	3
Garlic Dill New Potatoes LF	140	3	1	120	24	3	2	3
Green Beans	60	3.5	1.5	180	7	3	1	2
Macaroni & Cheese	300	11	7	1100	35	2	6	11
Mashed Potatoes	270	11	5	820	36	4	2	5
Poultry Gravy (4 oz)	50	2	0.5	690	7	0	2	0
Beef Gravy (3 oz)	35	1.5	0.5	500	4	0	0	1
Potato Salad	390	29	7	640	26	3	1	3
Seasonal Fresh Fruit Salad LF	60	0	0	20	15	1	13	1
Sweet Corn	170	4	1	95	37	2	10	6

Description & Serving	Cal	Fat	Sfat	Sod	Carb	Fiber	Sugar	Prot
Southern Style Squash Casserole	300	19	7	1390	23	3	10	10
Sweet Potato Casserole	460	16	4.5	270	77	3	39	4

Sandwich

	Cal	Fat	Sfat	Sod	Carb	Fiber	Sugar	Prot
Roasted Sirloin Open-Faced Sandwich	410	15	6	1640	32	1	3	35
Rotisserie Chicken Open-Faced Sandwich	320	8	2.5	1630	34	1	6	27
Roasted Turkey Open-Faced Sandwich	330	6	1.5	1480	43	1	14	26
Meatloaf Open-Faced Sandwich	670	38	17	1760	48	1	7	34
Classic Chicken Salad Sandwich	800	41	7	1900	65	4	5	40
Smokehouse BBQ Chicken Sandwich	850	29	9	2810	101	4	38	44
BBQ Brisket Sandwich	800	30	6	1840	90	3	21	43
Boston Chicken Carver, half	375	14.5	4	980	32	1	2	28
Boston Turkey Carver, half	350	13	4	850	32	2	2	25
Boston Meatloaf Carver	980	46	21	2350	92	4	12	47
Crispy Country Chicken Carver	1020	42	7	2210	114	4	23	45
Brisket Dip Carver	890	51	9	1350	63	3	3	43
Boston Sirloin Dip Carver, half	450	23	6.5	805	31	1	1	28
Beef Au jus	20	0.5	0	760	3	0	0	1

Salad

	Cal	Fat	Sfat	Sod	Carb	Fiber	Sugar	Prot
Caesar Salad Entrée	420	38	10	930	9	2	6	12
Caesar Salad Entrée w/o Dressing	140	8	5	270	7	2	4	10
Market Chopped Salad	480	40	8	1640	24	7	13	9
Market Chopped Salad Dressing	360	39	6	1710	2	0	1	0
Rotisserie Chicken (5 oz)	180	3	1	620	0	0	0	39
Roasted Turkey (3 oz)	110	2	0.5	370	0	0	0	23
Roasted Sirloin (3 oz)	160	6	2	170	0	0	0	26
Crispy Country Chicken	220	11	2	480	16	1	1	16
Lite Ranch Dressing	70	4	0.5	310	8	0	3	1

Dessert

	Cal	Fat	Sfat	Sod	Carb	Fiber	Sugar	Prot
Apple Gallette	420	22	12	280	54	3	25	3
Chocolate Chip Fudge Brownie	320	13	3	220	49	3	36	5
Chocolate Cupcake	350	17	6	210	48	2	36	3
Cornbread	180	5	1.5	320	31	0	12	2

Boston Pizza

Appetizer

	Cal	Fat	Sfat	Sod	Carb	Fiber	Sugar	Prot
Baked French Onion Soup	310	14	6	2400	35	3	9	17
Boston's Chili	320	20	9	820	16	5	5	18
Oven Roasted Wings, starter	430	30	10	1200	6	1	1	37
Oven Roasted Wings, double order	870	61	20	2400	12	2	2	73
Breaded Wings, starter	510	33	8	1510	20	2	4	34
Breaded Wings, double order	1020	65	16	3010	40	4	8	67
Three Cheese Toast, full order	730	34	18	1620	71	0	0	33
Three Cheese Toast, single order	370	17	9	820	36	0	0	17
Sun-Dried Tomato Bruschetta	400	18	4	960	52	4	5	9
Boston's Pizza Bread	500	12	3	660	84	0	5	15
Bandera Pizza Bread	950	53	16	1820	87	0	8	32

Description & Serving	Cal	Fat	Sfat	Sod	Carb	Fiber	Sugar	Prot
Twist Bread, full order	1140	39	9	2810	165	1	13	32
Twist Bread, single order	570	20	5	1410	82	0	6	16
Nachos	1130	67	27	1970	91	9	4	49
Cactus Cut Potatoes	830	70	9	950	38	4	2	10
Chicken Fingers	330	19	3	1040	14	5	2	31
Oven-Roasted Chicken Quesadilla	960	47	15	1770	91	9	6	45
Thai Chicken Bites	520	20	3	2050	59	7	41	32
Cracked Pepper Dry Ribs	240	25	0	1880	3	1	1	42
Calamari	480	24	5	830	22	0	2	43
Yam Fries w/ Chipotle Dip	670	55	5	650	43	4	18	2
Appie Platter	2150	150	38	4440	117	5	4	104
Spinach & Artichoke Dip	690	38	22	1140	74	6	6	20

Pizza

Description & Serving	Cal	Fat	Sfat	Sod	Carb	Fiber	Sugar	Prot
Pepperoni Pizza, indv	750	27	13	1650	89	2	6	40
Pepperoni Pizza, med	200	7	4	450	24	0	2	10
Pepperoni & Mushrooms Pizza, indv	750	27	13	1650	90	2	7	41
Pepperoni & Mushrooms Pizza, med	200	7	4	460	24	1	2	11
Hawaiian Pizza, indv	780	21	10	2480	101	2	16	49
Hawaiian Pizza, med	210	5	3	710	28	0	5	13
Deluxe Pizza, indv	850	29	14	2880	93	2	7	55
Deluxe Pizza, med	220	7	4	750	25	1	2	14
Bacon Double Cheeseburger Pizza, indv	910	39	19	2020	92	2	8	50
Bacon Double Cheeseburger Pizza, med	250	10	5	570	25	1	2	14
Tuscan Pizza, indv	940	37	19	1690	106	5	16	50
Tuscan Pizza, med	250	10	5	470	29	2	5	13
Szechuan Pizza, indv	750	20	9	800	101	1	15	41
Szechuan Pizza, med	200	5	2	210	27	0	4	11
BBQ Pulled Pork Pizza, indv	750	18	10	1540	109	1	27	39
BBQ Pulled Pork Pizza, med	200	5	3	430	30	0	8	10
Tropical Chicken Pizza, indv	890	35	16	1420	95	1	14	47
Tropical Chicken Pizza, med	250	11	5	430	26	0	4	14
BBQ Chicken Pizza, indv	730	24	13	1430	92	1	8	39
BBQ Chicken Pizza, med	190	6	3	400	25	0	2	10
Cajun Shrimp Pizza, indv	1050	59	20	2070	86	9	4	51
Cajun Shrimp Pizza, med	290	16	5	590	23	2	1	14
The Meateor Pizza, indv	960	39	18	2530	91	1	7	60
The Meateor Pizza, med	260	11	5	690	25	0	2	16
Great White North Pizza, indv	960	39	22	2930	91	1	6	62
Great White North Pizza, med	240	9	5	800	24	0	2	16
Spicy Perogy Pizza, indv	930	42	15	1010	93	1	5	45
Spicy Perogy Pizza, med	260	13	5	300	25	0	1	13
Boston Royal Pizza, indv	830	27	12	2520	98	3	9	53
Boston Royal Pizza, med	210	6	3	640	26	1	2	13
Rustic Italian Pizza, indv	860	35	17	3860	101	3	14	38
Rustic Italian Pizza, med	240	10	5	1160	28	1	4	11
The Pepper Pizza, indv	820	31	16	1460	95	4	8	41
The Pepper Pizza, med	220	9	4	410	25	3	2	11
Zorba, The Greek Pizza, indv	800	29	16	1400	96	4	9	43

Description & Serving	Cal	Fat	Sfat	Sod	Carb	Fiber	Sugar	Prot
Zorba, The Greek Pizza, med	210	8	4	390	26	1	3	11
Vegetarian Pizza, indv	680	16	9	1160	99	4	13	37
Vegetarian Pizza, med	170	4	2	320	26	1	3	9
Bruschetta Pizza, indv	870	37	19	930	99	3	8	37
Bruschetta Pizza, med	250	11	6	280	27	1	2	11

Salad

Description & Serving	Cal	Fat	Sfat	Sod	Carb	Fiber	Sugar	Prot
Garden Greens, starter	300	28	3	260	10	3	4	3
Garden Greens, regular	400	37	7	740	13	4	9	10
Caesar Salad, starter	210	19	4	370	7	3	5	5
Citrus Chicken	780	16	4	1080	119	6	21	30
Chipotle Chicken & Bacon, starter	640	41	8	1100	41	6	7	29
Chipotle Chicken & Bacon, regular	460	40	8	920	10	3	6	15
Spinach, starter	250	21	5	520	6	2	4	9
Baja Salad	410	30	10	1340	39	7	11	15
Crispy Chicken Pecan	1150	93	15	1950	32	12	12	57
Greek Salad, starter	590	54	13	4440	25	4	16	10
Greek Salad, regular	1040	105	23	2260	26	6	13	16

Delicious Alternatives

Description & Serving	Cal	Fat	Sfat	Sod	Carb	Fiber	Sugar	Prot
Spicy Garlic Chicken Pizza	650	12	6	860	101	8	6	36
Garden Greens	90	5	0	150	12	1	10	2
Delicious Alternatives Citrus Chicken Salad	360	7	3	590	47	6	13	27
Pollo Pomodoro Linguini	510	11	3	820	73	12	1	30
Chicken Stromboli	620	13	5	470	96	6	19	30
Lemon Baked Salmon Filet	310	7	1	260	14	3	11	48

Sandwich/Wrap/Stromboli/Burger

Description & Serving	Cal	Fat	Sfat	Sod	Carb	Fiber	Sugar	Prot
Boston Brute Sandwich	810	21	9	3200	116	3	6	42
Beef Dip Sandwich	860	27	8	3350	108	0	1	46
Ciabatta Chicken Sandwich	750	42	7	1620	58	3	3	33
Buffalo Chicken Sandwich	910	33	5	4310	118	6	9	42
New York Striploin Steak Sandwich	560	34	13	730	20	1	1	42
Boston Cheesesteak Sandwich	1140	49	19	3900	113	1	4	62
Chicken Parmesan Sandwich	850	45	10	2460	66	5	8	43
BBQ Pulled Pork Sandwich	780	15	5	2600	131	1	28	30
Chipotle Chicken Caesar Wrap	530	25	5	1070	53	6	7	26
Smoked Ham and Chicken Stromboli	770	25	11	1610	86	1	5	52
Chicken Santa Fe Stromboli	600	13	2	680	92	2	5	30
Sun-Dried Tomato, Cheese & Spinach Stromboli	710	22	10	690	104	3	6	27
BP's Prime Rib Burger w/ Cheddar	1050	77	28	2130	47	3	6	46
The Original Burger	940	68	23	1900	47	3	6	39
BP's Prime Rib Burger w/ Bacon	1000	73	24	2050	47	3	7	43
BP's Prime Rib Burger w/ Cheddar & Bacon	1110	82	30	2270	47	3	7	50

Pasta

Description & Serving	Cal	Fat	Sfat	Sod	Carb	Fiber	Sugar	Prot
Whole Wheat Linguini	610	3	1	0	122	16	8	24
Fettuccini	590	2	0	2	123	7	2	20
Spaghetti	590	2	0	2	123	7	2	20
Penne	450	2	0	1	95	5	2	15
Homestyle Lasagna	930	48	22	2280	68	5	14	59

Description & Serving	Cal	Fat	Sfat	Sod	Carb	Fiber	Sugar	Prot
Baked Seven Cheese Ravioli	490	26	15	850	34	2	2	30
Chicken Cannelloni	490	40	15	1550	11	3	5	22
Boston's Lasagna	670	19	9	1700	90	6	12	35
Chicken & Mushroom Fettuccini	1460	79	20	1990	139	11	9	52
Tuscan Linguini	1100	33	5	2610	170	29	39	38
Scallop & Prawn Fettuccini	1390	72	18	1900	138	12	7	46
Baked Shrimp & Feta Penne	1150	55	21	2040	110	11	10	56
Boston's Smokey Mountain Spaghetti & Meatballs	1800	63	30	3360	232	19	20	81
Spicy Italian Penne	1530	88	20	2670	137	10	10	53
Jambalaya Fettuccini	1510	80	18	3460	140	12	11	61
Roasted Vegetable Lasagna	700	19	6	940	105	2	4	23
Entrée								
Baked Salmon Filet	590	37	6	660	16	4	7	39
Certified Angus Beef Top Sirloin Steak	790	55	15	670	14	3	6	59
Cajun Rice Bowl	1000	43	5	2050	97	9	10	50
Teriyaki Rice Bowl	1320	42	7	3260	187	8	61	48
The Ribber	320	18	7	720	23	1	21	16
Slow-Roasted Pork Back Ribs	720	52	13	970	36	4	27	31
Dessert								
Chocolate Explosion	870	49	28	530	98	5	59	11
New York Cheesecake	600	32	16	460	76	1	44	11
Chocolate Brownie Addiction	250	9	3	130	41	1	25	2
Apple Crisp	740	19	5	190	138	6	84	7
Chocolate Lava Cake	520	11	4	480	98	2	65	6
Kids								
Pint-Sized Pizza	430	10	5	620	64	1	4	23
Super Spaghetti	290	1	0	1	62	3	1	10
Lovely Linguini	310	2	0	0	61	8	4	12
Bugs N' Cheese	500	24	9	760	53	4	4	19
Mighty Plump Perogies	480	17	5	920	64	6	9	19
Chicken Fingers	250	10	1	870	29	2	13	15
Baked Salmon	140	4	1	70	1	0	0	18
Gooey Grilled Cheese	390	15	8	830	47	1	0	11
BP Kids Cheeseburgers	480	23	9	1030	45	1	18	22
Grape Pop Rocks!	80	0	0	40	19	0	19	0
Orange Iceberg Slush	210	0	0	35	52	0	24	0
Shirley Temple	190	0	0	60	46	0	43	0
Bite-Sized Brownie	250	9	3	130	41	1	25	2
Pint-Sized Sundae	480	22	7	105	68	1	24	5
Worms & Dirt	420	13	13	280	69	0	50	7

Bruegger's

Breakfast								
Asiago Parmesan Bagel	330	20	3	670	61	4	7	14
Blueberry Bagel	320	2	0	530	67	4	14	11

Description & Serving	Cal	Fat	Sfat	Sod	Carb	Fiber	Sugar	Prot
Chocolate Chip Bagel	350	5	1.5	570	64	4	14	12
Cinnamon Raisin Bagel	330	2	0	510	69	4	17	11
Cinnamon Sugar Bagel	350	2	0	540	73	6	16	12
Cranberry Orange Bagel	330	2	0	510	68	4	17	11
Everything Bagel	310	2	0	790	31	4	7	12
Fortified Multi-Grain Bagel	350	4	0	550	69	6	10	13
Garlic Bagel	320	2	0	560	65	4	8	12
Honey Grain Bagel	330	3	0	510	65	5	10	13
Jalapeno Bagel	320	2	0	560	64	4	8	12
Onion Bagel	320	2	0	560	64	4	8	12
Plain Bagel	300	2	0	620	60	4	7	12
Poppy Bagel	310	2.5	0	620	61	4	7	12
Pumpernickel Bagel	330	2.5	0	620	67	5	11	12
Rosemary Olive Oil Bagel	350	7	0	540	64	4	10	12
Sesame Bagel	310	3	0	620	61	4	7	13
Sourdough Bagel	310	2	0	570	63	4	7	12
Sundried Tomato Bagel	320	2	0	640	64	4	11	12
Whole Wheat Bagel	390	6	0	680	73	9	8	22
Asiago Parmesan Square Bagel	360	4.5	1.5	740	66	4	11	15
Everything Square Bagel	320	2	0	740	64	4	8	12
Plain Square Bagel	350	2.5	0	670	70	4	11	13
Sesame Square Bagel	360	2.5	0	660	68	4	11	13
Breakfast Bagel w/ No Meat & Plain Bagel	420	18	6	1090	71	4	9	23
Breakfast Bagel w/ Bacon & Plain Bagel	460	23	8	980	65	4	9	28
Breakfast Bagel w/ Ham & Plain Bagel	460	18	6	1270	73	4	11	31
Breakfast Bagel w/ Sausage & Plain Bagel	640	30	11	1360	63	4	8	29
Classic Wrap w/ Bacon	520	45	15	1120	52	4	4	36
Classic Wrap w/ Ham	510	41	14	1630	54	4	5	40
Classic Wrap w/ Sausage	590	53	19	1100	15	4	3	35
Rio Grande Wrap w/ Bacon	560	49	16	1380	55	4	6	34
Rio Grande Wrap w/ Ham	630	34	10	1450	55	4	7	31
Rio Grande Wrap w/ Sausage	510	47	15	960	53	4	4	27
Smoked Salmon/Plain Bagel	460	10	4.5	780	65	5	9	27
Spinach & Cheddar Omelet/Plain Bagel	500	16	7	1070	64	4	8	24
Spinach, Cheddar & Bacon Omelet on Sesame Bagel	550	22	8	1290	60	3	8	28
Spinach, Cheddar & Ham Omelet on Sesame Bagel	540	17	7	1140	65	4	10	30
Spinach, Cheddar & Sausage Omelet on Sesame Bagel	660	32	12	970	64	4	8	29
Western/Plain Bagel	760	56	12	1580	66	4	10	27

Sandwich

BLT on Plain Bagel	570	23	5	1060	72	5	10	20
Chicken Breast on Plain Bagel	660	11	2.5	780	87	5	26	47
Garden Veggie on Plain Bagel	400	2.5	0	620	82	7	14	16
Ham on Plain Bagel	410	5	1	1780	66	4	12	27
Roast Beef on Plain Bagel	730	39	5	1280	71	5	10	30
Tuna Salad on Plain Bagel	620	27	3.5	990	73	5	10	23

Description & Serving	Cal	Fat	Sfat	Sod	Carb	Fiber	Sugar	Prot
Turkey on Plain Bagel	510	14	1.5	1290	70	5	9	26
Four Cheese & Tomato Panini on Hearty White	700	35	19	1320	57	3	4	42
Ham & Swiss Panini on Honey Wheat	600	18	8	1650	71	2	22	39
Primo Pesto Chicken Panini on Hearty White	700	32	10	1870	56	2	3	49
Tuna & Cheddar Melt Panini on Honey Wheat	1020	67	15	1560	61	3	9	42
Turkey Toscana Panini on Hearty White	710	37	10	1970	59	3	4	41
Herby Turkey Sandwich on Sesame Bagel	600	14	4.5	1420	80	5	14	43
Leonardo da Veggie on Asiago Softwich	590	17	9	1120	83	7	19	28
Tarragon Chicken Salad on Hearty White	770	41	6	1370	73	3	5	59
Thai Peanut Chicken on Plain Bagel	580	11	3.5	1190	91	7	17	28
Turkey Chipotle Club on Honey Wheat	800	51	7	1840	57	3	8	31
Roma Roast Beef on Hearty White	770	44	12	1740	62	3	6	46

Salad

	Cal	Fat	Sfat	Sod	Carb	Fiber	Sugar	Prot
Build Your Own Salad Base	30	0.5	0	5	5	2	3	2
Caesar, no dressing	160	8	2.5	220	14	2	3	7
Caesar w/ Caesar Dressing	270	17	4.5	900	22	2	5	9
Caesar w/ Chicken & Caesar Dressing	380	20	6	1420	23	2	5	28
Mandarin Medley, no dressing	220	8	4.5	300	29	70	21	8
Mandarin Medley w/ Balsamic Vinaigrette	340	17	5	660	36	7	27	8
Mandarin Medley w/ Chicken & Balsamic Vinaigrette	450	21	6	1180	37	7	27	26
Sesame Salad, no dressing	120	4.5	0	75	12	2	3	4
Sesame Salad w/ Asian Sesame Dressing	380	26	2.5	270	29	2	18	23
Sesame Salad w/ Chicken & Asian Sesame Dressing	490	29	3.5	790	30	2	18	42

Soup/Chili

	Cal	Fat	Sfat	Sod	Carb	Fiber	Sugar	Prot
Butternut Squash Soup	240	17	9	650	21	1	2	4
Chicken Spaetzle Soup	140	5	2.5	1200	15	1	3	8
Chicken Wild Rice Soup	280	22	10	840	12	1	2	8
Fire Roasted Tomato Soup	130	6	3	920	17	2	10	2
Four Cheese Broccoli Soup	260	20	10	1240	12	1	2	9
New England Clam Chowder	230	14	4.5	600	16	<1	12	23
Spinach & Lentil Soup	110	3.5	1	570	16	7	2	7
Beef Chili	190	8	3	880	18	6	3	10
White Chicken Chili	240	9	0	630	26	7	2	14

Dessert

	Cal	Fat	Sfat	Sod	Carb	Fiber	Sugar	Prot
Chocolate Chunk Brownies	330	18	7	150	40	2	27	4
Marshmallow Chew	280	6	3	330	55	0	29	2
Seven Layer Bar	650	43	23	280	58	5	42	10
Toffee Almond Bar	400	19	8	340	53	1	34	4
Chocolate Chip Cookie	390	17	8	150	52	2	32	5
Double Chocolate Cookie	390	19	9	160	51	3	33	5
Everything Cookie	380	18	9	260	49	2	29	5
Blueberry Muffin	400	17	3.5	330	57	2	26	7
Chocolate Muffin	460	24	6	250	57	3	38	6

Description & Serving	Cal	Fat	Sfat	Sod	Carb	Fiber	Sugar	Prot
Bread								
Bagel Bowl	720	9	0.5	1500	133	8	22	30
Ciabatta	250	2.5	0	730	48	2	2	9
Hearty White	260	0	0	620	54	2	2	10
Honey Wheat	280	3	0	520	54	2	6	12
White Wrap	180	1.5	1	420	32	3	1	6
Dressing/Condiment/Syrup								
Asian Sesame Ginger Dressing, 2 oz	260	21	2	190	17	0	15	0
Balsamic Vinaigrette, 2 oz	110	9	1	360	8	0	6	0
Caesar Dressing, 2 oz	110	9	2	680	8	0	2	2
Ranch Dressing, 2 oz	190	21	3	510	2	0	2	0
Chipotle Sauce, 0.5 oz	100	11	1.5	120	0	0	0	0
Cranberry Horseradish Relish, 0.7 oz	35	0.5	0	20	8	0	5	0
Cranberry Sauce, 2.5 oz	110	0	NP	10	27	1	22	0
Dijon Mustard, 0.5 oz	0	0	0	180	0	0	0	0
Honey Mustard, 0.5 oz	45	0	0	45	9	0	9	0
Horseradish Mayo, 1.1 oz	140	13	2	280	6	0	5	0
Hummus, 1.9 oz	110	6	1	120	10	0	0	5
Jelly/Jam - Grape, 0.7 oz	50	0	NP	5	13	NP	12	0
Jelly/Jam - Strawberry, 0.7 oz	50	0	NP	0	13	NP	12	0
Mayo, 0.5 oz	100	11	1.5	100	1	0	0	0
Peanut Butter, 1.1 oz	190	16	3	150	7	2	3	7
Pesto, 0.5 oz	100	10	2	70	0	NP	NP	1
Sundried Tomato Mayo, 0.7 oz	140	15	2.5	130	1	0	0	2
Sundried Tomato Spread, 0.6 oz	79	6	2	46	5	0	1	1
Thai Peanut Sauce, 0.6 oz	45	2.5	0	240	4	0	3	1
Bacon Scallion Cream Cheese, 1.5 oz	140	12	7	150	5	0	2	3
Garden Veggie Cream Cheese, 1.5 oz	130	11	6	140	5	1	2	3
Honey Walnut Cream Cheese, 1.5 oz	150	12	6	125	8	<1	3	3
Jalapeno Cream Cheese, 1.5 oz	140	13	8	150	4	0	2	3
Light Garden Veggie Cream Cheese, 1.5 oz	90	6	4	105	3	0	2	6
Light Herb Garlic Cream Cheese, 1.5 oz	100	6	3.5	125	4	0	2	6
Light Plain Cream Cheese, 1.5 oz	100	6	3	130	4	<1	3	6
Olive Pimiento Cream Cheese, 1.5 oz	140	13	6	130	3	0	1	3
Onion & Chive Cream Cheese, 1.5 oz	140	13	8	105	3	0	2	3
Plain Cream Cheese, 1.5 oz	130	11	7	125	6	<1	2	3
Smoked Salmon Cream Cheese, 1.5 oz	150	13	6	150	3	<1	2	3
Strawberry Cream Cheese, 1.5 oz	140	13	7	100	4	0	2	3
Almond Flavored Syrup, 1 oz	90	0	0	0	23	0	23	0
Caramel Flavored Syrup, 1 oz	100	0	0	0	24	0	24	0
Chocolate Syrup, 1 oz	88	0.7	0.5	12	20	<1	15	<1
Hazelnut Flavored Syrup, 1 oz	90	0	0	7	22	0	21	0
Vanilla Flavored Syrup, 1 oz	100	0	0	0	25	0	25	0
Topping								
American Cheese	80	7	4	320	0	0	0	5
Asiago Cheese, Shredded	50	4	2.5	35	0	0	0	4

Description & Serving	Cal	Fat	Sfat	Sod	Carb	Fiber	Sugar	Prot
Blue Cheese	80	5	4	290	0	0	0	5
Cheddar Cheese	80	6	3.5	120	0	0	0	5
Muenster Cheese	60	4.5	3	115	0	0	0	4
Provolone Cheese	50	4	2	125	0	0	0	4
Swiss Cheese	50	4	2	125	0	0	0	4
Bacon	70	6	2	220	1	0	1	4
Chicken Breast	140	4	1.5	700	1	0	0	25
Ham	80	2.5	1	910	3	0	3	12
Roast Beef	70	3.5	1	360	1	0	0	16
Salmon	80	2.5	1	737	0	0	0	13
Sausage	220	20	8	310	1	0	0	8
Tarragon Chicken Salad	300	24	3.5	440	10	0	0	29
Tuna Salad	330	30	4.5	460	3	0	1	12
Turkey	69	4	1	519	0	1	0	13
Capers	0	0	0	65	0	0	0	0
Cucumbers	5	0	0	0	0	0	0	0
Green Peppers	6	0	0	1	1	0	1	0
Jalapenos	5	0	0	290	1	1	0	0
Lettuce	1	0	0	1	0	0	0	0
Pickles	0	0	0	330	1	0	0	0
Red Onions	0	0	0	0	0	0	0	0
Roasted Red Peppers	15	0	0	200	3	0	2	1
Sprouts	1	0	0	0	0	0	0	0
Tomatoes	0	0	0	0	2	0	1	0
Almonds, sliced	25	2.5	0	0	1	0	0	20
Chow Mein Noodles	40	1.5	0	70	6	0	0	1
Cranberries, dried	60	0	0	0	15	2	13	0
Croutons	70	3	0	170	8	0	0	1
Mandarin Oranges	20	0	0	0	5	1	4	0
Sesame Seeds	40	3.5	0	0	2	1	0	1
Beverage								
Brueggaccino, 16 oz	460	28	18	150	43	0	43	8
Café au Lait, 16 oz	NP	NP	6	11	15	0	15	11
Café Latte, 16 oz	NP	12	6.7	11	17	0	17	12
Café Mocha, 16 oz	NP	12	6.7	11	31	0	28	12
Cappuccino, 16 oz	NP	9.3	5.3	11	15	0	15	9
Espresso, 3 oz	8	0	0	15	2	0	2	0
Flavored Coffee, 16 oz	5	0	0	11	0	0	0	0
French Roast Coffee, 16 oz	5	0	0	11	0	0	0	0
House Blend Coffee, 16 oz	5	0	0	11	0	0	0	0
House Decaf Coffee, 16 oz	5	0	0	11	0	0	0	0
Iced Coffee, 16 oz	5	0	0	11	0	0	0	0
Hot Tea, Regular, 8 oz	0	0	0	0	0	0	0	0
Hot Tea, Herbal, 8 oz	0	0	0	0	0	0	0	0
Hot Tea, Decaf, 8 oz	0	0	0	0	0	0	0	0
Iced Tea, Brewed, 12 oz	0	0	0	0	0	0	0	0
Oregon Chai Tea, 12 oz	117	0	0	12	29	0	27	0
Hot Chocolate, 8 oz	140	1.5	1.5	190	31	1	26	2

Description & Serving	Cal	Fat	Sfat	Sod	Carb	Fiber	Sugar	Prot

Bruster's Real Ice Cream

Ice Cream

Description & Serving	Cal	Fat	Sfat	Sod	Carb	Fiber	Sugar	Prot
Vanilla Ice Cream, 100 g	210	12	8	55	24	0	18	3
Chocolate Ice Cream, 100 g	210	12	7	60	23	1	19	3
NSNF Chocolate Ice Cream, 90 g	100	0	0	100	26	1	6	4
NSNF Cinnamon Ice Cream, 90 g	100	0	0	90	23	1	7	5
NSNF Vanilla Ice Cream, 90 g	110	0	0	90	23	1	7	4
NSNF Caramel Swirl Ice Cream, 92 g	110	0	0	100	30	1	6	0
NSNF Chocolate Caramel Ice Cream, 92 g	120	0	0	105	31	1	6	4
NSNF Chocolate Fudge Ice Cream, 92 g	120	0	0	120	31	1	6	4
NSNF Chocolate Raspberry Ice Cream, 92 g	110	0	0	85	31	1	6	4
NSNF Coffee Ice Cream, 92 g	100	0	0	95	24	1	7	5
NSNF Coffee Caramel Swirl, 92 g	120	0	0	100	30	1	6	4
NSNF Coffee Ripple, 92 g	110	0	0	110	30	1	6	4
NSNF Fudge Ripple, 92 g	110	0	0	110	30	1	6	4
NSNF Raspberry Swirl, 92 g	110	0	0	80	29	1	6	4

Yogurt/Sorbet

Vanilla Yogurt, 100 g	150	4	2.5	105	24	0	19	4
Chocolate Yogurt, 100 g	150	4.5	2.5	105	24	1	18	4
Strawberry Sorbet, 99 g	210	0	0	15	53	0	49	0
Orange Sherbet, 99 g	210	1	0	20	50	0	45	0

Buffalo Wild Wings

Appetizer

The Sampler	1520	76	20	3120	128	8	20	76
Crispy Southwest Dippers	630	25	10	1974	78	8	10	24
Mini Corn Dogs	713	24	5	1270	49	2	16	13
Chips & Salsa	500	30	14	1180	46	2	0	4
Cheeseburger Slammers	1559	92	34	1451	98	7	10	66
Pulled Pork Slammers	1167	51	13	1867	105	4	17	61
Roasted Garlic Mushrooms	360	18	3	1240	44	2	4	6
Ultimate Nachos	960	52	14	1680	108	8	8	24
Ultimate Nachos w/ Chicken	1120	52	14	3200	108	8	8	52
3/4 lb Popcorn Shrimp	880	44	6	2900	88	4	6	34
Mozzarella Sticks	560	22	15	1800	52	0	2	30
Queso Chili Fries	862	40	15	2654	92	10	10	26
Chicken Quesadilla	800	35	18	1810	70	5	6	51
Chili Con Queso Dip	920	48	14	2240	100	8	8	28
Naked Tenders, 6	260	12	1	3420	34	2	10	10
Pepperoni Kickers w/ Sauce	563	30	16	1910	53	0	9	28
Twisted Chicken w/ Sauce	1023	54	10	6440	99	3	27	36
BBQ Nachos	1245	52	14	3200	108	8	8	52

Entrée

Naked Tenders, 1	43	2	1	74	2	0	0	2
Breaded Tenders, 1	170	11	3	573	15	1	5	5
1/2 lb Popcorn Shrimp	587	29	4	1933	59	3	4	23

Description & Serving	Cal	Fat	Sfat	Sod	Carb	Fiber	Sugar	Prot
Wings w/ Sauce, 1	72	5	1	66	0	0	0	6
Boneless Wings w/ Sauce, 1	88	6	2	178	3	0	0	5
Ribs & Chicken Tenders	1860	118	38	2980	112	8	30	88
Ribs & Popcorn Shrimp	1480	92	32	2980	84	4	20	80
Ribs & Boneless Wings	1960	126	40	4380	88	6	16	102
Chicken Tenders & Popcorn Shrimp	1120	62	12	3220	110	10	30	24
Ribs & Traditional Wings	1860	124	40	3800	74	6	16	108
Ribs & More Ribs	2380	158	58	5320	88	6	28	144
Boneless Wings & Traditional Wings	1480	98	20	7940	68	6	2	66
Popcorn Shrimp & Fish	820	36	6	2520	70	4	6	50
Grilled Chicken Buffalitos	380	9	6	1240	44	4	4	40

Burger/Sandwich/Wrap

Description & Serving	Cal	Fat	Sfat	Sod	Carb	Fiber	Sugar	Prot
Black & Bleu Burger	770	51	20	860	44	3	4	37
Bacon Cheddar Burger	860	57	24	1170	44	3	4	46
Honey BBQ Bacon Burger	890	57	24	1340	51	3	10	46
Chili Queso Burger	880	57	26	1270	49	3	5	49
Big Jack Daddy Burger	900	56	23	1630	53	3	9	50
Cheeseburger	780	51	22	870	44	3	4	42
Veggie Burger	250	5	2	1060	63	3	7	40
Buffalo Ranch Chicken Sandwich	800	49	13	1460	60	3	5	32
Jerk Chicken Sandwich	530	10	3	1140	56	3	16	51
Pulled Pork Sandwich	570	25	7	3160	61	2	15	30
Honey BBQ Chicken Sandwich	530	18	9	890	42	3	4	50
Grilled Chicken Sandwich	470	7	3	750	50	3	10	51
Crispy Fish Sandwich	550	22	6	760	22	3	1	8
Buffalo Chicken Wild Flatbread Sandwich	934	52	26	2866	58	4	1	52
Honey BBQ Chicken Wild Flatbread Sandwich	874	32	23	2226	89	4	28	51
Parmesan Garlic Wild Flatbread Sandwich	974	56	27	2906	57	4	4	55
Southwest Chicken Queso Wrap	490	7	4	2660	73	6	6	39
Buffalo Ranch Chicken Wrap	1020	59	18	2120	97	8	16	28
Chicken Tender Wrap	1040	46	17	2800	125	11	25	37
Chicken Caesar Wrap	560	15	6	1770	68	5	4	39
Grilled Chicken Wrap	600	14	9	1980	68	6	4	54

Side

Description & Serving	Cal	Fat	Sfat	Sod	Carb	Fiber	Sugar	Prot
Potato Wedges Basket	560	28	7	2147	79	9	5	9
Potato Wedges Basket w/ Cheese	780	46	19	2507	81	9	5	23
Potato Wedges Regular	280	14	4	1073	40	5	2	5
Potato Wedges Regular w/ Cheese	390	23	10	1253	41	5	2	12
French Fries Basket	560	20	6	1320	84	8	4	8
French Fries Regular	280	10	3	660	42	4	2	4
Onion Rings Basket	1100	55	10	2200	130	10	20	10
Onion Rings Regular	460	26	5	960	52	4	8	4
Buffalo Chips Basket	514	9	2	70	93	9	5	9
Buffalo Chips Basket w/ Cheese	734	27	14	430	95	9	5	23
Buffalo Chips Regular	257	5	1	35	47	5	2	5
Buffalo Chips Regular w/ Cheese	367	14	7	215	48	5	2	12
Coleslaw	170	15	0	390	6	0	6	0
Side Salad	210	15	5	385	14	4	4	6
Tortilla Chips & Salsa	250	15	7	590	23	1	0	2

Description & Serving	Cal	Fat	Sfat	Sod	Carb	Fiber	Sugar	Prot
Salad								
Honey BBQ Chicken Salad w/o dressing	479	17	17	1645	49	6	24	35
Grilled Blackened Chicken Salad w/o dressing	608	30	11	1107	48	6	10	30
Grilled Chicken Salad w/o dressing	409	17	17	1245	31	6	10	35
Chicken Tender Salad w/o dressing	793	37	12	2560	79	8	24	39
Garden Salad w/o dressing	275	12	6	540	30	6	10	12
Chicken Caesar Salad w/ dressing	756	55	22	2382	35	4	10	34
Dessert								
New York Cheesecake	460	28	16	20	47	1	39	6
Deep-Dish Apple Pie	590	18	9	260	105	4	66	7
Chocolate Fudge Cake	820	33	13	95	127	3	108	11
Kids								
Kids Cheeseburger Slammer	400	26	10	400	20	1	3	21
Boneless Wings, 4	288	20	5	264	0	0	0	24
Chicken Tenders, 3	510	32	8	1720	44	4	15	14
Traditional Wings, 4	384	28	7	352	1	0	0	31
Naked Tenders, 3	130	7	2	222	7	0	0	7
Macaroni & Cheese	380	13	5	1240	49	3	9	16
Mini Corn Dogs, 5	357	12	3	735	25	1	5	7
Kids' Ice Cream	210	8	5	95	33	1	30	3
Sauce/Dressing								
Sweet BBQ Sauce, 1 oz	40	0	0	460	8	0	8	0
Teriyaki Sauce, 1 oz	70	0	0	1100	14	0	12	0
Mild Sauce, 1 oz	50	5	0	1040	2	0	0	0
Parmesan Garlic Sauce, 1 oz	120	12	2	740	2	0	2	2
Medium Sauce, 1 oz	40	4	0	1160	2	0	0	0
Honey BBQ Sauce, 1 oz	70	0	0	400	18	0	14	0
Spicy Garlic Sauce, 1 oz	50	4	0	1220	4	0	0	0
Asian Zing Sauce, 1 oz	90	0	0	580	22	0	20	0
Caribbean Jerk Sauce, 1 oz	80	3	0	500	12	0	12	0
Hot Sauce, 1 oz	50	4	0	1200	2	0	0	0
Hot BBQ Sauce, 1 oz	40	2	0	740	6	0	4	0
Mango Habanero Sauce, 1 oz	80	0	0	460	20	0	14	0
Wild Sauce, 1 oz	50	4	0	1160	4	0	0	0
Blazin' Sauce, 1 oz	60	5	0	1280	2	0	0	0
Honey Mustard Dressing, 1 oz	80	6	0	320	6	0	6	0
Bleu Cheese Dressing, 1 oz	150	16	3	220	1	0	1	1
Ranch Dressing, 1 oz	170	18	3	250	1	0	1	0
Southwestern Ranch Dressing, 1 oz	160	17	3	370	1	0	1	0

California Pizza Kitchen

Appetizer								
Cabo Crab Cakes	527	NP	NP	NP	NP	NP	NP	NP
Singapore Shrimp Rolls	528	NP	NP	NP	NP	NP	NP	NP
Tuscan Hummus	861	NP	NP	NP	NP	NP	NP	NP

Description & Serving	Cal	Fat	Sfat	Sod	Carb	Fiber	Sugar	Prot
Spinach Artichoke Dip	873	NP	NP	NP	NP	NP	NP	NP
Sonora Egg Rolls	1050	NP	NP	NP	NP	NP	NP	NP
Avocado Club Egg Rolls	1180	NP	NP	NP	NP	NP	NP	NP
Garlic Cheese Foccacia w/ Checca	704	NP	NP	NP	NP	NP	NP	NP
Herb Onion Foccacia w/ Checca	809	NP	NP	NP	NP	NP	NP	NP
Mediterranean Tortilla Spring Rolls, ea	336	NP	NP	NP	NP	NP	NP	NP
Baja Chicken Tortilla Spring Rolls, ea	326	NP	NP	NP	NP	NP	NP	NP
Thai Chicken Tortilla Spring Rolls, ea	454	NP	NP	NP	NP	NP	NP	NP
Lettuce Wraps w/ Chicken	912	NP	NP	NP	NP	NP	NP	NP
Lettuce Wraps w/ Shrimp	896	NP	NP	NP	NP	NP	NP	NP
Lettuce Wraps w/ Chicken & Shrimp	1055	NP	NP	NP	NP	NP	NP	NP
Sesame Ginger Chicken Dumplings	326	NP	NP	NP	NP	NP	NP	NP

Salad

Description & Serving	Cal	Fat	Sfat	Sod	Carb	Fiber	Sugar	Prot
The Original BBQ Chicken Chopped Salad, half	643	NP	NP	NP	NP	NP	NP	NP
Grilled Vegetable Salad, half	520	NP	NP	NP	NP	NP	NP	NP
Original Chopped Salad, half	446	NP	NP	NP	NP	NP	NP	NP
Moroccan Chicken Salad, half	421	NP	NP	NP	NP	NP	NP	NP
Waldorf Chicken Salad, half	822	NP	NP	NP	NP	NP	NP	NP
Thai Crunch Salad, half	1057	NP	NP	NP	NP	NP	NP	NP
CPK Cobb Salad, half	574	NP	NP	NP	NP	NP	NP	NP
Classic Caesar, half	400	NP	NP	NP	NP	NP	NP	NP
Miso Salad, half	618	NP	NP	NP	NP	NP	NP	NP
Miso Salad w/ Chilled Grilled Chicken Breast, half	616	NP	NP	NP	NP	NP	NP	NP
Chinese Chicken Salad, half	503	NP	NP	NP	NP	NP	NP	NP
Field Greens, half	686	NP	NP	NP	NP	NP	NP	NP

Soup/Sandwich

Description & Serving	Cal	Fat	Sfat	Sod	Carb	Fiber	Sugar	Prot
Asparagus Soup, cup	106	NP	NP	NP	NP	NP	NP	NP
Adobe Chicken Chowder, cup	340	NP	NP	NP	NP	NP	NP	NP
Dakota Smashed Pea & Barley Soup, cup	184	NP	NP	NP	NP	NP	NP	NP
Sedona Tortilla Soup, cup	271	NP	NP	NP	NP	NP	NP	NP
Grilled Vegetable Focaccia Sandwich	732	NP	NP	NP	NP	NP	NP	NP
Grilled Dijon Chicken Focaccia Sandwich	791	NP	NP	NP	NP	NP	NP	NP
Grilled Chicken Caesar Focaccia Sandwich	995	NP	NP	NP	NP	NP	NP	NP

Entrée

Pizza , 1 slice

Description & Serving	Cal	Fat	Sfat	Sod	Carb	Fiber	Sugar	Prot
Tricolore Salad Pizza	193	NP	NP	NP	NP	NP	NP	NP
Cheeseburger Pizza	236	NP	NP	NP	NP	NP	NP	NP
Buffalo Chicken Pizza	189	NP	NP	NP	NP	NP	NP	NP
Pear & Gorgonzola Pizza	188	NP	NP	NP	NP	NP	NP	NP
Chipotle Chicken Pizza	204	NP	NP	NP	NP	NP	NP	NP
Chipotle Steak Pizza	245	NP	NP	NP	NP	NP	NP	NP
Thai Chicken Pizza	203	NP	NP	NP	NP	NP	NP	NP
Italian Tomato & Basil Pizza	158	NP	NP	NP	NP	NP	NP	NP
The Meat Cravers Pizza	239	NP	NP	NP	NP	NP	NP	NP
The Works Pizza	222	NP	NP	NP	NP	NP	NP	NP
White Pizza	177	NP	NP	NP	NP	NP	NP	NP
The Greek Pizza	231	NP	NP	NP	NP	NP	NP	NP

Description & Serving	Cal	Fat	Sfat	Sod	Carb	Fiber	Sugar	Prot
The Greek Pizza - Vegetarian	234	NP	NP	NP	NP	NP	NP	NP
Vegetarian w/ Japanese Eggplant Pizza	175	NP	NP	NP	NP	NP	NP	NP
The Original BBQ Chicken Pizza	175	NP	NP	NP	NP	NP	NP	NP
The Hawaiian BBQ Chicken Pizza	179	NP	NP	NP	NP	NP	NP	NP
BBQ Chicken w/ Applewood Smoked Bacon Pizza	205	NP	NP	NP	NP	NP	NP	NP
Jamaican Jerk Pizza	212	NP	NP	NP	NP	NP	NP	NP
Shrimp Scampi Pizza	173	NP	NP	NP	NP	NP	NP	NP
California Club Pizza	246	NP	NP	NP	NP	NP	NP	NP
Wild Mushroom Pizza	198	NP	NP	NP	NP	NP	NP	NP
Pepperoni Pizza	176	NP	NP	NP	NP	NP	NP	NP
Carne Asada Pizza	220	NP	NP	NP	NP	NP	NP	NP
Mushroom Pepperoni Sausage Pizza	219	NP	NP	NP	NP	NP	NP	NP
Tostada Pizza	240	NP	NP	NP	NP	NP	NP	NP
BLT Pizza	213	NP	NP	NP	NP	NP	NP	NP
Hawaiian Pizza	165	NP	NP	NP	NP	NP	NP	NP
Hawaiian Pizza w/ Pepperoni	181	NP	NP	NP	NP	NP	NP	NP
Roasted Garlic Chicken Pizza	173	NP	NP	NP	NP	NP	NP	NP
Sweet & Spicy Italian Sausages Pizza	209	NP	NP	NP	NP	NP	NP	NP
Five-Cheese & Fresh Tomato Pizza	176	NP	NP	NP	NP	NP	NP	NP
Traditional Cheese Pizza	152	NP	NP	NP	NP	NP	NP	NP
Santa Fe Chicken Pizza	186	NP	NP	NP	NP	NP	NP	NP
Goat Cheese w/ Roasted Peppers Pizza	176	NP	NP	NP	NP	NP	NP	NP
Pesto Chicken Thin Crust Pizza	155	NP	NP	NP	NP	NP	NP	NP
Tricolore Salad Thin Crust Pizza	193	NP	NP	NP	NP	NP	NP	NP
Sicilian Thin Crust Pizza	197	NP	NP	NP	NP	NP	NP	NP
Margherita Thin Crust Pizza	177	NP	NP	NP	NP	NP	NP	NP
Pepperoni Supremo Thin Crust Pizza	160	NP	NP	NP	NP	NP	NP	NP
Pasta								
Four Cheese Ravioli	1045	NP	NP	NP	NP	NP	NP	NP
Asparagus & Spinach Spaghettini	1116	NP	NP	NP	NP	NP	NP	NP
Asparagus & Spinach Spaghettini w/ Grilled Chicken Breast	1341	NP	NP	NP	NP	NP	NP	NP
Asparagus & Spinach Spaghettini w/ Shrimp	1223	NP	NP	NP	NP	NP	NP	NP
Asparagus & Spinach Spaghettini w/ Sauteed Salmon	1346	NP	NP	NP	NP	NP	NP	NP
Sausage & Pepper Penne	1011	NP	NP	NP	NP	NP	NP	NP
Sausage & Pepper Penne w/ Bolognese Meat Sauce	1171	NP	NP	NP	NP	NP	NP	NP
Pesto Cream Penne	1348	NP	NP	NP	NP	NP	NP	NP
Pesto Cream Penne w/ Chicken	1433	NP	NP	NP	NP	NP	NP	NP
Pesto Cream Penne w/ Shrimp	1455	NP	NP	NP	NP	NP	NP	NP
Pesto Cream Penne w/ Chicken & Shrimp	1539	NP	NP	NP	NP	NP	NP	NP
Spaghetti Bolognese	850	NP	NP	NP	NP	NP	NP	NP
Kung Pao Spaghetti	1125	NP	NP	NP	NP	NP	NP	NP
Kung Pao Spaghetti w/ Chicken	1229	NP	NP	NP	NP	NP	NP	NP
Kung Pao Spaghetti w/ Shrimp	1251	NP	NP	NP	NP	NP	NP	NP
Kung Pao Spaghetti w/ Chicken & Shrimp	1355	NP	NP	NP	NP	NP	NP	NP
Thai Linguini	1421	NP	NP	NP	NP	NP	NP	NP

Description & Serving	Cal	Fat	Sfat	Sod	Carb	Fiber	Sugar	Prot
Thai Linguini w/ Chicken	1505	NP	NP	NP	NP	NP	NP	NP
Thai Linguini w/ Shrimp	1528	NP	NP	NP	NP	NP	NP	NP
Thai Linguini w/ Chicken & Shrimp	1612	NP	NP	NP	NP	NP	NP	NP
Jambalaya	1190	NP	NP	NP	NP	NP	NP	NP
Chicken Tequila Fettuccine	1308	NP	NP	NP	NP	NP	NP	NP
Portobello Mushroom Ravioli	957	NP	NP	NP	NP	NP	NP	NP
Portobello Mushroom Ravioli w/ Garlic-Parmesan Cream Sauce	976	NP	NP	NP	NP	NP	NP	NP
Tomato Basil Spaghettini	1223	NP	NP	NP	NP	NP	NP	NP
Tomato Basil Spaghettini w/ Grilled Chicken Breast	1448	NP	NP	NP	NP	NP	NP	NP
Garlic Cream Fettuccine	1537	NP	NP	NP	NP	NP	NP	NP
Garlic Cream Fettuccine w/ Chicken	1621	NP	NP	NP	NP	NP	NP	NP
Garlic Cream Fettuccine w/ Shrimp	1644	NP	NP	NP	NP	NP	NP	NP
Garlic Cream Fettuccine w/ Chicken & Shrimp	1728	NP	NP	NP	NP	NP	NP	NP
Broccoli Sun-Dried Tomato Fusilli	742	NP	NP	NP	NP	NP	NP	NP
Broccoli Sun-Dried Tomato Fusilli w/ Grilled Chicken Breast	972	NP	NP	NP	NP	NP	NP	NP

Chicken/Fish

Description & Serving	Cal	Fat	Sfat	Sod	Carb	Fiber	Sugar	Prot
Chicken Piccata	1535	NP	NP	NP	NP	NP	NP	NP
Chicken Milanese	781	NP	NP	NP	NP	NP	NP	NP
Chicken Marsala	1408	NP	NP	NP	NP	NP	NP	NP
Ginger Salmon w/ Wok-Stirred Mandarin Noodles, Snow Peas, & Sesame Seeds	1345	NP	NP	NP	NP	NP	NP	NP
Ginger Salmon w/ Wok-Stirred Mixed Vegetables	979	NP	NP	NP	NP	NP	NP	NP
Blue Crab Cakes w/ Grilled Asparagus & Spaghettini	1567	NP	NP	NP	NP	NP	NP	NP
Blue Crab Cakes w/ Wok-Stirred Mixed Vegetables	1037	NP	NP	NP	NP	NP	NP	NP
Pan-Sauteed Salmon w/ Grilled Asparagus & Spaghettini	1310	NP	NP	NP	NP	NP	NP	NP
Pan-Sauteed Salmon w/ Wok-Stirred Mixed Vegetables	780	NP	NP	NP	NP	NP	NP	NP
Pan-Sauteed Mahi Mahi w/ Asparagus & Spinach Spaghettini	1214	NP	NP	NP	NP	NP	NP	NP
Pan-Sauteed Mahi Mahi w/ Wok-Stirred Mixed Vegetables	560	NP	NP	NP	NP	NP	NP	NP

Dessert

Description & Serving	Cal	Fat	Sfat	Sod	Carb	Fiber	Sugar	Prot
Sticky Toffee Cake	311	NP	NP	NP	NP	NP	NP	NP
Sticky Toffee Cake a la Haagen-Dazs	527	NP	NP	NP	NP	NP	NP	NP
Red Velvet Cake	743	NP	NP	NP	NP	NP	NP	NP
Red Velvet Cake a la Haagen-Dazs	959	NP	NP	NP	NP	NP	NP	NP
Chocolate Souffle Cake	676	NP	NP	NP	NP	NP	NP	NP
Chocolate Souffle Cake a la Haagen-Dazs	892	NP	NP	NP	NP	NP	NP	NP
Key Lime Pie	835	NP	NP	NP	NP	NP	NP	NP
Hot Fudge Brownie Sundae	1065	NP	NP	NP	NP	NP	NP	NP
Turtle Sundae	1538	NP	NP	NP	NP	NP	NP	NP
Chocolate Banana Royale Cake	650	NP	NP	NP	NP	NP	NP	NP

Description & Serving	Cal	Fat	Sfat	Sod	Carb	Fiber	Sugar	Prot
Chocolate Banana Royale Cake a la Haagen-Dazs	866	NP	NP	NP	NP	NP	NP	NP
Apple Crisp	510	NP	NP	NP	NP	NP	NP	NP
Apple Crisp a la Haagen-Dazs	726	NP	NP	NP	NP	NP	NP	NP
Tiramisu	530	NP	NP	NP	NP	NP	NP	NP

Beverage

Alcoholic

Almond Joy Coffee	210	NP	NP	NP	NP	NP	NP	NP
B-52 Coffee	170	NP	NP	NP	NP	NP	NP	NP
Chip Shot Coffee	130	NP	NP	NP	NP	NP	NP	NP
French Kiss Coffee	380	NP	NP	NP	NP	NP	NP	NP
Irish Coffee	160	NP	NP	NP	NP	NP	NP	NP
Keoke Coffee	160	NP	NP	NP	NP	NP	NP	NP
Nutty Irishman Coffee	130	NP	NP	NP	NP	NP	NP	NP
Winter Wonderland Coffee	190	NP	NP	NP	NP	NP	NP	NP

Nonalcoholic

Café Latte	150	NP	NP	NP	NP	NP	NP	NP
Café Mocha	250	NP	NP	NP	NP	NP	NP	NP
Espresso, single	0	NP	NP	NP	NP	NP	NP	NP
Espresso, double	0	NP	NP	NP	NP	NP	NP	NP
Cappuccino	150	NP	NP	NP	NP	NP	NP	NP
Café au Lait	150	NP	NP	NP	NP	NP	NP	NP
Coffee	0	NP	NP	NP	NP	NP	NP	NP

Captain D's Seafood Kitchen

Appetizer

Cheesesticks, 4 pc	220	12	6	535	16	0	2	10
Jalapeño Poppers, 5 pc	194	11	6	467	20	2	3	3

Entrée

Seafood/Chicken

Fish & Fries	910	55	24	2010	81	5	3	22
Catfish Feast	1050	63	24	2090	87	7	12	28
Fish Dinner, 2 pc	1080	67	26	2320	94	7	13	23
Fish Dinner, 3 pc	1240	77	30	2810	104	7	15	30
Fish Dinner, 4 pc	1400	87	34	3290	114	7	16	38
Country Style Fish Dinner	1180	68	28	2020	99	7	12	39
Seasoned Tilapia Dinner	608	13	5	1364	84	6	12	35
Coastal Fried Flounder	1530	93	37	2980	115	8	12	63
Wild Alaskan Salmon Dinner	618	11	3	1254	84	6	13	44
Shrimp Skewers Dinner	678	10	3	2404	83	6	12	55
Bite Size Shrimp Dinner	1140	61	24	1930	120	9	18	22
Ultimate Premium Shrimp Platter	1290	65	26	2390	69	8	12	35
Shrimp Lover's Trio	936	30	13	1904	89	6	13	47
1/2 lb Clam Platter	1450	87	23	2540	133	13	14	28
Gulf Coast Oysters	1000	58	23	1800	100	8	12	16
Chicken Dinner, 3 pc	1190	70	29	2380	102	7	12	33

Description & Serving	Cal	Fat	Sfat	Sod	Carb	Fiber	Sugar	Prot
Combination								
Classic Fish & Chicken Dinner	1250	77	30	2750	105	7	13	32
Classic Fish & Shrimp Dinner	1285	75	30	2750	94	7	13	33
Seafood Scampi Platter	668	13	5	1604	84	6	12	42
Deluxe Seafood Platter	1485	85	34	3190	112	7	15	43
10 pc Fish or Chicken Only	690	47	21	2190	45	0	1	23
Fish & Chicken	600	32	13	1420	53	6	10	26
Fish & Shrimp	635	30	13	1420	42	6	10	28
Captain's Value Pack	880	54	24	2468	72	6	10	28
Seafood Feast	1103	61	26	2305	293	8	14	36
Sandwich								
Fish Snack Smacker	440	26	8	835	41	0	7	12
Chicken Snack Smacker	570	30	11	1820	49	0	7	25
Chicken Ranch Sandwich	710	36	11	1540	69	2	4	27
Deluxe Classic Fish Sandwich	700	37	10	1520	67	2	5	26
Wild Alaskan Salmon Sandwich	520	18	2	980	48	2	5	42
Salad								
Fried Chicken Salad	215	10	4	455	20	2	6	11
Bite Size Shrimp Salad	275	10	4	445	35	3	9	10
Wild Alaskan Salmon Salad	185	1	0	435	10	2	7	35
Side								
Breadsticks	300	11	3	300	42	2	6	6
Fries	310	15	7	450	38	4	0	3
Hush Puppies	400	26	11	650	36	3	4	5
Broccoli	40	1	0	30	5	2	1	2
Home-Style Cole Slaw	170	12	2	310	13	2	10	1
Macaroni & Cheese	160	7	2	570	17	0	2	6
Lemon Herb Rice	228	4	1	574	43	0	1	4
Fried Okra	230	14	6	410	23	2	2	3
Southern-Style Green Beans	60	2	0	400	10	3	2	1
Roasted Red Peppers	170	7	4	1200	25	3	1	3
Corn-on-the-Cob	190	2	0	10	37	4	5	5
Side Salad	65	0	0	90	15	4	8	2
Baked Potato	240	0	0	25	54	6	3	6
Kids								
Kids Mac & Cheese	414	12	4	728	66	0	33	9
Kids Chicken	684	31	14	1053	86	4	29	13
Kids Fish	674	31	14	1098	85	4	30	12
Kids Shrimp	744	31	14	1043	101	5	32	12
Dressing/Condiment								
Ranch Dressing, 23 g	120	12	2	210	1	0	1	0
Thousand Island Dressing, 28 g	120	11	2	320	5	0	3	0
Fat Free Italian Dressing, 28 g	10	0	0	440	2	0	1	0
Honey Mustard Dressing, 28 g	160	16	2	125	5	0	3	0
Blue Cheese Dressing, 43 g	230	24	4	440	2	0	2	2
Scampi Butter Sauce, 57 g	120	10	6	360	5	0	1	2

Description & Serving	Cal	Fat	Sfat	Sod	Carb	Fiber	Sugar	Prot
Ginger Teriyaki Sauce, 68 g	60	0	0	1300	13	0	9	2
Sweet Chili Sauce, 68 g	100	0	0	960	25	0	23	0

Dessert

Chocolate Cake	300	11	2	270	49	2	35	3
Pineapple Cream Cheese Pie	320	14	6	300	43	0	33	6
Pecan Pie	470	26	4	270	56	2	25	5
Cheesecake w/ Strawberries	430	26	9	220	45	1	27	6

Beverage

Iced Tea, Unsweetened	0	0	0	15	0	0	0	0
Iced Tea, Sweetened	90	0	0	15	23	0	23	0
Lemonade	180	0	0	80	49	0	49	0

Carino's Italian

Appetizer

Italian Nachos	1047	48	19	3403	94	9	2	59
Bruschetta Bread	1288	86	15	1878	105	7	7	25
Hand-Breaded Calamari	1233	26	6	5264	176	7	5	68
Mozzarella w/ Marinara	743	43	19	2234	57	2	9	33
Shrimp Scampi w/ Garlic Toast	2031	159	91	1817	91	5	8	40
Baked Stuffed Mushrooms	463	37	23	1095	20	2	4	13
Sicilian Fire Sticks	1564	94	32	4601	115	13	9	58

Pizza

Create Your Own Pizza - no toppings	467	21	12	2068	72	6	5	34
The Classic Pizza Margherita	481	21	12	2071	75	7	7	35

Salad & Soup

Pecan Crusted Chicken Salad	972	50	16	3417	86	6	16	41
Honey Pecan Crusted Salmon Salad	794	45	7	1661	52	7	38	45
Classic Grilled Chicken Caesar Salad	726	54	8	1928	35	6	6	32
Italian Wedge Salad	794	66	15	1392	34	6	25	18
Shrimp & Artichoke Caesar Salad	521	34	6	1280	23	4	6	33
Chicken Gorgonzola & Sun Dried Tomato Salad	655	41	10	1584	47	6	14	30
Caesar Salad	264	21	3	649	15	2	2	6
House Salad	171	7	1	908	22	2	7	6
Garlic Potato Soup	549	35	19	1796	38	2	3	19
Italian Chili Soup	246	12	4	879	23	4	6	11
Minestrone Soup	159	1	1	1720	30	7	7	10
Tuscan Bean Soup	188	8	3	1162	16	5	1	11

Lunch Portion

Pasta

Homemade 16-Layer Lasagna	902	46	23	2252	62	6	19	57
Create Your Own Pasta - Alfredo	506	16	10	781	70	4	4	18
Create Your Own Pasta - Spicy Marinara	355	3	0	338	68	5	7	13
Create Your Own Pasta - Meat Sauce	384	4	1	458	71	4	10	15
Create Your Own Pasta - Italian Sausage	577	23	7	796	63	4	3	29

Description & Serving	Cal	Fat	Sfat	Sod	Carb	Fiber	Sugar	Prot
Homemade Parmigiana - Chicken	630	20	7	1514	74	4	9	39
Homemade Parmigiana - Eggplant	646	27	14	1126	67	9	14	34
Angel Hair w/ Artichokes	457	9	1	1035	77	7	10	15
Skilletini - Chicken, Sausage, or Combo	1191	70	15	2218	94	6	10	45
Spaghetti & Handmade Meatballs	739	25	8	1700	91	8	14	37
Baked Cheese Tortelloni	741	35	21	2245	61	5	10	43
Chicken & Seafood								
Spicy Shrimp & Chicken	969	56	21	1395	73	3	8	42
Spicy Romano Chicken	920	55	20	1482	74	4	10	33
Angel Hair w/ Artichokes & Chicken	578	15	2	1392	77	7	10	30
Grilled Chicken Bowtie Festival	989	60	23	1485	72	4	6	38
Chicken Fettuccine	709	29	16	1655	73	3	5	35
Chicken Scallopini	1367	112	48	1241	52	3	4	33
Jalapeno Garlic Tilapia	1255	101	45	932	51	3	3	32
Sandwich								
Italian Meatball Panini w/ Parmesan Shoestring Fries	1740	71	33	2851	221	6	127	53
Chicken Parmesan Panini w/ Parmesan Shoestring Fries	1831	79	33	2556	223	4	123	56
Smoked Turkey & Bacon Panini w/ Parmesan Shoestring Fries	1635	64	31	2525	205	4	124	60

Entrée (Dinner Portion)

Description & Serving	Cal	Fat	Sfat	Sod	Carb	Fiber	Sugar	Prot
Pasta								
Homemade 16-Layer Lasagna	902	46	23	2252	62	6	19	57
Create Your Own Pasta - Alfredo Sauce	766	25	15	1200	105	5	6	27
Create Your Own Pasta - Marinara Sauce	532	5	0	508	102	7	10	20
Create Your Own Pasta - Meat Sauce	575	6	1	687	107	7	15	23
Create Your Own Pasta - Italian Sausage	1004	46	15	1591	95	6	5	53
Homemade Parmigiana - Chicken	1124	48	15	2863	102	6	14	72
Homemade Parmigiana - Eggplant	689	32	15	1226	67	9	14	34
Homemade Parmigiana - Veal	1167	56	21	2068	97	6	14	67
Angel Hair w/ Artichokes	673	14	1	1780	113	11	14	22
Skilletini - Chicken	1215	72	12	2195	94	6	10	47
Skilletini - Sausage	1406	95	22	2615	95	7	10	43
Skilletini - Shrimp	1189	62	10	1655	114	7	11	44
Skilletini - Combo	1258	67	11	1935	115	7	11	49
Spaghetti & Handmade Meatballs	1108	37	12	2551	136	11	21	55
Baked Cheese Tortelloni	1004	45	27	2979	87	7	13	57
Five Meat Tuscan Pasta	1167	68	17	1902	99	7	13	38
Stuffed Vegetable Rigatoni	907	42	14	2708	96	12	15	32
Carino's Favorites Combo	1408	59	25	3408	128	10	23	89
Timballo - Chicken, Sausage, or Combo	1621	100	28	3456	115	10	13	64
Beef								
Grilled Italian Sirloin	1020	81	37	864	3	1	0	65
Chicken & Seafood								
Spicy Shrimp & Chicken	1294	73	26	1805	106	5	9	53
Spicy Romano Chicken	1248	71	25	2081	110	7	15	42
Angel Hair w/ Artichokes & Chicken	794	21	2	2137	114	11	14	37

Description & Serving	Cal	Fat	Sfat	Sod	Carb	Fiber	Sugar	Prot
Grilled Chicken Bowtie Festival	1243	72	25	1745	104	6	8	43
Chicken Fettuccine	958	37	20	2199	107	5	7	43
Chicken Scallopini	1806	149	60	2144	55	3	6	57
Chicken Penne Gorgonzola	1420	89	37	2114	107	6	8	47
Chicken Milano	1418	92	34	3447	65	3	6	79
Chicken Balsamico	868	34	7	1588	85	4	24	54
Chicken Marsala	1427	101	30	2244	64	3	5	51
Lemon Rosemary Chicken	687	21	4	2290	69	8	16	53
Grilled Chicken Diavolo	600	19	4	1764	57	5	10	51
Jalapeno Garlic Tilapia	1607	126	54	1608	58	3	3	56
Lobster Ravioli	933	62	29	1905	64	5	7	26
Grilled Citrus Balsamic Salmon	1373	95	30	1509	76	5	28	49
Angel Hair w/ Artichokes & Shrimp	738	15	1	1876	114	11	14	35
Shrimp Scampi	2015	149	83	1157	115	7	10	46

Kids

Description & Serving	Cal	Fat	Sfat	Sod	Carb	Fiber	Sugar	Prot
Bigger Kid Create Your Own Pizza - no toppings, 1 slice	70	3	2	235	11	1	0	5
Bigger Kid Margherita Pizza, 1 slice	71	3	2	236	12	1	1	5
Kids Pizza, 1 slice	70	3	2	235	11	1	0	5
Kids Cheese Tortelloni	273	7	4	733	38	3	6	13
Kids Chicken Strips w/ Fries	1377	57	20	1694	180	2	136	34
Kids Fettuccine Alfredo	341	8	5	359	55	3	3	12
Kids Grilled Chicken w/ Italian Green Beans	231	9	2	1075	14	4	6	24
Kids Grilled Chicken w/ Spaghetti	439	11	2	668	56	3	5	30
Kids Pepperoni Mac & Cheese	407	18	10	1508	41	2	5	17
Kids Spaghetti w/ Butter & Cheese	478	25	5	310	52	3	3	11
Kids Spaghetti w/ Meatball	469	13	4	851	66	5	8	22
Kids Spaghetti w/ Tomato Sauce	277	2	0	192	55	3	5	9
Kids Ice Cream	180	8	6	75	21	0	21	5
Kids Ice Cream Sundae	335	8	6	97	58	0	51	5
Kids Apple Juice	145	0	0	18	36	0	35	0
Kids Cranberry Juice	165	0	0	41	41	0	41	0
Kids Grapefruit Juice	164	0	0	18	40	0	38	0
Kids Milk	188	10	6	156	15	0	15	10
Kids Orange Juice	138	0	0	19	34	0	30	0
Kids Pineapple Juice	164	0	0	18	40	0	38	0

Dessert

Description & Serving	Cal	Fat	Sfat	Sod	Carb	Fiber	Sugar	Prot
Mascarpone Bread Pudding	1678	96	56	1619	175	3	103	29
Italian Chocolate Cake	591	19	11	395	94	3	77	10
Mini Chocolate Cake	141	4	2	95	23	1	18	2
Tiramisu	773	54	29	84	59	0	42	12
Mini Tiramisu	311	25	14	37	16	0	13	5
Turtle Cheesecake	1033	63	38	771	105	2	84	12
Mini Cheesecake w/ Amerena Cherries	228	13	8	160	25	0	21	3
Apple Skilletini	832	41	16	649	105	4	76	9

Beverage

Description & Serving	Cal	Fat	Sfat	Sod	Carb	Fiber	Sugar	Prot
Bellini, 14 oz	344	0	0	16	46	0	39	0
Margarita Primo Italiano	263	1	0	483	27	0	20	0

Description & Serving	Cal	Fat	Sfat	Sod	Carb	Fiber	Sugar	Prot
Italian Sangria, 1 glass	259	0	0	13	35	0	30	0
Amalfi Strawberry Lemonade	320	1	0	21	54	2	51	0
Italian Margarita, 14 oz	216	0	0	486	26	0	25	0
Italian Margarita on the rocks w/ Sauza Gold Tequila	257	1	0	483	35	0	28	0
Pomegranate Granita	461	0	0	1	74	0	62	0
Italian Soda w/o Cream	101	0	0	10	26	0	25	0
Italian Soda w/ Cream	116	10	1	21	27	0	26	0

Carl's Jr.

Breakfast

Breakfast Burger	780	41	15	1460	64	3	13	38
Steak & Egg Burrito	650	36	14	1750	43	1	4	41
Loaded Breakfast Burrito	780	49	16	1480	51	3	3	36
Sourdough Breakfast Sandwich	450	21	8	1470	38	1	3	29
Bacon & Egg Burrito	550	32	10	990	37	1	2	29
Sunrise Croissant Sandwich	590	44	17	810	27	1	4	20
French Toast Dips w/o syrup, 5 pc	460	21	4	570	60	3	16	9
Hash Brown Nuggets	350	23	4	440	32	3	0	3

Burger

Famous Star w/ Cheese	660	39	13	1300	53	3	10	27
Super Star w/ Cheese	920	58	23	1640	54	3	11	47
Western Bacon Cheeseburger	710	33	13	1410	69	3	15	32
Double Western Bacon Cheeseburger	960	52	23	1750	70	3	15	52
Chili Cheeseburger	780	41	19	1650	58	4	9	41
Jalapeno Burger	720	46	15	1340	50	3	9	27
The Original Six Dollar Burger	890	54	20	2040	58	3	18	45
The Guacamole Bacon Six Dollar Burger	1040	70	25	2240	53	4	10	49
The Western Bacon Six Dollar Burger	1020	53	22	2520	81	3	19	53
The Low Carb Six Dollar Burger	570	43	18	1480	7	1	5	38
The Bacon Cheese Six Dollar Burger	950	62	23	1980	49	3	9	51
The Jalapeno Six Dollar Burger	930	61	22	2190	52	3	9	45
Big Hamburger	460	17	8	1090	54	3	14	24

Chicken/Fish

Charbroiled Chicken Club Sandwich	560	27	7	1280	44	2	9	39
Charbroiled Santa Fe Chicken Sandwich	630	35	8	1410	44	2	9	36
Charbroiled BBQ Chicken Sandwich	380	7	1.5	1010	49	2	12	34
Bacon Swiss Crispy Chicken Sandwich	750	40	9	1990	62	4	9	36
Spicy Chicken Sandwich	420	27	5	930	33	2	3	12
Chicken Strips, 3	370	26	4	620	19	2	0	14
Carl's Catch Fish Sandwich	710	37	6	1280	74	4	11	20
Fish & Chips	730	39	7	1630	72	6	0	22

Salad

Side Salad	50	2.5	1.5	55	4	2	3	3
Green Burrito Taco Salad w/o dressing	970	58	19	1850	76	17	7	42
Charbroiled Chicken Salad w/o dressing	250	9	3.5	590	14	4	8	29

Description & Serving	Cal	Fat	Sfat	Sod	Carb	Fiber	Sugar	Prot
Kids								
Kid's Hamburger	230	10	3.5	550	24	1	5	9
Kid's Cheeseburger	290	15	7	830	24	1	5	12
Kid's Chicken Stars, 4	210	16	4	310	10	1	0	8
Natural-Cut Fries, kid's	220	11	2	580	29	2	0	3
Side								
Natural-Cut Fries, sml	320	15	3	830	42	4	0	4
Natural-Cut Fries, med	460	22	4.5	1180	60	5	0	5
Natural-Cut Fries, lrg	500	24	5	1290	65	5	0	6
Chili Cheese Fries	990	56	19	2380	89	8	1	28
CrissCut Fries	450	29	5	900	42	4	0	5
Onion Rings	530	28	4.5	590	61	3	6	8
Fried Zucchini	330	18	3	610	36	2	7	6
Dressing								
House Dressing, 2 oz	220	22	3.5	440	3	0	2	1
Blue Cheese Dressing, 2 oz	320	34	7	410	1	0	1	2
Thousand Island Dressing, 2 oz	240	23	3.5	460	7	0	3	0
Low Fat Balsamic Dressing, 2 oz	35	1.5	0	480	5	0	3	0
Dessert								
Chocolate Chip Cookie	370	19	10	350	48	2	27	3
Strawberry Swirl Cheesecake	290	16	9	230	32	0	21	6
Chocolate Cake	300	12	3	350	48	1	36	3
Vanilla Shake	710	33	23	240	86	0	76	14
Chocolate Shake	710	33	23	300	86	1	71	14
Strawberry Shake	700	33	23	250	85	0	75	14
Oreo Cookie Shake	730	38	25	360	81	1	64	15
Vanilla Malt	780	34	24	320	101	0	87	15
Chocolate Malt	780	34	24	270	100	1	82	15
Strawberry Malt	770	34	24	320	99	0	86	15
Oreo Cookie Malt	790	38	25	440	95	1	76	17

Carvel

Ice Cream/Italian Ice

Description & Serving	Cal	Fat	Sfat	Sod	Carb	Fiber	Sugar	Prot
Vanilla Ice Cream, sml cup (4.5 oz)	270	15	10	130	28	0	24	4
Chocolate Ice Cream, sml cup (4.5 oz)	250	13	8	130	29	1	25	6
No Fat Vanilla Ice Cream, sml cup (4.5 oz)	160	0	0	75	33	0	29	5
No Fat Chocolate Ice Cream, sml cup (4.5 oz)	160	0	0	55	37	0	33	3
No Sugar Added Vanilla Ice Cream, sml cup (4.5 oz)	180	4	2.5	115	34	0	10	7
Sherbet Ice Cream	180	1.5	1	70	40	0	30	1
Lemon Italian Ice, sml (4 oz)	150	0	0	50	37	0	34	0
Mango Italian Ice, sml (4 oz)	120	0	0	10	34	0	31	0
Cherry Italian Ice, sml (4 oz)	120	0	0	10	35	0	33	0
Passion Fruit Italian Ice, sml (4 oz)	120	0	0	15	35	0	33	0
Guava Italian Ice, sml (4 oz)	120	0	0	10	33	0	30	0
Bubble Gum Italian Ice, sml (4 oz)	130	0	0	10	32	0	30	0

Description & Serving	Cal	Fat	Sfat	Sod	Carb	Fiber	Sugar	Prot
Strawberry Italian Ice, sml (4 oz)	120	0	0	10	30	0	27	0
Sour Blue Raspberry Italian Ice, sml (4 oz)	150	0	0	10	38	0	35	0

Cone with Ice Cream

Description & Serving	Cal	Fat	Sfat	Sod	Carb	Fiber	Sugar	Prot
Small waffle cone w/ Vanilla	350	16	11	160	46	1	30	5
Small waffle cone w/ Chocolate	330	13	8	160	47	2	31	7
Small sugar cone w/ Vanilla	320	15	10	160	39	0	28	5
Small sugar cone w/ Chocolate	300	13	8	160	40	1	29	7
Small cake cone w/ Vanilla	280	16	10	135	31	0	24	4
Small cake cone w/ Chocolate	260	13	8	135	32	1	25	6

Sundae

Description & Serving	Cal	Fat	Sfat	Sod	Carb	Fiber	Sugar	Prot
Hot Fudge Sundae, reg	670	38	24	280	73	1	62	8
Bittersweet Fudge Sundae, reg	690	38	27	280	77	1	64	8
Strawberry Sundae, reg	580	33	23	210	63	1	54	7
Caramel Sundae, reg	670	34	24	360	81	0	60	8
Olde Fashioned Sundae	340	15	11	150	47	0	34	4
Mini Sundae w/ Chocolate Syrup	220	10	8	95	29	0	22	3
No Fat Classic Fudge Sundae, reg	380	0	1.5	180	81	0	46	8
No Fat Classic Strawberry Sundae, reg	320	0	0	150	69	1	59	8
No Fat Olde Fashioned Sundae	300	0	1.5	150	67	0	33	6
No Fat Miniature Sundae	190	0	1.5	95	45	0	20	4
No Sugar Added Olde Fashioned Sundae	360	4.5	3	220	76	0	11	8
No Sugar Added Miniature Sundae	200	2.5	2	125	42	0	6	5
Sprinkle Cup	260	14	10	85	31	0	17	3
Bananas Foster Dasher	640	27	17	370	94	2	64	7
Mint Chocolate Chip Dasher	800	42	25	390	96	3	74	10
Peanut Butter Cup Dasher	1060	60	20	670	95	7	76	22
Strawberry Shortcake Dasher	630	31	19	190	82	2	63	8
Fudge Brownie Dasher	850	45	21	420	102	4	84	10
Banana Barge Dasher	970	46	24	290	128	7	95	19

CARVELANCHE

Description & Serving	Cal	Fat	Sfat	Sod	Carb	Fiber	Sugar	Prot
Carvelanche Butterfinger, 16 oz	730	38	24	340	92	1	72	10
Carvelanche Cookies & Cream, 16 oz	610	33	19	310	70	0	54	8
Carvelanche Cake Mix, 16 oz	770	31	20	500	110	0	77	10
Carvelanche M&M, 16 oz	760	39	18	230	88	0	75	11
Carvelanche Reese's, 16 oz	750	39	28	320	85	0	74	14
No Fat Carvelanche, Strawberry, 16 oz	430	0	0	160	91	1	81	12

Frozen Drink

Description & Serving	Cal	Fat	Sfat	Sod	Carb	Fiber	Sugar	Prot
Thick Chocolate Shake, 16 oz	650	27	16	320	93	2	69	14
Thick Vanilla Shake, 16 oz	660	31	20	280	86	0	79	11
Thick Strawberry Shake, 16 oz	600	31	20	280	70	1	61	11
Thick Shake Float, Vanilla, 16 oz	810	39	26	350	102	0	92	13
Thick Shake Float, Chocolate, 16 oz	790	34	20	390	109	3	83	17
Thick Shake Float, Strawberry, 16 oz	750	39	26	340	85	1	74	13
No Fat Chocolate Shake, 16 oz	440	0	0	190	104	0	59	5
No Fat Mocha Shake, 16 oz	440	0	0	230	97	0	52	10
No Fat Vanilla Shake, 16 oz	300	0	0	135	62	0	55	9
Ice Cream Soda Float, Vanilla Ice Cream & Coke, 16 oz	380	17	11	150	53	0	48	4

Description & Serving	Cal	Fat	Sfat	Sod	Carb	Fiber	Sugar	Prot
Ice Cream Soda Float, Chocolate Ice Cream & Coke, 16 oz	360	14	8	150	54	1	49	6
Ice Cream Soda Float, Vanilla Ice Cream & Soda Water, 16 oz	440	18	11	220	68	0	46	4
Ice Cream Soda Float, Chocolate Ice Cream & Soda Water, 16 oz	420	15	8	220	69	1	47	6
Caramel Macchiato Freeze, 16 oz	680	27	17	420	97	0	74	11
Light Caramel Macchiato Freeze, 16 oz	450	2.5	1.5	270	96	0	74	8
Coffee Freeze, 16 oz	670	32	20	340	84	0	73	14
Light Coffee Freeze, 16 oz	390	0.5	0	150	84	0	73	10
Mocha Freeze, 16 oz	610	25	15	280	88	0	70	10
Light Mocha Freeze, 16 oz	390	1	0	135	87	0	69	7
Broadway Banana Smoothie, 16 oz	320	0	0	25	78	2	67	0
Rockefeller Raspberry Smoothie, 16 oz	300	0	0	35	75	1	69	0
Berry Times Square Smoothie, 16 oz	330	0	0	35	80	2	66	0
Cherry Swirl Italian Ice, 16 oz	490	12	8	120	93	0	85	3
Passion Fruit Swirl Italian Ice, 16 oz	500	12	8	125	93	0	86	3
Mango Swirl Italian Ice, 16 oz	490	12	8	120	93	0	85	3

Frozen Treat

Description & Serving	Cal	Fat	Sfat	Sod	Carb	Fiber	Sugar	Prot
Cookie Dough Arctic Blender, 16 oz	880	44	18	460	113	1	93	11
Light Cookie Dough Arctic Blender, 16 oz	660	19	3.5	320	112	0	93	8
Fried Ice Cream Arctic Blender, 16 oz	850	29	18	590	132	1	87	12
Light Fried Ice Cream Arctic Blender, 16 oz	630	5	3	450	132	1	87	9
Peanut Butter Arctic Blender, 16 oz	700	37	18	390	79	2	61	14
Light Peanut Butter Arctic Blender, 16 oz	470	13	3	250	79	1	61	11
Chipster	350	17	9	230	45	4	27	4
Flying Saucer, Vanilla	240	11	6	170	33	1	19	4
Flying Saucer, Chocolate	230	10	5	170	33	1	20	4
Deluxe Flying Saucer w/ Sprinkles	350	17	9	170	49	1	20	3
98% Fat Free Flying Saucer, Vanilla	180	2.5	0	170	35	1	20	5
98% Fat Free Flying Saucer, Chocolate	180	2.5	0.5	160	34	1	19	5

Casey's General Store

Breakfast

Description & Serving	Cal	Fat	Sfat	Sod	Carb	Fiber	Sugar	Prot
Bacon & Egg Croissant	375	28	NP	890	27	1	NP	17
Ham & Egg Croissant	368	23.9	NP	830.7	19.2	1	NP	19.7
Sausage & Egg Biscuit	584	58.1	NP	1531.6	27.2	2	NP	26.2
Sausage & Egg Croissant	544	57.1	NP	891.6	19.2	3	NP	25.2
Jelly Donut, unfrosted	280	11	NP	340	40	1	NP	4
Long John, unfrosted	230	13	NP	170	22	1	NP	4
Maple Cinnamon Stick, unfrosted	340	16	NP	330	45	2	NP	6
Plain Chocolate Cake Donut, unfrosted	297	4.5	NP	861.6	58	1	NP	7.8
Plain Deluxe Cake Donut, unfrosted	302	4.4	NP	798.2	59	1	NP	7.4

Burger/Sandwich/Sausage

Description & Serving	Cal	Fat	Sfat	Sod	Carb	Fiber	Sugar	Prot
Bacon Cheeseburger	691	48.4	NP	1338	26.1	1.05	NP	32.9
Cheeseburger	601	40.4	NP	1088.3	26.1	1.05	NP	28.9
Hamburger	491	31.4	NP	644.3	25.1	1.05	NP	23.9

Description & Serving	Cal	Fat	Sfat	Sod	Carb	Fiber	Sugar	Prot
BBQ Beef	604	30.1	NP	1596	66.4	2.6	NP	32.4
Breaded Chicken	500	8.5	NP	880	79	4	NP	29
Breaded Pork	630	17.5	NP	1000	88	4	NP	30
Ham & Cheese	356	17.7	NP	1271	53.4	4	NP	25.1
Hot Sausage	594	43.1	NP	1721.3	50.2	4	NP	27.4
Mild Sausage	567	39.3	NP	1714.5	49.2	4	NP	30.1
Side/Snack								
Hashbrowns	130	3.5	NP	190	15	2	NP	2
Potato Cheese Bites	420	23	NP	1050	42	7	NP	12
Potato Wedges	327	14	NP	886.7	44.3	4.7	NP	4.7
Chicken Pot Pie Bites	462	18.2	NP	924	51.8	1.4	NP	19.6
Chicken Tenders, 3 pc	350	10.5	NP	700	24.5	0	NP	35
Popcorn Chicken	342	16.7	NP	1257.5	25.6	0.9	NP	21.6
Pizza								
Bacon Breakfast Pizza, 1 med slice	479	20.8	NP	1498.3	49.9	1.85	NP	23.5
Bacon Cheeseburger Pizza, 1 med slice	491	19.9	NP	1168.5	50	1.9	NP	22.4
Beef Pizza, 1 med slice	409	14.7	NP	834.8	47.9	2.1	NP	18.7
Cheese Pizza, 1 med slice	351	12.3	NP	516.3	48.8	2.12	NP	14.5
Hot Sausage Pizza, 1 med slice	421	16.8	NP	768.1	48.3	2.1	NP	17.5
Mild Sausage Pizza, 1 med slice	421	16.8	NP	768.1	48.3	2.1	NP	17.5
Pepperoni Pizza, 1 med slice	393	14.4	NP	683.8	48.1	2.1	NP	16.2
Sausage Breakfast Pizza, 1 med slice	443	14.9	NP	790.3	47.9	1.85	NP	19
Supreme Pizza, 1 med slice	463	17.1	NP	961.2	49.6	2.29	NP	20.7
Taco Pizza, 1 med slice	472	14.7	NP	619.4	63.6	2.12	NP	15.7
Beverage								
Fat Free French Vanilla Cappuccino, 12 oz	210	0	NP	255	46.5	0	NP	4.5
French Vanilla Cappuccino, 12 oz	210	6	NP	195	34.5	0	NP	4.5
Hot Chocolate, 12 oz	195	2.3	NP	330	42	0	NP	4.5
Dessert								
Apple Fritter, unfrosted	380	23	NP	400	39	1	NP	6
Brownie, unfrosted	360	15	NP	270	53	2	NP	4
Caramel Chocolate Pecan Cookie, unfrosted	310	16	NP	270	38	1	NP	3
Chocolate Chunk Cookie, unfrosted	300	10	NP	290	48	2	NP	3
Cinnamon Buns, unfrosted	298	15	NP	24	24	1	NP	5
Mini Chocolate Chip Cookies (10), unfrosted	550	30	NP	475	70	0	NP	5
Pinwheel, unfrosted	150	13	NP	95	5	0	NP	1
Premium Rings, unfrosted	230	13	NP	250	24	1	NP	4
Pull-A-Part, unfrosted	190	10	NP	220	22	1	NP	3
Raspberry Cheese Flips, unfrosted	430	25	NP	240	46	0	NP	5
S'mores Bar, unfrosted	530	28	NP	250	68	0	NP	5
Strawberry Cream Cheese Turnover, unfrosted	310	15	NP	310	39	3	NP	5

Charley's Grilled Subs

Breakfast								
2 Eggs Scrambled	367	26	8	616	5	0	NP	24
Toast (white), 2 pc	160	4	0	320	30	2	NP	4

Description & Serving	Cal	Fat	Sfat	Sod	Carb	Fiber	Sugar	Prot
Ham Omelet	497	33	10.5	1400	9.5	0	NP	37
Bacon Omelet	547	39	12.5	1440	9	0	NP	36
Sausage Omelet	601	44	15	1666	10	0	NP	38
Veggie Omelet	490.5	32	10	1183	15	1	NP	34
Western Omelet	520.5	33	10.5	1403	15.5	1	NP	38
Egg & Cheese Sandwich	477	18	6.5	1072	56	2	NP	24
Bacon Egg & Cheese Sandwich	557	25	9	1332	56	2	NP	28
Ham Egg & Cheese Sandwich	507	19	7	1292	56.5	2	NP	29
Sausage Egg & Cheese Sandwich	611	30	11.5	1558	57	2	NP	30
Steak Egg & Cheese Sandwich	627	26	9.5	1382	57	2	NP	43
Hash Browns	350	20	5	870	35	5	NP	0

Sandwich

Philly Cheesesteak Sandwich, reg	526	19	7.5	1449	58	3	NP	36
Deluxe Philly Sandwich, reg	533.5	19	7.5	1450	60	3	NP	37
BBQ Cheddar Sandwich, reg	586	11	3.5	1819	70	3	NP	36
Bacon 3 Cheese Sandwich, reg	645	30	10	1757	54.5	2	NP	43
Sicilian Sandwich, reg	620	28	11.5	1907	54.5	2	NP	41
Philly Chicken Sandwich, reg	523.5	16	6.5	1290	60	3	NP	42
Buffalo Chicken Sandwich, reg	531	16	6.5	1704	60.5	4	NP	42
Teriyaki Chicken Sandwich, reg	527	16	7.5	1232	60	3	NP	43
Cordon Bleu Sandwich, reg	530	17	NP	NP	NP	NP	NP	NP
Chicken Bacon Club Sandwich, reg	580	23	10	1367	54	2	NP	45
Turkey Cheddar Sandwich, reg	462	12	5.5	1422	54.5	2	NP	31
Ultimate Club Sandwich, reg	517	20	8.5	1586	54.5	2	NP	32
Italian Deli Sandwich, reg	555	26	11	1660	54.5	2	NP	29
Philly Ham Sandwich, reg	443.5	13	6.5	1013	60	3	NP	28
Philly Veg Sandwich, reg	462	15	7.5	1192	65.5	4	NP	23
Chicken Parmesan Sandwich, reg	500	16	6.5	1287	54	2	NP	40
Chicken California Sandwich, reg	500	16	6.5	1287	54	2	NP	40
Mushroom Swiss Steak Sandwich, reg	520.5	19	8.5	1269	57	2	NP	38
Philly Steak & Bleu Sandwich, reg	476	15	6.5	1399	57	3	NP	32

Salad

Grilled Chicken Salad	281	5	0	14	4.75	31	NP	NP
Chicken Teriyaki Salad	292	5	0	16	4.75	31.5	NP	NP
Buffalo Chicken Salad	296	5	0	16.5	5.75	31.5	NP	NP
Grilled Steak Salad	291	6	0	14	4.75	26	NP	NP
Fresh Garden Salad	141	3	0	13	4.75	7	NP	NP

Side

Fries, kids	366	27	4	290	25	1	NP	3
Fries, reg	611	45	7.5	483	41	2	NP	5
Bacon Ranch Fries	1149	95	18.5	1392	51	2	NP	15
Ultimate Fries	1249	103	20.5	2092	57	2	NP	16
Large Fries	733	55	11	579	50.5	2	NP	6
Cheddar Fries	1054	84	17	1652	55	2	NP	14
Cheddar Bacon Fries	1089	87	18	1762	55	2	NP	16
Chicken Fingers, 3	200	12	3	660	10	1	NP	13

Description & Serving	Cal	Fat	Sfat	Sod	Carb	Fiber	Sugar	Prot
Dressing/Condiment/Topping								
Tomatoes, 1 oz	7	0	0	0	1.5	1.5	NP	0.5
Lettuce, 1 oz	4	0	0	0	1	0.5	NP	0.5
Black Olives, 2 tbsp	30	25	0	100	0.5	0	NP	0
Banana Peppers, 12 rings	5	0	0	470	0	0	NP	0
Mayo, 1 tbsp	100	11	1.5	75	0	0	NP	0
Honey Mustard, 1 tsp	10	0	0	30	1	0	NP	0
Spicy Brown Mustard, 1 tsp	0	0	0	120	1	0	NP	0
Ketchup, 1 tbsp	15	0	0	180	4	0	NP	0
Italian Dressing, 2 tbsp	170	19	3	360	1	0	NP	0
Ranch Dressing, 2 tbsp	160	16	2.5	270	1	0	NP	0

Chester's

	Cal	Fat	Sfat	Sod	Carb	Fiber	Sugar	Prot
Entrée								
One Chicken Leg	260	15	3.5	640	12	1	0.21	19
Chicken Breast	250	14	3	720	12	<1	<0.10	20
Chicken Tenders	230	9	1.5	560	13	1	<0.10	25
Chicken Breaster Sandwich	270	10	2	610	29	2	3.05	16
Side								
Potato Wedges	190	7	1.5	10	27	3	0.55	4
Green Beans	60	3	0.5	720	7	3	1.33	0
Coleslaw	110	7	1	360	11	2	8.73	<1
Biscuit	400	21	5	1260	45	5	3.82	8

Chick-fil-A

	Cal	Fat	Sfat	Sod	Carb	Fiber	Sugar	Prot
Breakfast								
Bacon, Egg & Cheese Biscuit	490	26	12	1350	43	2	6	21
Plain Biscuit	310	13	6	700	41	2	4	5
Biscuit & Gravy	420	20	8	1370	51	2	5	8
Chick-n-Minis, 3	260	10	2.5	590	29	1	6	13
Chicken Biscuit	450	20	8	1310	48	3	5	19
Chicken Breakfast Burrito	420	18	7	890	41	4	3	22
Chicken, Egg, & Cheese Bagel	500	20	6	1280	49	3	9	30
Cinnamon Cluster	400	15	6	280	61	3	28	8
Hash Browns	280	19	4	410	25	2	0	3
Sausage Biscuit	590	41	16	1250	42	4	2	16
Sausage Breakfast Burrito	480	27	11	870	38	4	3	21
Sandwich/Strips/Wrap/Nugget								
Chargrilled Chicken Club Sandwich	380	12	5	1650	34	7	10	36
Chargrilled Chicken Sandwich	260	3	0.5	1300	33	7	9	27
Chicken Salad Sandwich	500	20	3.5	1220	53	4	13	29
Chicken Sandwich	430	17	3.5	1370	39	3	7	31
Chick-n-Strips, 1 pc	120	6	1	350	6	1	1	11
Chick-n-Strips, 4 pc	470	23	4.5	1390	22	3	4	44
Chargrilled Chicken Cool Wrap	410	12	4	1510	49	9	7	33

Description & Serving	Cal	Fat	Sfat	Sod	Carb	Fiber	Sugar	Prot
Chicken Caesar Cool Wrap	460	15	6	1720	46	8	6	39
Nuggets, 12	400	19	4	1250	15	3	4	40

Salad

Chargrilled & Fruit Salad	220	6	3.5	860	21	4	16	22
Chargrilled Chicken Garden Salad	170	6	3.5	860	10	4	5	22
Chick-n-Strips Salad	450	22	6	1160	26	6	7	39
Southwest Chargrilled Salad	240	9	4	750	17	5	6	25
Garlic & Butter Croutons	60	2	0	150	9	0	1	1
Harvest Nut Granola	60	2	0	10	10	2	3	1
Honey Roasted Sunflower Kernels	90	7	1	55	4	1	1	2
Tortilla Strips	80	4	0	50	8	1	1	1

Side

Side Salad	70	4.5	3	110	5	2	2	5
Carrot & Raisin Salad, sml	260	12	1.5	160	39	4	31	2
Carrot & Raisin Salad, lrg	390	18	2.5	230	59	5	47	2
Chicken Salad Cup	350	24	4	1100	6	1	6	27
Cole Slaw, sml	360	31	5	280	19	3	16	2
Cole Slaw, lrg	580	50	8	450	31	5	26	3
Fruit Cup, sml	50	0	0	0	13	1	11	0
Fruit Cup, med	70	0	0	0	17	2	14	0
Fruit Cup, lrg	100	0	0	0	27	3	22	1
Hearty Breast of Chicken Soup, sml	150	4	1.5	1060	19	2	2	9
Hearty Breast of Chicken Soup, lrg	240	7	2	1670	30	2	4	15
Waffle Potato Fries, sml	280	16	3.5	80	31	4	0	3
Waffle Potato Fries, med	370	21	4.5	105	41	5	0	4
Waffle Potato Fries, lrg	420	24	5	120	46	6	0	5

Dressing/Condiment

Barbecue Sauce	45	0	0	180	11	0	9	0
Blue Cheese Dressing	150	16	3	300	1	0	1	1
Buffalo Sauce	10	0	0	420	1	0	0	0
Buttermilk Ranch Dressing	160	17	2.5	280	1	0	1	0
Buttermilk Ranch Sauce	110	12	2	200	1	0	1	0
Caesar Dressing	160	17	2.5	240	1	0	0	1
Chick-fil-A Sauce	140	13	2	170	6	0	6	0
Fat Free Honey Mustard Dressing	60	0	0	210	14	1	11	0
Honey Mustard Sauce	45	0	0	150	10	0	10	0
Honey Roasted BBQ Sauce	60	5	1	70	2	0	2	0
Light Italian Dressing	15	0.5	0	580	2	0	2	0
Polynesian Sauce	110	6	1	210	14	0	5	0
Reduced Fat Berry Balsamic Vinaigrette	70	2	0	150	12	0	9	0
Spicy Dressing	140	14	2	130	2	0	1	0
Thousand Island Dressing	150	14	2	250	5	0	4	0
Apple Jelly	35	0	0	0	9	0	6	0
Grape Jelly	35	0	0	0	9	0	6	0
Ketchup	10	0	0	105	2	0	2	0
Light Mayonnaise	40	4	0.5	85	1	0	0	0
Mayonnaise	90	10	1.5	70	1	0	0	0

Description & Serving	Cal	Fat	Sfat	Sod	Carb	Fiber	Sugar	Prot
Mixed Fruit Jelly	35	0	0	0	9	0	6	0
Mustard	5	0	0	60	1	0	0	0

Dessert

Description & Serving	Cal	Fat	Sfat	Sod	Carb	Fiber	Sugar	Prot
Cheesecake	310	23	13	280	22	1	14	5
Chocolate Milkshake, sml	600	23	14	410	88	1	85	13
Chocolate Milkshake, lrg	740	28	17	520	112	1	107	16
Cookies & Cream Milkshake, sml	570	26	14	430	80	0	75	14
Cookies & Cream Milkshake, lrg	700	33	17	550	98	1	92	17
Fudge Nut Brownie	370	19	6	180	45	3	28	5
Icedream, cup	290	7	4.5	200	50	0	49	8
Icedream, cone	170	4	2	115	31	0	25	5
Lemon Pie	360	13	6	290	58	1	21	6
Peach Milkshake, sml	720	19	11	450	125	1	118	13
Peach Milkshake, lrg	850	21	13	540	153	1	144	15
Strawberry Milkshake, sml	610	23	13	410	92	1	83	13
Strawberry Milkshake, lrg	760	28	16	520	117	1	105	16
Vanilla Milkshake, sml	540	23	13	400	74	0	73	13
Vanilla Milkshake, lrg	660	27	16	510	90	0	89	16

Beverage

Description & Serving	Cal	Fat	Sfat	Sod	Carb	Fiber	Sugar	Prot
Café Blends Coffee, sml	5	0	0	5	0	0	0	0
Café Blends Coffee, med	5	0	0	10	0	0	0	1
Café Blends Coffee, lrg	5	0	0	10	0	0	0	1
Diet Lemonade, kids	15	0	0	5	5	0	1	0
Diet Lemonade, sml	15	0	0	10	6	0	2	0
Diet Lemonade, med	20	0	0	10	8	0	2	0
Diet Lemonade, lrg	30	0	0	15	11	1	3	0
Lemonade, kids	150	0	0	5	39	0	36	0
Lemonade, sml	170	0	0	5	46	0	43	0
Lemonade, med	240	0	0	10	63	0	58	0
Lemonade, lrg	350	0	0	15	92	0	85	0

Chili's

Appetizer

Description & Serving	Cal	Fat	Sfat	Sod	Carb	Fiber	Sugar	Prot
Southwestern Eggrolls w/ Avocado Ranch	910	57	14	1960	72	7	NP	27
Skillet Queso w/ chips	940	77	32	3870	42	7	NP	32
Bottomless Tostada Chips w/ Hot Sauce	470	39	5	2790	26	5	NP	4
Hot Spinach & Artichoke Dip w/ chips	930	77	34	3130	39	3	NP	24
Onion String & Crispy Jalapeno Stack w/ Jalapeno Ranch	2130	213	31	1320	34	5	NP	6
Texas Cheese Fries w/ Jalapeno Ranch, full order	1920	147	63	3570	67	7	NP	84
Triple Dipper Big Mouth Bites w/ Jalapeno Ranch, 2	780	51	15	1440	46	2	NP	30
Triple Dipper Southwestern Eggrolls w/ Avocado Ranch, 2	640	42	10	1370	48	5	NP	18
Triple Dipper Chicken Crisper Bites, 2	690	40	9	1970	58	2	NP	20
Triple Dipper Buffalo Chicken Crisper Bites, 2	620	34	8	2380	54	2	NP	23
Triple Dipper Chicken Crispers w/o dressing, 3	600	42	7	1300	20	2	NP	34

Description & Serving	Cal	Fat	Sfat	Sod	Carb	Fiber	Sugar	Prot
Triple Dipper Hot Spinach & Artichoke Dip w/ chips	460	38	17	1560	20	2	NP	12
Kickin' Jack Nachos, 8 chips	820	62	31	1820	43	6	NP	37
Kickin' Jack Nachos w/ Fajita Beef, 8 chips	1010	66	33	2760	44	6	NP	63
Kickin' Jack Nachos w/ Fajita Chicken, 8 chips	960	64	31	2740	45	6	NP	65

Wings

Description & Serving	Cal	Fat	Sfat	Sod	Carb	Fiber	Sugar	Prot
Triple Dipper Boneless Sweet Chile Glazed Wings w/ Ranch, 5	760	50	9	1640	49	1	NP	25
Triple Dipper Boneless Buffalo Wings w/ Bleu Cheese, 5	740	60	10	2070	26	1	NP	24
Triple Dipper Wings Over Buffalo w/ Bleu Cheese, 5	800	72	15	1730	1	0	NP	34
Boneless Sweet Chile Glazed Wings w/ Ranch	1300	80	14	2880	95	2	NP	46
Boneless Buffalo Wings w/ Bleu Cheese	1200	91	15	3750	48	1	NP	44
Wings Over Buffalo w/ Bleu Cheese	1330	116	26	1880	2	0	NP	66

Salad

Description & Serving	Cal	Fat	Sfat	Sod	Carb	Fiber	Sugar	Prot
Quesadilla Explosion Salad w/ dressing	1270	76	23	2650	86	10	NP	61
Spicy Garlic and Lime Grilled Shrimp Salad w/ dressing	630	40	11	1850	43	9	NP	29
Boneless Buffalo Chicken Salad w/ dressing	1070	77	15	4380	46	5	NP	44
Mesquite Chicken Salad w/ dressing	960	62	18	2680	45	10	NP	54
Chicken Caesar Salad w/ dressing	900	71	13	1740	28	6	NP	37
Southwestern Cobb Salad w/ dressing	1080	71	16	2650	57	9	NP	55
Side Salad House w/o dressing	210	12	6	310	17	3	NP	10
Side Salad Caesar w/ dressing	350	31	6	550	13	2	NP	6

Soup

Description & Serving	Cal	Fat	Sfat	Sod	Carb	Fiber	Sugar	Prot
Baked Potato Soup, cup	250	18	10	890	13	1	NP	9
Baked Potato Soup, bowl	510	35	21	1790	26	2	NP	18
Broccoli Cheese Soup, cup	120	8	3.5	650	9	1	NP	5
Broccoli Cheese Soup, bowl	250	16	7	1310	18	2	NP	11
Chicken Enchilada Soup, cup	220	13	5	690	9	1	NP	15
Chicken Enchilada Soup, bowl	430	27	10	1390	19	2	NP	29
Chicken Noodle Soup, cup	60	0.5	0	580	10	1	NP	3
Chicken Noodle Soup, bowl	120	1.5	0	1150	20	1	NP	7
Chicken Tortilla Soup, cup	130	7	2.5	1030	10	1	NP	7
Chicken Tortilla Soup, bowl	260	15	5	2060	20	3	NP	14
Chili's Terlingua Chili w/ toppings, cup	210	14	5	620	9	1	NP	12
Chili's Terlingua Chili w/ toppings, bowl	420	28	10	1240	18	2	NP	25
New England Clam Chowder, cup	190	13	7	390	11	1	NP	6
New England Clam Chowder, bowl	370	26	15	780	23	1	NP	12
Southwestern Vegetable Soup, cup	100	4	1.5	630	13	2	NP	4
Southwestern Vegetable Soup, bowl	210	8	3	1250	26	5	NP	9

Burger/Sandwich/Pita

Description & Serving	Cal	Fat	Sfat	Sod	Carb	Fiber	Sugar	Prot
Bacon Burger	1090	69	21	1800	57	3	NP	56
Big Mouth Bites	1580	97	28	2930	104	6	NP	61
Mushroom-Swiss Burger	1070	67	18	1670	65	4	NP	52
Old Timer	820	44	12	1310	59	3	NP	45
Old Timer w/ Cheese	900	51	16	1450	59	3	NP	50

Description & Serving	Cal	Fat	Sfat	Sod	Carb	Fiber	Sugar	Prot
Jalapeno Smokehouse Bacon Bigmouth Burger	1690	120	39	4050	68	4	NP	84
Southern Smokehouse Bacon Bigmouth Burger	1630	108	36	4170	80	4	NP	84
Smokehouse Bacon Triple Cheese Bigmouth Burger	1750	123	44	3860	66	3	NP	94
Guiltless Black Bean Burger	610	11	2	1790	91	18	NP	37
Chicken Crisper Bites	1410	79	18	3990	126	6	NP	42
Buffalo Chicken Crisper Bites	1620	100	21	5380	123	49	NP	6
Cajun Chicken Sandwich	930	49	12	2400	70	4	NP	47
Chili's Cheesesteak Sandwich	880	44	17	1820	61	3	NP	40
Smoked Turkey Sandwich	960	55	14	1790	57	2	NP	39
Chicken Ranch Sandwich	1170	71	11	2910	86	4	NP	45
Guiltless Buffalo Chicken Sandwich	390	7	2	2300	46	9	NP	36
Guiltless Grilled Chicken Sandwich	360	5	2	1390	44	9	NP	36
Grilled Chicken Sandwich	850	45	10	1920	62	2	NP	47
Spicy Chicken Cool Wrap	400	12	4	1320	47	9	NP	35
Fajita Pita Beef	490	21	4	1540	51	3	NP	30
Fajita Pita Chicken	460	13	2	1400	52	3	NP	31
Chicken Caesar Pita	700	41	8	1570	45	4	NP	39

Entrée

Spicy Garlic & Lime Grilled Chicken	170	11	2	1090	7	0	NP	12
Chili's Classic Sirloin	370	27	7	1270	5	1	NP	31
Guiltless Carne Asada Steak	370	10	8	1440	11	6	NP	46
Guiltless Cedar Plank Tilapia	200	4	2	690	8	5	NP	34
Guiltless Honey-Mustard Glazed Salmon	420	20	6	610	13	2	NP	50
Guiltless Grilled Salmon	400	20	6	420	8	3	NP	51
Guiltless Chicken Platter	370	2	1	1940	49	7	NP	39
Original Ribs	990	68	25	4100	33	2	NP	57
Honey-Chipotle Ribs	1270	67	25	4560	110	0	NP	55
Honey BBQ Ribs	1120	68	25	4780	66	2	NP	57
Memphis Dry Rub Ribs	1040	73	26	4410	33	4	NP	58
Original Ribs, 1/2 rack	490	34	12	2050	17	1	NP	28
Honey-Chipotle Ribs, 1/2 rack	700	34	12	2540	72	0	NP	28
Honey BBQ Ribs, 1/2 rack	600	34	13	2690	43	1	NP	29
Memphis Dry Rub Ribs	570	39	13	2480	23	2	NP	29
Chicken Crispers	1780	123	19	2910	107	10	NP	65
Crispy Honey-Chipotle Chicken Crispers	1930	108	17	4390	181	8	NP	61
Crispy Sweet Chile Glazed Chicken Crispers	1860	108	17	4160	158	8	NP	63
Country-Fried Chicken Crispers, no sauce	1490	90	15	3000	110	8	NP	60
Cajun Chicken Pasta	1340	68	37	3650	106	6	NP	67
Monterey Chicken	860	43	15	3060	57	9	NP	63
Margarita Grilled Chicken	680	14	2	2430	82	9	NP	53
Crispy Chicken Crisper Tacos, 3	1990	104	25	5790	195	13	NP	32
Chicken Club Tacos, 3	1500	76	21	4970	137	13	NP	67
Chicken Tacos, 3	1200	45	17	4430	144	16	NP	61
Grilled Shrimp Alfredo	1320	76	38	3560	105	6	NP	51
Grilled Salmon with Garlic and Herbs	630	28	7	1050	50	5	NP	47
Southwest Cedar Plank Tilapia	600	31	4.5	1750	55	7	NP	30
Flame-Grilled Ribeye w/ toast	990	79	31	1810	19	2	NP	50

Description & Serving	Cal	Fat	Sfat	Sod	Carb	Fiber	Sugar	Prot
Chili's Classic Sirloin w/ toast	540	38	10	1560	20	2	NP	33
Cajun Ribeye w/ toast	1000	79	31	1570	19	3	NP	50
Country-Fried Steak w/ toast & sides	1430	82	15	2950	122	9	NP	52

Fajita/Quesadilla

Description & Serving	Cal	Fat	Sfat	Sod	Carb	Fiber	Sugar	Prot
Flour Tortillas, 3	380	10	2.5	1000	62	3	NP	10
Fajita Condiments, 1 ea	230	19	10	360	7	2	NP	10
Mushroom Jack	720	41	13	3370	36	6	NP	58
Classic Steak	470	25	5	2520	25	4	NP	45
Classic Chicken	370	11	1.5	2000	25	4	NP	39
Classic Combo	420	18	3.5	2260	25	4	NP	42
Steak and Portobello	790	56	9	3430	33	6	NP	46
Buffalo Chicken Fajitas	1090	77	17	5240	50	5	NP	48
Fajita Trio	560	27	5	3060	29	4	NP	54
Fire Grilled Chicken Fajita Quesadilla	1480	96	35	3510	99	6	NP	69
Fire Grilled Jalapeno Beef Quesadilla	1780	126	42	4540	98	6	NP	68
Fire Grilled Bacon Chicken Ranch Quesadilla	1750	122	40	4270	95	5	NP	77

Kids

Description & Serving	Cal	Fat	Sfat	Sod	Carb	Fiber	Sugar	Prot
Pepper Pals Cheese Pizza	560	24	9	1130	67	3	NP	23
Pepper Pals Cheese Quesadilla	460	24	12	1000	42	2	NP	20
Pepper Pals Corndog	280	17	3.5	650	25	2	NP	5
Pepper Pals Country-Fried Chicken Crispers	560	37	5	1600	25	1	NP	31
Pepper Pals Grilled Cheese Sandwich	510	41	12	990	28	0	NP	10
Pepper Pals Grilled Chicken Platter	150	1	0	690	4	0	NP	27
Pepper Pals Grilled Chicken Sandwich	230	3.5	1	650	26	1	NP	22
Pepper Pals Little Chicken Crispers	600	42	7	1300	20	2	NP	34
Pepper Pals Little Mouth Burger	440	23	8	420	24	1	NP	33
Pepper Pals Little Mouth Cheeseburger	510	29	12	740	25	1	NP	36
Pepper Pals Macaroni & Cheese	500	18	6	930	69	3	NP	16
Pepper Pals Side Cinnamon Apples	190	7	2.5	65	34	4	NP	0
Pepper Pals Side Corn on the Cob w/o butter	150	1.5	0	5	32	3	NP	5
Pepper Pals Side Homestyle Fries	240	15	2.5	140	24	2	NP	2
Pepper Pals Side Kernel Corn	130	2	0	0	23	6	NP	4
Pepper Pals Side Mandarin Oranges	70	0	0	10	17	0	NP	0
Pepper Pals Side Kettle Black Beans	110	1	0	670	19	6	NP	6
Pepper Pals Side Rice	190	1	0	570	42	1	NP	4
Pepper Pals Side Seasonal Veggies	35	0	0	30	6	3	NP	3
Pepper Pals Chocolate Shake	490	24	14	140	67	0	NP	6

Side

Description & Serving	Cal	Fat	Sfat	Sod	Carb	Fiber	Sugar	Prot
Rice & Kettle Black Beans	300	1.5	0	1270	62	7	NP	11
Spicy Garlic & Lime Shrimp, 3	70	4.5	1	400	2	0	NP	6
Cinnamon Apples w/ butter	190	7	2.5	65	34	4	NP	0
Corn on the Cob	190	7	1	120	32	3	NP	5
Homestyle Fries	410	25	4.5	240	41	4	NP	4
Kettle Black Beans	110	1	0	690	20	6	NP	6
Loaded Mashed Potatoes	390	25	8	910	29	5	NP	14
Mashed Potatoes w/ Black Pepper Gravy	280	15	1.5	1050	33	5	NP	5

Description & Serving	Cal	Fat	Sfat	Sod	Carb	Fiber	Sugar	Prot
Portobello Mushroom	90	8	1	75	3	0	NP	1
Rice	190	1	0	570	42	1	NP	4
Seasonal Veggies	60	4	1	170	7	3	NP	3
Dressing/Condiment/Topping								
Ancho Chile Ranch	170	17	3.5	390	3	0	NP	1
Avocado Ranch	110	11	2	210	2	1	NP	1
BBQ Sauce	60	0	0	560	14	1	NP	1
Bleu Cheese	240	25	5	310	1	0	NP	1
Caesar	260	27	4.5	390	2	0	NP	2
Citrus Balsamic Vinaigrette	250	25	3.5	220	6	0	NP	0
Fire Roasted Tomato Vinaigrette	90	9	1.5	320	2	0	NP	0
Honey Mustard	180	21	3	380	1	0	NP	0
Honey Mustard No Fat	70	0	0	510	11	0	NP	0
Jalapeno Ranch	150	15	3	340	2	0	NP	1
Low Fat Ranch	45	3	0	440	4	0	NP	1
Low Fat Vinaigrette	60	2	0	230	8	0	NP	0
Ranch	170	18	3.5	340	2	0	NP	1
Gravy	35	1.5	0	350	4	0	NP	1
Guacamole	40	4	0	70	2	2	NP	1
Honey BBQ Sauce	80	0	0	600	20	1	NP	0
Honey Chipotle Sauce	140	0	0	530	35	0	NP	0
Sour Cream	60	6	3.5	55	2	0	NP	1
Hot Sauce	30	0	0	1120	6	2	NP	1
Salsa Ranch	250	24	4.5	1010	5	1	NP	2
Bacon, 2	50	4	1.5	220	0	0	NP	3
Cheese, American, 1 slice	70	6	3.5	320	1	0	NP	3
Cheese, Cheddar, 1 slice	80	7	4	135	0	0	NP	5
Cheese, Provolone, 1 slice	40	3	2	95	0	0	NP	3
Cheese, Swiss, 1 slice	50	4	2.5	35	0	0	NP	4
Dessert								
Cheesecake	700	42	26	460	67	0	NP	12
Chocolate Chip Paradise Pie	1140	66	32	530	129	5	NP	14
Frosty Chocolate Shake	740	35	21	210	100	0	NP	8
Chocolate Chip Cookie Molten Cake	1110	55	26	670	141	3	NP	13
Molten Chocolate Cake	1010	51	27	760	131	5	NP	11
White Molten Chocolate Cake	1260	67	25	460	149	0	NP	15
Sweet Shot Warm Cinnamon Roll	1280	13	8	95	38	1	NP	3
Sweet Shot Double Chocolate Fudge Brownie	420	24	14	25	51	1	NP	1
Sweet Shot Key Lime Pie	240	12	8	75	30	0	NP	4
Sweet Shot Red Velvet Cake	250	9	4.5	200	39	1	NP	3

Chipotle Mexican Grill

Shell/Wrap/Chips

Description & Serving	Cal	Fat	Sfat	Sod	Carb	Fiber	Sugar	Prot
Flour Tortilla (burrito), 1	290	9	3	670	44	2	0	7
Flour Tortilla (taco), 1	90	2.5	1	200	13	<1	0	2
Crispy Taco Shell, 1	60	2	0.5	10	9	1	<1	<1
Chips, 4 oz	570	27	3.5	420	73	8	4	8

Description & Serving	Cal	Fat	Sfat	Sod	Carb	Fiber	Sugar	Prot
Meat, 4 oz								
Barbacoa	170	7	2.5	510	2	0	<1	24
Chicken	190	6.5	2	370	1	0	1	32
Carnitas	190	8	2.5	540	1	0	0	27
Steak	190	6.5	2	320	2	0	1	30
Rice/Beans								
Cilantro-Lime Rice, 3 oz	130	3	0.5	150	23	0	0	2
Black Beans, 4 oz	120	1	0	250	23	11	<1	7
Pinto Beans, 4 oz	120	1	0	330	22	10	<1	7
Topping								
Fajita Vegetables, 2.5 oz	20	0.5	0	170	4	1	2	1
Tomato Salsa, 3.5 oz	20	0	0	470	4	<1	3	1
Corn Salsa, 3.5 oz	80	1.5	0	410	15	3	4	3
Red Tomatillo Salsa, 2 oz	40	1	0	510	8	4	4	2
Green Tomatillo Salsa, 2 oz	15	0	0	230	3	1	2	1
Cheese, 1 oz	100	8.5	5	180	0	0	0	8
Sour Cream, 2 oz	120	10	7	30	2	0	2	2
Guacamole, 3.5 oz	150	13	2	190	8	6	1	2
Romaine Lettuce (salad), 2.5 oz	10	0	0	5	2	1	1	1
Romaine Lettuce (tacos), 1 oz	5	0	0	0	1	1	0	0
Vinaigrette, 2 oz	260	24.5	4	700	12	1	11	0

Chuck E. Cheese

Description & Serving	Cal	Fat	Sfat	Sod	Carb	Fiber	Sugar	Prot
Appetizer/Side								
Breadsticks, 1	175	9	2	412	18	1	NP	6
Mozzarella Sticks w/ Marinara, 1	93	6	2	211	6	0	NP	4
French Fries	420	20	2	929	55	6	NP	6
Buffalo Wings, 4	300	20	4	1308	16	4	NP	16
Side Fruit Garnish	65	0	0	2	9	1	NP	0
Side Pasta Salad	150	4	0.5	280	24	1	NP	4
Side Celery & Bleu Cheese	269	26	5	606	6	2	NP	3
Mandarin Oranges	56	0	0	6	15	1	NP	0
Carrot Sticks w/ Ranch	183	15	2	451	12	2	NP	2
Pizza								
Individual Cheese Pizza	540	19	8	1255	69	3	NP	21
Small Pizza, 1 slice								
All Meat Combo Pizza	180	9	3	508	19	1	NP	9
BBQ Chicken Pizza	150	5	2	394	21	1	NP	7
Cheese Pizza	130	4	2	308	19	1	NP	5
Super Combo Pizza	160	7	3	393	19	1	NP	6
Veggie Combo Pizza	135	5	2	319	20	1	NP	5
Medium Pizza, 1 slice								
All Meat Combo Pizza	215	11	4	608	21	1	NP	9
BBQ Chicken Pizza	185	6	2	460	24	1	NP	8
Cheese Pizza	155	5	2	360	21	1	NP	6

Description & Serving	Cal	Fat	Sfat	Sod	Carb	Fiber	Sugar	Prot
Super Combo Pizza	185	8	3	453	22	1	NP	7
Veggie Combo Pizza	160	6	2	366	22	2	NP	6
Large Pizza, 1 slice								
All Meat Combo Pizza	240	11	4	566	24	1	NP	10
BBQ Chicken Pizza	205	7	3	447	27	1	NP	7
Cheese Pizza	170	6	3	404	23	1	NP	7
Super Combo Pizza	205	9	3	508	24	1	NP	8
Veggie Combo Pizza	175	6	2	402	24	1	NP	10
Sandwich								
Chicken Ciabatta Sandwich	715	28	7	1940	80	3	NP	44
Ham & Cheese Sandwich	685	27	8	2206	79	3	NP	33
Italian Sub Sandwich	790	39	12	2374	78	3	NP	34
Hot Dog	310	19	7	1084	35	2	NP	11
Sandwich Platter, 1/12 of sandwich	183	8	2	543	20	1	NP	9
Dessert								
Cinnamon Sticks, 1	70	2	1	87	11	0	NP	1
Apple Dessert Pizza, 1 slice	192	5	2	164	33	1	NP	2
Vanilla Buttercream Cake, 1 slice	310	18	6	230	35	0	NP	2
Chocolate Cake, 1 slice	290	13	4	220	41	2	NP	3
Chocolate Sheet Cake, 1/4 of cake	310	14	5	200	41	2	NP	3

Church's Chicken

Entrée, 1 piece								
Original Chicken Wing	300	19	5	540	7	3	0	27
Original Chicken Leg	110	6	2	280	3	0	0	10
Original Chicken Thigh	330	23	6	680	8	1	0	21
Original Chicken Breast	200	11	3	450	3	1	0	22
Spicy Chicken Wing	430	27	7	1020	17	2	0	29
Spicy Chicken Leg	180	11	3	470	8	1	0	12
Spicy Chicken Thigh	480	35	9	1035	20	2	0	22
Spicy Chicken Breast	320	20	5	760	12	2	0	21
Crunchy Tenders	120	6	2	440	6	<0.5	0	12
Spicy Crunchy Tenders	135	7	2	480	7	4	0	11
Spicy Fish Fillet	160	9	2	350	13	1	1	7
Chicken Fried Steak w/ White Gravy	470	28	7	1620	36	1	4	21
Sandwich								
Bigger Better Chicken Sandwich w/ Cheese	510	27	7	1070	46	4	4	20
Spicy Fish Sandwich	320	20	4	560	25	2	3	10
Chicken Fried Steak Sandwich	490	32	8	880	38	2	4	13
Side								
Honey Butter Biscuit	240	12	3	540	28	1	4	3
Mashed Potatoes & Gravy	70	2	0	480	12	1	2	2
Okra	350	22	7	590	36	5	3	3
Corn on the Cob, 1	140	3	0	15	24	9	2	4
Whole Jalapeno Peppers, 2	10	0	0	390	2	1	<1	0
Jalapeno Bombers, 4	240	10	6	970	29	3	5	8

Description & Serving	Cal	Fat	Sfat	Sod	Carb	Fiber	Sugar	Prot
Cole Slaw	150	10	2	170	15	2	7	1
French Fries	290	14	3	320	38	4	1	3
Cajun Rice	130	7	3	260	16	<1	0	1
Sweet Corn Nuggets	600	29	2	1260	72	5	14	7
Collard Greens	25	0	0	170	5	2	0	2
Macaroni & Cheese	210	11	4	690	23	1	6	8

Dessert

	Cal	Fat	Sfat	Sod	Carb	Fiber	Sugar	Prot
Edward's Double Lemon Pie	300	14	6	160	39	0	29	5
Edward's Strawberry Cream Cheese Pie	280	15	8	130	32	2	22	4
Apple Pie	260	11	4	250	39	1	15	2

Dressing/Condiment, 1 packet

	Cal	Fat	Sfat	Sod	Carb	Fiber	Sugar	Prot
BBQ Sauce	30	0	0	180	7	0	2	0
Creamy Jalapeno Sauce	100	11	1.5	140	1	0	0	0
Honey Mustard Sauce	110	11	1.5	130	4	0	1	0
Sweet & Sour Sauce	30	0	0	120	8	0	2	0
Purple Pepper Sauce	45	0	0	26	12	0	6	0
Ketchup	18	0	0	190	5	0	4	0
Hot Sauce	18	0	0	210	0	0	0	0
Honey	27	0	0	0	7	0	7	0
Ranch Sauce	130	13	2	320	1	0	0	0

CiCi's Pizza

Pizza, 12", 1 slice

	Cal	Fat	Sfat	Sod	Carb	Fiber	Sugar	Prot
Alfredo Pizza	120	3.5	1.5	270	18	<1	NP	4
Bacon Cheddar Pizza	110	4.5	1.5	340	19	<1	NP	5
Bar-B-Que Pizza	150	2.5	1	380	25	1	NP	6
Beef Pizza	140	4.5	2	340	20	<1	NP	6
Cheese Pizza	150	4	2	330	19	<1	NP	6
Ham & Pineapple Pizza	150	3.5	1.5	350	21	<1	NP	6
Ole Pizza	110	3	1	290	20	1	NP	5
Pepperoni Pizza	160	4.5	2	370	20	<1	NP	6
Pepperoni & Jalapeno Pizza	150	4.5	2	390	20	<1	NP	6
Sausage Pizza	140	5	2	420	20	1	NP	6
Spinach Alfredo Pizza	120	3.5	1.5	270	19	<1	NP	4
Tomato Alfredo Pizza	120	3	1	280	19	<1	NP	4
Zesty Ham & Cheddar Pizza	120	4	1	340	19	<1	NP	5
Zesty Pepperoni Pizza	150	6	2	370	19	<1	NP	6
Zesty Veggie Pizza	130	4	1	320	20	<1	NP	4
Classic Chicken Pizza	140	5	1.5	350	19	<1	NP	5
Buffalo Chicken Pizza	140	4.5	1.5	460	19	<1	NP	6
Macaroni & Cheese Pizza	170	3	1	260	29	1	NP	6
Ham Pizza	150	3.5	1.5	370	19	<1	NP	6
Pepperoni Flip Pizza	120	6	1.5	250	13	0	NP	3
Deep Dish Pizza	170	6	3	330	19	<1	NP	7

Side/Dessert

	Cal	Fat	Sfat	Sod	Carb	Fiber	Sugar	Prot
Garlic Bread, 1 pc	100	5	1.5	120	10	0	NP	4
Apple Pizza, 1 slice	150	3.5	1	190	26	<1	NP	3

Description & Serving	Cal	Fat	Sfat	Sod	Carb	Fiber	Sugar	Prot
Brownies, 1	140	6	1	95	22	0	NP	1
Cinnamon Rolls, 1	140	5	1	100	20	0	NP	2

Cinnabon

Dessert

Cinnamon Filled Churro	281	11.3	1.7	NP	39.4	NP	NP	5.3
Classic Cinnabon	813	32	8	801	117	4	55	15
Minibon	339	13	3	337	49	2	22	6
Caramel Pecanbon	1100	47	12	570	156	3	63	14
Cinnabon Stix	410	23	6	420	46	1	16	6
Cinnabon Pretzel	750	6	2	860	156	8	46	19
Cinnabon Bites, 6	520	16	4	530	78	2	25	8
Pecanbon Bites, 4	670	28	7	640	97	3	51	9
Frosting, 1.4 oz	180	11	3	109	20	0	18	1

Beverage

Orange Juice (Vareva), 8 oz	110	0	0	55	26	2	24	0
Strawberry Lemonade (Sun Orchard), 8 oz	100	0	3	0	25	0	24	0
Tropical Blast Chillata, 16 oz	330	7	4	50	69	0	48	2

The Coffee Bean & Tea Leaf

Cold Beverage

Hazelnut Iced Blended, 12 oz	330	NP	14	180	50	NP	NP	NP
Extreme NSA Mocha Iced Blended, 12 oz	80	NP	0	140	16	NP	NP	NP
Pomegranate Blueberry Ice Blended, 12 oz	350	NP	6	270	68	NP	NP	NP
Pomegranate Blueberry Ice Blended NSA Powder, 12 oz	170	NP	0.5	170	37	NP	NP	NP
Mocha Ice Blended, 12 oz	280	NP	4.5	340	52	NP	NP	NP
Mocha Ice Blended NSA Powder, 12 oz	110	NP	0	180	19	NP	NP	NP
Vanilla Ice Blended, 12 oz	290	NP	6	300	50	NP	NP	NP
Vanilla Ice Blended NSA Powder, 12 oz	110	NP	0.5	200	20	NP	NP	NP
Caramel Ice Blended, 12 oz	380	NP	7	350	68	NP	NP	NP
Caramel Ice Blended NSA Powder, 12 oz	200	NP	1	250	37	NP	NP	NP
Ultimate Mocha Ice Blended, 12 oz	320	NP	6	340	57	NP	NP	NP
Ultimate Mocha Ice Blended NSA Powder, 12 oz	150	NP	1.5	180	23	NP	NP	NP
Ultimate Vanilla Ice Blended, 12 oz	330	NP	7	310	55	NP	NP	NP
Ultimate Vanilla Ice Blended NSA Powder, 12 oz	150	NP	2	210	24	NP	NP	NP
White Chocolate Ice Blended, 12 oz	360	NP	11	410	58	NP	NP	NP
Black Forest Ice Blended, 12 oz	340	NP	6	340	69	NP	NP	NP
Black Forest Ice Blended NSA Powder, 12 oz	210	NP	1.5	180	35	NP	NP	NP
Banana Caramel Ice Blended, 12 oz	400	NP	7	320	78	NP	NP	NP
Banana Caramel Ice Blended NSA Powder, 12 oz	220	NP	1	220	47	NP	NP	NP
Pure Chocolate Ice Blended, 12 oz	300	NP	4.5	370	55	NP	NP	NP
Pure Chocolate Ice Blended NSA Powder, 12 oz	130	NP	0	210	21	NP	NP	NP
Pure Vanilla Ice Blended, 12 oz	320	NP	6	340	53	NP	NP	NP
Pure Vanilla Ice Blended NSA Powder, 12 oz	140	NP	0.5	240	22	NP	NP	NP
Malibu Dream Ice Blended, 12 oz	340	NP	6	260	63	NP	NP	NP

Description & Serving	Cal	Fat	Sfat	Sod	Carb	Fiber	Sugar	Prot
Malibu Dream Ice Blended NSA Powder, 12 oz	160	NP	0.5	160	32	NP	NP	NP
Green Tea Ice Blended, 12 oz	310	NP	6	330	52	NP	NP	NP
Chai Mate Ice Blended, 12 oz	310	NP	6	260	56	NP	NP	NP
Chai Mate Ice Blended NSA Powder, 12 oz	130	NP	0.5	160	26	NP	NP	NP
Pomegranate FruTea, 12 oz	150	NP	0	45	43	NP	NP	NP
Mucho Mango FruTea, 12 oz	180	NP	0	30	45	NP	NP	NP
Frozen Lemonade FruTea, 12 oz	240	NP	0	510	62	NP	NP	NP
Iced Coffee, 12 oz	5	NP	0	10	1	NP	NP	NP
Iced Tea, 12 oz	0	NP	0	5	1	NP	NP	NP
Tea Latte Over Ice Vanilla Powder, 12 oz	130	NP	3	130	23	NP	NP	NP
Tea Latte Over Ice NSA Vanilla Powder, 12 oz	45	NP	0	85	8	NP	NP	NP
Tea Latte Over Ice Chocolate Powder, 12 oz	120	NP	2	150	24	NP	NP	NP
Tea Latte Over Ice NSA Chocolate Powder, 12 oz	40	NP	0	75	7	NP	NP	NP
Cappuccino Over Ice, 12 oz	50	NP	1.5	45	5	NP	NP	NP
Cappuccino Over Ice Nonfat Milk, 12 oz	30	NP	0	45	5	NP	NP	NP
Latte Over Ice, 12 oz	100	NP	3	85	9	NP	NP	NP
Latte Over Ice Nonfat Milk, 12 oz	60	NP	0	85	9	NP	NP	NP
Mocha Latte Over Ice, 12 oz	170	NP	2	220	31	NP	NP	NP
Mocha Latte Over Ice NSA Powder, 12 oz	90	NP	0	150	15	NP	NP	NP
Vanilla Latte Over Ice, 12 oz	180	NP	3	200	30	NP	NP	NP
Vanilla Latte Over Ice NSA Powder, 12 oz	100	NP	0	170	16	NP	NP	NP
Caramel Latte Over Ice, 12 oz	200	NP	2	180	36	NP	NP	NP
Caramel Latte Over Ice NSA Powder, 12 oz	160	NP	1	170	30	NP	NP	NP
Hazelnut Latte Over Ice, 12 oz	200	NP	7	150	30	NP	NP	NP
White Chocolate Latte Over Ice, 12 oz	210	NP	6	260	33	NP	NP	NP

Hot Beverage

Brewed Coffee, 12 oz	5	NP	0	5	0	NP	NP	NP
Single Espresso	5	NP	0	0	0	NP	NP	NP
Double Espresso	5	NP	0	10	1	NP	NP	NP
Single Espresso Macchiato Whole Milk	10	NP	0	10	1	NP	NP	NP
Single Espresso Macchiato Nonfat Milk	10	NP	0	10	1	NP	NP	NP
Double Espresso Macchiato Whole Milk	15	NP	0	15	2	NP	NP	NP
Double Espresso Macchiato Nonfat Milk	10	NP	0	15	2	NP	NP	NP
Cappuccino Single Whole Milk, 12 oz	130	NP	4	115	11	NP	NP	NP
Cappuccino Single Nonfat Milk, 12 oz	80	NP	0	115	11	NP	NP	NP
Cappuccino Double Whole Milk, 12 oz	110	NP	3.5	100	10	NP	NP	NP
Cappuccino Double Nonfat Milk, 12 oz	70	NP	0	100	10	NP	NP	NP
Americano, 12 oz	5	NP	0	10	1	NP	NP	NP
Latte Whole Milk, 12 oz	210	NP	7	180	18	NP	NP	NP
Latte Nonfat Milk, 12 oz	130	NP	0	180	18	NP	NP	NP
Mocha Latte, 12 oz	270	NP	3	350	47	NP	NP	NP
Mocha Late NSA Powder, 12 oz	170	NP	0	260	26	NP	NP	NP
Vanilla Latte, 12 oz	280	NP	4	330	46	NP	NP	NP
Vanilla Latte NSA Powder, 12 oz	170	NP	0	280	27	NP	NP	NP
Caramel Latte, 12 oz	280	NP	2.5	300	49	NP	NP	NP
Caramel Latte NSA Powder, 12 oz	230	NP	1	270	40	NP	NP	NP
White Chocolate Latte, 12 oz	330	NP	8	400	52	NP	NP	NP
Hazelnut Latte, 12 oz	310	NP	9	250	46	NP	NP	NP

Description & Serving	Cal	Fat	Sfat	Sod	Carb	Fiber	Sugar	Prot
Café Au Lait Whole Milk, 12 oz	80	NP	2.5	70	7	NP	NP	NP
Café Au Lait Nonfat Milk, 12 oz	45	NP	0	70	7	NP	NP	NP
Café Mocha, 12 oz	190	NP	3	240	35	NP	NP	NP
Café Mocha NSA Powder, 12 oz	90	NP	0	150	15	NP	NP	NP
Café Vanilla, 12 oz	200	NP	4	220	34	NP	NP	NP
Café Vanilla NSA Powder, 12 oz	100	NP	0	170	15	NP	NP	NP
Café Caramel, 12 oz	200	NP	2.5	180	37	NP	NP	NP
Café Caramel NSA Powder, 12 oz	150	NP	1	160	28	NP	NP	NP
Café Hazelnut, 12 oz	230	NP	9	130	34	NP	NP	NP
Café White Chocolate, 12 oz	250	NP	8	290	41	NP	NP	NP
Tea Latte Vanilla Powder, 12 oz	200	NP	4	220	35	NP	NP	NP
Tea Latte NSA Vanilla Powder, 12 oz	100	NP	0	170	16	NP	NP	NP
Tea Latte Chocolate Powder, 12 oz	190	NP	3	240	36	NP	NP	NP
Tea Latte NSA Chocolate Powder, 12 oz	90	NP	0	150	15	NP	NP	NP
Hot Chocolate, 12 oz	280	NP	3	370	48	NP	NP	NP
Hot Chocolate NSA Powder, 12 oz	180	NP	0	280	28	NP	NP	NP
Hot Vanilla, 12 oz	290	NP	4	340	47	NP	NP	NP
Hot Vanilla NSA Powder, 12 oz	180	NP	0	290	28	NP	NP	NP

Beverage Add-On

Soy Milk, 8 oz	80	NP	0	115	11	NP	NP	NP
Half & Half, 1 oz	40	NP	2	15	1	NP	NP	NP
Caramel Swirl, .5 oz	65	NP	0.5	37.5	14.5	NP	NP	NP
Cherry	10	NP	0	0	2	NP	NP	NP
Fudge Swirl, .5 oz	65	NP	0.5	35	14	NP	NP	NP
Extra Chocolate Powder, approx 1/4 cup	164	NP	3	193	31	NP	NP	NP
Extra Vanilla Powder, approx. 1/4 cup	171	NP	4	171	30	NP	NP	NP
Shot of Espresso, 1 oz	5	NP	0	0	0	NP	NP	NP

Snack

Chocolate Covered Espresso Beans, 8 pc	53	NP	7	6	2	NP	NP	NP

Cold Stone Creamery

Ice Cream

Amaretto Ice Cream, Like It (approx. 5 oz)	330	20	12	80	33	0	29	5
Banana Ice Cream, Like It (approx. 5 oz)	310	18	12	70	33	0	28	5
Black Cherry Ice Cream, Like It (approx. 5 oz)	330	19	12	75	36	0	32	5
Blueberry Muffin Ice Cream, Like It (approx. 5 oz)	330	19	12	120	38	0	32	5
Butter Pecan Ice Cream, Like It (approx. 5 oz)	320	19	12	105	32	0	28	5
Cake Batter Ice Cream, Like It (approx. 5 oz)	340	19	12	180	41	0	32	5
Cheesecake Ice Cream, Like It (approx. 5 oz)	330	18	11	75	37	0	31	5
Chocolate Ice Cream, Like It (approx. 5 oz)	320	20	12	95	33	1	30	6
Chocolate Cake Batter Ice Cream, Like It (approx. 5 oz)	340	19	11	210	42	1	33	5
Chocolate Raspberry Truffle Ice Cream, Like It (approx. 5 oz)	320	17	12	100	39	1	36	4
Cinnamon Ice Cream, Like It (approx. 5 oz)	330	20	12	80	34	<1	29	5
Cinnamon Bun Ice Cream, Like It (approx. 5 oz)	370	21	12	100	43	0	36	4
Coconut Ice Cream, Like It (approx. 5 oz)	330	20	12	80	33	0	28	5

Description & Serving	Cal	Fat	Sfat	Sod	Carb	Fiber	Sugar	Prot
Coffee Ice Cream, Like It (approx. 5 oz)	330	20	12	80	34	0	29	5
Cookie Batter Ice Cream, Like It (approx. 5 oz)	380	20	11	240	44	0	34	5
Cotton Candy Ice Cream, Like It (approx. 5 oz)	330	19	12	75	34	0	28	5
Dark Chocolate Ice Cream, Like It (approx. 5 oz)	340	20	12	95	32	3	29	7
Dark Chocolate Peppermint Ice Cream, Like It (approx. 5 oz)	340	20	12	95	32	3	29	7
Egg Nog Ice Cream, Like It (approx. 5 oz)	260	15	10	65	26	0	21	5
French Toast Ice Cream, Like It (approx. 5 oz)	330	19	12	150	35	0	30	5
French Vanilla Ice Cream, Like It (approx. 5 oz)	340	19	14	80	37	0	33	5
Ghirardelli Chocolate Ice Cream, Like It (approx. 5 oz)	330	20	12	75	37	4	27	7
Ginger Bread Ice Cream, Like It (approx. 5 oz)	320	18	12	55	36	0	31	5
Irish Cream Ice Cream, Like It (approx. 5 oz)	330	20	13	80	33	0	29	5
Jell-O Banana Pudding Ice Cream, Like It (approx. 5 oz)	350	17	11	230	46	0	40	5
Jell-O Butterscotch Pudding Ice Cream, Like It (approx. 5 oz)	340	17	11	280	46	0	40	5
Jell-O Chocolate Pudding Ice Cream, Like It (approx. 5 oz)	340	17	12	220	45	1	39	5
Jell-O Vanilla Pudding Ice Cream, Like It (approx. 5 oz)	350	17	11	230	46	0	40	5
Macadamia Nut Ice Cream, Like It (approx. 5 oz)	330	20	12	75	34	0	29	5
Mango Ice Cream, Like It (approx. 5 oz)	310	18	12	70	33	0	28	5
Marshmallow Ice Cream, Like It (approx. 5 oz)	330	17	12	50	41	0	35	5
Mint Ice Cream, Like It (approx. 5 oz)	330	19	12	75	36	0	31	5
Mocha Ice Cream, Like It (approx. 5 oz)	320	20	12	95	33	1	29	6
Nutter Butter Ice Cream, Like It (approx. 5 oz)	390	24	13	210	41	0	35	6
Oatmeal Cookie Batter Ice Cream, Like It (approx. 5 oz)	340	19	12	110	36	0	28	5
Orange Dreamsicle Ice Cream, Like It (approx. 5 oz)	320	19	12	75	35	0	28	5
Peanut Butter Ice Cream, Like It (approx. 5 oz)	370	24	13	130	33	<1	28	7
Pecan Praline Ice Cream, Like It (approx. 5 oz)	330	19	12	90	37	0	31	5
Pistachio Ice Cream, Like It (approx. 5 oz)	330	20	12	85	34	0	29	5
Pumpkin Ice Cream, Like It (approx. 5 oz)	290	15	10	105	33	1	28	4
Raspberry Ice Cream, Like It (approx. 5 oz)	330	19	12	75	36	0	31	5
Sinless Sans Fat Sweet Cream, Like It (approx. 5 oz)	140	0	0	110	34	<1	9	6
Sinless Cake Batter Ice Cream, Like It (approx. 5 oz)	190	1	0	190	43	0	14	7
Strawberry Ice Cream, Like It (approx. 5 oz)	320	18	12	75	35	0	30	5
Sweet Cream Ice Cream, Like It (approx. 5 oz)	330	20	13	80	33	0	29	5
Vanilla Bean Ice Cream, Like It (approx. 5 oz)	330	19	12	75	32	0	28	5
White Chocolate Ice Cream, Like It (approx. 5 oz)	320	19	12	75	33	0	28	5

Mix-In

	Cal	Fat	Sfat	Sod	Carb	Fiber	Sugar	Prot
Butterfinger Candy, 1/2 bar	140	6	3	65	22	<1	15	2
Chocolate Chips, 1 oz	130	7	4.5	0	16	1	14	1
Chocolate Shavings, .5 oz	90	5	3	0	9	2	8	<1
Nestle Crunch Bar, 1/2 bar	130	7	4	35	16	<1	14	2
Gummy Bears, 1 oz	120	0	0	15	30	0	13	0
Heath Candy Bar, 1 bar	110	7	3.5	75	12	0	12	<1
Kit Kat Candy Bar, 1/2 bar	110	5	3.5	15	13	0	10	1

Description & Serving	Cal	Fat	Sfat	Sod	Carb	Fiber	Sugar	Prot
M&M's Candy, 1 oz	170	7	4.5	20	25	<1	22	2
Reese's Peanut Butter Cup, 1 pc	190	11	4	110	19	1	17	4
Snickers Candy, 1/2 bar	170	9	3	95	21	<1	17	3
White Chocolate Chips, 1 oz	160	9	8	45	18	0	18	2
Almond Joy Candy, 1 pc	170	9	6	50	21	2	16	1
Gumballs, 1 oz	90	0	0	0	23	<1	24	0
Ghirardelli Caramel Square, 1 ea	70	4	2.5	20	9	0	8	1
Peanut M&M's, 1 oz	150	8	3.5	30	18	<1	4	3
Reese's Pieces, 1 oz	180	9	2	70	21	1	19	4
Twix Candy, 1 pc	150	7	2.5	60	20	0	14	1
Whoppers Candy, 1 oz	120	4	3.5	85	19	0	15	1
York Peppermint Patties, 2 pc	120	2	1.5	10	24	<1	18	<1
Apple Pie Filling, .75 oz	60	0	0	25	16	<1	14	0
Bananas, 1/2	50	0	0	0	14	2	9	<1
Blackberries, .75 oz	10	0	0	0	2	<1	2	0
Black Cherries, .75 oz	80	0	0	10	8	0	17	0
Blueberries, .75 oz	10	0	0	0	2	0	2	0
Cherry Pie Filling, .75 oz	50	0	0	10	13	0	0	0
Maraschino Cherries, 1	5	0	0	0	1	0	1	0
Pineapple Chunks, .75 oz	15	0	0	0	4	0	4	0
Raspberries, .75 oz	25	0	0	0	5	1	2	0
Strawberries, .75 oz	20	0	0	0	7	<1	4	0
Peach Pie Filling, 1 oz	60	0	0	25	16	<1	14	0
Raisins, 1 oz	70	0	0	0	20	<1	16	<1
Coconut, .5 oz	80	5	4.5	40	7	<1	6	0
Cookie Dough, 1 pc	180	8	2.5	150	26	0	26	1
Graham Cracker Pie Crust, 1 oz	130	6	2.5	135	17	1	7	1
Brownies, 1 pc	170	3.5	1	180	32	1	22	2
Marshmallows, 1 oz	100	0	0	10	24	0	24	<1
Oreo Cookies, 2 cookies	120	5	1.5	140	18	<1	10	1
Peanut Butter, .75 oz	150	13	2.5	125	5	1	2	6
Yellow Cake, 1 pc	80	2.5	0.5	140	13	0	8	2
Granola, 1 oz	120	2	0	30	23	2	0	2
Nilla Wafers, 3 cookies	70	2.5	0	50	11	0	6	<1
Toasted Coconut, .5 oz	90	7	6	5	7	<1	6	<1
Oreo Pie Crust, 1 oz	180	8	1.5	190	19	0	10	0
Macadamia Nuts, 1 oz	180	19	3	65	3	2	<1	<1
Pecan Pralines, 1 oz	210	21	1.5	230	5	2	1	1
Pecans, 1 oz	140	15	1.5	80	3	2	<1	<1
Roasted Almonds, 1 oz	150	14	1	85	4	3	1	1
Walnuts, 1 oz	130	13	1	0	3	1	0	0
Cashews, 1 oz	170	14	2.5	90	9	1	2	2
Peanuts, 1 oz	210	18	3	110	5	3	0	0
Pistachio Nuts, 1 oz	200	16	2	0	10	4	<1	<1
Sliced Almonds, 1 oz	210	20	2	0	6	4	0	0
Cinnamon, 1/8 tsp	0	0	0	0	0	0	0	0
Honey, 1 oz	90	0	0	0	25	0	25	25
Rainbow Sprinkles, 1 oz	25	0	0	0	6	0	6	6
Reddi Whip Original, 1 dollop	45	2.5	1	15	5	0	2	2

Description & Serving	Cal	Fat	Sfat	Sod	Carb	Fiber	Sugar	Prot
Caramel, 1 oz	90	1	0.5	50	21	0	13	13
Fudge, 1 oz	90	2	2	80	18	0	16	16
Chocolate Sprinkles, 1 oz	25	0	0	0	6	0	2	6
Marshmallow Crème, 1 oz	100	0	0	20	24	0	20	20
Butterscotch Fat Free, 1 oz	80	0	0	85	19	0	15	5
Caramel Fat Free, 1 oz	80	0	0	85	19	0	14	14
Fudge Fat Free, 1 oz	80	0	0	15	20	0	16	16
Waffle Cone or Bowl, 1 ea	160	4	1	70	29	0	14	4
Dipped Waffle, 1 ea	310	15	7	70	46	2	31	31
Sugar Cone, 1 ea	50	0	0	20	11	0	3	3
Whipped Topping, 24 g	80	6	6	0	6	0	6	0

Sorbet/Yogurt

Description & Serving	Cal	Fat	Sfat	Sod	Carb	Fiber	Sugar	Prot
Countrytime Pink Lemonade Sorbet, Like It (approx. 5 oz)	240	0	0	25	59	0	59	0
Lemon Sorbet, Like It (approx. 5 oz)	150	0	0	15	40	0	34	0
Raspberry Sorbet, Like It (approx. 5 oz)	160	0	0	15	42	0	36	0
Watermelon Sorbet, Like It (approx. 5 oz)	160	0	0	15	41	0	35	0
Tart & Tangy Yogurt, Like It (approx. 5 oz)	140	0	0	70	33	0	24	3
Tart & Tangy Berry Yogurt, Like It (approx. 5 oz)	150	0	0	65	36	0	27	3

Milkshake

Description & Serving	Cal	Fat	Sfat	Sod	Carb	Fiber	Sugar	Prot
Cake 'n Shake Milkshake, Like It (16 oz)	1140	60	36	700	140	<1	106	18
Cherry Cheesecake Milkshake, Like It (16 oz)	1090	54	34	260	135	<1	92	16
Cream De Menthe Milkshake, Like It (16 oz)	1160	67	42	240	124	4	109	17
Lotta Caramel Latte Milkshake, Like It (16 oz)	1320	62	39	430	175	0	134	19
Milk & Cookies Milkshake, Like It (16 oz)	1090	63	38	370	117	<1	97	18
Oh Fudge! Milkshake, Like It (16 oz)	1250	70	45	460	141	4	127	22
PB&C Milkshake, Like It (16 oz)	1280	82	45	470	119	5	104	27
Savory Strawberry Milkshake, Like It (16 oz)	1000	55	35	240	116	2	98	16
Very Vanilla Milkshake, Like It (16 oz)	1180	57	40	370	149	0	121	16
Sinless Cake 'n Shake Milkshake, Like It (16 oz)	670	7	2	780	140	1	57	24
Sinless Oh Fudge! Milkshake, Like It (16 oz)	490	2	2	360	110	0	44	23
Sinless Milk & Cookies Milkshake, Like It (16 oz)	510	4.5	1	400	109	1	37	23
Sinless Very Vanilla Milkshake, Like It (16 oz)	500	1	0.5	330	113	0	41	22

Smoothie

Description & Serving	Cal	Fat	Sfat	Sod	Carb	Fiber	Sugar	Prot
2 to Mango Smoothie, Like It (16 oz)	220	0	0	25	55	1	43	0
Berry Lemony Smoothie, Like It (16 oz)	150	0.5	0	20	39	3	30	1
Berry Trinity Smoothie, Like It (16 oz)	110	1	0	25	28	6	15	2
Citrus Sunsation Smoothie, Like It (16 oz)	190	0	0	40	48	1	42	0
Man-Go Bananas Smoothie, Like It (16 oz)	240	0	0	20	59	2	42	1
On The YoGo Smoothie, Like It (16 oz)	210	1	0	20	54	2	40	1
Strawberry Bonanza Smoothie, Like It (16 oz)	140	1	0	30	37	4	24	2
Banana Banana Smoothie, Like It (16 oz)	340	3.5	2.5	150	78	5	46	3
Banana Strawberry Smoothie, Like It (16 oz)	280	4	2	150	64	4	40	3
Blueberry Banana Smoothie, Like It (16 oz)	250	3	2	150	57	3	36	2
Blueberry Pineapple Smoothie, Like It (16 oz)	230	3	2	150	49	2	34	1
Raspberry Banana Smoothie, Like It (16 oz)	290	3	2	150	65	6	38	2
Mango Pineapple Smoothie, Like It (16 oz)	390	3	2	150	90	1	67	1

Description & Serving	Cal	Fat	Sfat	Sod	Carb	Fiber	Sugar	Prot
Mango Strawberry Smoothie, Like It (16 oz)	380	3.5	2	150	89	2	65	2
Pineapple Coconut Orange Smoothie, Like It (16 oz)	370	12	11	170	64	3	47	2
Strawberry Raspberry Smoothie, Like It (16 oz)	250	3.5	2	150	55	4	35	2

Supplement

Nrgize Whey Protein Supplement, 15 g	60	1	0.5	25	4	2	1	10
Nrgize Energy Supplement, 4 g	4	0	0	0	2	2	0	0
Nrgize Anti-Stress, 4 g	4	0	0	0	2	2	0	0
Nrgize Anti-Oxidant/Immune Supplement, 4 g	4	0	0	0	2	2	0	0

Latte

Iced Sweet Cream Latte, Like It (16 oz)	230	12	8	70	25	0	23	6
Iced Milk Caramel Latte, Like It (16 oz)	280	11	7	110	41	0	31	6
Iced Rich Mocha Latte, Like It (16 oz)	270	12	8	140	38	0	34	6
Iced Raspberry Truffle Mocha Latte, Like It (16 oz)	300	12	8	150	45	1	40	6
Iced Vanilla Crème Latte, Like It (16 oz)	280	12	8	70	38	0	35	6
Iced Lite Sweet Cream Latte, Like It (16 oz)	60	0	0	75	9	0	8	6
Iced Lite Milk Caramel Latte, Like It (16 oz)	140	1	1	110	28	0	19	5
Iced Lite Rich Mocha Latte, Like It (16 oz)	140	2	2	140	25	0	22	6
Iced Lite Raspberry Truffle Mocha Latte, Like It 16 oz)	170	2	2	150	32	1	28	6
Iced Lite Vanilla Crème Latte, Like It (16 oz)	110	0	0	75	22	0	20	6
Sweet Cream Latte, w/o whip cream, Like It (16 oz)	230	12	8	70	25	0	23	6
Milk Caramel Latte, w/o whip cream, Like It (16 oz)	280	11	7	110	41	0	31	6
Rich Mocha Latte, w/o whip cream, Like It (16 oz)	270	12	8	140	38	0	34	6
Raspberry Truffle Mocha Latte, w/o whip cream, Like It (16 oz)	300	12	8	140	45	1	40	6
Vanilla Crème Latte, w/o whip cream, Like It (16 oz)	280	12	8	70	38	0	35	6
Lite Sweet Cream Latte, w/o whip cream, Like It (16 oz)	60	0	0	70	9	0	8	6
Lite Milk Caramel Latte, w/o whip cream, Like It (16 oz)	140	1	1	110	28	0	19	5
Lite Rich Mocha Latte, w/o whip cream, Like It (16 oz)	140	2	2	140	25	0	22	6
Lite Raspberry Truffle Mocha Latte, w/o whip cream, Like It (16 oz)	170	2	2	150	32	1	28	6
Lite Vanilla Crème Latte, w/o whip cream, Like It (16 oz)	110	0	0	70	22	0	20	6

Cake

A Cheesecake Named Desire, 6" round, serves 8, 1 slice	420	22	11	320	55	1	40	5
Cake Batter Confetti Cake, 6" round, serves 8, 1 slice	440	21	14	260	58	1	41	5
Chocolate Chipper Cake, 6" round, serves 8, 1 slice	470	28	12	230	53	2	42	7
Coffeehouse Crunch Cake, 6" round, serves 8, 1 slice	540	31	12	310	61	2	50	7
Cookie Dough Delirium Cake, 6" round, serves 8, 1 slice	520	26	15	220	62	1	46	6
Cookies & Creamery Cake, 6" round, serves 8, 1 slice	400	20	12	300	48	1	37	6
Dark Peppermint Pleasure Cake, 6" round, serves 8, 1 slice	480	26	11	200	58	3	44	6

Description & Serving	Cal	Fat	Sfat	Sod	Carb	Fiber	Sugar	Prot
Midnight Delight Cake, 6" round, serves 8, 1 slice	510	29	13	250	58	3	47	6
MMMMMM Chip Cake, 6" round, serves 8, 1 slice	400	21	13	250	47	1	38	6
Peanut Butter Playground Cake, 6" round, serves 8, 1 slice	550	34	13	340	59	3	46	9
Strawberry Passion Cake, 6" round, serves 8, 1 slice	440	22	11	310	57	1	41	6
Birthday Cake, 6" round, serves 8, 1 slice	310	18	12	125	34	0	30	4
Birthday Cake, sml rectangle, serves 25, 1 slice	320	18	12	140	35	0	30	5
Pumpkin Pie, 9" round, serves 10, 1 slice	270	15	9	140	33	1	25	3
Double Chocolate Devotion Cupcake	360	19	13	160	45	2	40	4
Cake Batter Delux Cupcake	380	19	14	170	50	2	42	4
Sweet Cream Cupcake	390	21	15	135	48	2	44	5

Così

Breakfast

	Cal	Fat	Sfat	Sod	Carb	Fiber	Sugar	Prot
Western Omelette Croissant	713	40	NP	1527	56	3	NP	29
Così Club Omelette Bagel	682	28	NP	980	64	2	NP	38
T.B.M. Omelette Bagel	652	28	NP	1015	66	3	NP	34
Garden Pesto Omelette Croissant	740	45	NP	1401	56	3	NP	26
Etruscan Whole Grain Bagel	339	3	NP	215	65	4	NP	13
Plain Bagel	309	1	NP	228	61	2	NP	12
Cinnamon Raisin Bagel	451	2	NP	236	88	7	NP	14
Poppy Seed Bagel	361	3	NP	242	69	3	NP	14
Everything Bagel	377	4	NP	1149	71	3	NP	14
Asiago Cheese	453	8	NP	513	75	3	NP	20
Cranberry Orange Bagel	418	1	NP	238	87	3	NP	13
Sesame Bagel	363	3	NP	241	69	3	NP	14
Banana Nut Muffin	510	25	NP	330	62	3	NP	9
Blueberry Muffin	440	19	NP	440	61	3	NP	8
Carrot Muffin	500	25	NP	380	61	4	NP	9
Chocolate Chocolate Chip Muffin	530	27	NP	420	66	3	NP	8
Corn Muffin	470	24	NP	620	58	2	NP	7
Lowfat Raisin Bran Muffin	350	7	NP	420	72	10	NP	9
Blueberry Scone	410	17	NP	380	60	2	NP	8
Cranberry Scone	400	15	NP	350	61	3	NP	7
Così Oatmeal	101	0	NP	98	16	2	NP	2
Quiche Lorraine	673	48	NP	1140	29	2	NP	30
Veggie Quiche	522	36	NP	702	30	2	NP	18
Così Break Bar	359	18	NP	18	44	4	NP	8
Così Harvest Mix	388	20	NP	23	47	7	NP	9
Fresh Fruit Yogurt Parfait - Strawberry	331	5	NP	223	62	3	NP	12
Fresh Fruit Yogurt Parfait - Bananas Foster	389	5	NP	224	77	4	NP	13
Apple Empanada	279	15	NP	176	32	1.2	NP	3.3
Croissant - Almond	315	17	NP	334	37	2.1	NP	5.2
Croissant - Butter	289	14	NP	450	36	1.3	NP	4.3
Croissant - Chocolate	324	17	NP	332	41	0.99	NP	3.2
Palmier (Elephant Ears)	365	25	NP	373	32	0.87	NP	3.1
Sticky Bun	314	18	NP	371	37	1.3	NP	3.1
Apple Crumb Cake	540	30	NP	510	62	1	NP	7

Description & Serving	Cal	Fat	Sfat	Sod	Carb	Fiber	Sugar	Prot
Plain Crumb Cake	600	36	NP	550	61	1	NP	8
Biscotti Chocolate	240	8	NP	75	34	0	NP	4
Biscotti Amaretto	240	8	NP	70	34	0	NP	5
Fruit Salad	83	1	NP	17	21	2	NP	2

Appetizer

Spinach Artichoke Shareable	192	13	NP	389	26	2	NP	7
Brie & Fruit Shareable	616	41	NP	582	36	3	NP	23
Hummus Dip Shareable	232	5	NP	375	41	4	NP	7

Salad

Signature Salad Light	371	19	NP	485	45	5	NP	9
Così Cobb Light Salad	519	34	NP	1347	17	2	NP	39
Bombay Chicken Light Salad	188	2	NP	810	21	4	NP	23
Shanghei Chicken Salad	305	13	NP	824	25	3	NP	25
Signature Salad	611	45	NP	664	44	5	NP	12
Wild Alaskan Salmon Salad	457	27	NP	1372	24	7	NP	35
Salad Bruschetta	645	14	NP	591	79	28	NP	54
Shanghai Chicken Salad	305	13	NP	824	25	3	NP	25
Greek Salad	517	47	NP	1480	19	4	NP	11
Bombay Chicken Salad	481	32	NP	1094	17	4	NP	25
Così Cobb Salad	708	55	NP	1328	16	2	NP	39
Caesar Salad	488	40	NP	1459	20	2	NP	18
Grilled Chicken Caesar Salad	621	44	NP	1670	20	2	NP	39
Tuscan Steak Salad	532	34	NP	1542	26	6	NP	30
Mixed Greens Salad	39	0	NP	21	8	3	NP	3

Soup

Pollo E Pasta, cup (10 oz)	162	4	NP	1100	14	1	NP	11
Tomato Basil Aurora, cup (10 oz)	225	15	NP	1088	20	4	NP	5
Beef w/ Winter Garden Vegetable Soup, cup (10 oz)	150	8	NP	1350	14	1	NP	9
Moroccan Lentil Soup, cup (10 oz)	199	3	NP	1159	32	7	NP	13
Three Bean Chili, cup (10 oz)	150	1	NP	1012	36	11	NP	10
Chicken Tortilla Soup, cup (10 oz)	138	2	NP	475	21	2.5	NP	7.5
New England Clam Chowder, cup (10 oz)	440	29	NP	625	24	1	NP	22

Sandwich

Chicken T.B.M. Light Sandwich	563	20	NP	961	54	4	NP	43
T.B.M. Light Sandwich	403	14	NP	819	53	3	NP	19
Tandoori Chicken Light Sandwich	445	8	NP	660	71	27	NP	17
Turkey Light Sandwich	390	5	NP	827	62	2	NP	26
Hummus & Fresh Veggies Sandwich	397	7	NP	532	72	7	NP	13
Sesame Ginger Chicken Sandwich	480	7	NP	1272	69	4	NP	35
Fire-Roasted Veggie Sandwich	328	8	NP	259	44	4	NP	11
Turkey Rustica Sandwich	619	27	NP	1673	60	4	NP	37
Grilled Chicken T.B.M. Sandwich	722	40	NP	845	51	4	NP	43
T.B.M. Sandwich	563	34	NP	703	50	3	NP	20
Steak T.B.M. Sandwich	831	49	NP	656	48	3	NP	51
Così Club Sandwich	447	6	NP	677	46	2	NP	30
Tuna Sandwich	539	6	NP	948	52	4	NP	53
Buffalo Blue Sandwich	565	25	NP	923	47	3	NP	36

Description & Serving	Cal	Fat	Sfat	Sod	Carb	Fiber	Sugar	Prot
Roasted Turkey & Brie Sandwich	687	32	NP	1186	62	2	NP	38
Tuscan Pesto Chicken Sandwich	510	18	NP	452	49	4	NP	39
Turkey Light Sandwich	390	5	NP	827	62	2	NP	26
Tandoori Chicken Sandwich	609	27	NP	590	68	27	NP	17
Fire-Roasted Veggie Sandwich	328	8	NP	259	44	4	NP	11
Italiano Sandwich	747	42	NP	2210	49	3	NP	42
Sesame Ginger Chicken Sandwich	480	7	NP	1272	69	4	NP	35
Wasabi Roast Beef Sandwich	556	27	NP	1351	49	2	NP	29
Hummus & Fresh Veggies Sandwich	397	7	NP	532	72	7	NP	13
Meatball Aurora Sandwich	558	25	NP	1178	53	5	NP	31
Grilled Chicken T.B.M. Melt	740	35	NP	1287	55	5	NP	55
T.B.M. Melt	707	39	NP	1546	58	5	NP	39
Bacon Turkey Cheddar Melt	572	24	NP	1101	48	2	NP	45
Steakhouse Gorgonzola Melt	752	47	NP	963	49	2	NP	30
Grilled Chicken Parmesan Melt	621	25	NP	1256	54	4	NP	49
Pesto Chicken Melt	671	31	NP	995	52	5	NP	50
Tuna Melt	874	40	NP	1154	51	4	NP	65

Pizza

Smoky BBQ Chicken Pizza, indv size	887	21	NP	1396	123	4	NP	49
Margherita Pizza, indv size	702	31	NP	1007	96	5	NP	35
Meat Trio Pizza, indv size	874	44	NP	1578	95	5	NP	46
Pepperoni Pizza, indv size	806	40	NP	1423	94	5	NP	39
Traditional Cheese Pizza, indv size	664	28	NP	886	94	5	NP	33
Meatball Pesto Pizza, indv size	992	57	NP	1766	102	7	NP	47
Smoky BBQ Chicken Pizza, dinner size	1774	42	NP	2792	246	8	NP	98
Margherita Pizza, dinner size	1404	62	NP	2014	192	10	NP	70
Meat Trio Pizza, dinner size	1748	88	NP	3156	190	10	NP	92
Pepperoni Pizza, dinner size	1614	80	NP	2843	190	10	NP	78
Traditional Cheese Pizza, dinner size	1330	56	NP	1774	190	5	NP	66
Meatball Pesto Pizza, dinner size	1984	114	NP	3532	204	14	NP	94

Signature Flatbread

Cosi Rustic Flatbread, 1 slice	214	1	NP	82	43	2	NP	8
Etruscan Whole Grain Flatbread, 1 slice	235	2	NP	72	46	3	NP	9

Kids

Kids Fruit Salad Side	27	0	NP	6	7	1	NP	0
Gooey Grilled Ham & Cheese	320	18	NP	688	22	1	NP	21
Peanut Butter & Jelly	343	15	NP	185	45	3	NP	11
Turkey Sandwich	151	1	NP	262	22	1	NP	13
Tuna Sandwich	256	3	NP	375	22	1	NP	25
Gooey Grilled Cheese	269	15	NP	314	22	1	NP	16
Pepperoni Pizza, kids size	403	20	NP	710	47	2	NP	19
Traditional Cheese Pizza, kids size	332	14	NP	441	47	2	NP	16
Shirley Temple, 12 oz	259	0	NP	50	67	0	NP	0
Hot Chocolate, 12 oz	274	11	NP	175	34	1	NP	11

Dressing/Condiment

Pesto Vinaigrette, 1 oz	260	26	NP	400	6	>2	NP	2
Cosi Vinaigrette, 2 oz	357	39	NP	169	2	0	NP	0

Description & Serving	Cal	Fat	Sfat	Sod	Carb	Fiber	Sugar	Prot
Fat-Free Balsamic Vinaigrette, 2 oz	28	0	NP	302	8	0	NP	0
Roasted Sherry Shallot Vinaigrette, 2 oz	283	26	NP	151	9	0	NP	0
Reduced-Fat Roasted Sherry Shallot, 2 oz	94	6	NP	170	11	0	NP	0
Caesar Dressing, 2 oz	265	28	NP	794	4	0	NP	4
Italian Dressing, 2 oz	246	26	NP	378	2	0	NP	2
Lowfat Ginger Soy Dressing, 2 oz	76	5	NP	491	11	0	NP	0
Pepperanch Dressing, 2 oz	340	32	NP	620	4	0	NP	2
Plain Cream Cheese, 2 oz	189	19	NP	229	0	0	NP	3
Fruit Trio Cream Cheese, 2 oz	182	12	NP	111	14	0	NP	2
Low Fat Plain Cream Cheese, 2 oz	106	8	NP	266	4	0	NP	5
Low Fat Veggie Cream Cheese, 2 oz	113	9	NP	246	2	0	NP	4

Dessert

S'Mores	361	10	NP	234	61	2	NP	5
S'Mores w/ Oreo	350	11	NP	294	59	2	NP	5
Extra Chocolate Bar	230	13	NP	35	24	1	NP	3
Blondie Brownie	570	36	NP	460	57	2	NP	6
Cheesecake Brownie	470	26	NP	260	55	1	NP	5
Rocky Road Brownie	550	33	NP	410	49	2	NP	13
Chocolate Chunk Cookie	480	20	NP	460	72	0	NP	8
White Chocolate Mac Cookie	520	24	NP	360	72	0	NP	8
Oatmeal Raisin Cookie	440	14	NP	380	76	3	NP	8
Crème Brulee Cheesecake, 1 pc	644	46	NP	391	48	1	NP	8
Cinnamon Apple Pie	964	41	NP	667	145	4	NP	11
Mississippi Mud Pie	777	50	NP	1065	80	2	NP	9
Double Trouble Brownie Sundae	1594	95	NP	1039	163	4	NP	25
Medium Sundae	408	24	NP	74	43	1	NP	6
Large Sundae	520	31	NP	101	55	1	NP	8
Double Scoop Ice Cream	225	14	NP	52	22	0	NP	4
Triple Scoop Ice Cream	338	20	NP	79	34	0	NP	7

Beverage

Hot

Latte, Tall (11 oz)	160	6	NP	171	16	0	NP	11
Cappuccino, Tall (7 oz)	97	3	NP	104	10	0	NP	7
Café Americano, Tall (11 oz)	5	0	NP	16	1	0	NP	0
Mocha, Tall (11 oz)	288	5	NP	137	13	0	NP	9
Caramel Mocha, Tall (11 oz)	308	4	NP	135	18	0	NP	9
Mint Mocha, Tall (11 oz)	310	4	NP	136	20	0	NP	9
Café Au Lait, Tall (11 oz)	90	3	NP	95	9	0	NP	6
House Coffee, Tall (11 oz)	6	0	NP	6	1	0	NP	0
Espresso, Solo (1 oz)	3	0	NP	4	0	0	NP	0
Espresso, Doppio (2 oz)	5	0	NP	8	1	0	NP	0
Hot Chocolate, Tall (11 oz)	366	4	NP	133	12	0	NP	9
Mint Hot Chocolate, 10 oz	10	10	NP	10	10	10	NP	10
Hot Apple Cider, Tall (11 oz)	165	0	NP	82	41	0	NP	0
Chai Tea Latte, Tall (11 oz)	140	3	NP	97	22	0	NP	6

Cold

Arctic Latte, Tall (11 oz)	330	10	NP	125	59	0	NP	4
Arctic Mocha, Tall (11 oz)	341	8	NP	111	65	1	NP	4

Description & Serving	Cal	Fat	Sfat	Sod	Carb	Fiber	Sugar	Prot
Double Oh! Arctic, Tall (11 oz)	708	19	NP	316	135	1	NP	5
Strawberry Banana Smoothie, Tall (12 oz)	246	2	NP	147	56	2	NP	1
Pineapple Mango Smoothie, Tall (12 oz)	261	2	NP	190	58	0	NP	0
Mixed Berry Smoothie, Tall (12 oz)	202	2	NP	153	43	0	NP	0
Chocolate Covered Strawberry Smoothie, Tall (12 oz)	238	2	NP	171	52	1	NP	1
Iced Tea, 14 oz	33	0	NP	12	9	0	NP	0
Soy Milk, 8 oz	75	4	NP	27	4	3	NP	6

Country Style

Breakfast

Cruller/Donut/Country Bits

	Cal	Fat	Sfat	Sod	Carb	Fiber	Sugar	Prot
French Cruller	160	11	5	130	15	0	5	1
Plain Cruller	250	13	6	300	30	1	14	3
Cherry Cruller	340	18	9	380	39	1	17	4
Orange Cruller	340	18	9	380	39	1	17	4
Chocolate Cruller	330	20	6	310	33	2	14	7
Sour Cream Cruller	310	19	9	250	31	1	15	3
Glazed Yeast Donut	210	10	4	280	26	1	7	4
Chocolate Raised Yeast Donut	230	10	4.5	280	33	1	13	4
Vanilla Raised Yeast Donut	230	10	4	280	33	1	13	4
Maple Raised Yeast Donut	230	10	4	280	33	1	13	4
Sprinkled Yeast Donut	240	11	5	290	33	1	13	4
Cherry Filled Yeast Donut	290	11	5	330	43	1	21	5
Lemon Filled Yeast Donut	290	11	5	350	42	1	19	5
Strawberry Filled Yeast Donut	290	11	5	330	42	1	19	5
Banana Filled Yeast Donut	290	11	5	330	41	1	18	5
Boston Crème Yeast Donut	280	11	5	340	40	1	15	5
Apple & Spice Yeast Donut	290	12	5	360	41	1	17	5
Dutchie Yeast Donut	260	11	5	320	37	1	11	5
Fritter Yeast Donut	300	12	5	350	42	1	19	5
Cinnamon Ring Yeast Donut	370	17	7	490	52	5	9	8
Glazed White Cake Donut	220	11	5	270	27	1	13	3
Chocolate Iced White Cake Donut	250	11	5	270	34	1	19	3
White Iced White Cake Donut	250	11	5	270	34	1	19	3
Marble Iced White Cake Donut	250	11	5	270	34	1	19	3
Sprinkled White Cake Donut	250	12	6	270	33	1	18	3
Toasted Coconut White Cake Donut	260	15	8	270	30	1	14	3
Coconut White Cake Donut	270	16	9	270	28	2	14	4
Glazed Chocolate Cake Donut	220	10	5	270	28	1	13	3
Chocolate Iced Chocolate Cake Donut	250	10	5	270	35	1	18	3
White Iced Chocolate Cake Donut	250	10	5	270	35	1	19	3
Marble Iced Chocolate Cake Donut	250	10	5	270	35	1	19	3
Sprinkled Chocolate Cake Donut	250	11	6	270	35	1	18	3
Toasted Coconut Chocolate Cake Donut	260	14	8	270	31	1	14	4
Coconut Chocolate Cake Donut	270	15	9	270	30	2	14	4
Yeast Glazed Country Bits	60	3	1	80	8	0	3	1
Yeast Filled Country Bits	70	3	1	80	11	0	5	1
Yeast Sprinkled Country Bits	70	3	1.5	80	10	0	5	1

Description & Serving	Cal	Fat	Sfat	Sod	Carb	Fiber	Sugar	Prot
Yeast Coconut Country Bits	80	4	2.5	80	9	0	3	1
White Cake Glazed Country Bits	70	3	1.5	75	8	0	4	1
White Cake Sprinkled Country Bits	80	3.5	2	75	11	0	6	1
White Cake Coconut Country Bits	80	4.5	2.5	75	10	0	5	1
Chocolate Cake Glazed Country Bits	70	3	1.5	80	9	0	4	1
Chocolate Cake Sprinkled Country Bits	80	3.5	1.5	80	11	0	6	1
Chocolate Cake Coconut Country Bits	80	4.5	2.5	80	10	0	5	1
Muffin/Danish								
Carrot Muffin	470	23	3.5	150	61	5	33	7
Morning Glory Muffin	440	18	3.5	80	64	5	38	7
Lemon Cranberry Muffin	400	16	3.5	290	58	5	27	9
Banana Muffin	470	22	3.5	125	65	5	36	8
Chocolate Chunk Muffin	400	13	1.5	200	70	2	36	6
Blueberry Muffin	400	16	1	200	59	2	25	6
Reduced Fat Apple Oatmeal Muffin	360	11	1	320	58	3	24	6
Raisin Bran Muffin	380	16	2.5	160	57	9	27	10
Reduced Fat Fruit & Fibre Muffin	350	8	0.5	310	63	9	33	7
Very Berry Muffin	450	21	3.5	200	57	5	26	8
Strawberry Banana Yogurt Muffin	400	20	3.5	350	54	1	32	4
Double Chocolate Muffin	470	23	4.5	150	61	1	33	5
Corn Muffin	500	19	1.5	490	75	0	33	9
Pomegranate Bran Muffin	340	17	2.5	450	47	8	24	7
Banana Mango Muffin	440	16	2.5	90	62	2	35	7
Whole Wheat Blueberry Muffin	380	18	2	340	47	5	23	7
Twelve Grain Muffin	380	14	1.5	300	57	6	26	8
Fruit & Flax Fibre Muffin	320	12	1	240	49	8	23	8
Spinach & Cheese Danish	310	14	4	390	37	2	4	7
Strawberry Cheese Danish	360	16	5	340	47	2	15	6
Bagel/Breakfast Sandwich								
Breakfast Bagel Deluxe	500	14	6	1410	67	2	4	26
Plain Bagel	210	2	0.5	310	40	1	2	6
Cheddar Bagel	230	6	3	330	34	1	2	8
Asiago Bagel	220	5	2.5	390	36	1	2	8
Pumpernickel Bagel	210	2.5	0.5	500	41	3	2	7
Whole Wheat Bagel	200	2	0.5	300	40	2	2	6
Sesame Bagel	220	3	1	300	40	2	2	7
Sundried Tomato Bagel	210	2	0.5	420	40	2	3	7
Poppy Seed Bagel	220	3.5	0	290	39	2	2	7
Multigrain Bagel	230	4	1	400	41	3	1	7
Honey Cinnamon Raisin Bagel	210	3.5	1	350	38	3	5	6
Everything Bagel	210	2	0.5	300	42	1	2	7
Cranberry Walnut Flax Bagel	240	6	1	260	39	3	2	7
Blueberry Bagel	220	1.5	0.5	270	46	2	9	6
BLT Breakfast Sandwich	250	12	5	420	28	2	4	8
Ham & Swiss Breakfast Sandwich	320	15	8	530	27	1	2	17
Sausage & Egg Breakfast Sandwich	380	18	11	560	26	1	2	16
Western Breakfast Sandwich	400	23	10	700	29	4	4	17
Sunriser Breakfast Sandwich	320	17	9	410	28	1	3	14

Description & Serving	Cal	Fat	Sfat	Sod	Carb	Fiber	Sugar	Prot
Sandwich/Wrap								
Smoked Ham & Cheese Sandwich	410	16	5	1380	51	3	9	18
Smoked Turkey & Cheese Sandwich	380	13	4	1210	46	3	8	21
Veggie & Cheese Sandwich	300	8	3.5	510	46	3	8	11
Stacked Club Sandwich	420	16	4.5	1350	49	2	8	19
Italian Deli Sandwich	450	18	6	1540	49	3	9	23
Grilled Chicken Bistro w/ Bacon Sandwich	510	20	6	1170	49	3	9	31
Original Philly Steak & Cheese Sandwich	450	17	7	810	48	2	9	24
Tuna Salad Sandwich	340	8	0.5	960	44	3	7	24
Egg Salad Sandwich	370	14	3	520	44	3	7	16
Chicken Salad Sandwich	360	10	1.5	1170	45	2	7	21
Stacked Club Sandwich	500	19	5	1500	56	3	2	22
Bistro Deli Classic	500	19	6	1530	58	3	4	23
BLT	420	15	3	840	61	3	14	13
Smokey Turkey	450	15	4	1220	57	3	10	20
Traditional Tuna	440	13	3.5	1120	56	3	9	26
Traditional Egg	470	18	6	710	56	4	9	20
Grilled Chicken Bistro	590	25	7	1270	58	3	10	30
Mediterranean Chicken	530	20	2.5	1060	57	3	3	27
Meatball Deluxe	550	21	7	1200	60	3	4	28
Chicken Parm	600	19	2	1650	79	4	8	25
The Original Steak & Cheese	530	21	6	980	59	2	12	24
Tuna Melt Griller	490	10	3	1210	71	5	4	29
Spicy Buffalo Chicken Griller	630	17	4.5	1430	91	6	7	27
Tuscan Bacon Turkey Griller	540	11	2.5	1430	78	5	10	30
The Clubhouse Griller	620	22	7	1820	74	5	6	30
Chicken Caesar Wrap	330	13	3.5	970	30	1	1	24
Greek Wrap	260	16	2.5	960	33	2	2	20
Cranberry Chicken Wrap	360	11	3	1040	40	2	10	24
Mango Turkey Wrap	250	10	1	900	32	2	1	10
Salad								
Country Salad	40	0.5	0.1	20	9	3	6	3
Tuna Salad	110	3.5	0.3	390	9	4	6	13
Egg Salad	130	7	1.5	95	10	4	6	9
Chicken Salad	110	4	0.5	440	10	3	6	10
Fruit Salad	340	0	0	55	88	4	80	4
Garden Salad	120	8	0.1	310	11	4	8	3
Caesar Salad	140	9	3	300	8	2	4	8
Cranberry Chicken Salad	200	2.5	1	640	26	4	19	18
Mediterranean Salad	150	12	5	530	6	3	4	7
Soup/Chili								
Cheddar Cauliflower Soup	130	6	2	1070	15	5	3	4
Cream of Asparagus Soup	150	8	6	920	17	4	4	4
Cream of Potato Soup	190	9	2.5	860	24	3	3	5
Vegetable Beef Barley Soup	100	2.5	1	990	15	4	3	5
Italian Wedding Soup	120	4	1.5	950	14	2	1	5
Corn Chowder	220	8	2.5	940	30	4	7	6

Description & Serving	Cal	Fat	Sfat	Sod	Carb	Fiber	Sugar	Prot
Tomato Basil & Raviolini Soup	120	1	0.5	750	23	1	5	4
Minestrone Soup	90	2.5	0.4	1150	14	4	4	4
Garden Vegetable Soup	80	0.5	0.2	640	14	3	5	5
Chicken Gumbo Soup	90	2	0.5	1280	13	2	4	6
Cream of Broccoli & Cheese Soup	190	11	1.5	960	16	3	5	6
Cream of Mushroom Soup	230	12	4.5	1190	15	0	4	4
Turkey Vegetable & Rice Soup	110	2	0.5	830	19	2	2	4
Chicken Noodle Soup	120	2.5	0.5	860	18	1	4	7
Chili	190	9	4	890	17	3	6	10
Chili w/ Cheddar Cheese	230	13	6	930	17	3	6	12
Chicken Stew	190	9	4	890	17	3	6	10

Dessert

Description & Serving	Cal	Fat	Sfat	Sod	Carb	Fiber	Sugar	Prot
Plain Tea Biscuit	170	5	1	540	26	1	4	4
Cheese Tea Biscuit	190	7	2.5	540	24	1	4	5
Raisin Tea Biscuit	180	4.5	1	480	30	1	6	4
Blueberry Tea Biscuit	160	4.5	1	480	24	1	4	4
White Chocolate Macadamia Cookie	200	10	2.5	135	23	1	15	2
Peanut Butter Cookie	190	11	2	150	20	1	10	4
Oatmeal Raisin Cookie	170	6	1	125	24	1	13	3
Triple Chocolate Cookie	190	9	3	120	24	1	16	2
Chocolate Chunk Cookie	190	9	2.5	150	24	1	14	2
Butter Croissant	260	15	10	350	26	2	2	5
Butter Cheese Croissant	320	20	13	450	26	2	2	8
Chocolatine Croissant	280	18	11	160	25	3	3	5
Raisin Butter Tart	350	16	4	180	49	1	28	4
Pecan Butter Tart	370	19	4	180	45	1	25	4

Beverage

Description & Serving	Cal	Fat	Sfat	Sod	Carb	Fiber	Sugar	Prot
Coffee w/ 1 cream & 1 sugar, 10 oz	50	2.5	1.5	5	7	0	7	0.4
Decaffeinated Coffee w/ 1 cream & 1 sugar, 10 oz	50	2.5	1.5	5	7	0	7	0.4
Tea w/ milk & sugar, 10 oz	30	0.2	0	15	7	0	7	0.4
Hot Chocolate, 10 oz	110	2	0.5	190	24	1	21	1
French Vanilla Frothy Coffee, 10 oz	110	3.5	3.5	5	20	0	14	1
Espresso, 40 ml	10	0	0	5	0	0	0	0.2
Cappuccino, 10 oz	80	3	2	15	6	0	5	5
Latte, 10 oz	70	2.5	1.5	20	5	0	4	4
Mocha Latte, 10 oz	70	1.5	1	25	8	0	6	3
Belgian Hot Chocolate, 10 oz	80	1.5	1	20	14	1	13	3
Green Tea Latte, 10 oz	190	3.5	2.5	120	30	0	27	8
Vanilla Latte, 10 oz	160	6	2.5	95	20	0	16	4
Caramel Latte, 10 oz	200	7	3.5	140	27	0	22	4
Country Style Orange Juice, 300 ml	140	0.2	0.1	5	31	1	26	2
Country Style Apple Juice, 284 ml	140	0	0	7	33	0	30	0.3
Country Style Cranberry Cocktail, 300 ml	170	0.3	0	5	43	0	38	0
Country Style Lemonade, 300 ml	140	0	0	13	36	0	32	0
Tropical Drinks, 10 oz	100	0	0	40	24	0	24	0
Polar Cappuccino, 10 oz	150	3	0	40	30	0	26	2
Lemon Cherry Freeze, 10 oz	160	0	0	30	40	0	40	0

Description & Serving	Cal	Fat	Sfat	Sod	Carb	Fiber	Sugar	Prot
### *Cousins Subs*								

Sandwich

Description & Serving	Cal	Fat	Sfat	Sod	Carb	Fiber	Sugar	Prot
5" Mini BLT	298	19	4	559	24	1	NP	9
5" Mini Chicken Cheddar Deluxe	329	19	5	775	26	1	NP	16
5" Mini Chicken Salad	280	11	2	572	32	1	NP	12
5" Mini Club	326	17	4	963	26	1	NP	18
5" Mini Club (Better Bunch) w/o mayo, cheese, or added salt	188	2	0	792	26	1	NP	15
5" Mini Garden Veggie	216	7	4	463	26	1	NP	11
5" Mini Garden Veggie (Better Bunch) w/o mayo, cheese, or added salt	136	1	0	263	26	1	NP	6
5" Mini Ham & Provolone	311	17	4	828	26	1	NP	14
5" Mini Ham (Better Bunch) w/o mayo, cheese, or added salt	173	2	0	657	26	1	NP	12
5" Mini Hot Veggie	254	10	6	641	28	1	NP	13
5" Mini Hot Veggie (Better Bunch) w/o mayo, cheese, or added salt	144	1	0	371	27	1	NP	6
5" Mini Italian Special	403	25	7	1012	25	1	NP	16
5" Mini Meatball & Provolone	361	19	9	853	27	1	NP	20
5" Mini Pepperoni Melt	345	21	6	861	25	1	NP	14
5" Mini Pizza Sub	336	18	9	964	28	1	NP	15
5" Mini Seafood w/ Crab	323	19	3	720	31	1	NP	10
5" Mini Three Cheese	363	23	8	598	25	1	NP	15
5" Mini Tuna	313	18	3	531	25	1	NP	15
5" Mini Turkey Breast	275	14	2	840	26	1	NP	14
5" Mini Turkey Breast (Better Bunch) w/o mayo, cheese, or added salt	173	2	0	662	26	1	NP	14
7.5" Cheese Steak	503	19	9	1209	49	1	NP	31
7.5" Chicken Breast	569	27	4	1248	50	1	NP	35
7.5" Chicken Breast (Better Bunch) w/o mayo, cheese, or added salt	366	2	0	1086	50	1	NP	35
7.5" Double Cheese Steak	747	36	18	1704	49	1	NP	52
7.5" Gyro	710	41	18	1692	61	2	NP	32
7.5" Philly Cheese Steak	531	19	9	1237	55	2	NP	32
7.5" Roast Beef	607	30	6	973	50	1	NP	35
7.5" Roast Beef (Better Bunch) w/o mayo, cheese, or added salt	405	6	2	617	50	1	NP	35

Salad

Description & Serving	Cal	Fat	Sfat	Sod	Carb	Fiber	Sugar	Prot
Chef Salad (Better Bunch) w/o croutons, cheese, or dressing	125	3	0	900	9	2	NP	18
Garden Salad (Better Bunch) w/o croutons, cheese, or dressing	34	0	0	22	7	2	NP	2
Garden Salad w/ Chicken Breast (Better Bunch) w/o croutons, cheese, or dressing	148	1	0	589	9	2	NP	25
Side Salad (Better Bunch) w/o croutons, cheese, or dressing	19	0	0	13	4	1	NP	1
Chef Salad	327	14	6	1465	25	2	NP	29

Description & Serving	Cal	Fat	Sfat	Sod	Carb	Fiber	Sugar	Prot
Garden Salad	235	11	5	587	23	2	NP	13
Garden Salad w/ Chicken Breast	349	12	5	1154	25	2	NP	37
Italian Salad	403	24	10	1740	24	2	NP	23
Seafood Salad	315	11	5	1262	34	2	NP	22
Side Salad	135	6	3	339	14	1	NP	7
Tuna Salad	623	46	11	1205	23	2	NP	35

Soup

Description & Serving	Cal	Fat	Sfat	Sod	Carb	Fiber	Sugar	Prot
Beef Steak & Noodle Soup, reg (198 g)	105	3	2	683	12	0	NP	7
Cheddar Cauliflower Soup, reg (198 g)	114	5	2	936	13	4	NP	4
Cheddar Cheese Soup, reg (198 g)	201	11	6	1085	18	1	NP	7
Chicken & Dumplings Soup, reg(198 g)	149	4	2	849	17	3	NP	10
Chicken Noodle Soup, reg (198 g)	114	4	1	910	16	2	NP	6
Chicken w/ Wild Rice Soup, reg (198 g)	219	9	2	901	13	4	NP	12
Chili, reg (198 g)	219	8	4	1076	26	16	NP	16
Cream of Broccoli w/ Cheese Soup, reg (198 g)	166	7	4	823	13	3	NP	5
Cream of Mushroom Soup, reg (198 g)	193	11	4	1006	13	0	NP	4
Cream of Potato Soup, reg (198 g)	166	8	2	753	21	3	NP	4
Eight Bean Soup w/ Ham, reg (198 g)	105	1	0	945	18	5	NP	7
Fiesta Tortilla Soup w/ Chicken, reg (198 g)	114	5	1	604	11	2	NP	6
New England Clam Chowder, reg (198 g)	149	3	2	928	25	2	NP	6
Tomato Basil w/ Raviolini, reg (198 g)	96	1	0	630	19	0	NP	4
Vegetable Beef, reg (198 g)	70	2	0	884	11	2	NP	4

Side

Description & Serving	Cal	Fat	Sfat	Sod	Carb	Fiber	Sugar	Prot
French Fries, sml	251	13	3	150	30	2	NP	4
French Fries, med	367	19	5	219	43	3	NP	5
French Fries, lrg	483	25	7	288	57	4	NP	7

Dessert

Description & Serving	Cal	Fat	Sfat	Sod	Carb	Fiber	Sugar	Prot
Chocolate Chip Cookie	210	11	4	120	26	0	NP	2
Chocolate Chip Cookie w/ M&M's	190	9	3	125	26	0	NP	2
Coconut Toffee Chip Cookie	200	9	4	140	23	0	NP	2
Double Chocolate Chip Cookie	190	9	3	135	25	1	NP	2
Oatmeal Cranberry Walnut Cookie	170	7	2	100	26	1	NP	2
Oatmeal Raisin Cookie	170	7	2	110	25	1	NP	2
Peanut Butter w/ Reese's Pieces Cookie	210	11	4	140	22	0	NP	4
Snickerdoodle Cookie	190	9	4	60	25	0	NP	2
Sugar Cookie	180	8	2	150	26	0	NP	2
White Chunk Macadamia Nut Cookie	200	11	4	125	24	0	NP	2

Bread

Description & Serving	Cal	Fat	Sfat	Sod	Carb	Fiber	Sugar	Prot
5" Mini Garlic Herb Bread	120	1	0	257	22	0	NP	5
5" Mini Italian Bread	120	1	0	257	22	0	NP	5
5" Mini Parmesan-Asiago Bread	124	1	0	269	22	0	NP	5
5" Mini Wheat Bread	120	2	0	257	22	2	NP	5
7.5" Garlic Herb Bread	240	2	0	513	44	0	NP	10
7.5" Italian Bread	240	2	0	513	44	0	NP	10
7.5" Parmesan-Asiago Bread	248	2	0	538	45	0	NP	11
7.5" Wheat Bread	240	3	0	513	44	3	NP	10
Flour Tortilla Wrap	210	5	2	460	36	3	NP	6

Description & Serving	Cal	Fat	Sfat	Sod	Carb	Fiber	Sugar	Prot
Culver's								
Burger/Hot Dog								
Culver's ButterBurger Original, Single	346	15	6	700	35	1	NP	19
Culver's ButterBurger Original, Double	480	23	9	730	36	1	NP	33
Culver's ButterBurger Original, Triple	613	31	12	841	37	1	NP	47
ButterBurger Cheese, Single	398	20	8	955	36	1	NP	22
ButterBurger Cheese, Double	580	32	14	1240	37	1	NP	38
ButterBurger Cheese, Triple	763	45	19	1606	38	1	NP	55
The Culver's ButterBurger Deluxe, Single	494	31	14	857	34	1	NP	22
The Culver's ButterBurger Deluxe, Double	671	43	20	1061	34	1	NP	39
The Culver's ButterBurger Deluxe, Triple	851	56	25	1346	34	1	NP	55
Bacon ButterBurger Deluxe, Single	573	38	17	1067	34	1	NP	26
Bacon ButterBurger Deluxe, Double	751	50	22	1351	34	1	NP	43
Bacon ButterBurger Deluxe, Triple	931	63	28	1636	34	1	NP	59
ButterBurger, Low Carb	443	32	14	862	1	0	NP	37
Cheddar Burger, Single	421	22	10	580	31	1	NP	24
Cheddar Burger, Double	641	37	18	750	31	1	NP	43
Cheddar Burger, Triple	861	52	25	920	31	1	NP	62
Cheddar Burger w/ Bacon	871	48	22	1405	56	2	NP	52
Mushroom & Swiss Burger, Single	417	21	10	497	33	1	NP	25
Mushroom & Swiss Burger, Double	633	35	17	584	35	1	NP	45
Mushroom & Swiss Burger, Triple	849	49	24	671	37	1	NP	65
Sourdough Melt, Single	413	20	10	600	33	0	NP	25
Sourdough Melt, Double	636	35	17	770	33	0	NP	44
Sourdough Melt, Triple	858	50	25	941	34	0	NP	63
Wisconsin Swiss Melt, Single	403	20	9	575	33	2	NP	26
Wisconsin Swiss Melt, Double	616	34	16	660	34	2	NP	46
Wisconsin Swiss Melt, Triple	828	48	23	746	35	2	NP	66
Beef Frank w/ Bun	392	22	8	1441	38	1	NP	13
Cheese Dog w/ Bun	461	31	13	1230	27	1	NP	20
Chili Dog w/ Bun	379	24	9	1210	28	1	NP	15
Sandwich/Wrap								
Grilled Reuben Melt	588	31	13	1950	41	2	NP	39
Angus Philly Steak Sandwich	518	20	10	1173	46	2	NP	38
Beef Pot Roast Sandwich	363	16	8	948	33	1	NP	24
Blackened Chicken Sandwich	369	8	4	1386	48	2	NP	31
Crispy Chicken Fillet Sandwich	625	29	10	1782	68	3	NP	26
Grilled Ham 'n Swiss on Rye	497	25	13	1892	33	2	NP	37
North Atlantic Cod Filet Sandwich	740	42	9	1224	58	3	NP	33
Pork Tenderloin Sandwich	593	29	7	1431	62	2	NP	26
Turkey Sourdough BLT	562	31	15	1923	36	0	NP	34
Turkey, Stacked, Sandwich	450	19	9	1642	47	2	NP	26
Chicken Salad Wrap	518	26	7	1133	39	4	NP	32
Tuna Salad Wrap	485	24	7	1084	39	4	NP	29
Salad								
Avocado Pecan Bleu w/ Blackened Chicken	557	41	11	1339	16	8	NP	36
Chicken Cashew w/ Grilled Chicken	441	25	8	1135	17	3	NP	38
Classic Caesar w/ Grilled Chicken	358	14	7	1419	15	2	NP	43

Description & Serving	Cal	Fat	Sfat	Sod	Carb	Fiber	Sugar	Prot
Cobb Salad	531	31	11	2026	19	6	NP	44
Crispy Chicken Salad	616	42	9	1043	34	6	NP	32
Garden Fresco	225	11	5	355	25	7	NP	16
Side Caesar	82	4	2	196	5	1	NP	7
Side Salad	86	5	3	139	6	1	NP	5

Soup/Chili

Description & Serving	Cal	Fat	Sfat	Sod	Carb	Fiber	Sugar	Prot
Baja Chicken Enchilada Soup	352	23	11	1487	21	4	NP	16
Bean w/ Ham Soup	190	3	1	1262	33	9	NP	9
Black Bean Soup	188	3	0	1125	32	11	NP	9
Boston Clam Chowder	252	11	3	1344	25	1	NP	12
Broccoli Cheese w/ Florets Soup	240	14	7	1380	16	1	NP	11
California Medley Soup	204	11	7	1608	18	2	NP	9
Cauliflower Cheese Soup	252	14	6	1128	23	1	NP	8
Cheesy Chicken Tortilla Soup	180	7	4	1764	16	1	NP	12
Chicken & Dumpling Soup	300	22	9	1248	19	1	NP	9
Chicken Gumbo	120	6	2	1224	13	1	NP	5
Chicken Noodle Soup	112	2	1	1550	14	1	NP	9
Chicken Tortilla Soup	168	3	1	1212	26	1	NP	10
Corn Chowder	276	13	3	996	35	4	NP	7
Cream of Asparagus Spears Soup	250	11	3	1344	26	1	NP	11
Cream of Broccoli Soup	185	10	5	1548	16	1	NP	8
Cream of Potato Soup	288	13	7	1032	26	1	NP	7
Creamy Garden Vegetable Soup	188	11	4	1275	19	4	NP	4
Creamy Tomato Bisque Soup	180	9	2	1560	20	2	NP	6
Creamy Turkey Vegetable Soup	216	9	3	996	19	1	NP	12
Fire Roasted Vegetable Soup	72	2	0	1368	12	2	NP	2
French Onion Soup	155	8	3	2029	12	0	NP	10
George's Chili	336	18	6	768	27	6	NP	18
George's Chili Supreme	456	30	15	823	27	5	NP	23
Harvest Grain w/ Portobello Mushrooms Soup	185	7	1	1404	26	4	NP	5
Italian Style Wedding Soup	275	6	3	1475	44	2	NP	11
Lumberjack Mixed Vegetable Soup	150	6	3	1662	21	7	NP	4
Minestrone Soup	100	1	0	1175	19	4	NP	4
Mushroom Medley Soup	252	16	4	1512	20	1	NP	6
Oven Roasted Turkey Noodle Soup	175	5	2	1312	21	1	NP	11
Pasta Fagioli Soup	172	3	1	1262	28	5	NP	8
Potato Au Gratin Soup	350	22	11	1237	28	1	NP	11
Potato w/ Bacon Soup	225	9	2	1288	28	4	NP	8
Seven Bean Medley Soup	150	2	0	1363	25	6	NP	8
Split Pea w/ Ham Soup	262	9	3	1462	32	12	NP	13
Stuffed Green Pepper w/ Beef Soup	150	3	1	1300	25	1	NP	6
Tomato Basil Ravioletti Soup	112	3	1	650	18	1	NP	4
Tomato Florentine Soup	112	1	0	1325	21	1	NP	4
Vegetable Beef & Barley Soup	112	4	1	1300	14	3	NP	7
Wild & Brown Rice w/ Chicken Soup	452	22	7	1200	27	1	NP	37
Wisconsin Cheese Soup	375	24	11	1487	29	1	NP	11

Side

Description & Serving	Cal	Fat	Sfat	Sod	Carb	Fiber	Sugar	Prot
Chili Cheddar Fries	661	34	11	572	73	5	NP	18
Cole Slaw	350	21	4	690	37	2	NP	1

Description & Serving	Cal	Fat	Sfat	Sod	Carb	Fiber	Sugar	Prot
Dinner Roll	140	6	2	200	19	0	NP	4
French Fries, junior	275	12	2	40	38	3	NP	4
French Fries, reg	385	17	3	56	53	4	NP	5
French Fries, lrg	495	22	4	72	68	5	NP	7
Green Beans	203	18	10	151	12	3	NP	2
Mashed Potatoes	120	1	0	204	24	2	NP	2
Mashed Potatoes & Gravy	140	2	0	394	26	2	NP	3
Onion Rings, Breaded	630	36	4	1070	70	3	NP	7
Wisconsin Dairyland Cheese Curds	670	38	15	1740	54	3	NP	28

Entrée

Beef/Steak

Description & Serving	Cal	Fat	Sfat	Sod	Carb	Fiber	Sugar	Prot
Beef Pot Roast Dinner	635	24	13	1572	74	5	NP	33
Chopped Steak Dinner	683	29	12	923	67	6	NP	40

Chicken

Description & Serving	Cal	Fat	Sfat	Sod	Carb	Fiber	Sugar	Prot
Breaded Chicken Tenders, 4 pc	440	20	4	1152	32	4	NP	36
Grilled Chicken Breast	374	8	3	1406	47	2	NP	32
Chicken, 2 pc	1755	94	21	3226	140	6	NP	87

Fish

Description & Serving	Cal	Fat	Sfat	Sod	Carb	Fiber	Sugar	Prot
Fish n' Chips, 6 pc	1381	83	17	1050	104	4	NP	45
North Atlantic Cod Filet, 2 pc	1831	116	18	2118	135	8	NP	54
Breaded Shrimp, approx. 8 pc	1250	61	11	2056	148	9	NP	28
Crispy Shrimp Basket, 8 pc	760	34	5	1166	92	7	NP	23

Kids

Description & Serving	Cal	Fat	Sfat	Sod	Carb	Fiber	Sugar	Prot
ButterBurger	346	15	6	700	35	1	NP	19
Cheese ButterBurger	396	20	8	955	36	1	NP	22
Breaded Chicken Tenders, 2 pc	220	10	2	576	16	2	NP	18
Corn Dog	260	14	4	540	26	0	NP	6
French Fries	275	12	2	40	38	3	NP	4
Grilled Cheese on Sourdough	290	14	7	860	33	0	NP	11
Hot Dog w/ Bun	366	22	8	1310	30	1	NP	13

Dressing/Condiment

Description & Serving	Cal	Fat	Sfat	Sod	Carb	Fiber	Sugar	Prot
BBQ Sauce, 0.99 oz	48	0	0	215	12	0	NP	0
Honey Mustard, 1.9 oz	130	6	1	410	20	0	NP	0
Horseradish Sauce, 1.23 oz	150	14	3	220	6	0	NP	0
Ketchup, 0.6 oz	15	0	0	190	4	0	NP	0
Mayonnaise, 0.49 oz	100	11	6	76	0	0	NP	0
Mustard, Mild, 0.35 oz	0	0	0	140	0	0	NP	0
Spicy Brown Mustard, 0.35 oz	0	0	0	120	0	0	NP	0
Picante Sauce, Mild & Medium, 1.13 oz	10	0	0	220	2	0	NP	0
Shrimp Cocktail Sauce, 1.5 oz	50	0	0	400	12	2	NP	0
Steak Sauce, 0.42 oz	10	0	0	150	2	0	NP	0
Sweet & Sour Dipping Sauce, 1.9 oz	90	0	0	320	23	0	NP	0
Tartar Sauce, 0.99 oz	188	18	3	136	1	0	NP	0
Bleu Cheese, Fancy, Chunky, 1.76 oz	310	33	6	480	2	0	NP	1
Caesar Dressing, 1.76 oz	220	23	5	580	2	0	NP	2
French Dressing, 1.76 oz	190	13	2	320	19	0	NP	0
French, Reduced Calorie Dressing, 1.76 oz	140	9	2	400	16	0	NP	0

Description & Serving	Cal	Fat	Sfat	Sod	Carb	Fiber	Sugar	Prot
Ranch, Buttermilk, Gourmet, 1.76 oz	230	24	4	500	3	0	NP	1
Ranch, Reduced Calorie, 1.76 oz	130	12	2	280	5	0	NP	1
Raspberry Vinaigrette, 1.9 oz	45	0	0	170	11	0	NP	0
Sesame Ginger Dressing, 1.9 oz	70	0	0	400	16	0	NP	1
Thousand Island, Gourmet, 2.12 oz	220	18	2	460	14	0	NP	0

Dessert

Concrete Mixer

Description & Serving	Cal	Fat	Sfat	Sod	Carb	Fiber	Sugar	Prot
Chocolate Concrete Mixer, short	807	40	25	290	99	0	NP	13
Turtle Concrete Mixer, short	911	59	26	342	83	2	NP	15
Vanilla Concrete Mixer, short	679	40	25	186	67	0	NP	12

Milkshake/Malt

Description & Serving	Cal	Fat	Sfat	Sod	Carb	Fiber	Sugar	Prot
Chocolate Malt, short	738	36	22	275	89	0	NP	14
Chocolate Shake, short	742	36	22	287	93	0	NP	13
Vanilla Malt, short	674	36	22	223	73	0	NP	13
Vanilla Shake, short	614	36	22	183	61	0	NP	12

Sundae

Description & Serving	Cal	Fat	Sfat	Sod	Carb	Fiber	Sugar	Prot
Banana Split, 2 scoop	1081	64	28	339	115	6	NP	16
Bananas Foster Sundae, 1 scoop	420	20	11	170	53	2	NP	6
Caramel Cashew, 1 scoop	585	33	15	274	58	1	NP	11
Strawberry Shortcake Sundae, 1 scoop	577	28	15	710	73	1	NP	9
Turtle Sundae, 1 scoop	605	41	15	258	53	2	NP	10

Ice Cream Cone/Dish

Description & Serving	Cal	Fat	Sfat	Sod	Carb	Fiber	Sugar	Prot
Baby Scoop Chocolate Cake Cone	193	8	5	77	25	1	NP	4
Baby Scoop Vanilla Cake Cone	200	10	6	63	22	0	NP	3
Chocolate Cake Cone, 1 scoop	319	14	9	123	40	1	NP	6
Chocolate Dipped Waffle Cone, 1 scoop	533	24	17	191	72	3	NP	9
Chocolate Dish, 1 scoop	294	14	9	108	35	1	NP	6
Chocolate Waffle Cone, 1 scoop	384	15	9	143	55	2	NP	8
Vanilla Cake Cone, 1 scoop	332	18	11	99	35	0	NP	6
Vanilla Chocolate Dipped Waffle Cone, 1 scoop	546	28	19	167	67	2	NP	9
Vanilla Dish, 1 scoop	307	18	11	84	30	0	NP	6
Vanilla Waffle Cone, 1 scoop	397	19	11	119	50	1	NP	8
Lemon Ice	140	0	0	0	35	0	NP	0

Topping

Description & Serving	Cal	Fat	Sfat	Sod	Carb	Fiber	Sugar	Prot
Almond	84	8	1	0	3	2	NP	3
Andes Crème De Menthe Thins	151	10	9	15	16	1	NP	2
Apple	23	0	0	11	6	0	NP	0
Black Sherry	18	0	0	1	5	0	NP	0
Blackberry	14	0	0	1	4	0	NP	0
Blueberry	17	0	0	4	4	0	NP	0
Brownie Pieces	361	16	3	90	52	2	NP	3
Butterfinger	110	5	3	55	18	1	NP	1
Butterscotch	43	0	0	36	10	0	NP	0
Cashew	90	7	1	58	4	1	NP	3
Cherry	20	0	0	1	5	0	NP	0
Chocolate Chip Cookie Dough	120	5	3	32	17	0	NP	1
Crème De Menthe	45	1	0	37	10	0	NP	0

Description & Serving	Cal	Fat	Sfat	Sod	Carb	Fiber	Sugar	Prot
Culver's Chocolate Syrup	64	0	0	52	16	0	NP	0
Heath Toffee Chunks	155	9	5	103	17	0	NP	1
Hershey's Take Five	141	7	4	119	17	1	NP	3
M&M Minis	140	7	4	0	18	2	NP	2
Marshmallow Crème	39	0	0	10	10	0	NP	0
Milk Chocolate Flakes	142	9	8	1	17	2	NP	2
Nestle Crunch	140	7	5	42	19	1	NP	1
Novelty Coating	87	7	5	1	6	1	NP	0
Oreo Cookie Crumbs	62	2	1	74	9	1	NP	1
Peach	15	0	0	1	4	0	NP	0
Peanut Butter	179	15	2	132	6	1	NP	6
Pecan Halves	100	11	1	56	2	1	NP	2
Pineapple	20	0	0	1	5	0	NP	0
Raspberry	18	0	0	0	4	1	NP	0
Reese's Pieces Minis	142	7	4	55	16	1	NP	4
Reese's Peanut Butter Cups	150	9	3	88	16	1	NP	3
Snickers Candy Bar Pieces	67	4	1	36	8	1	NP	1
Spanish Peanuts	160	14	2	110	5	2	NP	8
Sprinkles, Blue & White	140	7	0	0	21	0	NP	0
Strawberry	13	0	0	2	3	0	NP	0

Beverage

Old Fashioned Cherry Soda	516	25	16	133	63	0	NP	9
Culver's Root Beer Float	467	18	11	108	70	0	NP	6
Lemon Ice Smoothie	403	16	10	72	61	0	NP	5
Mocha Iced Coffee, short	172	9	6	55	19	0	NP	3
Vanilla Iced Coffee, short	175	10	6	48	17	0	NP	3

Dairy Queen

Breakfast

Biscuits & Gravy	820	47	13	2590	87	0	6	13
Sausage Biscuit Sandwich	540	37	10	1180	37	0	3	15
Bacon Biscuit Sandwich	480	31	8	1210	37	0	3	15
Ham Biscuit Sandwich	460	28	7	1420	38	0	4	16
Sausage Biscuit Twin Pack	940	24	16	2020	71	0	5	17
Ultimate Hashbrowns w/ Bacon	750	49	17	1470	45	5	2	31
Ultimate Hashbrowns w/ Sausage	880	62	21	1480	45	5	2	32
Ultimate Hashbrowns w/ Ham	740	45	15	1960	47	5	4	35
Country Platter w/ Bacon	170	66	16	2500	92	2	5	30
Country Platter w/ Sausage	1360	91	24	2250	95	3	5	36
Country Platter w/ Ham	1100	64	15	3030	97	3	7	34
Pancake Platter w/ Sausage	530	25	7	1040	57	3	9	16
Pancake Platter w/ Bacon	400	13	3.5	1030	57	3	9	14
Pancake Platter w/ Ham	380	8	2	1510	59	3	11	18
Ultimate Breakfast Burrito	660	36	12	1180	59	5	2	22
Sausage, 1 patty	110	10	3	150	0	0	0	4
Bacon, 3 slices	80	6	2	290	0	0	0	6
Ham, 1 slice	35	1	0	390	1	0	1	5
Hashbrowns	190	12	2.5	210	18	2	0	2

Description & Serving	Cal	Fat	Sfat	Sod	Carb	Fiber	Sugar	Prot
Salad								
Crispy Chicken Salad	460	19	6	1230	31	6	8	29
Grilled Chicken Salad	280	11	5	890	14	4	8	31
Sandwich/Wrap								
Iron Grilled Turkey Sandwich	530	25	7	1550	42	2	2	29
Iron Grilled Classic Club Sandwich	580	29	9	1750	43	2	3	32
Iron Grilled Supreme BLT Sandwich	590	33	9	1560	42	2	3	26
Crispy Chicken Sandwich	560	28	3.5	980	48	3	5	20
Crispy Chicken Sandwich w/ Cheese	610	32	6	1230	48	3	6	22
Grilled Chicken Sandwich	370	16	2.5	780	32	1	5	24
Crispy Flamethrower Chicken Sandwich	860	55	11	1760	51	3	6	30
Grilled Flamethrower Chicken Sandwich	590	36	9	1480	34	1	6	34
Barbeque Beef Sandwich	270	4.5	1	830	43	1	15	16
Barbeque Pork Sandwich	340	12	1.5	840	41	1	9	18
Crispy Fish Sandwich	430	18	2.5	1150	51	2	7	16
Crispy Fish Sandwich w/ Cheese	480	22	5	1390	52	2	7	18
Iron Grilled Cheese Sandwich	320	13	8	1020	30	1	2	13
Pork Tenderloin Sandwich	610	35	6	1330	58	3	6	19
Shredded Chicken Sandwich	290	7	1.5	560	30	1	5	30
Crispy Chicken Wrap	290	16	3	620	17	2	1	11
Grilled Chicken Wrap	200	12	3	450	9	1	1	12
Crispy Chicken Flamethrower Chicken Wrap	310	19	4	620	17	2	1	11
Burger/Hot Dog								
1/4 pound Bacon Cheddar Grillburger	650	35	15	1410	41	2	11	36
1/4 pound Flamethrower Grillburger	780	52	16	1450	41	2	9	34
1/2 pound Flamethrower Grillburger	1060	75	26	1980	41	2	9	54
Original Cheeseburger	400	18	9	920	34	1	9	19
Original Hamburger	350	14	7	680	33	1	8	17
Original Double Cheeseburger	640	34	18	1230	34	1	9	34
Original Double Hamburger	540	26	13	740	33	1	8	29
Original Bacon Double Cheeseburger	730	41	21	1550	35	1	9	41
Classic Grillburger	470	21	8	950	42	2	11	24
1/4 pound Classic Grillburger w/ Cheese	560	28	12	1090	42	2	11	30
1/2 pound Classic Grillburger w/ Cheese	910	54	25	1540	42	2	12	52
1/2 pound Grillburger	720	40	15	1240	42	2	12	42
1/2 pound Grillburger w/ Cheese	870	51	23	1440	42	2	12	51
California Grillburger	620	39	11	830	39	2	8	25
Deluxe Cheeseburger	400	18	9	930	35	1	9	20
Deluxe Hamburger	350	14	7	680	34	1	9	17
Deluxe Double Cheeseburger	640	34	18	1240	35	1	10	34
Deluxe Double Hamburger	540	26	13	750	34	1	9	29
DQ Ultimate Burger	780	48	22	1390	33	1	8	41
Mushroom Swiss Grillburger	620	37	12	910	39	2	8	29
All-Beef Hot Dog	250	14	5	770	21	1	4	9
All-Beef Cheese Dog	290	19	8	690	19	1	2	12
All-Beef Chili Dog	290	17	6	930	24	1	5	11
All-Beef Chili Cheese Dog	430	22	10	1010	39	2	5	18
Corn Dog	460	19	5	970	56	1	55	17

Description & Serving	Cal	Fat	Sfat	Sod	Carb	Fiber	Sugar	Prot
Side								
French Fries, kids	190	8	1	400	27	2	0	2
French Fries, reg	310	13	2	640	43	3	0	4
French Fries, lrg	500	21	3.5	1040	70	5	0	6
Chili Cheese Fries	1240	71	28	2550	119	9	4	34
Onion Rings	360	16	2	840	47	2	3	6
Side Salad	45	0	0	50	11	3	6	2
Breaded Mushrooms	250	9	1	500	36	2	1	7
Spicy Chili Cup	470	16	7	2600	54	2	2	29
Entrée								
Chicken Strip Basket, 4 pc w/ country gravy	1360	63	11	2910	103	8	6	39
Popcorn Shrimp Basket	990	49	26	3630	115	8	3	18
Iron Grilled Chicken Quesadilla Basket	1070	50	18	2310	117	5	8	34
Iron Grilled Veggie Quesadilla Basket	1020	49	19	2470	114	9	7	26
Kids								
All-Beef Hot Dog Kids Meal w/ French Fries	470	25	8	1270	48	3	4	12
Cheeseburger Kids Meal w/ French Fries	590	27	10	1290	61	3	9	22
Chicken Strip Kids Meal w/ French Fries	470	18	2.5	1170	44	4	0	18
Hamburger Kids Meal w/ French Fries	540	23	8	1050	60	3	8	19
Iron Grilled Cheese Kids Meal w/ French Fries	510	21	9	1410	57	3	2	15
All-Beef Hot Dog Kids Meal w/ Applesauce	380	18	7	930	47	2	4	11
Cheeseburger Kids Meal w/ Applesauce	500	18	9	930	59	3	9	20
Chicken Strip Kids Meal w/ Applesauce	350	10	1	780	39	3	0	15
Hamburger Kids Meal w/ Applesauce	450	14	7	690	59	3	8	17
Iron Grilled Cheese Kids Meal w/ Applesauce	420	13	8	1050	56	3	2	13
Vanilla Cone, kids size	140	4	2.5	60	22	0	16	4
Chocolate Cone, kids size	150	4.5	3	70	23	0	15	4
Dipped Cone, Chocolate, kids size	190	8	3.5	65	25	0	18	4
Dipped Cone, Butterscotch, kids size	190	9	4.5	65	24	0	18	4
Dipped Cone, Cherry, kids size	190	9	6	65	24	0	18	4
Dessert								
BLIZZARD, small								
Banana Cream Pie Blizzard	580	22	13	290	84	0	63	11
Banana Split Blizzard	440	13	9	190	71	0	58	11
Butterfinger Blizzard	470	16	10	220	71	0	56	11
Cappuccino Heath Blizzard	600	24	14	310	86	0	75	11
Cherry CheeseQuake Blizzard	500	20	13	280	68	0	54	11
Choco Cherry Love Blizzard	500	21	10	190	68	0	57	11
Chocolate Chip Blizzard	590	29	12	190	70	1	59	11
Cookie Dough Blizzard	710	27	14	350	103	1	76	13
Chocolate Xtreme Blizzard	660	29	15	340	88	1	75	13
French Silk Pie Blizzard	680	31	18	260	88	1	68	12
Georgia Mud Fudge Blizzard	690	35	12	400	82	2	69	13
Hawaiian Blizzard	440	15	10	180	67	1	55	10
Heath Blizzard	600	25	16	310	84	1	73	11
M&M's Chocolate Candy Blizzard	660	22	14	230	101	1	86	13

Description & Serving	Cal	Fat	Sfat	Sod	Carb	Fiber	Sugar	Prot
Mint Oreo Blizzard	580	20	10	410	89	1	69	12
Mocha Chip Blizzard	570	24	18	200	78	1	66	12
Oreo CheeseQuake Blizzard	590	25	14	410	78	1	58	12
Oreo Cookies Blizzard	550	20	10	410	81	1	61	12
Peanut Butter Butterfinger Blizzard	670	32	13	400	83	2	61	14
Reese's Peanut Butter Cups Blizzard	530	21	11	260	74	1	62	13
Snickers Blizzard	670	25	13	310	99	1	83	14
Strawberry CheeseQuake Blizzard	510	21	13	280	69	0	54	12
Tropical Blizzard	500	24	10	220	62	3	48	11
Turtle Pecan Cluster Blizzard	680	32	11	320	86	2	66	13
Frozen Treat								
Vanilla Cone, sml	230	7	4.5	100	31	0	26	6
Chocolate Cone, sml	240	7	5	115	32	0	25	6
Dipped Cone, Chocolate, sml	330	15	6	105	36	0	31	6
Dipped Cone, Butterscotch, sml	340	16	8	110	35	0	31	6
Dipped Cone, Cherry, sml	330	16	11	105	35	0	30	6
Peanut Buster Parfait	700	30	16	360	94	2	72	16
Banana Split	520	13	10	160	94	3	73	9
Oreo Brownie Earthquake	760	27	16	400	117	2	88	11
Chocolate Coated Waffle Cone w/ Soft Serve	540	21	13	170	77	1	57	10
Plain Waffle Cone w/ Soft Serve	420	13	7	140	67	0	47	10
Strawberry Shortcake	480	17	13	370	75	1	62	8
Triple Chocolate Utopia	750	36	15	340	93	2	79	13
Pecan Mudslide Treat	300	10	7	135	45	0	38	8
Milkshake/Malt, small								
Chocolate Shake	570	15	10	250	92	0	79	13
Strawberry Shake	470	15	10	220	70	0	59	14
Marshmallow Shake	560	15	10	230	94	0	80	13
Caramel Shake	610	17	11	320	99	0	70	15
Hot Fudge Shake	610	22	15	300	87	0	71	15
Banana Shake	450	14	9	210	68	1	55	14
Cherry Shake	500	15	10	240	76	0	66	13
Pineapple Shake	480	15	10	220	71	0	62	13
Chocolate Malt	650	16	10	310	110	0	93	15
Strawberry Malt	570	15	10	290	93	1	80	15
Marshmallow Malt	650	16	10	290	112	0	94	15
Caramel Malt	690	18	12	380	116	0	84	16
Hot Fudge Malt	700	23	16	360	105	0	85	77
Banana Malt	540	15	10	260	86	1	68	16
Cherry Malt	590	16	10	300	94	0	80	15
Pineapple Malt	550	15	10	280	89	0	76	15
Sundae								
Chocolate Sundae, sml	280	7	4.5	115	48	0	41	5
Mashmallow Sundae, sml	280	7	4.5	110	49	0	42	15
Caramel Sundae, sml	300	7	5	150	51	0	36	6
Hot Fudge Sundae, sml	300	10	7	140	46	0	37	6
Banana Sundae, sml	230	7	4.5	90	37	1	29	6
Cherry Sundae, sml	250	7	4.5	110	40	0	34	5

Description & Serving	Cal	Fat	Sfat	Sod	Carb	Fiber	Sugar	Prot
Pineapple Sundae, sml	230	7	4.5	100	38	0	32	6
Strawberry Sundae, sml	260	7	4.5	105	44	0	36	6
Turtle Waffle Bowl Sundae, sml	810	34	18	320	116	2	76	12
Chocolate Covered Strawberry Waffle Bowl Sundae	790	40	27	180	99	2	78	10
Fab Fudge Waffle Bowl Sundae	750	30	21	230	108	1	79	10
Fudge Brownie Temptation Waffle Bowl Sundae	970	49	21	370	120	3	94	14
Nut & Fudge Waffle Bowl Sundae	880	47	21	420	99	4	68	17
Topping								
Almond Pieces, 14 g	90	8	0.5	110	2	1	0	3
Banana Slices, 28 g	25	0	0	0	6	1	3	0
Blackberry Topping, 28 g	60	0	0	10	14	0	13	0
Blueberry Topping, 28 g	60	0	0	10	15	1	12	0
Butterfinger Pieces, 28 g	110	4.5	2	55	18	0	11	1
Butterscotch Topping, 28 g	90	0	0	85	20	0	13	1
Caramel Topping, 28 g	90	0.5	0.5	60	20	0	11	1
Cheesecake Pieces, 28 g	100	6	3.5	80	10	0	6	2
Cherry Topping, 28 g	40	0	0	20	9	0	9	0
Chewy Baked Brownie Pieces, 28 g	130	6	1.5	130	17	0	16	2
Choco Chunks, 28 g	150	10	8	0	17	1	14	1
Chocolate Topping, 28 g	70	0	0	25	17	0	15	0
Cocoa Fudge, 28 g	160	10	2	50	15	1	12	2
Coconut Flakes, 14 g	80	7	6	35	7	2	14	1
Cookie Dough Pieces, 28 g	130	6	1.5	70	18	0	10	1
Heath Pieces, 28 g	150	9	5	95	17	0	17	1
Hot Fudge Topping, 28 g	90	3	2.5	45	15	0	11	1
M&M's Chocolate Candies, 28 g	140	6	3.5	20	20	1	18	1
Maple Walnut Topping, 28 g	130	8	0.5	5	14	1	11	2
Marshmallow Topping, 28 g	70	0	0	15	18	0	16	0
Oreo Cookie Pieces, 28 g	140	6	1.5	190	20	1	11	1
Peanut Butter Topping, 28 g	180	15	2	170	8	1	3	3
Peanuts, 14 g	80	7	1	55	3	1	1	4
Pecan Pieces, 14 g	100	11	1	55	2	1	1	1
Pineapple Pieces, 28 g	30	0	0	5	7	0	7	0
Rainbow Sprinkles, 14 g	70	2.5	1	0	10	0	5	0
Red Raspberry Topping, 28 g	50	0	0	5	14	2	11	0
Reese's Peanut Butter Cups Pieces, 28 g	150	9	3	85	16	1	13	3
Snickers Pieces, 28 g	130	7	2.5	70	17	1	14	2
Strawberry Topping, 28 g	25	0	0	5	6	0	5	0
Whipped Topping, 28 g	90	7	7	0	7	0	7	0
Cake								
8" DQ Cake, 1/8 slice	410	15	10	210	59	1	46	9
8" Cookie Dough Blizzard Cake, 1/8 slice	740	32	20	340	100	1	77	12
8" Chocolate Xtreme Blizzard Cake, 1/8 slice	780	36	22	410	101	2	82	13
8" Oreo Blizzard Cake, 1/8 slice	760	33	20	460	104	2	80	13
8" Reese's Peanut Butter Cups Blizzard Cake, 1/8 slice	720	33	20	340	94	2	76	13
8" Strawberry CheeseQuake Blizzard Cake, 1/8 slice	610	27	19	310	79	0	63	12

Description & Serving	Cal	Fat	Sfat	Sod	Carb	Fiber	Sugar	Prot
Beverage								
Cappuccino MooLatte, 16 oz	500	18	15	170	71	0	63	8
Caramel MooLatte, 16 oz	630	19	15	240	101	0	78	9
French Vanilla MooLatte, 16 oz	560	18	14	160	88	0	74	8
Mocha MooLatte, 16 oz	590	23	15	190	82	0	72	9
Arctic Rush - All Flavors, sml	240	0	0	0	48	0	48	0
Arctic Rush Freeze - All Flavors, sml	440	11	8	160	70	0	61	9
Arctic Rush Float - All Flavors, sml	360	7	4.5	95	60	0	55	6
Frozen Lemonade, sml	200	0	0	0	40	1	39	0
Frozen Limeade, sml	200	0	0	0	41	1	38	0
Diet Coke Float, sml	220	7	4.5	100	32	0	27	6
Root Beer Float, sml	370	7	4.5	130	74	0	68	6
Minute Maid Orange Float, sml	380	7	4.5	95	76	0	71	6

D'Angelo

Description & Serving	Cal	Fat	Sfat	Sod	Carb	Fiber	Sugar	Prot
Sandwich								
Baked Stuffed Lobster Sub, sml	640	33	4.5	1120	54	5	5	31
BLT & Cheese Sub, sml	500	23	11	1510	51	6	7	23
Capicola & Cheese Sub, sml	400	14	4	1410	46	4	3	25
Cheese Sub, sml	580	29	16	2000	52	4	7	31
Cheeseburger Sub, sml	530	25	10	1430	49	5	5	28
Chicken Club Sub, sml	620	32	7	1280	48	5	5	35
Chicken Honey Dijon Sub, sml	530	15	6	1300	56	6	10	43
Chicken Salad Sub, sml	670	43	7	1030	45	4	3	26
Chicken Stir Fry Sub, sml	470	12	6	1570	53	6	7	38
Classic Veggie Sub, sml	450	15	7	1180	60	7	9	22
Grilled Chicken Sub, sml	370	7	1	910	48	5	4	30
Ham Sub, sml	300	4	0	1210	49	2	6	19
Ham & Cheese Sub, sml	380	10	4.5	1680	49	1	5	24
Ham & Salami Sub, sml	450	19	6	1460	46	1	3	26
Hamburger Sub, sml	460	20	7	1120	48	5	4	24
Italian Sub, sml	530	26	8	1630	50	2	4	27
Lobster Sub, sml	560	27	4	1060	47	5	4	31
Lobster Roll Sub, sml	390	22	3.5	660	24	2	4	23
Meatball Sub, sml	670	34	13	2260	66	10	12	28
Meatball & Cheese Sub, sml	780	42	18	2520	67	10	13	36
Mortadella & Cheese Sub, sml	590	33	11	1710	47	4	4	29
Number 9 Sub, sml	600	24	11	1620	53	6	7	43
Pastrami & Cheese Sub, sml	610	34	14	1880	47	5	3	34
Pepperoni Sub, sml	600	34	11	1830	47	7	5	29
Roast Beef Sub, sml	320	5	1.5	990	46	4	4	26
Salad Sub, sml	280	3	0	510	56	8	10	10
Salami & Cheese Sub, sml	570	33	11	1750	45	4	3	27
Steak Sub, sml	500	17	6	1190	49	5	3	36
Steak & Cheese Sub, sml	590	24	11	1650	52	5	5	42
Steak Bomb Sub, sml	630	29	10	1780	51	6	5	45
Surf n' Turf Sub, sml	800	40	11	1380	55	5	6	54

Description & Serving	Cal	Fat	Sfat	Sod	Carb	Fiber	Sugar	Prot
Toasted Pastrami Reuben Sub, sml	750	47	14	2310	54	6	7	29
Toasted Roast Beef & Cheddar Sub, sml	600	27	10	1440	55	6	7	37
Toasted Spicy Meatball Sub, sml	860	49	18	2960	68	11	14	43
Toasted Tuna & Swiss Sub, sml	810	56	56	960	48	5	5	30
Toasted Turkey & Ham Sub, sml	570	26	7	1530	49	6	6	35
Toasted Turkey Thanksgiving Sub, sml	620	17	2	1220	81	6	11	35
Tuna Sub, sml	700	48	8	900	45	1	3	22
Turkey Sub, sml	330	3	0	540	45	4	3	30
Turkey Club Sub, sml	420	10	3	810	48	3	5	36
Number 9 One Pounder	1460	64	27	2630	105	6	13	117
Steak One Pounder	1180	52	19	1660	74	3	5	102
Steak & Cheese One Pounder	1300	61	25	2290	78	3	7	109
Steak Bomb One Pounder	1590	76	27	3030	101	6	11	130
Specialty Sandwich/Wrap								
BLT & Cheese Pokket Sandwich	440	22	11	1340	39	4	6	22
Caesar Salad Pokket Sandwich	560	37	8	1410	47	4	7	18
Capicola & Cheese Pokket Sandwich	330	12	4	1230	32	1	1	23
Cheese Pokket Sandwich	510	27	16	1830	38	1	5	30
Cheeseburger Pokket Sandwich	460	23	10	1260	35	2	3	27
Chicken Caesar Salad Pokket Sandwich	680	39	9	1980	48	4	8	40
Chicken Club Pokket Sandwich	550	30	7	1110	34	2	3	34
Chicken Honey Dijon Pokket Sandwich	460	14	6	1130	42	2	8	42
Chicken Salad Pokket Sandwich	600	41	7	850	31	1	1	24
Chicken Stir Fry Pokket Sandwich	400	10	6	1400	39	2	5	37
Classic Vegetable Pokket Sandwich	360	13	7	950	43	4	7	20
Classic Veggie Pokket Sandwich w/o cheese	200	1	0	320	40	4	6	9
Greek Pokket Sandwich	750	55	12	1720	46	4	8	19
Grilled Chicken Pokket Sandwich	300	5	1	740	35	2	3	29
Ham Pokket Sandwich	220	2	0	1040	33	1	2	17
Ham & Cheese Pokket Sandwich	310	8	4.5	1500	35	1	3	23
Ham & Salami Pokket Sandwich	380	18	6	1290	32	1	1	25
Hamburger Pokket Sandwich	390	18	7	940	34	2	2	23
Italian Pokket Sandwich	440	24	8	1420	32	1	2	25
Lobster Pokket Sandwich	490	26	4	890	34	2	2	30
Meatball Pokket Sandwich	600	32	13	2090	52	7	10	26
Mortadella & Cheese Pokket Sandwich	530	32	11	1530	33	1	2	28
Number 9 Pokket Sandwich	530	22	11	1440	39	3	5	41
Pastrami & Cheese Pokket Sandwich	540	33	14	1700	33	1	1	33
Pepperoni Pokket Sandwich	400	21	7	1140	32	2	2	22
Roast Beef Pokket Sandwich	250	4	1.5	820	32	1	2	24
Salad Pokket Sandwich	190	1	0	330	39	4	6	8
Salami & Cheese Pokket Sandwich	500	31	11	1580	31	1	1	26
Steak Pokket Sandwich	510	22	8	1010	32	1	1	46
Steak & Cheese Pokket Sandwich	500	22	11	1440	34	1	2	40
Steak Bomb Pokket Sandwich	590	28	10	1670	43	3	4	45
Tuna Pokket Sandwich	630	46	8	720	31	1	1	20
Turkey Pokket Sandwich	260	1	0	360	31	1	1	29
Turkey Club Pokket Sandwich	360	8	3	620	32	3	4	38

Description & Serving	Cal	Fat	Sfat	Sod	Carb	Fiber	Sugar	Prot
BLT & Cheese Wrap	590	30	13	1620	55	5	5	24
Buffalo Chicken Salad Wrap	810	45	9	2440	65	7	8	35
Caesar Salad Wrap	710	45	10	1690	64	5	7	19
Capicola & Cheese Wrap	480	21	6	1510	50	3	1	25
Cheese Wrap	670	36	18	2110	56	3	5	31
Cheeseburger Wrap	600	31	12	1530	52	3	2	28
Chicken Caesar Salad Wrap	830	48	11	2260	65	6	8	41
Chicken Club Wrap	710	39	9	1390	53	4	3	35
Chicken Cobb Wrap	910	54	15	1810	72	7	17	36
Chicken Filet & Bacon Wrap	710	39	9	1390	53	4	3	36
Chicken Honey Dijon Wrap	620	22	8	1410	61	4	9	44
Chicken Salad Wrap	760	49	9	1130	49	3	1	26
Chicken Stir Fry Wrap	550	19	8	1680	57	4	5	39
Classic Veggie Wrap	520	22	9	1250	61	6	7	22
Greek Wrap	910	64	14	2000	65	6	8	21
Grilled Chicken Wrap	440	13	3	1010	50	3	1	30
Ham & Cheese Wrap	470	17	7	1790	54	3	3	25
Ham & Salami Wrap	550	26	8	1720	50	3	2	29
Hamburger Wrap	600	31	11	1240	50	3	1	28
Italian Wrap	600	33	10	1700	50	3	2	27
Lobster Wrap	650	34	6	1170	52	3	2	32
Meatball Wrap	750	41	15	2370	70	9	10	28
Mortadella & Cheese Wrap	680	40	13	1810	52	3	2	30
Number 9 Wrap	680	31	13	1720	58	5	5	43
Pastrami Wrap	700	41	16	1980	52	3	1	34
Pepperoni Wrap	560	30	9	1420	50	4	2	23
Roast Beef Wrap	410	12	3.5	1100	50	3	2	26
Salad Wrap	360	9	2	620	60	8	8	11
Salami & Cheese Wrap	640	38	12	1790	49	3	1	27
Steak Wrap	670	30	10	1290	50	3	1	48
Steak & Cheese Wrap	660	31	13	1720	53	3	2	42
Steak Bomb Wrap	720	36	12	1890	55	5	3	46
Tuna Wrap	780	55	10	1010	49	3	1	22
Turkey Wrap	410	10	2	640	49	3	1	31
Turkey Club Wrap	510	17	5	920	53	5	4	36

Quesadilla

Description & Serving	Cal	Fat	Sfat	Sod	Carb	Fiber	Sugar	Prot
Chicken Stir Fry Quesadilla	360	15	7	1100	31	2	4	26
Number 9 Quesadilla	380	19	9	790	31	2	3	24
Veggie Quesadilla	290	13	7	750	33	3	4	14

Salad

Description & Serving	Cal	Fat	Sfat	Sod	Carb	Fiber	Sugar	Prot
Antipasto Salad	270	17	4.5	1190	18	8	9	16
Caesar Salad	620	54	11	1640	28	6	11	16
Chicken Caesar Salad	670	53	11	2070	21	5	11	36
Chicken Stir Fry Salad	170	4	1	590	11	4	6	25
Cobb Salad	330	18	8	800	14	6	8	30
Greek Salad	780	70	14	1550	23	6	12	14
Greek Salad w/o dressing	320	22	7	1130	20	6	9	14

Description & Serving	Cal	Fat	Sfat	Sod	Carb	Fiber	Sugar	Prot
Lobster Salad	380	25	4.5	580	12	4	5	26
Roast Beef Salad	140	4	1.5	520	11	4	6	21
Tossed Salad	60	0	0	25	13	5	8	3
Turkey Salad	170	1	0	75	10	4	5	29

Soup

Beef Stew, sml	220	8	3.5	820	23	2	6	12
Broccoli & Cheddar Soup, sml	250	19	11	840	12	2	3	9
Chicken Noodle Soup, sml	110	3	1	830	14	1	4	6
Hearty Vegetable Soup, sml	40	0	0	270	7	2	4	2
Italian Wedding Soup, sml	120	6	2	920	11	2	3	6
Lobster Bisque Soup, sml	360	29	18	820	16	1	3	8
NE Clam Chowder, sml	320	18	10	700	31	1	1	9
Portuguese Kale Soup, sml	130	5	1.5	630	16	3	5	8
Beef Stew, lrg	330	12	5	1230	34	3	9	18
Broccoli & Cheddar Soup, lrg	370	28	16	1260	18	3	4	13
Chicken Noodle Soup, lrg	160	5	1.5	1240	21	1	6	9
Hearty Vegetable Soup, lrg	60	1	0	400	10	3	6	3
Italian Wedding Soup, lrg	180	9	3	1380	16	3	4	9
Lobster Bisque Soup, lrg	540	43	27	1230	24	1	4	12
NE Clam Chowder, lrg	480	27	15	1050	46	1	1	13
Portuguese Kale Soup, lrg	190	7	2	940	24	4	7	12

Kids

Cheeseburger Sub	300	13	5	1080	32	4	3	15
Ham & Cheese Sub	230	5	1.5	1000	32	1	3	15
Kidz Tuna Sub	390	24	4	530	30	1	2	12
Meatball Sub	340	16	6	970	37	5	5	15
Chocolate Chip Cookie	170	6	2.5	85	26	0	16	3

Dressing/Condiment

Balsamic Dressing, 85 g	180	18	3	700	9	0	6	0
Bleu Cheese Dressing, 30 g	150	15	3	280	3	0	2	1
Caesar Dressing, 85 g	400	43	7	1190	6	0	6	6
Creamy Italian Dressing, 85 g	350	36	5	850	7	1	5	0
Fat Free Caesar Dressing, 85 g	60	0	0	1670	9	0	9	0
Greek Dressing, 85 g	230	26	4.5	770	6	0	3	0
Honey Mustard Dressing, 30 g	150	14	2	210	7	0	6	0
Lite Ranch Dressing, 85 g	240	19	3	960	6	1	4	2
Buffalo Sauce, 28 g	10	0	0	590	0	2	0	0
Fat Free Mayonnaise, 12 g	10	0	0	95	2	0	0	0
Honey Dijon Mustard, 36 g	70	2	0	170	17	1	14	2
Mayonnaise, 30 g	240	26	4.5	140	0	0	0	0
Olive Oil Blend, 27 g	240	27	3.5	0	0	0	0	0
Salsa, 57 g	20	0	0	320	0	0	2	0
Sour Cream, 57 g	110	9	7	20	2	0	2	2
Turkey Gravy, 85 g	460	38	10	1990	26	1	0	5
Vinegar, 28 g	10	0	0	0	0	0	0	0
Yellow Mustard, 30 g	20	1	0	340	2	1	0	1

Description & Serving	Cal	Fat	Sfat	Sod	Carb	Fiber	Sugar	Prot
Denny's								

Breakfast

Description & Serving	Cal	Fat	Sfat	Sod	Carb	Fiber	Sugar	Prot
Ultimate Omelette	670	54	18	1330	8	2	3	36
Ham & Cheddar Omelette	590	44	17	1330	4	0	1	40
Veggie-Cheese Omelette	500	37	12	940	10	2	4	29
Veggie-Cheese Omelette w/ Eggbeaters	410	22	7	1100	11	2	7	39
Lumberjack Slam	850	46	15	2770	60	3	11	45
French Toast Slam	940	53	17	1820	68	4	14	47
All American Slam	820	69	26	1520	5	1	1	42
Meat Lover's Scramble	1130	66	29	3180	80	6	12	51
Heartland Scramble	1150	66	20	2800	97	7	12	40
T-bone Steak & Eggs	780	36	19	1210	4	0	1	110
Top Sirloin Steak & Eggs	420	21	6	920	1	0	1	54
Country Fried Steak & Eggs	660	42	15	1620	29	3	0	39
Moons Over My Hammy	780	42	16	2580	50	2	3	46
Two Eggs Breakfast & More	480	39	13	1010	4	1	0	25
Two Eggs Breakfast	2	15	5	330	1	0	0	13
Fabulous French Toast Platter	1010	52	16	2000	93	5	16	43
Belgian Waffle Platter, 3 slices	650	50	24	1190	31	2	1	20
Pancakes	410	5	10	1420	82	3	14	9
Southwestern Sizzlin Skillet	990	61	21	2120	71	6	10	35
Flat Jack Sizzlin Skillet	1210	60	18	2590	126	7	48	45
Bacon, 4	180	13	5	700	2	0	1	14
Sausage, 4	370	34	13	660	4	3	0	9
Ham, grilled slice, Honey Smoked	110	3	1	940	6	0	1	14
One Egg	120	10	3	120	>1	0	0	6
Egg Beaters Egg Substitute (eqiv of 2 eggs)	56	0	0	186	2	0	0	11
Biscuit & Sausage Gravy	440	32	12	1650	53	0	3	9
Country Fried Potatoes	390	28	6	560	30	10	0	3
Hashed Browns	200	12	3	560	20	0	1	2
Hashed Browns w/ cheese	310	19	7	800	26	0	2	8
Hashed Browns w/ onions, cheese, gravy	480	22	8	3840	60	2	6	10
Toast, dry, 1	80	1	0	166	16	1	2	3
Bagel w/ cream cheese	330	9	5	580	53	2	8	11
Biscuit	150	10	4.5	530	23	0	1	3
English Muffin w/ margarine	180	3	1	300	25	1	1	4
Grits w/ margarine	260	5	1	840	47	1	0	5
Quaker Oatmeal w/ 8 oz milk	270	7	4	290	37	4	20	14
Cinnamon Apples	100	0.5	0	70	24	1	20	0
Banana, whole	110	0	0	0	29	4	14	1
Grapes	55	0	0	0	29	4	13	1
Maple-Flavored Syrup, 3 tbsp	143	0	0	26	36	0	28	0
Sugar-Free Maple-Flavored Syrup, 3 tbsp	23	0	0	71	9	0	1	0
Whipped Margarine, 1 tbsp	40	5	1	30	0	0	0	0
Cherry Topping, 3 oz	86	0	0	7	21	0	12	0

Appetizer

Description & Serving	Cal	Fat	Sfat	Sod	Carb	Fiber	Sugar	Prot
Sampler	1380	71	6	3710	139	6	11	53
Buffalo Chicken Strips, 5 (w/ celery sticks)	730	32	0	2940	53	1	1	57

Description & Serving	Cal	Fat	Sfat	Sod	Carb	Fiber	Sugar	Prot
Chicken Strips, 5 (w/ celery sticks)	700	30	0	1640	52	0	0	57
Buffalo Wings	300	21	5	1940	5	2	2	20
Smothered Cheese Fries	870		18	1240	75	7	3	27
Mozzarella Sticks, 8	750	40	17	2270	195	1	5	16
Nachos	1150	49	25	2080	138	11	11	46
Sweet & Tangy BBQ Chicken Wings	350	14	3	1390	37	3	10	17
Sweet & Tangy BBQ Chicken Strips	800	30	0	2400	73	1	17	58
Sweet & Tangy BBQ Shrimp	350	19	5	1410	21	1	16	21
Sweet & Tangy BBQ Bacon Burger	670	37	13	970	55	4	6	30
Crispy Chicken Sandwich	940	42	7	2690	96	5	17	44
Strips & Sticks	1070	73	14	2110	112	1	16	30
Nacho Cheese Fries	700	46	14	1540	52	6	2	17
Potachos	1460	110	53	2700	82	8	7	40

Soup/Salad

Description & Serving	Cal	Fat	Sfat	Sod	Carb	Fiber	Sugar	Prot
Chicken Noodle Soup	180	8	4	330	14	1	4	11
Clam Chowder Soup	170	11	7	260	10	0	1	4
Vegetable Beef Soup	140	5	0	1290	17	3	3	7
Grilled Chicken Salad Deluxe	290	10	5	770	15	4	8	36
Chicken Strip Salad Deluxe	590	29	5	1180	44	4	7	42
Fit-Fare Grilled Chicken Breast Salad	290	10	5	770	15	4	8	36

Dressing/Condiment

Description & Serving	Cal	Fat	Sfat	Sod	Carb	Fiber	Sugar	Prot
Blue Cheese Dressing, 1 oz	160	17	3	205	1	0	1	1
French Dressing, 1 oz	74	5	0	248	8	0	4	0
Ranch Dressing, 1 oz	129	14	2	189	1	0	4	0
Thousand Island Dressing, 1 oz	107	10	2	275	5	0	4	0
Caesar Dressing, 1 oz	100	10	2	300	0	0	0	1
Honey Mustard Dressing, 1 oz	160	15	3	140	5	0	4	0
Fat Free Ranch Dressing, 1 oz	25	0	0	230	5	1	1	0
Fat Free Italian, 1 oz	9	0	0	367	3	0	2	0
Pico de Gallo, 3 oz	21	0	0	125	5	1	3	1
Croutons (for salad), 0.25 oz	90	3	0	240	15	0	0	3
Sour Cream, 1.5 oz	91	9	6	23	2	0	0	1
BBQ Sauce, 1.5 oz	91	0	0	364	21	0	18	0

Sandwich/Burger

Description & Serving	Cal	Fat	Sfat	Sod	Carb	Fiber	Sugar	Prot
Philly Melt	730	41	13	1680	51	3	5	40
Chicken Ranch Melt	920	42	11	2800	79	4	2	53
Spicy Buffalo Chicken Melt	940	46	11	3870	81	4	2	46
The Super Bird Sandwich	560	27	60	2360	43	2	3	38
Club Sandwich	660	34	7	1640	55	4	9	29
Grilled Chicken Sandwich w/ Honey Mustard Dressing	970	58	10	2070	69	4	25	39
Fit-Fare Chicken Sandwich w/ applesauce	490	7	1.5	1460	67	5	24	38
Bacon, Lettuce & Tomato Sandwich	570	37	9	850	36	2	7	20
Western Burger	1300	82	30	2700	83	6	18	58
Mushroom Swiss Burger	900	54	22	2140	59	6	14	47
Bacon Cheddar Burger	1100	72	31	2660	55	6	12	61
Classic Burger w/ Cheese	930	58	25	2190	56	5	13	49
Double Cheeseburger	1540	116	52	3880	33	5	9	92

Description & Serving	Cal	Fat	Sfat	Sod	Carb	Fiber	Sugar	Prot
Classic Burger	770	45	17	1560	56	5	13	39
Boca Burger	500	15	4	1320	62	10	12	30
Fit Fare Boca Burger	410	8	3	770	60	17	12	25

Entrée

Grilled Shrimp Skewers w/ rice pilaf	370	10	2	1140	39	2	2	32
Mushroom Swiss Chop'd Steak w/ gravy	930	75	29	1930	18	1	4	46
Chicken Strips, 4	560	24	0	1300	41	0	2	45
Grilled Chicken Dinner	280	4	1	1190	4	0	2	55
Fit Fare Grilled Chicken Dinner	380	10	2	1280	12	2	6	56
Country Fried Steak	1000	65	22	2580	54	6	1	51
Meat Loaf Dinner	880	68	26	2450	17	0	6	49
T-bone Steak & Shrimp Skewer Dinner	830	60	26	900	0	0	0	72
T-bone Steak & Breaded Shrimp Dinner	930	64	27	1490	20	2	5	68
T-bone Steak	740	56	25	740	0	0	0	59
Top Sirloin Steak & Breaded Shrimp	440	15	4	1470	23	2	7	52
Top Sirloin Steak & Shrimp Skewers	310	9	3	760	1	0	1	55
Top Sirloin Steak	220	6	2	600	1	0	1	41
Fish & Chips (French Fries)	1080	49	9	1650	117	8	0	40
Grilled Tilapia w/ rice pilaf	550	19	4	1420	37	1	2	53
Fit Fare Grilled Tilapia w/ rice pilaf, corn, tomato slices	600	11	3	1560	66	3	7	58
Lemon Pepper Tilapia w/ rice pilaf	640	27	14	1520	41	2	3	55

Side

Seasoned Fries	510	33	6	1010	48	5	0	6
French Fries, salted	450	23	4	250	57	6	0	6
Onion Rings	520	36	2	980	48	6	5	53
Side Garden Salad w/o dressing	113	7	5	150	7	2	4	7
Coleslaw	260	22	3.5	520	15	3	12	2
Corn	130	3	0	250	26	1	3	4
Cottage Cheese	70	2	1	300	5	0	3	9
Country Fried Potatoes	390	28	6	560	30	10	0	3
Mashed Potatoes, plain	170	7	1	510	76	1	1	2
Mixed Vegetables	60	3	0.5	60	5	1	2	1
Onion Rings	520	36	2	980	48	3	5	6
Breaded Shrimp, 6	190	8	2	750	20	2	4	9
Grilled Shrimp Skewer, 1	90	3.5	1	160	0	0	0	14
Sliced Tomatoes, 3	10	0	0	3	2	1	2	1
Vegetable Rice Pilaf	200	3	0	820	37	1	2	4
Dinner Rolls	260	9	4	330	38	1	8	5
Garlic Dinner Bread, 2	170	9	2	350	21	1	0	4
Butter Roll, 2	260	9	5	330	38	1	8	5

Seniors

Senior Scrambled Egg & Cheddar w/ pancakes	800	47	18	2060	58	3	10	33
Senior French Toast Slam w/ 1 egg	300	14	4	530	31	1	6	14
Senior Belgian Waffle Slam w/ egg	450	31	16	640	29	0	1	15
Sr. Omelette	480	37	15	820	6	1	3	27
Sr. Starter	210	19	6	290	1	1	0	9

Description & Serving	Cal	Fat	Sfat	Sod	Carb	Fiber	Sugar	Prot
Sr. Bacon Cheddar Burger	630	41	17	890	29	2	7	36
Senior Club	580	33	6	1650	40	3	7	27
Grilled Cheese Deluxe Sandwich	540	30	12	1540	50	2	5	17
Shrimp Skewer w/ rice	290	6	2	980	39	2	2	18
Meatloaf w/ gravy	570	45	17	1330	9	0	3	32
Grilled Tilapia	260	5	2	490	0	0	0	49
Senior Grilled Chicken Breast	140	2	0	590	2	0	1	28
Senior Country Fried Steak w/ gravy	530	34	12	1460	30	3	1	26
Senior Fish & Chips	770	36	6	860	87	7	0	23

Kids

Description & Serving	Cal	Fat	Sfat	Sod	Carb	Fiber	Sugar	Prot
Smiley-Alien Hotcakes w/ meat	410	18	8	1080	50	2	15	13
Smiley-Alien Hotcakes w/o meat	320	11	6	730	49	1	15	6
Space Saucers	440	17	7	1060	59	2	19	11
Junior Grand Slam	380	18	6	1050	39	2	7	15
Big Dipper French Toastix w/ meat	450	27	9	800	36	2	9	17
Big Dipper French Toastix	310	15	5	460	34	1	9	11
Mini Hot Dog in a Bun	330	17	6	940	33	1	4	11
Little Dipper Sampler	420	23	8	1200	82	1	3	16
Cosmic Cheeseburger	370	20	9	550	26	1	6	21
Flying Saucer Pizza	320	14	3.5	470	38	2	3	11
Galactic Grilled Cheese	360	20	7	550	32	1	5	10
Moons & Stars Chicken Nuggets w/ BBQ sauce	290	11	2.5	830	33	0	19	14
Macaroni & Cheese	340	11	3	830	48	2	11	12
Moon Crater Mashed w/ brown gravy	140	6	1	650	52	1	2	2
Astronaut Applesauce	110	2	0	40	24	2	15	1
Goldfish Galaxy	140	5	1	260	20	1	1	4
Deep Space French Fries	450	23	4	250	57	6	0	6
Far Out Fruit Medley	80	0	0	1	20	2	13	1
Anti-Gravity Grapes	55	0	0	0	29	4	13	1
Orbits of Oreo Sundae	410	18	9	310	59	2	39	6
Delicious Dip Sundae	300	16	11	90	36	1	46	4
Solar S'Cream - all flavors	113	6	4	21	13	0	10	2
Cosmos Milkshake - all flavors	400-580	17-31	17-31	120-170	54-63	1	40-69	10

Beverage

Description & Serving	Cal	Fat	Sfat	Sod	Carb	Fiber	Sugar	Prot
Hot Chocolate, 8 oz	100	2	2	219	28	1	24	3
Cappuccino French Vanilla, 8 oz	100	3	3	220	28	1	24	3
Strawberry Mango Pucker, 15 oz	220	0	0	10	56	1	52	0
Pineapple Cream, 15 oz	190	0	0	40	50	1	29	0
Razzdango, 15 oz	190	0	0	30	49	1	15	0
Island Fizz, 15 oz	190	0	0	20	47	0	27	0
Very Double Berry, 14 oz	280	0	0	10	69	0	62	0
OJ Mango, 14 oz	240	0	0	5	60	0	55	0
Cherry Limeade, 12 oz	180	0	0	30	45	0	12	0

Dessert/Dessert Topping

Description & Serving	Cal	Fat	Sfat	Sod	Carb	Fiber	Sugar	Prot
Apple Pie	510	23	9	610	72	3	35	4
Coconut Cream Pie	630	39	24	370	65	1	43	6

Description & Serving	Cal	Fat	Sfat	Sod	Carb	Fiber	Sugar	Prot
French Silk Pie	770	57	30	400	59	2	38	6
Apple Crisp a la Mode	750	21	9	570	134	4	91	7
Cheesecake	640	41	26	350	58	0	44	9
Cheesecake (no sugar added)	290	23	14	340	23	0	2	6
Carrot Cake	820	45	16	660	100	2	77	9
Hershey's Chocolate Cake	580	28	15	400	75	2	55	6
Hot Fudge Brownie a la mode	970	45	19	610	139	6	106	11
Neutron Brownie	400	20	7	250	55	3	39	4
Banana Split	810	31	18	190	125	5	95	12
Double Scoop/Sundae	280- 370	12- 18	7- 12	80- 135	38- 50	1	32- 48	5
Single Scoop/Sundae (Delicious Dip)	300	16	11	90	36	1	16	4
Milkshake (vanilla/chocolate)	560	26	16	272	76	<1	NP	11
Float (root beer or cola)	430	17	9	120	69	0	NP	6
Oreo Sundae	760	37	21	470	103	3	76	9
Oreo Blender Blaster	890	44	20	580	113	3	77	15
Chocolate Topping	140	0.4	0.2	120	36	1	NP	1
Cherry Topping	86	0	0	7	21	0	12	0
Fudge Topping	200	8	7	80	32	1	29	2
Strawberry Topping	70	0	0	15	19	1	NP	0
Whipped Cream	23	2	0	3	2	0	NP	0

Domino's Pizza

Medium 1-Topping Pizza, 1 slice

	Cal	Fat	Sfat	Sod	Carb	Fiber	Sugar	Prot
Hand Tossed Cheese Pizza	170	5	2.5	360	25	1	2	7
Thin Crust Cheese Pizza	140	7	2.5	240	14	1	1	5
Deep Dish Cheese Pizza	220	10	3.5	530	27	3	1	8

Toppings, per medium slice

	Cal	Fat	Sfat	Sod	Carb	Fiber	Sugar	Prot
Extra Cheese	25	2	1	85	1	0	0	2
Pepperoni	40	3.5	1	140	0	0	0	2
Ham	10	0	0	100	0	0	0	1
Sausage	45	3.5	1.5	130	1	0	0	2
Beef	40	3	1.5	70	0	0	0	2
Onions	0	0	0	0	1	0	0	0
Green Peppers	0	0	0	0	0	0	0	0
Mushrooms	0	0	0	0	0	0	0	0
Black Olives	10	1	0	65	1	0	0	0
Pineapple	5	0	0	0	2	0	2	0
American Cheese	40	3	2	190	0	0	0	2
Cheddar Cheese	30	2.5	1.5	45	0	0	0	2
Provolone Cheese	45	3.5	0	110	0	0	0	3
Anchovies	0	0	0	35	0	0	0	0
Bacon	40	3	1	100	0	0	0	3
Chicken	15	0.5	0	90	0	0	0	3
Philly Meat	10	0	0	60	0	0	0	2
Green Olives	15	1.5	0	95	0	0	0	0

Description & Serving	Cal	Fat	Sfat	Sod	Carb	Fiber	Sugar	Prot
Garlic	10	0	0	0	1	0	0	0
Banana Peppers	0	0	0	40	0	0	0	0
Jalapeno	0	0	0	135	0	0	0	0
Green Chile Peppers	0	0	0	0	0	0	0	0

Large 1-Topping Pizza, 1 slice

Description & Serving	Cal	Fat	Sfat	Sod	Carb	Fiber	Sugar	Prot
Hand Tossed Cheese Pizza	240	8	3	490	34	2	3	10
Thin Crust Cheese Pizza	180	10	3.5	340	19	1	2	7
Deep Dish Cheese Pizza	330	14	5	760	40	5	2	12

Toppings, per large slice

Description & Serving	Cal	Fat	Sfat	Sod	Carb	Fiber	Sugar	Prot
Extra Cheese	30	2.5	1.5	120	1	0	0	2
Pepperoni	50	4.5	1.5	190	0	0	0	2
Ham	15	0.5	0	135	0	0	0	2
Sausage	60	5	2	180	2	1	0	2
Beef	50	4.5	2	100	0	0	0	3
Onions	0	0	0	0	1	0	0	0
Green Peppers	0	0	0	0	1	0	0	0
Mushrooms	5	0	0	0	1	0	0	1
Black Olives	15	1	0	90	1	0	0	0
Pineapple	10	0	0	0	3	0	3	0
American Cheese	45	4	2.5	220	0	0	0	2
Cheddar Cheese	35	3	2	55	0	0	0	2
Provolone Cheese	60	4.5	3	160	0	0	0	5
Anchovies	0	0	0	35	0	0	0	0
Bacon	60	4	1.5	150	0	0	0	4
Chicken	25	1	0	130	1	0	0	4
Philly Meat	15	0.5	0	85	0	0	0	2
Green Olives	20	2	0	125	1	0	0	0
Garlic	15	0	0	0	1	0	0	0
Banana Peppers	5	0	0	50	1	0	1	0
Jalapeno	5	0	0	180	1	0	1	0
Green Chile Peppers	0	0	0	0	0	0	0	0
Tomatoes	0	0	0	25	1	0	1	0

Large Specialty Pizza, 1 slice

Description & Serving	Cal	Fat	Sfat	Sod	Carb	Fiber	Sugar	Prot
America's Favorite Feast	170	13	6	640	5	1	1	9
Deluxe Feast	130	10	4.5	510	5	1	1	7
Extravaganzza	200	15	7	780	7	1	1	11
Hawaiian Feast	120	8	4.5	550	7	1	3	8
Meatzza Feast	200	15	7	780	5	1	1	12
Pepperoni Feast	180	15	7	730	5	1	1	10
Vegi Feast	110	8	4	480	6	1	1	7
Bacon Cheeseburger Feast	190	15	7	640	4	1	1	11
Barbeque Feast	170	11	6	550	11	0	5	8
Philly Cheesesteak Feast	130	9	6	470	2	0	1	9
Brooklyn Style Cheese	240	10	5	560	27	2	3	12
Brooklyn Style Extra Large Pepperoni	60	5	2	210	0	0	0	2
Honolulu Hawaiian	340	15	7	710	35	2	4	16

Description & Serving	Cal	Fat	Sfat	Sod	Carb	Fiber	Sugar	Prot
Buffalo Chicken	350	17	8	800	33	1	2	18
Cali Chicken Bacon Ranch	430	24	9	850	34	1	2	21
Fiery Hawaiian	340	15	7	790	36	2	4	16
Memphis Barbecue Chicken	360	16	7	700	38	2	6	18
TC Pacific Coast Veggie	230	13	6	440	20	2	2	11

Sandwich

Chicken Bacon Ranch Oven Baked Sandwich	890	45	16	2210	72	2	3	49
Chicken Parm Oven Baked Sandwich	770	30	16	2130	73	3	3	51
Italian Oven Baked Sandwich	880	45	22	2560	71	3	3	47
Philly Cheese Steak Oven Baked Sandwich	690	27	14	2080	72	3	4	41

Side

Breadsticks, 1	110	6	1.5	100	11	0	1	2
Cheesy Bread, 1	120	6	2	150	11	0	1	4
Cinna Stix, 1	120	6	1	85	14	1	3	2
Buffalo Chicken Kickers, 2	100	4.5	0.5	280	7	1	0	9
Barbeque Buffalo Wings, 2	230	14	3.5	410	6	0	4	17
Hot Buffalo Wings, 2	200	14	3.5	690	2	0	0	16
Garden Fresh Salad, 1/2	70	4	2.5	80	5	2	2	4
Grilled Chicken Caesar Salad, 1/2	100	4.5	2	310	6	2	2	10

Dressing/Condiment/Topping

Blue Cheese Dipping Sauce, 43 g	210	22	4	390	2	0	2	1
Garlic Dipping Sauce, 28 g	250	28	5	160	0	0	0	0
Hot Dipping Sauce, 43 g	50	4.5	0.5	1480	3	0	1	0
Italian Dipping Sauce, 57 g	25	0	0	270	5	1	4	1
Marinara Dipping Sauce, 57 g	25	0	0	270	5	1	4	1
Parmesan Peppercorn Dipping Sauce, 43 g	190	21	3	390	2	0	1	0
Ranch Dipping Sauce, 43 g	190	21	3	390	2	0	1	0
Sweet Icing Dipping Sauce, 71 g	250	2.5	0.5	0	57	0	55	0
Croutons	45	2	0	70	6	0	0	1
Blue Cheese Dressing, 43 g	230	24	5	450	2	0	2	2
Buttermilk Ranch Dressing, 43 g	220	24	4	420	2	0	2	1
Creamy Caesar Dressing, 43 g	210	22	3.5	510	2	0	1	1
Light Italian Dressing, 43 g	20	1	0	780	2	0	2	0
Golden Italian Dressing, 43 g	220	23	3.5	370	2	0	2	0

Pasta

Chicken Alfredo Pasta in Dish	600	29	16	1080	58	2	2	27
Chicken Alfredo BreadBowl Pasta	700	25	11	1070	93	3	4	26
Chicken Carbonara Pasta in Dish	670	35	18	1220	59	2	2	32
Chicken Carbonara BreadBowl Pasta	740	28	12	1140	94	3	4	28
Italian Sausage Marinara Pasta in Dish	670	32	15	1760	66	5	9	28
Italian Sausage Marinara BreadBowl Pasta	730	26	11	1410	97	4	9	26
3-Cheese Mac-N-Cheese Pasta in Dish	670	34	22	1780	61	2	4	29
3-Cheese Mac-N-Cheese BreadBowl Pasta	730	28	14	1420	95	3	5	27
Pasta Primavera Pasta in Dish	540	27	16	770	59	3	3	16
Pasta Primavera BreadBowl Pasta	670	24	11	910	94	4	5	20

Description & Serving	Cal	Fat	Sfat	Sod	Carb	Fiber	Sugar	Prot
Donatos								

Thin Crust Pizza, 1/4 of large

Description & Serving	Cal	Fat	Sfat	Sod	Carb	Fiber	Sugar	Prot
Pepperoni	627	34	15	1471	50	2	9	32
Serious Cheese	627	34	16	1543	51	2	9	34
The Works	689	37	15	1716	56	4	11	35
Vegy	544	24	11	1675	57	4	13	26
Founder's Favorite	702	38	16	2344	52	2	10	39
Classic Trio	674	37	15	1715	52	3	10	35
Mariachi Beef	630	32	15	1551	55	3	12	32
Mariachi Chicken	639	30	15	1723	56	3	12	35
Hawaiian	588	27	10	1541	56	4	14	32
Chicken Vegy Medley	497	20	8	1444	51	3	10	31
Serious Meat	736	42	17	1973	52	3	10	44
Spinach	611	34	16	1306	51	2	9	29
White	690	42	21	1531	49	1	8	34
BBQ Chicken	792	26	12	1928	66	2	24	34
Margherita	622	36	14	1164	48	2	12	30
Pepperoni Zinger	656	36	15	1386	50	2	13	34
Chicken Spinach Mozzarella	643	34	14	1367	49	2	10	36

Thicker Crust Pizza, 1/4 of large

Description & Serving	Cal	Fat	Sfat	Sod	Carb	Fiber	Sugar	Prot
Pepperoni	798	39	16	1740	76	4	4	37
Serious Cheese	798	38	17	1812	77	4	4	40
The Works	847	41	16	1948	81	6	6	40
Vegy	715	29	12	1944	83	6	7	32
Founder's Favorite	858	42	16	2522	78	4	5	44
Classic Trio	832	41	16	1947	78	5	5	40
Mariachi Beef	796	36	16	1814	81	5	6	37
Mariachi Chicken	806	35	16	1978	81	4	6	40
Hawaiian	758	32	11	1810	82	5	8	38
Chicken Vegy Medley	657	24	9	1599	75	3	3	37
Serious Meat	907	47	18	2241	78	4	5	50
Margherita	782	41	15	1280	71	3	6	36
Pepperoni Zinger	827	41	17	1655	76	4	8	40
Chicken Spinach Mozzarella	803	39	15	1482	73	3	4	42

Hand Tossed Pizza, 2 slices

Description & Serving	Cal	Fat	Sfat	Sod	Carb	Fiber	Sugar	Prot
Pepperoni	499	27	12	1439	65	5	20	23
Serious Cheese	597	25	14	1324	65	5	10	27
The Works	669	31	14	1622	68	6	11	28
Vegy	550	19	10	1489	70	6	12	22
Founder's Favorite	678	31	14	2069	66	5	10	30
Classic Trio	658	31	14	1621	66	5	10	27
Mariachi Beef	591	24	12	1361	68	5	11	24
Mariachi Chicken	617	24	12	1498	68	5	11	28
Hawaiian	578	22	9	1360	69	6	13	26
Chicken Vegy Medley	517	17	7	1038	63	5	6	24
Serious Meat	735	37	16	1907	66	5	10	35

Description & Serving	Cal	Fat	Sfat	Sod	Carb	Fiber	Sugar	Prot
BBQ Chicken	630	22	11	1564	73	4	17	29
Margherita	583	27	11	959	60	4	10	24
Pepperoni Zinger	645	30	14	1428	65	5	12	27
Chicken Spinach Mozzarella	587	25	10	1061	61	4	8	27
Fresh Mozzarella Trio	701	34	15	1541	66	5	13	30

No Dough Pizza, whole

Pepperoni	499	35	16	1226	17	2	3	31
Serious Cheese	457	31	17	1201	17	2	3	31
The Works	547	37	17	1416	21	4	5	34
Founders Favorite	558	38	17	2003	18	3	4	38
Classic Trio	532	37	17	1415	18	3	4	34
Mariachi Beef	528	34	18	1310	23	4	6	35
Mariachi Chicken	495	30	16	1498	21	4	6	38
Hawaiian	436	26	12	1199	22	4	8	30
Chicken Vegy Medley	495	29	15	1567	20	3	5	41
Serious Meat	653	46	21	1874	19	3	4	47
Pepperoni Zinger	584	42	19	1221	17	3	8	37
Fresh Mozzarella Meatball	502	33	14	1327	21	3	8	31

Flatbread Pizza, whole

3 Meat	689	31	13	1873	67	5	7	34
Cheese	693	31	15	1773	66	5	7	35
Deluxe	613	25	10	1588	68	5	8	28
Pepperoni	716	34	14	1775	67	5	7	34
Vegy	606	24	10	1877	69	5	7	27

Salad

Side Italian Salad	104	8	4	289	4	1	2	7
Side Harvest Salad	81	3	0	25	13	2	11	1
Entrée Italian Chef Salad	268	19	9	873	8	3	5	19
Entrée Chicken Harvest Salad	410	23	6	762	30	6	22	26

Sandwich

Big Don Italian Sub on White	717	34	13	2239	68	3	5	35
Big Don Italian Sub on White w/ Pizza Sauce	656	26	11	2168	70	4	6	36
Big Don Sausage Italian Sub on White	998	56	21	3001	69	3	6	53
Big Don Sausage Sub on White w/ Pizza Sauce	936	48	19	2928	71	4	6	54
Big Don Fresh Vegy Sub on White	540	19	7	1597	71	5	5	22
Big Steak Hoagie on White w/ Mushroom Gravy	801	39	17	2304	68	3	2	44
Big Steak Hoagie on White w/ Pizza Sauce	806	39	17	2273	69	3	4	45
Meatball Sub on White	1119	63	28	3108	78	8	8	60
Turkey Club Sub on White	743	30	10	2185	66	3	5	49
Chicken Bacon Cheddar Sub on White	818	37	15	1874	68	3	4	48
Roast Beef & Provolone Sub on White	803	39	14	1626	70	5	5	46
Big Steak Hoagie on White	801	39	17	2304	68	3	2	44
Big Don Italian Sub on Wheat	709	34	13	2170	68	6	5	35
Big Don on Wheat w/ Pizza Sauce	648	26	11	2099	69	7	7	36
Big Don Sausage Italian Sub on Wheat	990	56	21	2932	69	6	6	54
Big Don Sausage on Wheat w/ Pizza Sauce	928	48	19	2859	70	7	7	54
Big Ham & Cheese Sub on Wheat	612	23	8	2060	69	6	6	36

Description & Serving	Cal	Fat	Sfat	Sod	Carb	Fiber	Sugar	Prot
Turkey Club Sub on Wheat	735	30	10	2116	66	6	5	49
Chicken Bacon Cheddar Sub on Wheat	810	37	15	1805	68	6	4	48
Roast Beef & Provolone Sub on Wheat	796	40	14	1557	70	8	5	46
Fresh Vegy Sub on Wheat	532	19	7	1527	71	8	5	22
Meatball Sub on Wheat	1119	63	28	3108	78	8	8	60
Big Steak Hoagie on Wheat w/ Mushroom Gravy	794	39	17	2235	68	5	2	44
Big Steak Hoagie on Wheat w/ Pizza Sauce	798	39	17	2204	69	6	4	45

Sides/Wings

Breadsticks w/ Pizza Sauce, 2	261	9	2	513	38	3	4	7
Breadsticks w/ Nacho Cheese Sauce, 2	398	22	8	1032	39	2	2	13
3 Cheese Garlic Bread, 1/4 serving	174	9	4	390	16	1	1	8
Chicken Breast Strips, 2	125	4	1	612	12	0	0	11
Wedge Fries, side portion	261	13	3	486	34	6	0	4
Buffalo Wings - Plain, 5	552	43	10	1297	10	0	0	34
Buffalo Wings - Mild, 5	618	48	10	2355	13	0	2	34
Buffalo Wings - Hot, 5	597	48	11	2236	11	0	0	34
Buffalo Wings - BBQ, 5	595	43	10	1623	10	0	9	34
Buffalo Wings - Garlic, 5	669	56	12	1537	12	0	1	34
Buffalo Wings - Spicy, 5	713	60	13	2476	23	0	1	34

Dressing/Condiment/Topping

House Italian Dressing, 1.5 oz	230	24	4	460	1	0	1	0
Light Italian Dressing, 1.5 oz	20	1	0	770	2	0	2	0
Chicken Bacon Ranch Pizza Dip, 3 oz	450	47	7	790	4	0	3	1
Buttermilk Ranch Dressing, 1.5 oz	230	24	3.5	380	2	0	1	1
Fat Free Ranch Dressing, 1.5 oz	45	0	0	540	10	1	4	0
Tuscan Caesar Dressing, 1.5 oz	180	18	3	490	3	0	2	1
Dijon Honey Mustard Dressing, 1.5 oz	200	18	3	250	8	1	8	1
Blue Cheese Dressing, 1.5 oz	230	24	4.5	440	2	0	2	2
Honey French Dressing, 1.5 oz	220	18	3	310	14	0	13	0
Thousand Island Dressing, 1.5 oz	220	21	3	360	7	0	7	0
Roasted Red Pepper Croutons, 0.5 oz	50	3	0	85	5	0	0	1
Apple Cider Vinaigrette, 1.5 oz	140	12	2	40	8	0	8	0

Dessert

Chocolate Chunk Cookie	430	21	10	330	57	2	34	6
Apple Timpano, 2 slices	406	9	3	463	72	3	39	8
Cinnamon Timpano, 2 slices	523	22	8	478	73	2	36	9

Dunkin' Donuts

Cold Beverage

Watermelon Coolatta, 16 oz	250	0	0	55	60	0	59	0
Grape Coolatta, 16 oz	240	0	0	55	59	0	58	0
Vanilla Bean Coolatta, 16 oz	430	6	3.5	170	90	0	86	3
Coffee Coolatta, 16 oz	330	23	14	60	28	0	23	3
Coffee Coolatta w/ Milk, 16 oz	170	4	2.5	75	29	0	29	4
Coffee Coolatta w/ Skim Milk, 16 oz	140	0	0	75	30	0	29	4
Tropicana Orange Coolatta, 16 oz	220	0	0	35	52	0	50	1

Description & Serving	Cal	Fat	Sfat	Sod	Carb	Fiber	Sugar	Prot
Strawberry Fruit Coolatta, 16 oz	300	0	0	40	72	0	65	0
Frozen Cappuccino w/ Skim Milk, 16 oz	280	0	0	105	62	0	53	5
Frozen Cappuccino w/ Whole Milk, 16 oz	300	4	2.5	105	61	0	53	5
Iced Coffee, 16 oz	10	0	0	5	2	0	0	1
Iced Coffee w/ Skim Milk & Splenda, 16 oz	30	0	0	25	5	0	2	2
Iced Coffee w/ Cream, 16 oz	70	6	4	20	3	0	0	1
Iced Coffee w/ Cream & Sugar, 16 oz	120	6	4	20	20	0	17	1
Iced Coffee w/ Milk, 16 oz	30	1	1	20	3	0	1	2
Iced Coffee w/ Milk & Sugar, 16 oz	90	1	1	20	21	0	19	2
Iced Coffee w/ Skim Milk, 16 oz	20	0	0	25	3	0	2	2
Iced Coffee w/ Skim Milk & Sugar, 16 oz	80	0	0	25	21	0	19	2
Iced Coffee w/ Sugar, 16 oz	70	0	0	5	19	0	17	1
Mocha Spice Iced Latte, 16 oz	220	6	4	95	35	1	32	7
Iced Latte Lite, 16 oz	120	0	0	170	19	0	15	10
Mocha Raspberry Iced Latte, 16 oz	230	6	4	110	36	1	32	7
Iced Latte, 16 oz	120	6	3.5	105	10	0	10	6
Iced Latte w/ Sugar, 16 oz	170	6	3.5	100	27	0	27	6
Iced Caramel Swirl Latte, 16 oz	220	6	3.5	150	35	0	34	8
Iced Mocha Swirl Latte, 16 oz	220	6	4	115	35	1	32	7
Iced Latte w/ Skim Milk & Sugar, 16 oz	130	0	0	110	28	0	27	7
Iced Caramel Swirl Latte w/ Skim Milk, 16 oz	180	0	0	150	36	0	35	9
Iced Mocha Swirl Latte w/ Skim Milk, 16 oz	180	0	0	125	36	1	32	8
Iced Latte w/ Skim Milk, 16 oz	70	0	0	110	11	0	10	7
Iced Latte Lite, 16 oz	80	0	0	110	13	0	10	7
Vanilla Iced Latte Lite, 16 oz	90	0	0	110	14	0	10	7
Freshly Brewed Unsweetened Iced Tea, 16 oz	5	0	0	0	1	0	0	0
Freshly Brewed Sweetened Iced Tea, 16 oz	80	0	0	0	20	0	19	0
Raspberry Flavored Iced Tea, 16 oz	10	0	0	0	3	0	0	0
Peach Flavored Iced Tea, 16 oz	15	0	0	0	3	0	0	0
Raspberry Flavored Sweetened Iced Tea, 16 oz	90	0	0	0	22	0	19	0
Peach Flavored Sweetened Iced Tea, 16 oz	90	0	0	0	22	0	19	0

Hot Beverage

Description & Serving	Cal	Fat	Sfat	Sod	Carb	Fiber	Sugar	Prot
Coffee, 10 oz	5	0	0	5	1	0	0	0
Coffee w/ Skim Milk & Splenda, 10 oz	25	0	0	25	5	0	2	2
Coffee w/ Splenda, 10 oz	15	0	0	5	3	0	0	0
Coffee w/ Cream, 10 oz	60	6	4	20	2	0	0	1
Coffee w/ Cream & Sugar, 10 oz	120	6	4	20	19	0	17	1
Coffee w/ Milk, 10 oz	25	1	1	20	2	0	1	1
Coffee w/ Milk & Sugar, 10 oz	80	1	1	20	20	0	19	1
Coffee w/ Skim Milk, 10 oz	15	0	0	25	3	0	2	2
Coffee w/ Skim Milk & Sugar, 10 oz	70	0	0	25	20	0	19	2
Coffee w/ Sugar, 10 oz	60	0	0	5	18	0	17	0
Blueberry Coffee, 10 oz	15	0	0	5	2	0	0	0
Caramel Coffee, 10 oz	10	0	0	5	2	0	0	0
Cinnamon Coffee, 10 oz	15	0	0	5	2	0	0	0
Hazelnut Coffee, 10 oz	10	0	0	10	2	0	0	0
Raspberry Coffee, 10 oz	15	0	0	5	3	0	0	0
Toasted Almond Coffee, 10 oz	15	0	0	5	2	0	0	1

Description & Serving	Cal	Fat	Sfat	Sod	Carb	Fiber	Sugar	Prot
French Vanilla Coffee, 10 oz	10	0	0	10	2	0	0	0
Coconut Coffee, 10 oz	10	0	0	5	2	0	0	0
Mocha Spice Latte, 10 oz	220	6	4	95	35	1	32	7
Latte Lite, 16 oz	120	0	0	170	19	0	15	10
Vanilla Latte Lite, 16 oz	130	0	0	170	20	0	15	10
Mocha Raspberry Latte, 10 oz	230	6	4	110	36	1	32	7
Latte, 10 oz	120	6	3.5	105	10	0	10	6
Latte w/ Sugar, 10 oz	170	6	3.5	100	27	0	27	6
Caramel Swirl Latte, 10 oz	220	6	3.5	150	35	0	34	8
Mocha Swirl Latte, 10 oz	220	6	4	115	35	1	32	7
Cappuccino, 10 oz	80	4	2.5	70	7	0	7	4
Cappuccino w/ Sugar, 10 oz	140	4	2.5	70	24	0	24	4
Espresso, 1.75 oz	0	0	0	0	0	0	0	0
Espresso w/ Sugar, 1.75 oz	30	0	0	5	7	0	7	0
Latte Lite, 20 oz	80	0	0	110	13	0	10	7
Vanilla Latte Lite, 20 oz	90	0	0	110	14	0	10	7
Dunkaccino, 20 oz	230	11	9	190	35	1	24	2
Turbo Shot, 1.75 oz	0	0	0	0	0	0	0	0
Hot Chocolate, 10 oz	210	7	7	270	39	2	30	2
White Hot Chocolate, 10 oz	230	9	7	310	38	0	31	2
Sweet Tea, 16 oz	120	0	0	0	29	0	28	0
Earl Grey Tea, 10 oz	0	0	0	5	0	0	0	0
English Breakfast Tea, 10 oz	0	0	0	5	0	0	0	0
Decaffeinated Tea, 10 oz	0	0	0	5	0	0	0	0
Green Tea, 10 oz	0	0	0		0	0	0	0
Freshly Brewed Unsweetened Tea, 10 oz	0	0	0	5	0	0	0	0
Freshly Brewed Tea w/ Milk, 10 oz	20	1	0.5	20	1	0	1	1
Decaffeinated Tea w/ Milk, 10 oz	20	1	0.5	20	1	0	1	1
English Breakfast Tea w/ Milk, 10 oz	20	1	0.5	20	1	0	1	1
Earl Grey Tea w/ Milk, 10 oz	20	1	0.5	20	1	0	1	1
Green Tea w/ Milk, 10 oz	20	1	0.5	20	1	0	1	1
Freshly Brewed Tea w/ Milk & Sugar, 10 oz	80	1	0.5	20	19	0	19	1
Decaffeinated Tea w/ Milk & Sugar, 10 oz	80	1	0.5	20	19	0	19	1
English Breakfast Tea w/ Milk & Sugar, 10 oz	80	1	0.5	20	19	0	19	1
Earl Grey Tea w/ Milk & Sugar, 10 oz	80	1	0.5	20	19	0	19	1
Green Tea w/ Milk & Sugar, 10 oz	80	1	0.5	20	19	0	19	1
Freshly Brewed Tea w/ Skim Milk, 10 oz	10	0	0	20	2	0	2	1
Decaffeinated Tea w/ Skim Milk, 10 oz	10	0	0	20	2	0	2	1
English Breakfast Tea w/ Skim Milk, 10 oz	10	0	0	20	2	0	2	1
Earl Grey Tea w/ Skim Milk, 10 oz	10	0	0	20	2	0	2	1
Green Tea w/ Skim Milk, 10 oz	10	0	0	20	2	0	2	1
Freshly Brewed Tea w/ Skim Milk & Sugar, 10 oz	70	0	0	20	19	0	19	1
Decaffeinated Tea w/ Skim Milk & Sugar, 10 oz	70	0	0	20	19	0	19	1
English Breakfast Tea w/ Skim Milk & Sugar, 10 oz	70	0	0	20	19	0	19	1
Earl Grey Tea w/ Skim Milk & Sugar, 10 oz	70	0	0	20	19	0	19	1
Green Tea w/ Skim Milk & Sugar, 10 oz	70	0	0	20	19	0	19	1
Freshly Brewed Tea w/ Sugar, 10 oz	60	0	0	5	17	0	17	0
Decaffeinated Tea w/ Sugar, 10 oz	60	0	0	5	17	0	17	0
English Breakfast Tea w/ Sugar, 10 oz	60	0	0	5	17	0	17	0

Description & Serving	Cal	Fat	Sfat	Sod	Carb	Fiber	Sugar	Prot
Earl Grey Tea w/ Sugar, 10 oz	60	0	0	5	17	0	17	0
Green Tea w/ Sugar, 10 oz	60	0	0	5	17	0	17	0
Vanilla Chai, 14 oz	330	9	8	170	53	0	46	11

Donut

Description & Serving	Cal	Fat	Sfat	Sod	Carb	Fiber	Sugar	Prot
Pumpkin Donut	320	18	8	270	36	1	17	3
Apple Crumb Donut	460	14	8	330	80	2	49	4
Apple 'n Spice Donut	240	11	4.5	320	32	1	8	3
Bavarian Kreme Donut	250	12	5	330	31	1	9	3
Blueberry Cake Donut	330	18	8	460	38	1	19	3
Blueberry Crumb Donut	470	14	8	330	84	2	52	4
Boston Kreme Donut	280	12	5	350	38	1	16	3
Chocolate Coconut Cake Donut	400	22	11	410	49	2	30	3
Chocolate Frosted Cake Donut	340	19	8	330	38	1	19	3
Chocolate Frosted Donut	230	10	4	330	32	1	13	3
Chocolate Glazed Cake Donut	280	15	7	400	33	1	16	3
Chocolate Kreme Filled Donut	310	16	7	340	37	1	17	4
Cinnamon Cake Donut	290	18	8	310	30	1	12	3
Double Chocolate Cake Donut	290	16	7	410	34	1	17	3
Glazed Cake Donut	320	18	8	310	37	1	18	3
Glazed Donut	220	9	4	320	31	1	12	3
Jelly Filled Donut	260	11	5	330	36	1	6	3
Maple Frosted Donut	230	10	4	330	33	1	14	3
Marble Frosted Donut	230	10	4	330	32	1	13	3
Old Fashioned Cake Donut	280	18	8	310	27	1	9	3
Powdered Cake Donut	300	18	8	310	30	1	12	3
Strawberry Frosted Donut	230	10	4	330	33	1	14	3
Sugar Raised Donut	190	9	4	320	22	1	4	3
Vanilla Kreme Filled Donut	320	17	8	340	37	1	18	3
French Cruller	250	20	9	105	18	0	10	2
Apple Fritter	400	15	6	530	63	2	22	5
Chocolate Iced Bismark	350	14	5	460	53	1	22	4
Bow Tie Donut	310	15	7	400	39	1	15	4
Chocolate Frosted Coffee Roll	380	19	8	530	50	2	18	5
Coffee Roll	370	18	7	510	49	2	17	5
Éclair	350	14	5	460	53	1	22	4
Glazed Fritter	400	15	6	530	63	2	22	5
Maple Frosted Coffee Roll	380	18	8	520	50	2	19	5
Vanilla Frosted Coffee Roll	380	18	8	520	50	2	19	5
Cinnamon Cake Munchkin	60	3	1.5	60	6	0	2	1
Glazed Cake Munchkin	60	3	1.5	65	8	0	4	1
Plain Cake Munchkin	50	3	1.5	60	5	0	2	1
Powdered Cake Munchkin	60	3.5	1.5	60	6	0	3	1
Glazed Chocolate Cake Munchkin	60	3	1.5	90	8	0	4	1
Glazed Munchkin	50	2.5	1	65	7	0	3	1
Jelly Filled Munchkin	60	2.5	1	65	8	0	1	1
Sugar Raised Munchkin	40	2.5	1	65	5	0	1	1
Plain Cake Stick	300	20	9	300	26	1	9	3
Glazed Cake Stick	340	20	9	300	38	1	20	3
Jelly Stick	400	20	9	320	54	1	20	3

Description & Serving	Cal	Fat	Sfat	Sod	Carb	Fiber	Sugar	Prot
Powdered Cake Stick	320	20	9	300	31	1	13	3
Cinnamon Cake Stick	310	20	9	300	30	1	12	3
Glazed Chocolate Cake Stick	390	25	11	540	40	2	17	3
Danish/Muffin/Biscuit								
Apple Cheese Danish	330	16	7	270	41	1	18	4
Cheese Danish	330	17	8	270	39	1	17	5
Strawberry Cheese Danish	320	16	7	260	40	1	18	4
Blueberry Muffin	510	16	1.5	490	87	3	51	6
Reduced Fat Blueberry Muffin	450	10	1.5	670	86	3	45	6
Chocolate Chip Muffin	630	23	6	520	98	5	59	8
Coffee Cake Muffin	620	25	7	530	93	2	54	7
Corn Muffin	510	17	2	860	84	2	36	6
Honey Bran Raisin Muffin	500	14	1.5	450	86	9	48	7
English Muffin	160	1.5	0	340	31	2	2	6
Biscuit	280	14	8	620	32	1	2	5
Bagel/Croissant								
Plain Bagel	330	3	0.5	780	71	3	0	14
Sesame Bagel	370	7	0.5	780	72	3	0	16
Poppy Seed Bagel	370	6	0.5	780	73	3	0	15
Onion Bagel	340	3.5	0.5	660	65	3	4	12
Wheat Bagel	350	4	0.5	650	66	5	5	13
Multigrain Bagel	400	9	1	600	65	10	2	18
Everything Bagel	360	5	0.5	780	74	3	0	15
Garlic Bagel	350	3.5	0.5	780	76	4	0	15
Salt Bagel	330	3	0.5	3540	71	3	0	14
Cinnamon Raisin Bagel	370	4	0.5	530	72	3	7	13
Plain Croissant	310	16	7	350	35	1	4	7
Cream Cheese, 50 g								
Reduced Fat Smoked Salmon Cream Cheese	140	11	7	260	6	0	3	4
Reduced Fat Blueberry Cream Cheese	150	9	6	210	15	0	11	2
Reduced Fat Strawberry Cream Cheese	150	10	6	200	15	0	11	2
Reduced Fat Veggie Cream Cheese	120	10	6	240	6	0	2	2
Reduced Fat Onion & Chive Cream Cheese	130	11	7	250	6	0	3	3
Reduced Fat Cream Cheese	100	8	5	250	5	0	2	4
Plain Cream Cheese	150	15	9	250	3	0	3	3
Breakfast Entrée								
Hash Browns, 9	200	11	1.5	730	22	3	0	2
Egg & Cheese on English Muffin	320	13	5	730	34	2	3	14
Egg & Cheese on Bagel	480	15	5	1180	75	3	2	22
Egg & Cheese on Croissant	470	28	12	750	39	1	6	15
Egg & Cheese on Biscuit	430	26	13	1010	36	1	4	13
Ham, Egg & Cheese on English Muffin	350	15	6	1040	35	2	3	21
Ham, Egg & Cheese on Bagel	520	17	6	1480	75	3	2	28
Ham, Egg & Cheese on Croissant	510	30	12	1050	39	1	6	21
Ham, Egg & Cheese on Biscuit	470	28	14	1320	36	1	4	19
Bacon, Egg & Cheese on English Muffin	360	16	6	920	35	2	4	18
Bacon, Egg & Cheese on Bagel	530	18	6	1370	76	3	2	26
Bacon, Egg & Cheese on Croissant	510	31	13	930	39	1	6	18

Description & Serving	Cal	Fat	Sfat	Sod	Carb	Fiber	Sugar	Prot
Bacon, Egg & Cheese on Biscuit	470	29	14	1200	36	1	4	16
Sausage, Egg & Cheese on English Muffin	490	28	10	1130	35	2	3	22
Sausage, Egg & Cheese on Bagel	660	29	11	1590	76	3	2	30
Sausage, Egg & Cheese on Croissant	640	42	17	1150	40	1	6	22
Sausage, Egg & Cheese on Biscuit	600	40	18	1410	37	1	4	20
Supreme Omelet & Cheese on English Muffin	350	15	7	1040	36	3	3	19
Supreme Omelet & Cheese on Bagel	520	17	7	1480	77	3	2	26
Supreme Omelet & Cheese on Croissant	500	30	14	1050	41	2	6	19
Supreme Omelet & Cheese on Biscuit	470	28	15	1310	37	2	4	17
Ham, Supreme Omelet & Cheese on English Muffin	390	16	8	1340	36	3	4	25
Ham, Supreme Omelet & Cheese on Bagel	560	18	8	1780	77	3	2	32
Ham, Supreme Omelet & Cheese on Croissant	540	31	14	1360	41	2	6	25
Ham, Supreme Omelet & Cheese on Biscuit	510	29	16	1620	38	2	4	23
Bacon, Supreme Omelet & Cheese on English Muffin	390	18	8	1220	36	3	4	22
Bacon, Supreme Omelet & Cheese on Bagel	560	20	8	1670	77	3	2	30
Bacon, Supreme Omelet & Cheese on Croissant	550	33	15	1230	41	2	7	22
Bacon, Supreme Omelet & Cheese on Biscuit	510	31	16	1500	38	2	4	21
Sausage, Supreme Omelet & Cheese on English Muffin	520	29	12	1440	37	3	4	26
Sausage, Supreme Omelet & Cheese on Bagel	690	31	13	1890	78	3	2	34
Sausage, Supreme Omelet & Cheese on Croissant	680	44	19	1450	41	2	6	26
Sausage, Supreme Omelet & Cheese on Biscuit	640	42	20	1710	38	2	4	24
Wake-Up Wrap	170	10	4	450	14	1	1	7
Wake-Up Wrap w/ Bacon	190	12	4.5	540	14	1	2	9

Salad/Soup

Caesar Salad	320	29	6	790	11	3	2	6
Chicken Caesar Salad	440	33	7	1020	11	3	2	25
Garden Salad	180	6	3	500	21	4	6	8
Broccoli Cheddar Soup	190	11	6	990	14	2	5	10
Chicken Noodle Soup	130	3	1	970	19	1	1	7

Sandwich

Pressed Cuban Sandwich	680	33	13	2000	50	2	6	46
Chicken Bruschetta Sandwich	580	26	7	1200	49	2	4	37
Chipotle Chicken Sandwich	600	25	8	1380	50	3	5	43
Pastrami Supreme Sandwich	750	39	16	2060	51	3	4	48
Turkey & Cheese Sandwich	450	13	4.5	1500	52	3	4	35
Tuna (Albacore) Sandwich	660	19	2.5	1280	56	3	9	31
Tuna Melt Sandwich	770	30	7	1560	57	3	8	36
Toasted Italian Sandwich	560	25	9	2630	52	3	5	33
Steak & Cheese Sandwich	470	16	6	2040	50	2	3	31
Turkey & Bacon Club Sandwich	440	13	3	1800	51	3	5	35
Egg White Veggie Flatbrad Sandwich	290	9	4	680	39	3	4	11
Egg White Turkey Sausage Flatbread Sandwich	280	6	2.5	820	37	3	5	19
Chicken Parmesan Flatbread Sandwich	480	22	7	1220	47	3	4	23
Ham & Swiss Flatbread Sandwich	340	12	5	1030	36	1	2	21
Turkey Cheddar & Bacon Flatbread Sandwich	390	19	7	1090	34	1	2	21
Grilled Cheese Flatbread Sandwich	370	18	9	830	33	1	2	17

Description & Serving	Cal	Fat	Sfat	Sod	Carb	Fiber	Sugar	Prot
Dessert								
Chocolate Chunk Cookie	540	23	13	550	80	3	48	7
Oatmeal Raisin Cookie	480	14	7	310	83	5	51	8
Brownie	430	23	5	260	56	1	47	3
Cinnamon Twist	210	11	5	300	25	1	12	3

Eat'n Park

Breakfast

Baked Goods

Description & Serving	Cal	Fat	Sfat	Sod	Carb	Fiber	Sugar	Prot
Bear Claw	515	23.96	NP	2936	66.38	2.49	NP	8.88
Boston Brown Bread, 2 slices	279	8.85	NP	908	42.72	1.44	NP	7.42
Cinnamon Biscuit (Mini)	130	5.04	NP	300	19.42	0.69	NP	2.21
Cinnamon Bun	270	9.93	NP	602	42.1	1.33	NP	3.78
Crumby Bun	193	9.36	NP	530	24.16	0.84	NP	3.15
Honey Bun	172	8.24	NP	404	22.17	0.67	NP	2.51
Apple Raisin Muffin	249	7.3	NP	292	43.03	1.52	NP	4.1
Banana Nut Muffin	284	12.56	NP	291	39.3	1.71	NP	5.19
Blueberry Muffin	242	7.82	NP	312	39.4	1.49	NP	4.22
Chocolate Nut Muffin	313	13.48	NP	322	44.75	1.67	NP	5.6
Corn Muffin	212	7.74	NP	509	31.14	1.36	NP	4.18
Cranberry Muffin	266	9.58	NP	295	41.2	1.34	NP	4.38
Mocha Java Muffin	222	8.77	NP	213	33.87	2.35	NP	2.14
Oat Bran Apple Raisin Muffin	296	10.2	NP	268	45.84	2.12	NP	6.29
Oat Bran Muffin	333	12.67	NP	334	47.46	2.12	NP	7.6
Pumpkin Raisin Muffin	259	7.8	NP	314	43.75	1.59	NP	4.65
Strawberry Crème Muffin	273	9.44	NP	327	43.2	1.19	NP	4.58
Strawberry Filled Muffin	280	9.09	NP	363	45.43	1.47	NP	4.86
Sticky Loaf	293	12.78	NP	827	39.92	1.2	NP	4.74
Pastry Bite	114	6.93	NP	46	11.39	0.26	NP	1.38
Plain Bagel	312	1.81	NP	606	60.55	2.61	NP	11.91
Raisin Bagel	320	1.74	NP	541	65.36	3.91	NP	11.08
Croissant	258	14.88	NP	75	26.58	0.89	NP	4.56

Eggs

Description & Serving	Cal	Fat	Sfat	Sod	Carb	Fiber	Sugar	Prot
Fried Egg	102	8.12	NP	156	0.56	0	NP	6.29
Poached Egg	77	5.28	NP	62	0.56	0	NP	6.26
2 Poached Eggs w/ toast & margarine	352	19.51	NP	449	25.93	1.15	NP	16.69
Egg Beater Breakfast	76	0.1	NP	209	5.6	1.61	NP	13.2
Rib-Eye Eggs	936	58.28	NP	1355	26.88	1.82	NP	71.13
T-Bone Eggs	890	55.09	NP	1291	26.88	1.82	NP	67
Bacon & Cheese Omelette	500	38.99	NP	1013	2.38	0	NP	32.77
Cheese Omelette	390	29.61	NP	709	2.27	0	NP	26.97
Ham & Cheese Omelette	463	32.4	NP	1316	3.02	0	NP	37.53
Meat Lovers Omelette	716	54.82	NP	2023	3.56	0	NP	49.25
Supreme Omelette	418	29.87	NP	734	8.6	1.7	NP	27.99
Western Omelette	344	21.08	NP	794	6.71	1.02	NP	30.01

Description & Serving	Cal	Fat	Sfat	Sod	Carb	Fiber	Sugar	Prot
Pancakes/Waffles								
Apple Cinnamon Pancake	499	15.8	NP	754	84.85	3.64	NP	6.8
Pancake	223	2.84	NP	710	42.65	1.59	NP	5.91
Blueberry Pancake	286	3.6	NP	889	55.09	2.37	NP	7.48
Apple Cinnamon Waffle	901	44.55	NP	1261	11.72	4.09	NP	16.97
Apple Waffles	960	44.45	NP	1259	125.57	4.31	NP	17.5
Belgian Waffles	623	31.6	NP	1221	68.74	2.03	NP	16.11
Specialty Breakfast								
Cornbeef Hash, 7.5 oz	341	23.06	NP	838	16.27	1.36	NP	16.27
French Toast, 1 pc	128	4.81	NP	180	13.78	0.58	NP	6.69
Plain Oatmeal	154	2.53	NP	3	26.9	4.26	NP	6.42
Oatmeal w/ bananas	317	5.51	NP	499	58	6.93	NP	11.9
Oatmeal w/ fruit	424	9.79	NP	605	67.67	7.06	NP	19.27
Oatmeal w/ milk	224	5.02	NP	498	34.34	4.51	NP	10.86
Breakfast Side/Condiment								
Toast, 1 slice, buttered	262	13.66	NP	399	29.71	1.38	NP	5.04
Toast, 1 slice, dry	134	1.8	NP	269	24.75	1.15	NP	4.1
Raisin Toast, 1 slice, buttered	244	13.79	NP	279	27.2	2.24	NP	4.23
Rye Toast, 1 slice, buttered	267	13.61	NP	499	30.92	3.71	NP	5.56
Sourdough Toast, 1 slice, buttered	237	13.25	NP	368	25.01	1.35	NP	4.52
Whole Wheat Toast, 1 slice, buttered	259	14.19	NP	414	29.51	4.42	NP	6.33
Bacon, 1 slice	37	3.13	NP	101	0.04	0	NP	1.93
Fruit Cup	60	0.49	NP	12	14.51	1.24	NP	1.15
Ham, 3 oz	110	4.19	NP	911	1.14	0	NP	15.84
Hash Browns, 6 oz	237	11.94	NP	278	28.15	2.92	NP	5.39
Homefries, 6 oz	208	11.86	NP	178	24.2	2.35	NP	2.25
Sausage, 1 pc	132	12.14	NP	273	0	0	NP	5.32
Maple Syrup, 2 oz	221	0	NP	95	60.13	0	NP	0
Reduced Maple Syrup, 2 oz	34	0	NP	133	8.64	0.98	NP	0
Sugar-Free Syrup, 2 oz	43	0	NP	167	10.8	1.22	NP	0
Appetizer								
Breaded Zucchini	415	23.09	NP	393	39.33	3.01	NP	13.07
Buffalo Chicken Tenders	434	21.2	NP	2606	24.3	1.95	NP	34.62
Cheese Fries	878	49.67	NP	665	93.07	8.14	NP	18.16
Cheese Sticks	411	24.61	NP	675	16.92	0.45	NP	29.61
Onion Rings	209	12.99	NP	219	19.49	1.32	NP	4.21
Southwest Quesadilla	853	49.83	NP	829	55.97	6.85	NP	48.28
Wings (Hot or Barbeque)	400	27.96	NP	854	0.5	0.34	NP	34.36
Salad								
Arizona Chicken Salad	431	17.85	NP	546	38.11	6.06	NP	31.5
Buffalo Chicken Salad	606	42.25	NP	2365	42.25	7.47	NP	34.39
Chicken Caesar Salad	272	8.86	NP	589	15.6	4.15	NP	32.54
Chicken Portabella Salad	331	12.37	NP	486	21.67	5.24	NP	33.87
Chicken & Strawberry Salad	216	5.95	NP	135	12.97	5.72	NP	28.82
Grilled Chicken Salad	439	19.11	NP	194	29.64	5.18	NP	37.15
Fruit Salad w/ sherbet	308	3.03	NP	49	73.34	7.49	NP	4.57

Description & Serving	Cal	Fat	Sfat	Sod	Carb	Fiber	Sugar	Prot
Garden Salad	102	2.98	NP	198	16.49	3.65	NP	3.35
Spinach & Chicken Salad	329	15.26	NP	393	9.77	3.79	NP	38.49
Taco Salad	803	40.6	NP	2001	70.49	14.46	NP	43.07

Soup/Chili

Description & Serving	Cal	Fat	Sfat	Sod	Carb	Fiber	Sugar	Prot
Bean Soup, cup	145	4.06	NP	746	17.55	3.72	NP	9.83
Beef Noodle Soup, cup	111	4.87	NP	849	11.23	1.04	NP	5.38
Broccoli Soup, cup	197	11.23	NP	766	21.98	0.85	NP	3.74
Cheese Soup, cup	215	11.49	NP	756	27.14	0.28	NP	2.83
Chicken Noodle Soup, cup	130	4.53	NP	781	16.41	0.7	NP	5.57
Chicken Rice Soup, cup	76	1.36	NP	673	11.12	0.56	NP	4.36
Chili, cup	132	5.01	NP	646	13.16	3.67	NP	9.2
Clam Chowder, cup	159	8.36	NP	415	19.36	0.41	NP	2.92
Harvest Grain Soup, cup	450	18	NP	3300	69	9	NP	12
Minestrone Soup, cup	85	1.51	NP	801	14.56	2.47	NP	3.93
Mushroom Barley Soup, cup	69	0.8	NP	914	13.28	3.05	NP	2.9
Potato Soup, cup	214	9.83	NP	620	31.81	1	NP	1.59
Vegetable Beef Barley Soup, cup	103	3.42	NP	690	12.97	3.24	NP	5.59
Vegetarian Pasta Soup, cup	44	1.1	NP	391	8.53	0.97	NP	1.08
Wedding Soup, cup	110	3.48	NP	106	11.8	0.79	NP	5.26

Sandwich

Description & Serving	Cal	Fat	Sfat	Sod	Carb	Fiber	Sugar	Prot
Bacon, Turkey, Swiss Sandwich	526	37.31	NP	1883	16.19	1.01	NP	30.69
Buffalo Chicken Sandwich	786	40.9	NP	1986	70.81	5.43	NP	35.64
Chargrilled Chicken Sandwich	318	6.25	NP	595	32.15	1.4	NP	30.93
Breaded Chicken Sandwich	517	19.38	NP	1399	49.96	2.03	NP	33.34
Cheddar Chicken Sandwich	445	14.52	NP	1055	36.89	2.13	NP	39.27
Spicy Chicken Sandwich	331	6.37	NP	751	34.69	1.71	NP	31.29
Bacon Deluxe Chicken Sandwich	563	23.19	NP	1372	50.16	2.03	NP	36.04
Fiesta Chicken Sandwich	324	11.47	NP	537	20.94	2.06	NP	33.64
Tuscan Chicken Sandwich	453	19.56	NP	659	30.83	1.86	NP	37.09
Chicken Portabella Hoagie	836	55.17	NP	1753	45.69	2.7	NP	40.03
Chicken Salad Croissant	593	38.81	NP	736	35.97	2.18	NP	25.64
Tuna Croissant	582	39	NP	540	34.98	2.11	NP	23.65
Turkey Croissant	389	18.38	NP	1419	30.46	1.22	NP	24.55
Dutch Ham & Swiss Sandwich	572	30.57	NP	2049	35.26	5.53	NP	40.94
Grilled Cheese Sandwich	507	35.51	NP	1426	26.17	1.35	NP	20.66
Italian Hoagie	863	51.56	NP	3427	40.45	1.97	NP	57.42
Hot Roast Beef Sandwich	309	6.29	NP	1083	32.56	1.55	NP	28.73
Hot Turkey Sandwich	260	5.15	NP	1632	27.49	1.35	NP	24.13
Chicken Fajita Pita	619	18.54	NP	1281	68.48	3.56	NP	42.35
Tuna Pita	638	25.51	NP	924	71.87	3.91	NP	29.55
Turkey Pita	444	4.89	NP	1952	67.35	3.02	NP	30.45
Reuben Sandwich	720	48.98	NP	2192	31.14	3.72	NP	37.62
Santa Fe Turkey & Bacon Sandwich	854	59.59	NP	3291	43.74	2.39	NP	36.89
Shredded Pot Roast Sandwich	532	30.42	NP	1053	27.56	1.28	NP	35.44
Steak & Cheese Sandwich	765	50.45	NP	1095	42.62	2.73	NP	34.29
Tuna Melt	609	40.71	NP	1458	35.23	4.16	NP	26.03
Turkey Club	777	46.27	NP	2642	49.91	2.54	NP	38.98

Description & Serving	Cal	Fat	Sfat	Sod	Carb	Fiber	Sugar	Prot
Turkey Pastrami Sandwich	714	45.86	NP	1999	39.92	6.2	NP	38.53
Whale of a Cod Sandwich	866	39.63	NP	2796	75.97	2.62	NP	49.35
Breaded Whitefish Sandwich	788	35.49	NP	1888	68.77	3.36	NP	45.28

Burger

Description & Serving	Cal	Fat	Sfat	Sod	Carb	Fiber	Sugar	Prot
Bacon & Cheese Burger	614	35.92	NP	795	32.67	1.57	NP	37.25
Black Angus American Grill Burger	788	50.71	NP	665	30.96	2.6	NP	50.4
Black Angus Bacon & Cheddar Burger	1037	69.54	NP	2045	50.66	2.27	NP	51.92
Black Angus Classic Burger	815	50.51	NP	1189	40.7	1.53	NP	47.52
Black Angus Classic Cheeseburger	974	63.8	NP	1797	41.38	1.53	NP	56.94
Black Angus Mushroom & Onion Burger	885	56.21	NP	1502	44.49	2.3	NP	48.77
Black Bean Gardenburger	790	48.07	NP	1625	62.29	5.9	NP	22.94
Black Bean Gardenburger w/o cheese & mayo	473	16.17	NP	1288	62.29	5.9	NP	15.57
Cheese Burger	540	29.67	NP	593	32.59	1.57	NP	33.38
Classic Gardenburger	250	5.56	NP	805	40.53	4.72	NP	10.39
Hamburger 1/3 lb	495	25.86	NP	418	32.4	1.57	NP	30.68
Kansas City BBQ Burger	850	58.77	NP	908	24.41	0.88	NP	52.68
Provolone, Mushroom, & Onion Burger	874	55.02	NP	1358	44.41	2.3	NP	48.68
Superburger	707	49.03	NP	1140	37.62	2.59	NP	27.67
Swiss, Mushroom, & Onion Burger	878	54.95	NP	1208	44.82	2.3	NP	49.41
Swiss Burger	580	31.73	NP	475	34.43	1.89	NP	36.94
Turkey Burger	502	21.65	NP	805	37.6	3.21	NP	38.12

Entrée

Chicken/Turkey

Description & Serving	Cal	Fat	Sfat	Sod	Carb	Fiber	Sugar	Prot
Chargrilled Chicken, 4 oz	139	3.63	NP	264	0	0	NP	24.89
Stuffed Chicken Breast	369	16.6	NP	1288	27.31	1.26	NP	26.25
Chicken Fillets, 5 pc	529	26.18	NP	1353	27.84	0.99	NP	42.65
Chicken Milano	217	10.43	NP	565	3.69	0.13	NP	25.39
Chicken & Biscuits	494	20.02	NP	967	29.93	1.01	NP	46.21
Chicken Parmigiana Marinara	842	32.5	NP	3483	90.39	5.85	NP	47.45
Chicken Parmigiana Meat Sauce	898	38.16	NP	2589	86.03	5.44	NP	51.71
Chicken Stir-Fry	554	24.63	NP	670	47.27	7.65	NP	38.48
Country Fried Chicken Steak	789	40.44	NP	1966	42.45	1.41	NP	60.05
Turkey	332	13.3	NP	2198	26.9	1.13	NP	25.06

Fish/Shrimp

Description & Serving	Cal	Fat	Sfat	Sod	Carb	Fiber	Sugar	Prot
Baked Cajun Cod	306	16.71	NP	453	13.35	0.56	NP	24.43
Breaded Fish	926	45.35	NP	2806	56.28	1.99	NP	69.06
Chesapeake Crab Stuffed Cod	286	9	NP	671	20.12	0.74	NP	29.52
Island Cod	180	3.03	NP	249	13.02	0.67	NP	23.74
Mahi Mahi w/ tropical salsa	201	2.48	NP	149	9.75	1.29	NP	33.89
Nantucket Cod	290	16.91	NP	703	6.82	0.59	NP	26.94
Salmon	207	10.17	NP	76	0	0	NP	27.08
Scallops	398	25.54	NP	822	23.23	0.71	NP	19.69
Maryland Scrod	445	31.61	NP	461	10.92	0.73	NP	28.95
Baked Scrod, 8 oz	434	25.17	NP	705	5.94	0.21	NP	43.89
Floridian Scrod, 4 oz	120	1.5	NP	94	3.94	0.28	NP	21.73
Breaded Whitefish	788	35.49	NP	1888	68.77	3.36	NP	45.28
Baked Stuffed Shrimp	344	23.37	NP	925	7.51	0.16	NP	25.34
Fried Jumbo Shrimp	251	9.56	NP	800	28.08	1.18	NP	14.48

Description & Serving	Cal	Fat	Sfat	Sod	Carb	Fiber	Sugar	Prot
Pasta								
Chicken Broccoli Alfredo	604	19.14	NP	1003	60.82	4.03	NP	45.18
Spaghetti in Marinara	621	7.9	NP	1006	119.73	7.43	NP	19.08
Spaghetti in Meat Sauce	820	18.68	NP	1731	139.57	7.56	NP	25.83
Ziti in Marinara w/ meatballs	785	32.85	NP	1505	84.67	5.5	NP	38.63
Ziti in Meat Sauce w/ meatballs	959	42.28	NP	1719	102.02	5.61	NP	44.53
Pork/Steak								
Ham Steak	183	6.98	NP	1518	1.89	0	NP	26.4
Sesame Pork Chops	320	18.33	NP	1032	2.49	0.23	NP	34.13
Ground Sirloin	422	25.38	NP	107	0	0	NP	45.25
Rib-Eye	614	42.1	NP	842	1.01	0.67	NP	54.44
Salisbury Steak	442	23.52	NP	818	28	1.4	NP	27.54
T-Bone	568	38.91	NP	778	1.01	0.67	NP	50.31
Veal Parmigiana w/ marinara	599	15.3	NP	1375	81.56	5.71	NP	35.18
Veal Parmigiana w/ meat sauce	822	26.34	NP	1971	107.38	6.18	NP	41.08
Side								
Biscuit	214	12.62	NP	497	22.42	0.75	NP	3.22
Cheese Biscuit	127	6.32	NP	407	15.18	0.54	NP	2.76
Cornbread	108	3.95	NP	259	15.88	0.69	NP	2.13
Garlic Toast	465	19.27	NP	835	61.32	3.32	NP	10.88
Italian Bread, 1 slice	54	0.7	NP	117	10	0.54	NP	1.76
Applesauce	108	0.26	NP	4	28.22	1.7	NP	0.26
Coleslaw	200	17.52	NP	234	10.25	2.33	NP	1.56
Cottage Cheese	114	2.46	NP	518	4.63	0	NP	17.53
French Fries	347	18.25	NP	11	43.74	3.93	NP	3.74
Beef Gravy	21	0.48	NP	344	3.48	0.09	NP	0.78
Turkey Gravy	32	1.4	NP	333	2.86	0.24	NP	2.23
Macaroni & Cheese	146	2.21	NP	775	26.21	1.02	NP	4.79
Buttered Noodles	247	13.53	NP	356	25.65	1.3	NP	5.9
Nacho Chips	143	7	NP	172	18	1.68	NP	1.98
Onion Rings, 10 pc	105	6.49	NP	110	9.74	0.66	NP	2.1
Baked Potato	190	0.2	NP	10	43.96	3.06	NP	4
Scalloped Potato	230	7.89	NP	509	34.15	2.48	NP	6.27
Whipped Potato	280	23.05	NP	324	16.58	1.22	NP	2.78
Mexican Rice	111	1.93	NP	25	21.51	1.44	NP	2.58
White Rice	148	2.44	NP	397	27.98	0.4	NP	2.69
Rice Pilaf	137	3.57	NP	383	23.43	0.51	NP	3.55
Rice Pudding	163	1.69	NP	130	31.14	0.2	NP	5.31
Fresh Strawberries Cup	51	0.63	NP	2	11.94	3.91	NP	1.04
Sugar Snap Peas	29	0.17	NP	9	6.58	3.06	NP	1.52
Mixed Vegetables	29	0.19	NP	29	5.83	3.29	NP	2.54
Kids								
Breakfast								
Cereal w/ milk	615	16.37	NP	880	114.95	14.87	NP	15.32
French Toast (Bacon)	355	15.85	NP	390	34.72	1.14	NP	16.68
French Toast (Sausage)	546	33.89	NP	735	34.64	1.14	NP	23.46
Giggle (Bacon)	380	26.85	NP	581	20.44	0.92	NP	13.49
Giggle (Sausage)	571	44.89	NP	925	20.36	0.92	NP	20.27

Description & Serving	Cal	Fat	Sfat	Sod	Carb	Fiber	Sugar	Prot
Lunch/Dinner								
Burger	285	14.72	NP	265	21.43	1.28	NP	15.88
Cheeseburger	365	21.36	NP	569	21.77	1.28	NP	20.59
Grilled Cheese Sandwich	524	39.07	NP	1533	21.17	0.92	NP	22.18
Chicken Fillet	317	15.71	NP	812	16.7	0.59	NP	25.59
Fish Plank	315	14.93	NP	93	19.57	0.69	NP	24.02
Hot Dog	361	23.77	NP	1130	24.11	1.15	NP	11.71
Macaroni & Cheese	171	2.58	NP	904	30.58	1.19	NP	5.59
Peanut Butter & Jelly Sandwich	439	20.3	NP	500	54.79	3.78	NP	14.05
Pizza	413	12.56	NP	991	49.48	2.31	NP	24.89
Spaghetti	355	5.08	NP	802	69.23	3.79	NP	9.6
Seniors								
Breakfast								
French Toast	399	11.54	NP	241	79.01	0.13	NP	1.07
Lunch/Dinner								
Breaded Fish, 4 oz	463	22.86	NP	1403	28.14	1	NP	34.53
Chicken Fillets, 4 pc	423	20.95	NP	1082	22.27	0.79	NP	34.12
Fried Jumbo Shrimp	187	6.44	NP	758	23.88	1.03	NP	9.94
Hot Roast Beef Sandwich	183	5.5	NP	623	17.04	0.79	NP	15.39
Hot Turkey Sandwich	175	4.58	NP	1292	17.84	1.02	NP	15.25
Sesame Pork Chop, 4 oz	160	9.17	NP	516	1.28	0.12	NP	16.31
Pot Roast Sandwich	262	15.1	NP	452	13.03	0.62	NP	17.56
Baked Scrod, 4 oz	330	23.8	NP	338	5.81	0.19	NP	22.49
Spaghetti in Marinara	311	3.98	NP	503	59.87	3.71	NP	9.54
Spaghetti in Meat Sauce	410	9.34	NP	866	69.78	3.78	NP	12.91
Dressing/Condiment								
Cream Cheese	99	9.89	NP	84	0.75	0	NP	2.14
Jelly	34	0.03	NP	6	9.13	0.16	NP	0.1
Ketchup	23	0.08	NP	267	6.14	0.29	NP	0.34
Relish, .75 oz	40	0.14	NP	248	10.73	0.34	NP	0.11
Salsa, 2 oz	14	0.15	NP	168	3.21	1.23	NP	0.71
BBQ Sauce, 2 oz	84	0.04	NP	623	22	0.26	NP	0.24
Cheese Sauce, 2 oz	151	11.97	NP	154	3.89	0.05	NP	6.98
Cocktail Sauce, 2 oz	71	0.25	NP	809	18.63	0.89	NP	1.04
Lite Soy Sauce, 1 tbsp	8	0.01	NP	531	1.36	0.13	NP	0.82
Supreme Sauce, 2 oz	151	16	NP	176	2.08	0.07	NP	0.25
Sweet 'n Sour Sauce, 2 oz	81	1.57	NP	233	16.36	0.53	NP	0.32
Teriyaki Sauce, 2 tbsp	15	0	NP	690	2.87	0.02	NP	1.07
Chipotle BBQ Sauce, 2 oz	170	1	NP	1140	41	1	NP	1
Sweet Thai Sauce, 2 oz	140	0	NP	1350	36	0.99	NP	0
Bleu Cheese Dressing, 2 tbsp	92	6.87	NP	436	6.9	0	NP	1.03
Caesar Dressing, 2 tbsp	245	24.51	NP	725	7.53	0.03	NP	0.32
French Fat-Free Dressing, 2 tbsp	70	0.02	NP	528	17	0	NP	0.2
Fruit Salad Dressing, 2 tbsp	143	13.79	NP	91	5.39	0.06	NP	0.27
House Dressing, 2 tbsp	115	11.48	NP	271	2.31	0	NP	0.98
Fat-Free Italian Dressing, 2 tbsp	12	0.02	NP	300	3.1	0.09	NP	0.1
Italian Dressing, 2 tbsp	122	12.26	NP	235	3.77	0.01	NP	0.16

Description & Serving	Cal	Fat	Sfat	Sod	Carb	Fiber	Sugar	Prot
Poppyseed Dressing, 2 tbsp	240	16	NP	5	24	0	NP	0
Thousand Island Dressing, 2 tbsp	95	9.36	NP	291	3.12	0	NP	0.24

Topping

Mozzarella Cheese	226	17.46	NP	294	1.75	0	NP	15.31
Leaf Lettuce	1	0.01	NP	0	0.1	0.07	NP	0.05
Shredded Lettuce	3	0.05	NP	3	0.59	0.4	NP	0.29
Grilled Onions, 1 oz	21	1.18	NP	1	2.45	0.51	NP	0.33
Raw Onions	11	0.05	NP	1	2.45	0.51	NP	0.33
Pickle Chips, 3	3	0.03	NP	182	0.59	0.17	NP	0.09
Pickle Spear	4	0.04	NP	256	0.83	0.24	NP	0.12
Tomatoes, 2 slices	6	0.1	NP	3	1.39	0.33	NP	0.26
Tomatoes, 2 wedges	5	0.09	NP	2	1.21	0.29	NP	0.22

Dessert

Chocolate Chip Cookie	207	9.04	NP	170	28.4	0.74	NP	3.03
Macadamia Nut Cookie	240	16.2	NP	78	22	0.99	NP	2.47
Smiley Cookie	297	13.17	NP	190	42.18	0.75	NP	2.57
Banana Fudge Sensation	977	43.91	NP	307	147.3	5.44	NP	13.71
Caramel Nut Fudge Sensation	1065	54.96	NP	378	144.88	5.52	NP	12.65
Cheesecake	507	36.03	NP	311	39.55	0.17	NP	8.09
Cheesecake w/ strawberries	751	36.19	NP	410	105.31	1.14	NP	8.35
Cookie Fudge Fantasy	1195	60.12	NP	408	164.1	4.29	NP	15.04
Grilled Stickies a la Mode	728	38.58	NP	1267	80.59	1.61	NP	8.89
Grilled Stickies a la Mode Loaf	487	27.94	NP	1190	53.23	1.6	NP	6.38
Ice Cream, 2 scoops	285	15.59	NP	113	33.45	0	NP	4.96
Apple Cranberry Pie, 1 slice	655	36.24	NP	476	78.29	2.85	NP	5.35
Apple Pie, No Sugar Added, 1 slice	341	10.28	NP	462	61.32	3.73	NP	2.79
Apple Pie, 1 slice	489	24.11	NP	326	65.65	2.81	NP	4.22
Banana Crème Pie, 1 slice	439	22.11	NP	400	55.06	1.2	NP	6.49
Blackberry Pie, 1 slice	510	23.4	NP	312	73.26	5.07	NP	4.07
Blueberry Pie, 1 slice	439	23.44	NP	317	55.12	3.39	NP	4.11
Cherry Pie, 1 slice	457	24.01	NP	312	58.17	3.16	NP	4.65
Chocolate Peanut Butter Pie, 1 slice	566	39.31	NP	443	48.89	1.79	NP	8.83
Coconut Crème Pie, 1 slice	480	26.16	NP	469	55.45	0.6	NP	6.93
Lemon Meringue Pie, 1 slice	262	13.38	NP	217	31.33	0.52	NP	4.28
Oreo Cream Pie, 1 slice	495	28.08	NP	504	60.02	1.83	NP	4.54
Peach Pie, No Sugar Added, 1 slice	268	9.9	NP	462	50	1.75	NP	2.99
Peachberry Pie, 1 slice	389	18.84	NP	369	52.04	3.78	NP	4.44
Pecan Pie, 1 slice	679	39.82	NP	386	79.34	2.13	NP	6.7
Pumpkin Pie, 1 slice	395	19.27	NP	438	48.67	2.71	NP	8.48
Strawberry Pie, 1 slice	360	18.02	NP	165	49.4	4.71	NP	3.29
Sugar-Free Chocolate Pudding	90	2.69	NP	160	12.53	0.79	NP	4.46
Plain Sherbet	98	1.42	NP	33	21.55	0.35	NP	0.78
Strawberry Fudge Delight	1161	45.92	NP	425	191.48	3.22	NP	13.48
Strawberry Shortcake	687	26.43	NP	210	113.77	2.1	NP	6.61
Apple Sundae	569	21.46	NP	153	95.59	1.92	NP	6.19
Chocolate Sundae	525	21.95	NP	191	84.6	2.06	NP	7
Hot Fudge Sundae	625	31.45	NP	218	85.19	1.63	NP	8.92
Strawberry Sundae	606	21.43	NP	219	106.18	1.68	NP	5.83

Description & Serving	Cal	Fat	Sfat	Sod	Carb	Fiber	Sugar	Prot
Tin Roof Sundae	794	44.13	NP	384	95.29	6.77	NP	19
Frozen Yogurt, 2 scoops	65	0.69	NP	37	12.15	0	NP	2.79

Beverage

Cappuccino	114	3.04	NP	81	16.63	0.12	NP	5.39
Iced Chai	92	2.73	NP	73	12.34	0.06	NP	4.82
Chai, sml	112	3.29	NP	88	15.03	0.22	NP	5.8
Decaffeinated Coffee	4	0	NP	2	1.15	0.32	NP	0.23
Regular Coffee	4	0	NP	4	0.77	0.21	NP	0.19
Hot Chocolate	327	7.7	NP	190	63.19	1.87	NP	9.03
Hot Tea	2	0	NP	5	0.49	0	NP	0
Decaffeinated Hot Tea	2	0	NP	2	0.34	0	NP	0
Iced Tea	2	0	NP	7	0.67	0	NP	0
Iced Latte	167	3.81	NP	101	26.98	0.12	NP	6.72
Latte, sml	173	4.45	NP	118	25.91	0.14	NP	7.85
Lemonade	93	0.1	NP	3	24.19	0.21	NP	0.15
Milkshake, sml	583	27.16	NP	269	78.69	1.05	NP	12.8
Chai Tea Milkshake	579	32.33	NP	208	67.49	69	NP	9.44
Mocha Java Milkshake	631	32.57	NP	236	81.65	1.14	NP	10.04
Vanilla Latte Milkshake	631	32.57	NP	236	81.65	1.14	NP	10.04

Einstein Bros. Bagels

Breakfast

Asiago Cheese Bagel	330	5	3	660	59	2	5	15
Blueberry Bagel	290	1.5	0	480	64	3	11	9
Chocolate Chip Bagel	290	3	1	460	60	3	11	10
Garlic Dip'd Bagel	290	2.5	0	490	60	2	5	10
Onion Dip'd Bagel	270	1	0	460	59	2	5	9
Cinnamon Raisin Swirl Bagel	290	1	0	450	64	3	13	10
Cinnamon Sugar Bagel Chicago Style	310	2.5	0.5	510	66	3	12	10
Cranberry Bagel	290	1	0	450	64	3	13	9
Egg Bagel	300	6	1.5	480	52	2	6	12
Everything Bagel	270	2	0	610	56	2	5	10
Good Grains Bagel	290	2.5	0	480	62	4	9	10
Honey Whole Wheat Bagel	270	1	0	480	61	3	9	9
Onion Bagel	270	1.5	0	480	59	2	5	9
Plain Bagel	260	1	0	460	56	2	5	9
Poppy Dip'd Bagel	280	3	0	460	56	2	5	10
Potato Bagel	260	1	0	540	58	2	6	9
Power Bagel, Fruit & Nut	380	6	1	330	72	5	20	13
Pumpernickel Bagel	250	1.5	0	710	55	3	4	9
Sesame Dip'd Bagel	280	3	0	460	56	2	5	10
Sundried Tomato Bagel	270	1.5	0	570	58	3	4	10
Green Chile Bagel	370	8	4.5	710	62	2	6	16
Dutch Apple Bagel	340	7	1.5	540	66	2	15	8
Spinach Florentine Bagel	360	8	4	620	61	2	5	16
Six-Cheese Bagel	350	6	3.5	680	60	2	5	16
Double Topped - Apple Cream Cheese	550	17	9	780	89	4	32	11

Description & Serving	Cal	Fat	Sfat	Sod	Carb	Fiber	Sugar	Prot
Double Topped - Elvis' Favorite	700	30	6	730	98	8	34	24
Double Topped - Strawberry Cream Cheese	480	12	8	720	82	3	23	11
Braided Challah Roll	220	3.5	0.5	200	41	1	5	8
Ciabatta Bread	290	2.5	0	640	60	2	1	10
Multi Grain Bread, 1 slice	130	2.5	0	220	23	2	3	5
Asiago Cheese Bagel Pretzel	300	7	2.5	710	52	2	5	11
Cinnamon Sugar Bagel Pretzel	320	5	1	630	66	3	18	8
Plain Bagel Pretzel	270	5	1	630	52	2	5	8
Salt Bagel Pretzel	270	5	1	1740	52	2	5	8
Blueberry Muffin	480	22	4.5	480	65	2	36	6
Strawberry White Chocolate Muffin	550	25	7	510	78	1	49	7
Egg Way, Original Sandwich	530	20	9	840	62	2	7	30
Egg Way w/ Bacon Sandwich	580	24	11	1030	59	2	8	33
Egg Way w/ Black Forest Ham Sandwich	570	21	9	1270	62	2	7	37
Egg Way w/ Sausage Sandwich	600	24	10	1020	63	2	8	38
Egg Way, Spinach Mushroom & Swiss Omelette	540	20	8	860	65	3	8	29
Bacon & Spinach Panini	860	51	15	1610	66	6	5	27
Sausage Ranchero Panini	680	29	12	1360	64	4	5	32
Vegetable Breakfast Panini	730	36	17	1300	68	4	6	26
Spicy Elmo Wrap	720	41	17	1050	56	6	6	34
Santa Fe Wrap	720	37	14	1290	60	7	8	37

Sandwich/Wrap/Hot Dog

Description & Serving	Cal	Fat	Sfat	Sod	Carb	Fiber	Sugar	Prot
Deli Bacon Sandwich	830	52	14	1930	52	4	10	39
Deli Chicken Sandwich	460	18	4	890	47	4	7	28
Deli Ham Sandwich	520	26	5	1550	48	4	7	26
Deli Pastrami Sandwich	630	33	9	1860	53	5	8	34
Deli Tuna Salad Sandwich	440	15	2.5	920	50	4	7	29
Deli Turkey & Swiss Sandwich	690	41	9	1510	49	4	7	36
Ham Deli Melt	510	16	9	1700	62	3	7	36
Pastrami Deli Melt	540	17	9	1690	64	3	7	38
Tuna Salad Deli Melt	590	23	9	1140	64	3	7	38
Turkey Deli Melt	510	15	8	1430	62	3	7	38
Veggie Deli Melt	640	29	16	1350	76	5	12	24
Reuben, reg size	650	38	12	2360	47	3	9	34
Rachel, reg size	910	64	16	2210	51	2	15	36
Turkey Reuben, reg size	610	36	11	2040	45	3	8	36
Turkey Rachel, reg size	870	62	15	1860	49	1	14	38
Club Mex on Challah	750	49	11	1530	46	2	8	36
Grilled Chicken, Bacon & Swiss	750	46	11	1220	45	2	8	40
Roasted Turkey & Swiss	690	41	9	1460	49	4	7	35
Tasty Turkey on Asiago Bagel	580	20	11	1500	69	3	9	37
Veg Out on Sesame Seed Bagel	440	14	7	760	66	4	9	17
Lox & Bagels	520	21	11	980	66	3	11	25
Italian Chicken Panini	800	40	12	2450	66	5	3	35
Turkey Club Panini	790	41	11	2200	66	6	5	34
California Chicken Wrap	630	29	8	1170	63	8	6	33
Chipotle Turkey Wrap	730	37	12	1990	70	9	11	34
Original Bagel Dog	470	20	7	1190	56	2	7	20

Description & Serving	Cal	Fat	Sfat	Sod	Carb	Fiber	Sugar	Prot
Original Bagel Dog w/ Cheddar Cheese	550	26	11	1310	56	2	7	25
Original Asiago Bagel Dog	490	21	8	1230	56	2	7	22
Original Asiago Bagel Dog w/ Cheddar Cheese	560	27	12	1350	56	2	7	26

Pizza

Cheese Pizza Bagel	420	12	7	980	63	3	7	23
Pepperoni Pizza Bagel	470	16	8	1120	63	3	7	24
Spinach & Mushroom Pizza Bagel	580	25	13	1250	70	4	8	26
Cheesy Garlic & Herb Pizza Bagel	500	19	12	1010	65	2	7	24

Salad

Half Caesar Salad	280	27	6	680	7	2	2	6
Half Caesar Salad w/ Chicken	350	28	6	960	8	2	2	18
Half Bros Bistro Salad	410	34	5	160	19	3	15	7
Half Bros Bistro Salad w/ Chicken	480	36	6	440	19	3	15	19
Half Chipotle Salad	290	18	4	730	26	5	7	6
Half Chipotle Salad w/ Chicken	360	21	4.5	970	27	5	7	18

Soup

Chicken Noodle Soup, cup	120	3.5	1	770	14	1	1	5
Corn Crab Chowder, cup	280	18	15	940	18	1	7	8
Seafood Minestrone, cup	130	4.5	1	1010	16	2	4	8
Italian Wedding Soup, cup	160	6	1.5	1060	15	2	2	11
Turkey Chili, cup	220	7	1.5	930	24	5	5	20
Vegetarian Broccoli Cheese Soup, cup	290	20	10	990	16	2	6	14

Side

Fruit Salad	140	0	0	35	36	3	31	2
Fruit & Yogurt Parfait	230	1.5	0	200	42	4	25	12
Bagel Croutons	150	12	3	460	9	0	1	1
Traditional Potato Salad	355	28.5	4	550	20	2	1	3
Cole Slaw	230	21	3	135	12	3	8	2
Whole Kosher Pickle	5	0	0	650	1	1	0	0

Dessert

Fudge Brownie	510	25	13	115	74	2	62	6
Chocolate Chip Coffee Cake	760	34	13	270	110	2	58	6
Mixed Berry Coffee Cake	710	29	10	270	110	2	59	5
Chocolate Mudslide Cookie	320	17	9	75	46	1	38	4
Mini Chocolate Mudslide Cookie	160	8	4.5	40	23	1	19	2
Heavenly Chocolate Chunk Cookie	360	18	9	290	48	2	29	4
Mini Heavenly Chocolate Chunk Cookie	180	9	4.5	150	24	1	14	2
Iced Sugar Cookie	480	15	6	260	76	1	46	4
Mini Iced Sugar Cookie	230	7	3	130	39	1	24	2
Lemon Pound Cake	440	16	8	390	69	1	47	7
Marshmallow Crispy Treat	220	3.5	1	60	48	0	20	3
Oatmeal Raisin Cookie	320	11	5	310	54	2	31	5
Mini Oatmeal Raisin Cookie	160	5	2.5	160	27	1	16	2
Cinnamon Stix	370	21	10	125	41	2	18	5
Cinnamon Walnut Strudel	630	42	17	360	56	4	20	9

Description & Serving	Cal	Fat	Sfat	Sod	Carb	Fiber	Sugar	Prot
Dressing/Condiment								
Whipped Blueberry Reduced Fat Cream Cheese, 2 tbsp	70	5	3.5	50	6	0	5	1
Whipped Garlic Herb Reduced Fat Cream Cheese, 2 tbsp	60	5	3.5	100	3	0	1	1
Whipped Garden Vegetable Reduced Fat Cream Cheese, 2 tbsp	60	5	3.5	100	3	0	1	1
Whipped Honey Almond Reduced Fat Cream Cheese, 2 tbsp	70	5	3	45	6	0	4	1
Whipped Jalapeno Salsa Reduced Fat Cream Cheese, 2 tbsp	60	5	3.5	105	3	0	1	1
Whipped Onion & Chive Cream Cheese, 2 tbsp	70	6	4	60	3	0	1	1
Whipped Plain Cream Cheese, 2 tbsp	70	7	4.5	65	1	0	1	1
Whipped Plain Reduced Fat Cream Cheese, 2 tbsp	60	5	3.5	100	2	0	1	1
Whipped Smoked Salmon Cream Cheese, 2 tbsp	60	6	3.5	120	2	0	1	1
Whipped Strawberry Reduced Fat Cream Cheese, 2 tbsp	70	5	3.5	50	5	0	4	1
Whipped Sun Dried Tomato Basil Reduced Fat Cream Cheese, 2 tbsp	60	5	3.5	100	2	0	1	1
Blackberry Syrup, 2 tbsp	100	0	0	0	25	0	25	0
Caramel Syrup, 1 oz	100	0	0	0	25	0	25	0
Cherry Syrup, 2 tbsp	100	0	0	0	25	0	25	0
Chocolate Syrup, 2 tbsp	0	0	0	0	4	0	0	0
Hazelnut Syrup, 1 oz	100	0	0	0	25	0	25	0
Vanilla Syrup, 1 oz	100	0	0	0	25	0	25	0
Sugar Free Vanilla Syrup, 1 oz	0	0	0	0	4	0	0	0
Caesar Dressing, 2 tbsp	150	16	2.5	350	1	0	1	1
Raspberry Vinaigrette, 2 tbsp	160	14	2	0	8	0	8	0
Chile Lime Dressing, 2 tbsp	60	3.5	0	650	5	0	3	1
Ancho Mayo	310	34	5	240	1	0	1	0
Ancho Lime Salsa	15	0.5	0	270	2	0	1	0
Creamy Mustard Spread	270	29	4.5	220	1	0	1	0
Deli Mustard	5	0	0	65	0	0	0	0
Feta Pinenut Spread	70	5	3.5	190	2	0	0	4
Honey Butter	170	18	5	220	0	0	0	0
Hummus	70	3	0	150	6	4	0	4
Roasted Garlic Horseradish Spread	15	0	0	340	4	1	1	0
Spicy Roasted Tomato Spread	140	14	2	240	3	1	1	0
Topping								
Light Whipped Cream, 2 tbsp	35	2.5	2.5	0	2	0	2	0
On Top Reduced Fat Topping, 2 tbsp	20	1.5	1	5	2	0	2	0
Candied Walnuts	260	22	0	20	9	3	7	4
American Cheese	70	6	3.5	340	1	0	0	4
Swiss Cheese	70	6	3.5	85	0	0	0	5
Medium Cheddar Cheese	80	6	4	120	0	0	0	5
Monterey Jack Cheese w/ Jalapeno Peppers	70	5	3.5	160	0	0	0	5
Provolone Cheese	70	5	3	160	0	0	0	5

Description & Serving	Cal	Fat	Sfat	Sod	Carb	Fiber	Sugar	Prot
Gorgonzola Cheese	100	9	5	260	0	0	0	7
Cold Smoked Salmon	80	4.5	1	250	0	0	1	12
Chicken Salad	210	14	3	480	2	0	1	18
Chicken Breast	140	4.5	1	490	1	0	0	24
Pastrami	110	4	1.5	1020	2	0	1	17
Tuna Salad	170	10	2	470	2	1	1	18
Ham	90	3	1.5	1030	0	0	0	15
Oven Roasted Turkey	80	1.5	0	700	0	0	0	18
Turkey Sausage	70	4	1	180	1	0	1	8
Thick Cut Bacon	60	5	2	220	1	0	1	4
Beverage								
Café Latte, reg (12 oz)	140	5	3.5	140	13	0	0	9
Café Latte w/ Whole Milk, reg (12 oz)	200	10	6	140	16	0	0	10
Nonfat Café Latte, reg (12 oz)	100	1	0	150	14	0	0	10
Cappuccino, reg (12 oz)	90	3.5	2	95	9	0	0	6
Cappuccino w/ Whole Milk, reg (12 oz)	150	8	4.5	110	13	0	0	7
Cappuccino w/ Nonfat Milk, reg (12 oz)	60	0	0	95	9	0	8	6
Mocha, reg (12 oz)	230	6	4.5	135	34	0	32	8
Mocha w/ Whole Milk, reg (12 oz)	270	9	5	150	38	0	33	8
Low Fat Mocha, reg (11 oz)	240	10	6	135	29	0	27	7
Espresso, reg (2 oz)	1	0	0	0	0	0	0	0
Americano, reg (8 oz)	1	0	0	0	0	0	0	0
Chai Tea w/ 2% Milk, sml (12 oz)	220	2	1	65	47	0	45	3
Chai Tea w/ Skim Milk, sml (12 oz)	210	0	0	65	47	0	45	3
Chai Tea w/ Whole Milk, sml (12 oz)	230	3	1.5	55	47	0	45	3
Hot Chocolate w/ Whole Milk, reg (12 oz)	320	14	10	160	39	0	33	9
Hot Chocolate, reg (12 oz)	290	11	8	160	39	0	33	9
Iced Americano, 8 oz	1	0	0	0	0	0	0	0
Iced Coffee, 12 oz	0	0	0	0	0	0	0	0
Iced Latte, 16 oz	120	4.5	3	125	12	0	11	8
Iced Mocha, 16 oz	210	6	4	120	33	0	31	7
Iced Nonfat Latte, 16 oz	90	0	0	130	12	0	11	8
Low Fat Iced Mocha, 16 oz	180	2.5	2	115	32	0	30	7
Whole Milk Iced Latte, 16 oz	190	9	5	150	17	0	17	9
Whole Milk Iced Mocha, 16 oz	390	9	5	200	66	0	56	9
Café Latte Frozen Blended Drink, 18 oz	400	10	2.5	140	65	0	29	9
Café Mocha Frozen Blended Drink, 18 oz	510	8	2.5	160	102	0	64	7
Café Caramel Frozen Blended Drink, 18 oz	620	9	2.5	140	100	0	66	8
Cookies & Cream Frozen Blended Drink, 18 oz	680	36	25	200	101	1	89	11
Wild Berry Frozen Blended Drink, 18 oz	290	0	0	105	66	5	50	6
Strawberry Frozen Blended Drink, 18 oz	450	19	14	95	75	3	64	6
Vanilla Frozen Blended Drink, 18 oz	600	31	23	150	92	0	89	10

El Pollo Loco

Entrée								
Twice Grilled Burrito	840	39	18	2000	56	6	2	66
Ultimate Grilled Burrito	710	23	9	1690	86	8	1	39
Classic Chicken Burrito	550	17	6	1350	69	6	1	31

Description & Serving	Cal	Fat	Sfat	Sod	Carb	Fiber	Sugar	Prot
BRC Burrito	440	12	4.5	1000	68	6	0	15
Grilled Chicken Tortilla Roll, no sauce	390	16	6	1050	37	3	0	26
Chicken Breast, Skinless	180	3.5	1	560	0	0	0	35
Chicken Breast	220	9	2.5	620	0	0	0	36
Chicken Leg	90	4	1	170	0	0	0	12
Chicken Thigh	220	15	4.5	320	0	0	0	21
Chicken Wing	90	5	1.5	290	0	0	0	11
Chopped Chicken Breast Meat	100	1.5	0.5	330	0	0	0	21
The Original Pollo Bowl	690	10	2	1890	106	12	2	40
Ultimate Pollo Bowl	1050	34	14	2520	110	13	2	71
Chicken Caesar Bowl	490	22	4.5	1200	44	2	3	28
Chicken Taquito w/ Avocado Salsa, 1	230	12	2.5	590	20	2	0	10
Chicken Breast Meal	275	8	2	800	12	4	5	39
Chicken Soft Taco	260	12	6	580	18	2	2	16
Crunchy Chicken Taco	190	8	2.5	480	16	2	0	12
Taco al Carbon	150	5	1.5	290	17	1	1	11
Grilled Chicken Nachos	810	40	14	1990	70	10	4	39
Cheese Quesadilla	420	23	13	810	35	2	0	19

Salad, no dressing

Chicken Tostada Salad w/o dressing	839	42	12	1310	74	7	5	40
Chicken Caesar Salad w/o dressing	232	7	2	517	18	3	5	25
Small Garden Salad w/o dressing	72	3	1	173	8	2	3	2
Loco Salad w/o dressing	169	14	3	207	8	1	2	3

Side

Pinto Beans	200	4	0.5	370	29	8	1	11
Spanish Rice	220	2	0	650	45	1	0	4
Mashed Potatoes	110	1.5	0.5	400	23	2	1	2
Gravy	10	0	0	150	2	0	0	0
Refried Beans w/ cheese	270	7	1.5	730	36	10	2	14
Macaroni & Cheese	280	17	11	770	28	0	3	11
Fresh Vegetables w/o margarine	35	0	0	35	8	3	3	2
Fresh Vegetables w/ margarine	60	3	0	65	8	3	3	2
French Fries	330	17	3	660	42	4	0	4
BBQ Black Beans	200	3	0	520	36	4	16	7
Cole Slaw	130	10	1.5	220	9	2	7	1
Corn Cobbette	90	0.5	0	0	19	2	3	2
Chicken Tortilla Soup, sml	160	8	2.5	660	14	2	1	10
Chicken Tortilla Soup, reg	210	9	3	1050	18	2	2	16
Chicken Tortilla Soup, lrg	450	20	6	2290	37	5	4	34
6.5" Flour Tortillas	210	7	2.5	370	30	2	2	5
6" Corn Tortillas	120	2	0	60	24	2	0	2
Tortilla Chips	170	8	1	250	23	2	1	2
Chips & Guacamole	250	14	2	350	26	4	1	3

Dressing/Condiment

Regular Creamy Cilantro Dressing, 1.3 oz	190	20	3	260	1	0	1	1
Large Creamy Cilantro Dressing, 3 oz	440	46	7	590	3	0	3	3
Light Creamy Cilantro Dressing	70	5	1	400	6	0	3	1

Description & Serving	Cal	Fat	Sfat	Sod	Carb	Fiber	Sugar	Prot
Ranch Dressing	230	24	3.5	390	2	0	2	1
Thousand Island Dressing	220	21	3	350	6	0	6	0
Light Italian Dressing	20	1	0	770	2	0	2	0
House Salsa, 1.5 oz	10	0	0	160	2	0	1	0
Pico de Gallo, 1.5 oz	15	1	0	170	2	0	1	0
Avocado Salsa, 1.5 oz	40	3.5	0.5	290	2	1	0	0
Salsa de Arbol, 1.5 oz	10	0	0	290	2	0	1	0
Guacamole, 1.3 oz	70	6	1	100	3	2	0	1
Sour Cream, 1.3 oz	80	7	4.5	20	1	0	0	1
Queso Sauce, 1.3 oz	80	6	4	260	3	0	1	2
Ketchup, 0.3 oz	10	0	0	100	2	0	2	0
Jalapeno Hot Sauce, 0.3 oz	5	0	0	110	1	0	0	0
Kids								
Drumstick	90	4	1	170	0	0	0	12
Popcorn Chicken	200	12	2	550	10	3	0	14
French Fries	240	12	2	520	30	3	0	3
Vanilla Cone	190	5	3	100	32	0	27	5
Dessert								
Two Churros	300	18	4.5	210	32	2	10	3
Caramel Flan	260	12	10	125	34	0	34	5
Vanilla Soft Serve, cup	300	8	5	170	48	0	47	8
Vanilla Cone, reg	320	8	5	170	53	0	44	8
Vanilla Cone, lrg	490	13	8	270	81	0	72	13
Beverage								
Horchata, 20 oz	60	2	0	10	9	0	7	0
Horchata, 32 oz	90	3.5	0	15	15	0	12	0
Horchata, 44 oz	120	4.5	0	20	20	0	16	0

Fazoli's

Pasta

	Cal	Fat	Sfat	Sod	Carb	Fiber	Sugar	Prot
Tortellini & Sun-Dried Tomato Rustico	850	46	15	1380	81	6	9	30
Penne Rosa w/ Savory Chicken	660	16	6	1660	90	6	13	37
Creamy Chicken Basil	900	41	13	1640	87	4	9	39
Chicken Piccata	870	43	18	1530	86	5	7	36
Chicken Carbonara	800	27	13	1790	88	4	9	42
Ultimate Sampler Platter	1130	34	16	2740	153	12	22	49
Classic Sampler Platter	880	30	14	2200	110	9	16	39
Twice-Baked Lasagna	700	39	20	2420	47	6	11	41
Tortellini Robusto	1020	50	28	2580	80	5	10	59
Rigatoni Romano	880	44	20	2510	76	7	12	44
Penne w/ Creamy Basil Chicken	970	51	25	2340	73	4	9	52
Fazoli's Deep Dish Pasta	850	40	17	2320	85	8	17	39
Creamy Chicken Florentine	890	42	24	2250	73	5	9	52
Chicken Parmigiano	1000	39	15	2550	108	8	15	51
Chicken Broccoli Penne Bake	920	42	24	2310	77	6	11	52
Baked Spaghetti	640	22	12	1340	80	7	13	29

Description & Serving	Cal	Fat	Sfat	Sod	Carb	Fiber	Sugar	Prot
Baked Spaghetti w/ Meatballs	890	39	20	2040	86	7	13	41
Baked Spaghetti w/ Italian Sausage	950	46	20	2350	85	7	13	44
Spaghetti w/ Meat Sauce, sml	520	8	2.5	1100	87	7	12	21
Spaghetti w/ Meat Sauce, reg	780	12	3.5	1650	131	11	18	31
Spaghetti w/ Marinara, sml	440	2	0	650	86	6	12	15
Spaghetti w/ Marinara, reg	660	3	0	980	129	9	18	22
Sliced Italian Sausage	200	16	5	680	3	0	1	10
Ravioli w/ Meat Sauce	570	21	10	1530	70	8	12	27
Ravioli w/ Marinara Sauce	490	15	8	1080	69	7	13	21
Penne w/ Meat Sauce, sml	520	8	2.5	1100	87	7	12	21
Penne w/ Meat Sauce, reg	780	12	3.5	1650	131	11	18	31
Penne w/ Marinara, sml	440	2	0	650	86	6	12	15
Penne w/ Marinara, reg	660	3	0	980	129	9	18	22
Penne w/ Alfredo, sml	610	19	10	1040	84	4	8	21
Penne w/ Alfredo, reg	900	27	15	1500	126	5	12	29
Grilled Chicken	110	3.5	1	510	2	0	1	17
Fettuccine w/ Meat Sauce, sml	520	8	2.5	1100	87	7	12	21
Fettuccine w/ Meat Sauce, reg	780	12	3.5	1650	131	11	18	31
Fettuccine w/ Marinara, sml	440	2	0	650	86	6	12	15
Fettuccine w/ Marinara, reg	660	3	0	980	129	9	18	22
Fettuccine w/ Alfredo, sml	610	19	10	1040	84	4	8	21
Fettuccine w/ Alfredo, reg	900	27	15	1500	126	5	12	29
Pizza								
Pepperoni Pizza Slice	310	14	6	840	32	2	2	14
Cheese Pizza Slice	270	11	5	690	32	2	2	12
Salad								
Side Italian Salad	80	4.5	2	370	4	1	2	5
Side Garden Salad	30	0	0	20	6	2	4	2
Grilled Chicken Artichoke Salad	240	4.5	2.5	910	11	4	4	32
Crispy Chicken BLT Salad	480	26	7	1430	31	4	4	32
Cranberry & Walnut Chicken Salad	390	14	3.5	950	27	4	19	32
Chicken Caprese Salad	370	19	6	790	9	3	4	32
Caesar Salad	230	25	4	350	1	0	0	1
Caesar Side Salad	40	2	1	70	4	2	1	4
Antipasto Salad	260	15	7	1590	11	3	6	21
Sandwich								
Smoked Turkey Basil Submarino	750	37	10	2550	68	3	5	36
Italian Four Cheese & Tomato Submarino	690	35	18	1480	58	3	4	36
Italian Beef Gorgonzola Submarino	750	38	11	2280	72	4	7	35
Ham 'n' Swiss Supremo Submarino	690	31	8	2390	68	3	9	33
Fire-Roasted Red Pepper Chicken Submarino	640	21	8	1960	59	4	6	46
Fazoli's Original Submarino	880	50	14	2890	68	3	7	34
Club Italiano Submarino	780	36	10	2800	68	3	8	39
Side								
Garlic Breadstick, 1	150	7	1.5	290	20	1	1	3
Breadstick, Dry, 1	100	2	0	160	20	0	1	3

Description & Serving	Cal	Fat	Sfat	Sod	Carb	Fiber	Sugar	Prot
Kids								
Spaghetti w/ Meatballs	300	7	2.5	570	45	3	6	12
Spaghetti w/ Meat Sauce	260	4	1	560	44	4	6	10
Spaghetti w/ Marinara Sauce	220	1	0	330	43	3	6	7
Pepperoni Pizza	310	14	6	840	32	2	2	14
Meat Lasagna	260	13	6	910	21	3	4	14
Fettuccine Alfredo	290	8	4.5	470	42	2	4	8
Cheese Pizza	270	11	5	690	32	2	2	12
Dressing/Condiment/Topping								
Croutons	70	3	0	100	8	0	0	2
Red Wine Vinaigrette, 1.5 oz	110	10	1.5	410	3	0	2	0
Ranch Dressing, 1.5 oz	220	24	4	420	2	0	2	1
Lite Ranch, 1.5 oz	120	12	2	350	2	0	1	1
Lemon Basil Vinaigrette, 1.5 oz	110	11	1.5	380	5	0	3	0
Italian Dressing, 1.5 oz	160	14	2	760	7	0	7	0
Honey French Dressing, 1.5 oz	220	18	3	310	14	0	13	0
Fat Free Italian Dressing, 1.5 oz	25	0	0	390	6	0	3	0
Creamy Parmesan Peppercorn Ranch Dressing, 1.5 oz	230	24	4	380	2	0	2	1
Balsamic Vinaigrette, 1.5 oz	180	18	2.5	350	5	0	4	0
Dessert								
NY Style Cheesecake w/ Strawberry Topping	630	45	26	630	49	1	32	8
Italian Lemon Ice	170	0	0	15	46	0	46	0
Italian Lemon Ice w/ Strawberry	270	0	0	55	70	0	70	0
Chocolate Layer Cake	700	38	17	550	87	4	63	7
Chocolate Chunk Cookie	510	26	15	350	68	3	39	5
Chocolate Chip Cannolis	190	11	6	55	20	0	3	4
Choco-Lato Mousse	610	50	30	220	39	2	28	4

Firehouse Subs

Description & Serving	Cal	Fat	Sfat	Sod	Carb	Fiber	Sugar	Prot
Medium Sub (8")								
Hook & Ladder Sub	410	7	2	1360	68	3	9	19
Meatball Sub	740	42	16	1690	61	4	6	29
NY Steamer Sub	410	12	8	1940	48	2	4	25
Italian Sub	560	25	10	1870	55	3	10	24
Engine Company Sub	390	6	3	950	52	4	6	29
Engineer Sub	380	5	1	1600	55	4	8	28
Steak Sub	500	14	6	1300	62	4	8	29
Club On A Sub	510	16	4	1790	53	3	10	30
Hero Sub	430	7	4	1800	54	3	9	35
Turkey Sub	370	4	1	1390	54	3	7	28
Ham Sub	410	7	3	1330	58	3	12	18
Pastrami Sub	420	8	3	1690	58	2	6	31
Corned Beef Sub	400	13	6	1550	55	2	6	34
Roast Beef Sub	410	6	2	1370	48	3	5	30
Sliced Deli Chicken Sub	380	4	1	880	47	3	5	31

Description & Serving	Cal	Fat	Sfat	Sod	Carb	Fiber	Sugar	Prot
Veggie Sub	300	5	2	1020	56	4	6	12
Chicken Salad Sub	760	46	7	1330	63	2	8	27
Tuna Salad Sub	610	28	4	1170	62	2	10	32
Smokehouse Beef & Cheddar Sub	740	36	15	1820	63	3	16	41

Side

Chili	370	28	8	1520	17	4	5	14
Pickle Spear	5	0	0	240	1	0	0	0

Salad

Chef's Salad w/ Ham	360	18	3	900	16	3	17	26
Chef's Salad w/ Turkey	300	15	2	1120	12	3	4	34
Chef's Salad w/ Tuna Salad	610	40	9	720	16	3	9	40
Chef's Salad w/ Sliced Deli Chicken	320	14	1	1080	12	3	3	30
Chef's Salad w/ Chicken Salad	740	58	12	880	16	3	7	31

Kids

Turkey & Cheese	230	6	3	810	25	1	3	18
Ham & Cheese	240	8	4	800	28	1	6	13
Peanut Butter & Jelly	600	31	5	730	79	5	32	19
Grilled Cheese	380	25	8	640	23	2	1	11
Roast Beef & Cheese	385	15	5	780	42	2	9	20
Meatball & Cheese	450	30	11	880	28	1	3	19
Oreo Cookies, 2	110	5	1	150	15	0	13	1

Dessert

Chocolate Chip Cookie	290	14	5	240	37	2	13	5
Peanut Butter Cookie	360	26	6	300	25	3	5	10
Oatmeal Raisin Cookie	310	16	5	240	35	3	13	5
Macadamia Nut Cookie	330	17	7	170	41	1	26	4
Brownie	420	18	8	310	63	1	34	5

Dressing/Condiment/Topping

Italian Dressing, 1.5 oz	200	21	3	410	4	0	3	0
Ranch Dressing, 1.5 oz	260	28	4	240	2	0	2	1
Fat Free Ranch Dressing, 1.5 oz	40	0	0	550	11	1	4	0
Fat Free Raspberry Vinaigrette Dressing, 1.5 oz	45	0	0	110	12	0	10	0
Thousand Island Dressing, 1.5 oz	190	18	3	420	6	0	4	0
Balsamic Vinaigrette Dressing, 1.5 oz	160	17	3	400	2	0	1	0
Mayonnaise, 1 oz	200	22	3	130	1	0	0	0
White Bread, 8"	240	3	1	490	46	2	4	8
Wheat Bread, 8"	230	3	1	580	46	4	8	8
Provolone Cheese, 2 slices	100	8	5	250	1	0	0	7
Swiss Cheese, 2 slices	110	8	5	60	1	0	0	8
Monterey Jack Cheese, 2 slices	105	9	5	190	1	0	0	7
Cheddar Cheese, 2 slices	110	9	6	350	0	0	0	7

Five Guys Burgers and Fries

Burger/Sandwich

Hamburger	700	43	19.5	430	39	2	8	39
Cheeseburger	840	55	26.5	1050	40	2	9	47

Description & Serving	Cal	Fat	Sfat	Sod	Carb	Fiber	Sugar	Prot
Bacon Burger	780	50	22.5	690	39	2	8	43
Bacon Cheeseburger	920	62	29.5	1310	40	2	9	51
Little Hamburger	480	26	11.5	380	39	2	8	23
Little Cheeseburger	550	32	15	690	39.5	2	8.5	27
Little Bacon Burger	560	33	14.5	640	39	2	8	27
Little Bacon Cheeseburger	630	39	18	950	39.5	2	8.5	31
Veggie Sandwich	440	15	6	1040	60	2	14	16
Grilled Cheese	430	26	9	715	41	2.5	10	11

Hot Dog

	Cal	Fat	Sfat	Sod	Carb	Fiber	Sugar	Prot
Hot Dog	545	35	15.5	1130	40	2	8	18
Cheese Dog	615	41	19	1440	40.5	2	8.5	22
Bacon Dog	625	42	18.5	1390	40	2	8	22
Bacon Cheese Dog	695	48	22	1700	40.5	2	8.5	26

Side

	Cal	Fat	Sfat	Sod	Carb	Fiber	Sugar	Prot
One Serving of Fries	310	15	3	45	39	3	1	5
Regular Fries	620	30	6	90	78	6	2	10
Large Fries	1464	71	14	213	184	14	5	24

Topping/Dressing/Condiment

	Cal	Fat	Sfat	Sod	Carb	Fiber	Sugar	Prot
Cheese, 1 slice	70	6	3.5	310	<1	0	<1	4
Bacon, 2 slices	80	7	3	260	0	0	0	4
Mushrooms, 25 g	10	0	0	100	1	<1	0	1
Green Peppers, 25 g	5	0	0	1	2	<1	<1	0
Onions, 26 g	10	0	0	1	3	<1	1	0
Jalepenos, 11 g	3	0	0	184	<1	0	0	0
Lettuce, 30 g	4	0	0	3	1	<1	<1	0
Tomatoes, 52 g	9	0	0	3	2	<1	2	<1
Mayonnaise, 14 g	100	11	2	75	NP	NP	0	0
Ketchup, 1 tbsp	15	0	0	190	4	0	4	0
A.1. Original Steak Sauce, 1 tbsp	15	0	0	280	3	0	2	0
BBQ Sauce, 1 tbsp	60	0	0	400	16	0	10	0
Mustard, 1 tbsp	0	0	0	55	0	0	0	0
Hot Sauce, 1 tsp	0	0	0	0	0	0	0	0
Relish, 15 g	15	0	0	85	4	0	3	0
Pickles, 6 chips	5	0	0	265	1	0	0	0

Freshëns

Ice Cream

	Cal	Fat	Sfat	Sod	Carb	Fiber	Sugar	Prot
NF Vanilla Cup, 7 oz	241	0	0	148	48	0	35	7
NF Chocolate Cup, 7 oz	256	1	0	146	48	1	33	8
NF Vanilla Cake Cone	197	0	0	121	40	0	26	5
NF Chocolate Cake Cone	208	0.5	0	119	40	1	25	6
NF Vanilla Waffle Cone	297	1.5	0	162	62	1	37	8
NF Chocolate Waffle Cone	309	1.5	0	160	61	2	36	9

Frozen Treat

	Cal	Fat	Sfat	Sod	Carb	Fiber	Sugar	Prot
Chocolate Milkshake	533	4.5	2.5	316	103	0	79	15
Oreo Milkshake	643	9	3.5	528	121	1	88	16

Description & Serving	Cal	Fat	Sfat	Sod	Carb	Fiber	Sugar	Prot
Strawberry Milkshake	568	4	2.5	286	115	1	94	14
Vanilla Milkshake	506	4	2.5	279	99	0	79	14
Brownie Batter Microblast	724	25	13	317	115	1	79	15
Cookie Dough Microblast	630	16	8	304	108	1	75	13
Oreo Microblast	469	5	1	442	90	1	59	12
Reese's Peanut Butter Microblast	751	29	13	382	104	3	79	21
Tripple Berry Microblast	401	1	0	216	82	2	61	11

Smoothie

Description & Serving	Cal	Fat	Sfat	Sod	Carb	Fiber	Sugar	Prot
Acai Energy Smoothie, 21 oz	322	3	NP	19	72	3	67	1
All That Razz Smoothie, 21 oz	360	0	NP	179	79	3	69	12
Berry Breeze Smoothie, 21 oz	306	0	NP	24	77	3	70	1
Caribbean Craze Smoothie, 21 oz	288	0	NP	16	73	2	66	1
High Test Energizer Smoothie, 21 oz	299	0	NP	96	74	1	67	1
Jamaican Jammer Smoothie, 21 oz	355	0	NP	177	78	2	69	12
Mango Beach Smoothie, 21 oz	90	0	NP	23	48	1	5	0
Maui Mango Smoothie, 21 oz	292	0	NP	22	74	2	60	1
Mystic Mango Smoothie, 21 oz	357	3	NP	47	82	2	53	3
OJ Sunrise Smoothie, 21 oz	353	3	NP	41	81	2	59	3
Orange Passion Smoothie, 21 oz	133	3	NP	43	37	1	6	2
Peach Sunset Smoothie, 21 oz	268	0	NP	21	67	2	61	1
Peachy Pineapple Smoothie, 21 oz	337	0	NP	178	73	2	66	11
Peanut Butter Energizer Smoothie, 21 oz	474	10	NP	277	83	2	74	16
Pineapple Paradise Smoothie, 21 oz	331	4	NP	25	77	NP	72	0
Strawberry Oasis Smoothie, 21 oz	89	0	NP	17	49	1	9	1
Strawberry Shooter Smoothie, 21 oz	246	0	NP	15	64	1	59	1
Strawberry Squeeze Smoothie, 21 oz	313	0	NP	176	68	1	62	11
Strawberry Sunrise Smoothie, 21 oz	153	0	NP	162	35	1	6	10
Acai Energy Bowl Smoothie, 21 oz	361	7	NP	36	68	5	57	3
Energy Zone Acai Energy Smoothie, 21 oz	443	4	NP	13	98	4	93	2
Blueberry Bay Smoothie, 21 oz	305	0	NP	22	77	3	70	1
Mango Spirit Smoothie, 21 oz	291	0	NP	21	74	2	60	1
Mystical Mango Smoothie, 21 oz	362	3	NP	53	83	2	54	3
Orange Sunrise Smoothie, 21 oz	358	3	NP	47	83	2	60	3
Peach Paradise Smoothie, 21 oz	325	0	NP	180	70	2	63	11
Peach Passion Smoothie, 21 oz	267	0	NP	20	67	2	61	1
Raspberry Royale Smoothie, 21 oz	358	0	NP	178	79	3	69	12
Strawberry Karma Smoothie, 21 oz	245	0	NP	14	64	1	59	0
Strawberry Mirage Smoothie, 21 oz	287	0	NP	15	73	2	66	1
Strawberry Nirvana Smoothie, 21 oz	311	0	NP	176	68	1	63	11
Strawberry Spirit Smoothie, 21 oz	354	0	NP	177	78	2	69	12
Soulful Strawberry Smoothie, 21 oz	89	0	NP	19	49	1	9	0
Majestic Mango Smoothie, 21 oz	90	0	NP	26	48	1	5	0
Magical Strawberry Smoothie, 21 oz	154	0	NP	165	35	1	6	10
Mystic Mango 2Go Juice Smoothie, 8 oz	140	0	NP	5	35	1	29	1
Verry Berry 2Go Juice Smoothie, 8 oz	130	0	NP	10	33	NP	28	0
CitrusC 2Go Juice Smoothie, 8 oz	130	0	NP	10	32	NP	28	1
MegaGreen 2Go Juice Smoothie, 8 oz	150	0	NP	10	36	NP	33	0
Pomegranate Blueberry 2Go Juice Smoothie, 8 oz	140	0	NP	10	38	0	32	0

Description & Serving	Cal	Fat	Sfat	Sod	Carb	Fiber	Sugar	Prot
JavaBoost								
Mocha JavaBoost, 16 oz	462	9	7	172	87	1	68	8
Mocha Light JavaBoost, 16 oz	282	4	3.5	130	58	1	29	6
Caramel JavaBoost, 16 oz	475	10	7	242	88	0	67	8
Caramel Light JavaBoost, 16 oz	302	5	4	194	61	0	30	7
Java Chip JavaBoost, 16 oz	704	32	19	187	104	1	83	10
Strawberry Crème JavaBoost, 16 oz	471	9	7	167	89	1	73	8
Strawberry Crème Light JavaBoost, 16 oz	293	4	3.5	130	61	1	33	6
Vanilla Crème JavaBoost, 16 oz	419	9	7	157	78	0	63	8
Vanilla Crème Light JavaBoost, 16 oz	262	4	3.5	123	54	0	28	6
Double Chocolate JavaBoost, 16 oz	751	41	24	189	99	0	78	11
Snack								
Banana Nut Muffin	440	22	4	420	53	6	26	10
Whole Grain Blueberry Cranberry Muffin	460	22	4.5	460	58	7	31	10
Fudge Brownie	380	17	5	230	48	5	31	10
Yogurt Parfait w/ Granola	402	2.5	NP	177	402	4	48	10
Yogurt Parfait w/o Granola	295	1	NP	108	295	2	40	8
Freshëns Gummy Bear	140	0	NP	0	32	0	22	2
Freshëns CA/Aloha Mix	200	10	NP	30	24	2	13	3
Freshëns Dark Chocolate Covered Almonds	240	18	NP	0	16	3	11	5
Freshëns Yogurt Covered Pretzels	180	6	NP	150	30	0	13	3
Energy Sports Mix	170	8	NP	10	23	3	16	3
Super Antioxidant Mix	180	8	NP	0	21	3	15	4

Friendly's

Breakfast								
Super Sizzlin Combo	570	37	11	1020	43	4	1	16
Super Sizzlin Bacon	440	23	6	980	42	4	1	16
Super Sizzlin Sausage	690	50	17	1070	43	4	1	17
Super Sizzlin Ham	450	18	4	1800	45	4	4	26
3 Pancakes	930	17	8	2140	175	5	61	14
French Toast, 3 pc	760	20	9	1220	128	3	55	16
2 Sausage	200	19	7	270	0	0	0	6
Bacon, 2 slices	70	6	2	230	0	0	0	6
Hickory Smoked Ham	100	4	2	850	2	0	2	14
Tri-Tip Steak	350	19	8	850	0	0	2	44
2 Pancakes	500	17	7	1440	77	3	15	9
Pancake Syrup	240	0	0	30	58	0	38	0
Homefries	290	12	2	530	41	4	1	5
1 Egg Sunny	90	7	2	90	0	0	0	6
1 Egg Scrambled	110	8	2	80	1	0	1	7
1 Egg Poached	70	5	2	150	0	0	0	6
1 Eggbeater Scrambled	50	3	0	130	1	0	1	8
White Toast	200	10	5	320	23	2	1	4
Wheat Toast	200	10	5	300	22	2	3	5
Rye Toast	340	12	5	470	48	2	4	10

Description & Serving	Cal	Fat	SFat	Sod	Carb	Fiber	Sugar	Prot
English Muffin	310	11	5	460	45	2	2	8
Grape Jelly	60	0	0	0	14	0	14	0
Orange Marmalade	40	0	0	0	10	0	4	0
Cranberry Muffin	630	40	10	580	59	2	33	8
Blueberry Muffin	610	36	10	630	64	1	37	7
Bagel	350	11	5	520	55	5	5	10
Bagel w/ cream cheese	440	19	9	640	57	5	6	11
Strawberry Topping	190	0	0	40	48	4	44	1
Ham & Cheese Omelette w/ orange slice	580	43	16	1630	9	0	7	50
Western Omelette w/ orange slice	640	45	18	1150	12	1	8	45
4 Cheese & Bacon Omelette w/ orange slice	670	50	18	1110	8	0	5	46
Garden Omelette w/ orange slice	860	55	19	1170	52	5	7	40
Bacon Cheese Supermelt w/ orange slice	680	39	15	1350	52	3	7	33
Sausage Mushroom Swiss Supermelt w/ orange slice	910	58	24	1260	56	4	7	42
Ham & Cheese Supermelt w/ orange slice	660	35	14	1540	53	3	7	34

Appetizer

Towering Fronions	1430	90	13	2970	140	7	31	14
Munchie Mania	1670	108	36	3700	123	8	22	52
Loaded Waffle Fries	1660	112	28	4740	123	9	7	32
Mini Mozzarella Cheese Sticks	680	40	14	1870	55	4	5	24
Chicken Quesadilla	570	35	19	1340	29	3	6	33
Buffalo Chicken	1200	95	22	2920	45	5	5	41
Jumbo Fronions & Waffle Fries	1270	76	11	3140	134	8	24	12
Loaded Jumbo Fronions & Waffle Fries	1600	110	22	3750	129	8	16	23
Slider Munchie Mania - Mini Cheeseburger	1740	109	32	4420	141	12	14	49
Slider Munchie Mania - Chicken	1990	127	35	4690	161	14	24	52

Salad

Side Salad w/o dressing	60	1	0	100	10	2	3	2
Side Caesar Salad w/ dressing	410	36	7	640	15	1	5	9
Crispy Chicken Salad w/o dressing	710	42	12	820	45	6	6	37
Oriental Chicken Salad w/o dressing	500	21	3	1200	41	5	23	37
Chicken Caesar Salad w/ dressing	1030	84	16	2010	32	3	10	47
Kickin' Buffalo Chicken Salad w/o dressing	770	50	10	1350	48	6	6	31

Soup

Cup Chunky Chicken Noodle Soup	260	9	3	1880	27	2	4	19
Cup Minestrone Soup	60	1	0	530	11	2	2	3
Cup Broccoli Cheddar Soup	170	12	7	690	10	1	3	6
Cup Homestyle Clam Chowder Soup	240	17	10	800	13	1	3	10

Sandwich/Wrap

Crispy Chicken Tender Deluxe	800	46	10	1410	72	6	10	28
Grilled Chicken Deluxe	640	32	8	1580	54	5	9	38
Honey Mustard Chicken Sandwich	850	49	14	1410	74	6	12	33
Buffalo Chicken Sandwich	940	61	12	1950	69	6	7	30
Country Club Chicken Sandwich	940	57	16	1720	71	6	10	40
Chicken Parm Supermelt	830	43	13	1640	73	4	7	43

Description & Serving	Cal	Fat	Sfat	Sod	Carb	Fiber	Sugar	Prot
Turkey Club Supermelt	670	33	12	2090	54	3	10	42
Reuben Supermelt	800	42	17	2750	57	2	10	50
Tuna Supermelt	810	52	14	1540	50	3	6	35
Honey BBQ Chicken Supermelt	1080	62	21	2030	86	4	23	47
Friendly's BLT	680	45	12	980	51	3	8	20
Grilled Cheese	460	23	11	1120	48	2	4	16
Grilled Ham & Cheese	510	23	14	1880	49	2	6	28
Crispy Chicken Wrap	800	40	7	1450	84	6	14	27
Crispy Chicken Caesar Wrap	1180	80	17	2170	75	5	7	40
Buffalo Chicken Wrap	1180	80	18	2480	75	5	6	38

Burger

All American Burger	860	54	18	1010	55	4	12	39
Cheese add-on	90	7	5	380	1	0	0	4
Bacon add-on	70	6	2	230	0	0	0	6
Bacon Cheeseburger	940	61	23	1390	55	3	11	43
Deluxe Cheeseburger "Set-Up"	850	61	24	1150	35	3	5	40
Western BBQ Burger	1230	77	29	1860	86	4	21	51
Mushroom Swiss Bacon Burger	1240	87	32	1900	61	3	16	59
Swiss Patty Melt	1030	64	26	1600	62	4	12	52
Turkey Burger	140	78	26	1910	61	3	16	50
Ultimate Bacon Cheeseburger	1050	69	26	1730	55	3	11	52
Colossal Burger	1490	104	42	2320	56	4	12	82

Entrée

Beef

Friendly Frank	410	30	12	910	25	1	5	11
Steak Fajita Quesadilla	1220	79	39	2890	65	7	12	62
Sirloin Steak	510	28	9	1150	19	1	4	46
Southwest BBQ Steak	760	42	18	2230	37	2	13	57
Homestyle Meatloaf	850	49	18	2280	45	1	7	54
Sirloin Steak Tips	490	20	6	2580	31	5	17	46

Chicken

Chicken Quesadilla	1020	67	35	2280	56	4	8	29
Chicken Fajita Quesadilla	1220	77	37	2790	65	7	11	67
Chicken Strips Basket, 5 pc	540	32	5	910	32	3	1	32
Honey BBQ Chicken Strips, 5 pc	910	32	5	1450	126	3	79	32
Kickin' Buffalo Chicken Strips, 5 pc	810	59	5	2080	35	3	1	32
BBQ Chicken Platter	1010	42	18	3370	75	2	32	79
Cheddar Jack Chicken	640	34	17	2000	5	1	2	78

Seafood

Fishamajig	640	37	13	1360	51	3	5	26
Tuna Roll	580	43	9	920	25	2	5	24
Shrimp Basket	570	35	4	2310	42	4	2	12
Clamboat Basket	990	54	8	2610	104	6	5	24
New England Fish 'n Chips	660	44	7	1700	45	3	7	21
Grilled Flounder	520	32	6	1870	28	2	1	29

Vegetarian

Vegetable Fajita Quesadilla	1210	82	37	2920	77	12	14	43

Description & Serving	Cal	Fat	Sfat	Sod	Carb	Fiber	Sugar	Prot
Side								
Garlic Bread	130	6	1	190	18	0	1	3
Garden Vegetables	110	6	3	110	13	4	6	3
Corn	160	7	3	70	20	4	9	4
Broccoli	90	6	3	100	6	4	2	3
Rice	210	3	0	900	41	0	2	3
Spanish Rice	330	15	6	1200	41	0	2	7
Homestyle Mashed Potatoes	240	12	7	160	29	2	4	4
Golden Fries	350	16	2	130	47	4	0	5
Waffle Fries	590	33	5	1430	67	5	1	7
Cole Slaw	160	12	2	260	13	2	8	1
Applesauce	110	0	0	0	27	1	25	0
Mandarin Oranges	80	0	0	10	20	0	18	0
Portabella Mushrooms	40	1	0	240	5	2	0	2
Kids								
Breakfast								
2 Pancakes	760	17	7	1470	141	4	57	9
Funcake	600	19	9	930	100	2	48	8
Tie-Dyed Pancake	600	12	6	730	117	3	63	6
French Toast Stix	640	17	8	860	109	2	53	11
Sausage	200	19	7	270	0	0	0	6
Bacon	70	6	2	230	0	0	0	6
2 Eggs Sunny	220	17	4	290	1	0	1	13
2 Eggs Scrambled	220	16	3	290	3	0	3	14
Toast	200	10	5	320	23	2	1	4
Lunch/Dinner								
Beef								
Cheeseburger	450	27	12	1010	29	1	4	21
Hamburger	410	24	10	820	29	1	4	19
Cheeseburger Sliders	450	21	7	1270	46	6	6	21
Cheeseburger Sliders (Big Kids Meal)	720	32	11	2910	80	9	21	31
Friendly Frank	410	30	13	1000	25	1	4	10
Cheesy Mac & Frank	510	26	9	1470	50	2	1	18
Chicken								
Friendly's Chicken Fingers	330	19	3	730	19	2	1	19
Chicken Sliders	710	38	10	1340	65	7	16	24
Chicken Sliders (Big Kids Meal)	1030	52	14	2400	106	11	31	35
Chicken in the Garden, Crispy	510	30	9	820	33	5	5	29
Chicken in the Garden, Grilled	350	16	8	1000	15	4	5	38
Dippin' Chicken	750	40	6	1910	70	2	33	26
Wrap It Up, Crispy	950	49	13	2370	94	5	24	34
Wrap It Up, Grilled	790	35	12	2550	76	4	24	43
Vegetarian								
Mini Mozzarella Sticks	360	21	7	1250	30	2	4	12
Mini Mozzarella Sticks (Big Kids Meal)	730	41	15	2650	68	4	17	24
Mozzarella Sticks	430	26	9	1430	36	3	4	15
Mac & Cheese	340	11	3	1020	48	2	1	12

Description & Serving	Cal	Fat	Sfat	Sod	Carb	Fiber	Sugar	Prot
Grilled Cheese	290	17	9	890	24	2	1	8
Cheese Quesadilla	890	60	34	1580	51	3	7	37
Cotton Candy Drink	220	0	0	30	56	0	54	0
Side								
Side Salad	60	1	0	100	10	2	3	2
Fries	390	17	3	150	52	4	1	6
Waffle Fries	390	22	3	950	44	3	1	5
Homestyle Mashed Potatoes	240	12	7	160	29	2	4	4
Cole Slaw	160	12	2	260	13	2	8	1
Beverage/Dessert								
Royal Razz	220	0	0	30	56	0	54	0
Friendly's Shirley Temple	220	0	0	30	55	0	53	0
Vanilla Fribble	410	13	9	240	64	0	56	10
Chocolate Fribble	390	12	8	280	61	1	51	12
Strawberry Fribble	410	13	9	290	66	0	55	10
Kids Double Headed Cone	20	0	0	20	5	0	0	1
Kids Hot Fudge Sundae	330	17	11	100	41	1	30	4
Oreo Sundae	420	20	12	200	53	1	38	6
Monster Mash Sundae	430	22	12	160	51	1	41	8
Cone Head Sundae	430	20	13	170	56	1	39	7
Peanut Butter Cup Friend-Z Sundae	860	45	19	500	95	5	73	19
Birthday Cake Friend-Z	690	29	13	270	100	0	76	9
Jim Dandy Jr.	470	20	10	100	67	1	50	6
Seniors								
Turkey Club Supermelt	690	35	14	2290	53	3	10	45
Friendly's Big Beef Burger	860	54	18	1210	55	4	12	39
Cheddar Jack Chicken	320	17	9	1000	3	1	1	39
BBQ Chicken Platter	420	17	9	1330	28	0	15	39
Clamboat Platter	660	36	5	1740	70	4	4	16
Dressing/Condiment								
Honey Mustard Dressing (for side salad)	180	15	2	210	12	0	9	0
Sesame Oriental Dressing (for side salad)	130	7	1	480	18	0	15	0
Bleu Cheese Dressing (for side salad)	240	24	5	360	2	0	2	3
Ranch Dressing (for side salad)	160	17	3	380	2	0	2	2
Thousand Island Dressing (for side salad)	190	18	3	420	8	0	6	0
Italian Dressing (for side salad)	210	21	3	350	3	0	3	0
Fat-Free Italian Dressing (for side salad)	30	0	0	420	8	0	6	0
Dessert								
Frozen Drink								
Vanilla Double Thick Milkshake	650	26	17	220	91	0	80	13
Chocolate Double Thick Milkshake	590	26	17	260	74	1	63	18
Strawberry Double Thick Milkshake	600	23	13	310	84	0	74	13
Coffee Double Thick Milkshake	650	26	15	230	93	0	77	13
Vanilla Fribble Shake	620	19	12	360	100	0	88	16
Chocolate Fribble Shake	590	17	11	420	94	1	78	19
Strawberry Fribble Shake	610	19	12	420	93	0	78	16
Coffee Fribble Shake	630	19	12	360	102	0	85	16

Description & Serving	Cal	Fat	Sfat	Sod	Carb	Fiber	Sugar	Prot
Butterfinger Fribble Shake	990	33	20	520	155	2	125	19
Oreo Freeze	770	25	16	530	120	2	93	18
Barq's Float	580	19	14	150	98	0	89	6
Watermelon Slammer	450	4	3	80	100	0	76	3
Orange Slammer	600	4	3	80	138	0	115	3
Frozen Treat								
Jim Dandy	1080	46	27	270	156	2	121	14
Royal Banana Split	880	35	20	200	132	2	102	10
Forbidden Fudge Brownie	920	40	51	320	130	5	86	12
Fruit & Sherbet Happy Ending Sundae	240	5	3	50	47	0	36	2
Ultimate Cookies 'N Cream	680	32	20	320	85	1	60	11
Reese's Peanut Butter Cup Sundae	870	51	50	360	90	8	61	16
Strawberry Shortcake Sundae	580	26	16	190	79	2	63	8
Butterfinger Sundae	830	36	22	370	117	2	81	9
Reese's Pieces Sundae	1310	70	37	450	151	5	113	22
Caramel Fudge Brownie Sundae	1530	70	43	680	206	2	133	21
Friend-Z Heath	680	34	19	410	88	0	78	9
Friend-Z Oreo	580	23	12	470	84	2	62	9
Friend-Z M&M	560	23	52	260	80	2	70	10
Friend-Z Reese's Peanut Butter Cup	860	45	21	520	96	4	71	20
Friend-Z Strawberry/Banana	430	14	9	220	69	1	57	8
Friend-Z Butterfinger	820	32	19	430	122	3	90	11
Friend-Z Strawberry Shortcake	470	17	9	260	72	1	58	8
Birthday Cake Friend-Z	690	29	13	270	100	0	76	9
Giant Crowd Pleaser	2460	117	64	910	317	5	235	40
Mint Cookie Crunch	650	32	20	260	80	1	58	11
Ice Cream								
Vanilla Ice Cream, 1 scoop	120	6	4	35	14	0	11	2
Chocolate Ice Cream, 1 scoop	110	6	4	40	10	0	9	2
Strawberry Ice Cream, 1 scoop	110	5	3	35	14	0	12	2
Coffee Ice Cream, 1 scoop	110	6	4	35	13	0	11	2
Mint Chocolate Ice Cream, 1 scoop	130	7	4	35	15	0	12	2
Chocolate Chip Cookie Dough Ice Cream, 1 scoop	130	7	4	40	17	0	12	2
Black Raspberry Ice Cream, 1 scoop	120	5	4	35	15	0	13	2
Chocolate Almond Chip Ice Cream, 1 scoop	120	7	4	40	11	0	10	2
Chocolate Chip Ice Cream, 1 scoop	130	7	4	35	15	0	12	2
Cookies 'n Cream Ice Cream, 1 scoop	130	6	4	55	16	0	12	2
Pistachio Ice Cream, 1 scoop	130	7	4	35	14	0	11	3
Vienna Mocha Chunk Ice Cream, 1 scoop	140	8	5	35	16	0	14	2
Nuts Over Caramel Ice Cream, 1 scoop	150	8	4	50	18	0	11	2
Butter Pecan Ice Cream, 1 scoop	130	8	4	35	13	0	11	2
Maple Walnut Ice Cream, 1 scoop	130	8	4	35	13	0	11	2
Butter Crunch Ice Cream, 1 scoop	130	6	4	100	16	0	14	2
Forbidden Chocolate Ice Cream, 1 scoop	130	7	5	35	14	0	11	3
Hunka Chunka PB Fudge Ice Cream, 1 scoop	180	11	5	70	17	1	12	3
Mocha Mud Crunch Ice Cream, 1 scoop	160	9	5	60	18	1	13	2
Peanut Butter Cup Ice Cream, 1 scoop	150	9	4	70	16	1	13	3
Orange Sherbet, 1 scoop	80	1	1	15	17	0	12	1

Description & Serving	Cal	Fat	Sfat	Sod	Carb	Fiber	Sugar	Prot
Watermelon Sherbet, 1 scoop	80	1	1	15	17	0	13	1
Non Fat Vanilla Yogurt, 1 scoop	80	0	0	55	17	0	11	3
Non Fat Red Raspberry Swirl Yogurt, 1 scoop	90	0	0	45	19	0	14	3
No Sugar Added Vanilla Ice Cream, 1 scoop	100	7	5	25	11	3	2	2
Vanilla Soft Serve, 4 oz	180	7	4	100	25	0	21	3
Chocolate Soft Serve, 4 oz	170	6	4	120	24	0	21	4
Twist Soft Serve, 4 oz	170	7	4	110	25	0	21	4
Sugar Cone	50	0	0	50	11	0	4	1
Cake Cone	30	0	0	15	7	0	0	1
Waffle Cone	90	1	0	35	20	1	7	2
Topping								
No Sugar Added Fudge Topping	90	0	0	0	25	2	0	1
Hot Fudge Topping	110	4	4	45	18	1	10	1
Marshmallow Topping	100	0	0	10	24	0	18	0
Peanut Butter Topping	210	17	3	130	7	3	4	7
Caramel Topping	130	2	1	100	27	0	14	1
Strawberry Topping	40	0	0	10	10	1	9	1
Swiss Chocolate Topping	100	0	0	35	25	0	19	0
Whipped Topping	80	6	4	20	5	0	4	1
Chocolate Syrup	100	0	0	20	23	1	16	1
Roasted Sliced Almonds	110	10	1	60	3	2	1	4
Walnuts	100	10	0	0	2	0	1	0
Reese's Pieces	130	6	4	50	15	1	14	3
Peanut Butter Cup	90	5	2	60	10	1	9	2
Crushed Heath	170	10	5	100	19	0	18	1
Gummy Bears	90	0	0	10	21	0	14	1
M&M's	100	5	3	15	15	1	14	1
Crushed Oreos	60	2	1	65	9	0	5	1
Butterfinger Pieces	120	5	3	60	18	1	12	1
Chocolate Sprinkles	120	5	2	4	19	0	9	0
Rainbow Sprinkles	120	5	2	1	18	0	9	0
Cherry	10	0	0	2	2	0	1	0

Gatti's Pizza

Pizza, medium

Original Crust, 1 slice

Description & Serving	Cal	Fat	Sfat	Sod	Carb	Fiber	Sugar	Prot
Cheese Pizza	197	6	3	374	26	1	1	10
Pepperoni Pizza	203	7	3	405	26	NP	1	9
Canadian Bacon Pizza	188	5	2	408	26	1	1	10
Bacon Pizza	207	7	3	455	26	1	1	11
Burger Pizza	207	6	3	489	27	1	1	11
Sausage Pizza	217	7	3	498	27	1	1	11
Italian Sausage Pizza	230	9	4	513	27	1	1	11
Spicy Burger Pizza	212	6	3	460	27	1	1	11
Meat Market Pizza	238	9	4	599	27	1	1	12
Bacon Double Cheeseburger Pizza	264	10	5	631	29	1	4	14
BBQ Chicken Pizza	218	8	4	248	23	0	1	13
Sampler Pizza	231	8	3	612	28	1	2	11

Description & Serving	Cal	Fat	Sfat	Sod	Carb	Fiber	Sugar	Prot
Pan Perfect Crust, 1 slice								
Cheese Pizza	260	NP	4	410	30	1	1	12
Pepperoni Pizza	267	NP	4	442	30	NP	1	11
Canadian Bacon Pizza	251	NP	4	444	30	1	1	11
Bacon Pizza	271	NP	4	492	30	1	1	13
Burger Pizza	270	NP	4	525	31	1	1	13
Sausage Pizza	280	NP	5	534	31	1	1	12
Italian Sausage Pizza	293	NP	5	549	31	1	1	12
Spicy Burger Pizza	275	NP	4	496	31	1	1	13
Meat Market Pizza	302	NP	5	635	31	1	1	14
Bacon Double Cheeseburger Pizza	327	NP		667	33	1	4	16
BBQ Chicken Pizza	281	NP	5	284	27	0	1	14
Sampler Pizza	294	NP	5	648	32	1	2	13
Thin Crust, 1 slice								
Cheese Pizza	137	6	3	275	12	1	1	8
Pepperoni Pizza	143	7	3	307	12	1	1	7
Canadian Bacon Pizza	127	5	2	309	13	1	1	8
Bacon Pizza	147	7	3	257	12	1	1	9
Burger Pizza	147	6	3	390	13	1	1	9
Sausage Pizza	156	8	3	399	13	1	1	9
Italian Sausage Pizza	170	9	4	414	13	1	1	9
Spicy Burger Pizza	152	7	3	361	14	1	1	9
Meat Market Pizza	178	9	4	500	14	1	1	10
Bacon Double Cheeseburger Pizza	203	10	5	532	16	1	4	12
BBQ Chicken Pizza	158	8	4	149	10	0	1	11
Sampler Pizza	171	8	3	513	14	1	1	10

Pizza, large

Description & Serving	Cal	Fat	Sfat	Sod	Carb	Fiber	Sugar	Prot
Original Crust, 1 slice								
Cheese Pizza	177	5	2	332	24	1	1	9
Pepperoni Pizza	185	6	3	368	24	0	1	8
Canadian Bacon Pizza	167	4	2	361	24	0	1	8
Bacon Pizza	186	6	2	404	24	0	1	10
Burger Pizza	187	5	2	446	25	0	1	10
Sausage Pizza	197	6	3	455	25	0	1	10
Italian Sausage Pizza	210	8	3	470	25	0	1	9
Spicy Burger Pizza	192	6	3	418	25	0	1	10
Meat Market Pizza	213	8	3	528	25	0	1	11
Bacon Double Cheeseburger Pizza	241	9	4	574	27	1	4	13
BBQ Chicken Pizza	181	7	3	121	19	0	0	10
Sampler Pizza	204	7	3	530	25	1	1	10
Pan Perfect Crust, 1 slice								
Cheese Pizza	229	10	4	365	25	1	1	10
Pepperoni Pizza	237	11	4	401	25	1	1	10
Canadian Bacon Pizza	219	9	3	394	25	1	1	10
Bacon Pizza	238	10	4	437	25	1	1	11
Burger Pizza	239	10	4	480	26	1	1	11
Sausage Pizza	249	11	4	489	26	1	1	11

Description & Serving	Cal	Fat	Sfat	Sod	Carb	Fiber	Sugar	Prot
Italian Sausage Pizza	262	13	5	504	26	1	1	11
Spicy Burger Pizza	244	10	4	451	26	1	1	11
Meat Market Pizza	264	12	5	562	26	1	1	12
Bacon Double Cheeseburger Pizza	293	14	6	607	29	1	4	14
BBQ Chicken Pizza	233	12	5	155	20	0	0	12
Sampler Pizza	256	12	4	563	27	1	1	11
Thin Crust, 1 slice								
Cheese Pizza	121	5	3	240	11	1	1	7
Pepperoni Pizza	129	6	3	276	11	1	1	7
Canadian Bacon Pizza	111	4	2	269	11	1	1	7
Bacon Pizza	129	6	3	312	11	1	1	8
Burger Pizza	131	6	2	357	12	1	1	8
Sausage Pizza	140	7	3	364	12	1	1	8
Italian Sausage Pizza	154	8	3	379	12	1	1	8
Spicy Burger Pizza	136	6	3	326	12	1	1	1
Meat Market Pizza	156	8	3	437	12	1	1	9
Bacon Double Cheeseburger Pizza	184	9	4	482	15	1	3	11
BBQ Chicken Pizza	125	7	4	124	6	0	0	9
Sampler Pizza	147	7	3	438	13	1	1	8
Side								
Spaghetti, 1/2 cup	118	1	0	2	24	1	1	4
Chicken Wings HOT, 3 pc	150	11	3	280	1	0	1	14
Tossed Salad, 1 cup	9	0	0	6	2	1	1	1
Cheese Sticks, 1 slice	140	7	2	163	14	0	0	5
Jalapeno Cheese Sticks, 1 slice	141	7	2	208	15	0	0	5
Garlic Sticks, 1 slice	108	5	1	79	14	0	0	2
Dressing/Condiment								
Ranch Dressing, 2 tbsp	126	13	2	255	1	1	0	1
Meat Sauce, 1/2 cup	100	4	1	520	13	2	8	5
Marinara, 1/2 cup	50	0	0	630	11	1	6	2
Alfredo, 1/4 cup	130	12	7	380	3	0	1	4
Dessert Pizza, 1 slice								
Coconut Cream Dessert Pizza	211	7	2	181	32	1	3	4
Chocolate Dessert Pizza	260	9	2	190	39	1	7	5
Dutch Apple Dessert Pizza	280	10	2	181	43	1	9	5
Very Cherry Dessert Pizza	279	9	2	181	43	1	10	5

Godfather's Pizza

Pizza

Mini Size, 1 slice

	Cal	Fat	Sfat	Sod	Carb	Fiber	Sugar	Prot
Original Crust All Meat Combo Pizza	220	9	3.5	470	21	1	2	12
Original Crust Bacon Cheeseburger Pizza	210	9	4.5	540	21	1	2	11
Original Crust Cheese Pizza	150	4	2	250	20	1	1	7
Original Crust Combo Pizza	200	8	3	500	21	2	2	10
Original Crust Hawaiian Pizza	160	4	2	270	22	1	4	7

Description & Serving	Cal	Fat	SFat	Sod	Carb	Fiber	Sugar	Prot
Original Crust Hot Stuff Pizza	210	9	3.5	490	21	1	2	10
Original Crust Humble Pie Pizza	220	11	4	430	21	1	2	10
Original Crust Pepperoni Pizza	160	5	2	310	20	1	1	7
Original Crust Super Combo Pizza	220	9	4	520	22	2	2	11
Original Crust Super Hawaiian Pizza	170	5	2	270	21	1	3	9
Original Crust Super Taco Pizza	230	10	5	520	22	2	2	11
Original Crust Taco Pizza	210	9	4	490	22	2	2	11
Original Crust Veggie Pizza	160	4.5	2	300	21	1	2	7

Small Size, 1 slice

Golden Crust

	Cal	Fat	SFat	Sod	Carb	Fiber	Sugar	Prot
All Meat Combo Pizza	310	14	6	710	26	2	2	16
Bacon Cheeseburger Pizza	290	14	6	650	26	2	2	15
Cheese Pizza	200	6	2.5	360	25	1	2	9
Combo Pizza	300	14	5	750	27	2	2	14
Hawaiian Pizza	220	7	3	380	26	1	3	10
Hot Stuff Pizza	300	14	6	760	26	2	2	14
Humble Pie Pizza	320	16	6	630	26	2	2	13
Pepperoni Pizza	240	10	4	480	25	1	2	11
Super Combo Pizza	300	14	6	780	27	2	3	15
Super Hawaiian Pizza	240	9	3.5	380	27	1	3	11
Super Taco Pizza	290	14	7	650	27	2	3	14
Taco Pizza	280	12	6	600	26	2	3	14
Veggie Pizza	210	6	3	430	27	2	3	10

Original Crust

	Cal	Fat	SFat	Sod	Carb	Fiber	Sugar	Prot
All Meat Combo Pizza	240	14	6	760	32	2	2	18
Bacon Cheeseburger Pizza	320	14	7	700	32	2	3	17
Cheese Pizza	240	7	3	420	31	1	2	11
Combo Pizza	320	13	5	780	33	2	3	15
Hawaiian Pizza	240	7	3	430	32	2	3	11
Hot Stuff Pizza	330	14	6	810	32	2	3	15
Humble Pie Pizza	340	16	6	680	32	2	3	15
Pepperoni Pizza	270	9	4	530	31	2	2	12
Super Combo Pizza	330	14	6	850	33	2	3	17
Super Hawaiian Pizza	260	8	3.5	430	32	2	3	13
Super Taco Pizza	340	15	8	720	33	2	3	17
Taco Pizza	320	14	7	680	32	2	3	16
Veggie Pizza	250	7	3	490	32	2	3	11

Medium Size, 1 slice

Golden Crust

	Cal	Fat	SFat	Sod	Carb	Fiber	Sugar	Prot
All Meat Combo Pizza	300	14	5	670	26	2	2	15
Bacon Cheeseburger Pizza	270	12	5	640	26	2	2	13
Cheese Pizza	220	8	3	380	25	1	2	10
Combo Pizza	290	13	5	680	27	2	2	13
Hawaiian Pizza	230	8	3.5	450	27	1	3	11
Hot Stuff Pizza	290	14	6	670	27	2	2	13
Humble Pie Pizza	300	15	6	630	26	2	2	13
Pepperoni Pizza	250	11	4.5	500	26	1	2	11

Description & Serving	Cal	Fat	Sfat	Sod	Carb	Fiber	Sugar	Prot
Super Combo Pizza	320	15	8	760	28	2	2	16
Super Hawaiian Pizza	250	9	3.5	450	27	1	3	12
Super Taco Pizza	330	17	10	670	28	2	3	15
Taco Pizza	300	14	8	630	27	2	3	15
Veggie Pizza	230	8	3	430	27	2	2	10
Original Crust								
All Meat Combo Pizza	370	15	6	840	35	2	3	20
Bacon Cheeseburger Pizza	330	13	6	810	35	2	3	16
Cheese Pizza	260	7	3	470	34	2	2	12
Combo Pizza	350	14	6	890	36	3	3	17
Hawaiian Pizza	270	7	3	530	36	2	4	13
Hot Stuff Pizza	360	15	6	870	35	2	3	17
Humble Pie Pizza	360	16	6	780	35	2	3	16
Pepperoni Pizza	290	10	5	580	34	2	2	13
Super Combo Pizza	350	14	8	820	36	2	3	18
Super Hawaiian Pizza	290	9	4	530	36	2	4	15
Super Taco Pizza	390	18	9	880	36	3	4	19
Taco Pizza	360	16	8	830	36	2	4	18
Veggie Pizza	270	8	3.5	550	36	2	3	12
Thin Crust								
All Meat Combo Pizza	270	15	5	520	18	1	1	14
Bacon Cheeseburger Pizza	260	14	6	500	18	1	1	12
Cheese Pizza	170	8	3	230	15	1	1	8
Combo Pizza	240	13	3	530	17	1	1	11
Hawaiian Pizza	190	8	3	330	16	1	1	9
Hot Stuff Pizza	260	15	5	530	18	1	1	11
Humble Pie Pizza	260	15	5	480	16	1	1	11
Pepperoni Pizza	210	11	4	350	15	1	1	9
Super Combo Pizza	290	16	6	620	19	2	1	14
Super Hawaiian Pizza	220	10	3.5	330	19	1	2	11
Super Taco Pizza	300	18	8	530	19	1	2	13
Taco Pizza	260	15	7	480	16	1	2	13
Veggie Pizza	180	8	3	280	16	1	1	8
Large Size, 1 slice								
Golden Crust								
All Meat Combo Pizza	340	16	6	760	29	2	2	17
Bacon Cheeseburger Pizza	330	17	7	750	29	2	3	15
Cheese Pizza	250	9	3.5	440	28	1	2	11
Combo Pizza	330	15	6	740	30	2	2	15
Hawaiian Pizza	260	9	3.5	510	30	1	4	12
Hot Stuff Pizza	330	16	6	780	29	2	2	15
Humble Pie Pizza	340	17	7	730	29	2	2	15
Pepperoni Pizza	290	12	4.5	560	28	1	2	12
Super Combo Pizza	370	18	6	880	31	2	3	18
Super Hawaiian Pizza	280	11	4	510	30	2	4	14
Super Taco Pizza	370	20	10	780	30	2	3	17
Taco Pizza	350	17	8	740	30	2	3	17
Veggie Pizza	260	10	3.5	500	30	2	3	11

Description & Serving	Cal	Fat	Sfat	Sod	Carb	Fiber	Sugar	Prot
Original Crust								
All Meat Combo Pizza	410	17	7	920	37	2	3	22
Bacon Cheeseburger Pizza	390	17	8	890	37	2	3	21
Cheese Pizza	290	9	4	530	36	2	2	14
Combo Pizza	390	16	7	970	38	3	3	19
Hawaiian Pizza	300	9	4	600	37	2	4	15
Hot Stuff Pizza	400	18	7	960	37	2	3	19
Humble Pie Pizza	410	19	8	900	37	2	3	19
Pepperoni Pizza	330	12	5	650	36	2	2	15
Super Combo Pizza	430	19	9	1060	39	3	4	22
Super Hawaiian Pizza	330	11	4.5	600	38	2	4	17
Super Taco Pizza	450	22	12	980	39	3	4	22
Taco Pizza	420	19	10	930	38	3	4	22
Veggie Pizza	300	9	4	610	38	2	3	14
Thin Crust								
All Meat Combo Pizza	300	17	6	610	19	1	1	16
Bacon Cheeseburger Pizza	280	16	7	570	18	1	2	14
Cheese Pizza	210	10	3.5	270	17	1	1	9
Combo Pizza	280	16	6	630	20	2	1	13
Hawaiian Pizza	230	10	3	380	21	1	4	11
Hot Stuff Pizza	290	17	5	620	19	1	1	13
Humble Pie Pizza	300	18	6	570	19	1	1	13
Pepperoni Pizza	240	13	5	400	18	1	1	10
Super Combo Pizza	330	19	6	730	20	2	2	17
Super Hawaiian Pizza	240	11	4	380	19	1	3	13
Super Taco Pizza	330	21	8	620	20	2	2	15
Taco Pizza	300	18	7	580	19	2	2	15
Veggie Pizza	220	10	3.5	340	19	1	2	9
Jumbo Size, 1 slice								
All Meat Combo Pizza	500	21	9	1140	46	3	3	27
Bacon Cheeseburger Pizza	480	21	10	114	45	3	4	25
Cheese Pizza	350	10	5	650	44	2	3	17
Combo Pizza	480	20	8	1200	47	3	4	24
Hawaiian Pizza	370	11	5	740	46	2	5	18
Hot Stuff Pizza	490	22	9	1190	46	3	4	23
Humble Pie Pizza	510	24	9	1110	46	3	4	23
Pepperoni Pizza	400	15	6	800	44	2	3	19
Super Combo Pizza	520	23	10	1310	48	4	4	27
Super Hawaiian Pizza	410	13	6	740	47	2	6	21
Super Taco Pizza	530	26	13	1190	48	3	5	26
Taco Pizza	500	22	11	1120	47	3	5	25
Veggie Pizza	370	11	5	750	46	3	4	17
Gluten-Free, 1 slice								
Beef Pizza	170	7	3	500	18	1	2	7
Cheese Pizza	140	4.5	2	380	18	1	2	5
Classic Combo Pizza	180	8	3	570	19	1	2	7
Meat Combo Pizza	190	8	3.5	570	18	1	2	9
Pepperoni Pizza	170	7	3	480	18	1	2	6
Sausage Pizza	170	6	2.5	510	18	1	2	7

Description & Serving	Cal	Fat	Sfat	Sod	Carb	Fiber	Sugar	Prot
Calzone								
Cheese Calzone	1660	51	24	2920	200	9	11	81
Combo Calzone	1450	40	16	2900	199	10	12	63
Pepperoni Calzone	1410	39	16	2540	195	9	11	60
Side								
Monkey Bread - Cinnamon	830	24	4.5	970	139	4	37	18
Monkey Bread - Italian	690	23	4.5	970	105	4	5	19
Potato Wedges	690	32	8	1440	96	11	3	11
Breadsticks	110	2	0	160	20	1	1	3
Breadsticks w/ cheese	140	4	1.5	220	20	1	1	5
Garlic Toast	150	9	2	260	15	1	1	3
Garlic Toast w/ cheese	210	12	3.5	360	16	1	1	7
Cheesesticks, sml, 1	130	3.5	1.5	210	18	1	1	5
Cheesesticks, med, 1	200	7	2.5	300	24	1	1	8
Cheesesticks, lrg, 1	220	8	3	340	26	1	1	9
Hot Wings, breaded, 1	45	3	1	90	1	0	0	3
Dessert, 1 slice								
Apple Dessert, sml	150	2.5	0.5	160	28	1	4	3
Apple Dessert, med	200	4	1	220	38	1	6	4
Apple Dessert, lrg	230	4.5	1	240	42	1	6	5
Cherry Dessert, sml	150	2.5	0.5	160	28	1	1	3
Cherry Dessert, med	210	4	1	210	39	1	2	4
Cherry Dessert, lrg	230	4.5	1	230	43	1	2	5
Cinnamon Streusel, sml	160	3	0.5	160	29	1	4	3
Cinnamon Streusel, med	230	5	1	220	40	1	5	5
Cinnamon Streusel, lrg	260	6	1.5	250	45	1	6	5

Great Harvest Bread Company

Description & Serving	Cal	Fat	Sfat	Sod	Carb	Fiber	Sugar	Prot
Bread								
Apple Cherry Pecan Bread, 1 slice	140	2	NP	310	25	3	13	4
Apple Cinnamon Walnut Bread, 1 slice	150	1.5	NP	240	28	4	8	5
Apple Crunch Bread, 1 slice	130	2	NP	310	22	3	7	4
Apricot Almond Bread, 1 slice	130	2	NP	310	22	3	7	4
Asiago Pesto Bread, 1 slice	160	6	NP	470	20	1	3	5
Breakfast Blast Bread, 1 slice	130	1.5	NP	230	26	4	10	4
Burly Bread, 1 slice	140	2	NP	330	25	4	6	5
Caraway Rye Bread, 1 slice	120	0.5	NP	320	25	5	5	5
Carrot Poppyseed Bread, 1 slice	110	0.5	NP	310	21	3	5	4
Challa Bread, 1 slice	130	1	NP	270	26	2	5	5
Cheddar Garlic Bread, 1 slice	150	4.5	NP	410	21	1	4	6
Cherry Apple Berry Bread, 1 slice	130	0	NP	300	27	3	9	4
Cherry Walnut Bread, 1 slice	140	2	NP	290	26	3	11	4
Cinnamon Chip Bread, 1 slice	150	3	NP	300	26	3	11	4
Cinnamon Chip Bread w/ enriched white flour, 1 slice	150	3	NP	370	28	1	11	3
Cinnamon Raisin Walnut Bread, 1 slice	130	2	NP	330	25	3	8	4
Cinnamon Swirl Bread, 1 slice	160	3	NP	250	28	3	13	4

Description & Serving	Cal	Fat	Sfat	Sod	Carb	Fiber	Sugar	Prot
Cornbread-White, 1 slice	140	2.5	NP	290	27	1	5	3
Cornbread-Wheat, 1 slice	140	2.5	NP	290	25	3	5	4
Country Bread, 1 slice	120	0.5	NP	370	22	4	3	5
Cracked Pepper Parmesan Bread, 1 slice	140	3	NP	430	20	3	4	7
Cracked Pepper Swiss Bread, 1 slice	140	3	NP	310	20	3	4	7
Cranberry Orange Bread, 1 slice	120	0	NP	290	26	3	12	4
Dakota Bread, 1 slice	150	4	NP	570	22	3	5	6
Flax Oatbran Bread, 1 slice	130	4	NP	340	21	4	7	5
Focaccia Bread, 4 oz	280	2.5	NP	830	56	2	10	7
Focaccia-Italian Herb Bread, 4 oz	280	5	NP	630	52	2	4	7
Golden Wheat Apple, Cinnamon Chip, Walnut Bread, 1 slice	140	2.5	NP	320	26	3	9	4
Hearty Caraway Rye Bread, 1 slice	120	0.5	NP	350	24	4	2	4
High 5 Fiber Bread, 1 slice	140	3.5	NP	260	23	5	5	5
High Country Crunch Bread, 1 slice	140	4.5	NP	50	21	3	4	5
Honey Whole Wheat Bread, 1 slice	120	0	NP	350	24	3	7	5
Irish Soda Bread, 1 slice	130	0.5	NP	200	27	2	9	4
Low Carb Bread, 42 g slice	100	3	NP	200	12	3	3	6
Low Carb Dakota Bread, 42 g slice	120	5	NP	160	13	3	3	6
Low Carb Cinnamon Chip Bread, 42 g slice	110	4	NP	180	14	2	5	5
Mediterranean Olive Bread, 1 slice	130	2	NP	530	23	2	3	4
Merry Berry Bread, 1 slice	130	1.5	NP	310	27	3	10	4
Nine Grain Bread, 1 slice	130	0.5	NP	270	26	4	5	5
Oatmeal Poppyseed Bread, 1 slice	130	1	NP	330	24	4	6	5
Oregon Herb (Onion Dill Rye) Bread, 1 slice	120	0.5	NP	340	25	3	7	4
Panza Bread, 1 slice	130	2.5	NP	610	22	2	4	5
Pecan Swirl Bread, 1 slice	190	8	NP	220	26	4	12	4
Pizza Bread, 1 slice	140	4.5	NP	470	18	2	4	7
Popeye Bread, 1 slice	110	1	NP	390	22	2	4	4
Potato Chive Bread, 1 slice	110	0	NP	360	24	1	4	3
Pumpkin Nut & Spice Bread, 1 slice	120	1	NP	270	27	2	9	3
Pumpkin Swirl Bread, 1 slice	140	2	NP	210	28	2	12	3
Raisin Bread, 1 slice	120	0	NP	340	26	3	9	4
Raisin Cinnamon Chip Bread, 1 slice	150	3	NP	260	28	3	12	4
Red, White & Blueberry Bread, 1 slice	140	0	NP	340	26	3	9	4
Rosemary Garlic Bread, 1 slice	120	0.5	NP	350	24	4	6	5
Spinach Feta Bread, 1 slice	120	3.5	NP	420	18	2	5	5
Sprouted Wheat Bread, 1 slice	130	0.5	NP	350	24	4	2	6
Star Spangled Swirl Bread, 1 slice	150	1	NP	250	31	4	14	4
Sundried Tomato Spinach Bread, 1 slice	120	0	NP	420	24	3	6	4
Sunflower Whole Wheat Bread, 1 slice	140	2.5	NP	320	23	4	6	5
Swedish Rye Bread, 1 slice	130	0.5	NP	410	26	3	8	4
Tuscan Herb Bread, 1 slice	120	1	NP	280	22	4	5	5
Trail Bread, 1 slice	130	1.5	NP	310	25	3	9	4
White Bread, 1 slice	130	0	NP	440	27	1	5	3
Whole Grain Goodness Bread, 1 slice	130	3	NP	260	21	4	4	5

Sweet Bread

Apple Cream Cheese Cake Bread, 1 slice	190	11	NP	55	21	2	15	3
Apple Spice Cake Bread, 1 slice	170	9	NP	120	23	1	15	2

Description & Serving	Cal	Fat	Sfat	Sod	Carb	Fiber	Sugar	Prot
Banana Chocolate Chip Bread, 1 slice	160	7	NP	115	25	2	15	3
Banana Walnut Bread, 1 slice	160	6	NP	120	23	2	13	3
Carrot Bread, 1 slice	190	10	NP	180	23	20	16	3
Chocolate Brownie Bread, 1 slice	180	7	NP	150	29	1	19	2
Chocolate Cherry Bread, 1 slice	190	8	NP	120	27	2	17	4
Pumpkin Chocolate Chip Bread, 1 slice	180	9	NP	125	25	1	15	2
Zucchini Bread, 1 slice	130	3.5	NP	105	23	2	13	3

Muffin/Coffee Cake/Brownie

Description & Serving	Cal	Fat	Sfat	Sod	Carb	Fiber	Sugar	Prot
Apple Cream Cheese Muffin, half	308	17	NP	85	33	3	23	5
Blackberry Bran Muffin, half	130	1	NP	260	29	40	12	4
Cappuccino Chocolate Muffin w/ whole wheat & enriched white flour, half	220	11	NP	70	26	1	18	4
Cappuccino Chocolate Muffin w/ enriched white flour, half	230	12	NP	75	28	1	19	4
Oat Berry Muffin, half	180	6	NP	230	33	4	16	5
Rhubarb Streusel Muffin, half	390	19	NP	115	47	3	28	7
Apple Strussel Coffee Cake, 1 pc	160	6	NP	12	24	1	15	2
Blueribbon Blueberry Coffee Cake, 1 pc	170	7	NP	130	25	2	18	3
Whole Wheat Coffee Cake, 1 pc	300	15	NP	280	38	3	25	6
Brownie, 1 pc	370	22	NP	55	41	3	28	6

Roll/Bun

Description & Serving	Cal	Fat	Sfat	Sod	Carb	Fiber	Sugar	Prot
Cinnamon Roll, half	450	11	NP	460	81	4	47	8
Lemon Cream Roll, 1" slice	270	12	NP	180	36	1	24	5
Savory Breakfast Roll, half	170	10	NP	560	36	3	8	11
Breakfast Buns w/ frosting, 1 pc	270	11	NP	590	39	3	16	4

Cookie/Scone/Biscotti

Description & Serving	Cal	Fat	Sfat	Sod	Carb	Fiber	Sugar	Prot
Autumn Spice Cookie	450	18	NP	240	69	5	43	7
Chocolate Chip Oatmeal Walnut Cookie	510	27	NP	240	63	5	39	8
Chocolate Bliss Cookie	290	15	NP	80	41	3	35	4
Ginger Cookie	430	19	NP	440	59	1	27	5
Mint Chocolate Chip Cookie	510	27	NP	240	65	2	42	6
Peanut Butter Chocolate Chip Cookie	460	27	NP	310	31	5	36	9
Peanut Butter Cookie	460	27	NP	390	48	4	30	11
Turtle Cookie	510	27	NP	240	63	5	39	8
Oatmeal Raisin Cookie	460	18	NP	240	70	5	44	7
Snickerdoodle	420	18	NP	280	59	40	33	7
White Chocolate Cherry Cookie	480	22	NP	240	67	4	39	7
Berry Cream Cheese Scone, half	290	12	NP	290	41	1	17	5
Golden Berry Cream Cheese Scone, half	290	12	NP	590	39	3	17	7
Chocolate Chip Hazelnut Scone, half	310	15	NP	270	42	1	22	5
Cinnamon Chip Cream Cheese Scone, half	350	16	NP	640	48	1	23	5
Maple Oatmeal Scone, half	350	16	NP	250	49	2	25	5
Chocolate Chocolate Chip Biscotti, 1 pc	230	11	NP	190	30	3	13	7
Vanilla Almond Biscotti, 1 pc	200	7	NP	135	29	2	12	6

Bar/Granola

Description & Serving	Cal	Fat	Sfat	Sod	Carb	Fiber	Sugar	Prot
Cupid's Crunch, 1/2 cup	290	19	NP	10	24	4	18	8
Granola, 1/2 cup	220	7	NP	0	36	3	15	6

Description & Serving	Cal	Fat	Sfat	Sod	Carb	Fiber	Sugar	Prot
Kahuna Bar, half	810	35	NP	290	115	7	85	11
Mud Bar, half	380	21	NP	65	46	1	29	4
Pumpkin Oh's, 1" slice	260	12	NP	220	36	1	28	4
Savannah Bar, half	290	10	NP	115	46	4	29	5
Trek Bar, 1 pc	380	18	NP	115	49	6	28	12

The Great Steak & Potato Co.

Breakfast

Bacon, Egg & Cheese Sandwich	600	36	11	1300	39	2	2	29
Egg & Cheese Sandwich	500	29	9	890	39	2	2	23
Ham & Cheese Sandwich	430	22	6	1400	41	2	4	18
Ham, Egg & Cheese Sandwich	570	32	10	1540	42	2	4	31
Sausage, Egg & Cheese Sandwich	700	47	15	1300	39	2	2	30
Steak, Egg & Cheese Sandwich	600	34	10	990	40	2	3	34
Deluxe Home Potatoes	390	23	4	1460	44	7	3	4
Fresh Cut Home Potatoes	380	23	4	1460	42	6	2	3

Sandwich/Burger/Wrap

Buffalo Chicken (Upstate) Philly, 7"	660	24	10	2420	65	5	9	37
Chicagoland Cheesesteak, 7"	680	29	11	2480	63	5	9	43
Great Steak Cheesesteak, 7"	740	37	9	1270	62	5	8	41
Ham Delight, 7"	710	33	10	2190	71	5	16	36
Ham Explosion, 7"	710	34	10	2200	70	6	13	37
Kansas City (BBQ) Cheesesteak, 7"	680	26	10	1740	71	5	14	40
Original Philly Cheesesteak, 7"	650	26	10	2570	62	5	10	40
Original Chicken Philly, 7"	620	22	9	1670	62	5	10	37
Pastrami, 7"	790	41	16	1850	65	5	9	43
Reuben, 7"	690	33	11	2550	61	5	7	37
Super Steak Cheesesteak, 7"	750	37	9	1270	64	6	9	42
Teriyaki Chicken Philly, 7"	740	32	9	2280	65	5	11	40
Turkey Philly, 7"	670	30	8	1650	64	5	8	38
Ultimate Chicken Philly, 7"	730	33	11	1590	64	6	9	38
Veggie Delight, 7"	610	31	8	2040	66	6	10	20
Wisconsin Inside-Out, 7"	560	27	12	1360	57	4	5	24
Chicken Philly Slider	300	13	6	880	24	2	5	19
Steak Philly Slider	310	15	6	850	24	2	5	20
Hamburger	590	30	9	480	40	3	3	37
Cheeseburger	640	35	12	730	41	3	3	40
Philly Burger	820	50	15	820	47	4	6	46
Gyro	580	30	10	1550	52	5	8	29
Great Steak Cheesesteak Wrap	820	43	11	1400	67	5	6	40
Original Chicken Philly Wrap	700	28	11	1800	67	4	7	36
Super Steak Cheesesteak Wrap	930	54	13	1500	69	5	6	41
Ultimate Chicken Philly Wrap	810	39	13	1720	69	5	6	36

Potato

Broccoli & Cheese Baked Potato	400	24	10	1070	35	4	5	13
Cheese & Bacon Baked Potato	530	35	14	840	29	3	2	25
Sour Cream & Chive Baked Potato	350	23	10	160	32	3	2	5

Description & Serving	Cal	Fat	Sfat	Sod	Carb	Fiber	Sugar	Prot
The Great Potato - Chicken	600	33	13	1420	37	4	7	32
The Great Potato - Ham	520	28	12	2470	43	4	11	29
The Great Potato - Steak	620	38	13	1360	37	4	7	35
The Great Potato - Turkey	490	25	10	1930	39	4	7	31
The King Baked Potato	590	41	18	860	31	3	2	26
Plain Baked Potato	160	0	0	15	36	4	2	4

Salad

Chef Salad w/o dressing	260	11	6	1320	15	4	8	28
Garden Salad w/o dressing	60	1	0	40	13	5	7	3
Side Salad w/o dressing	30	0	0	20	6	2	4	2
Great Grilled Chicken Salad w/o dressing	380	18	8	460	18	5	9	31
Great Grilled Ham Salad w/o dressing	360	20	8	1520	24	5	13	28
Great Grilled Steak Salad w/o dressing	400	23	7	590	18	5	9	33
Great Grilled Turkey Salad w/o dressing	330	17	6	970	20	5	9	30
Grilled Chicken Wedge w/o dressing	270	12	4	610	11	3	6	24
Grilled Steak Wedge w/o dressing	290	16	4	550	11	3	6	28

Side

Great Fry, reg	440	20	3	1130	60	7	0	7
Great Fry, lrg	540	25	4	1360	72	8	0	8
Great Fry, ex lrg	930	40	6	2490	132	15	0	15
Wacker Fry, reg	490	27	9	1600	51	5	3	12
Wacker Fry, lrg	620	35	11	2060	63	7	3	15
Wacker Fry, ex lrg	1130	59	19	3890	126	13	6	28
Coney Island Fry, reg	570	30	10	2030	61	12	5	18
Coney Island Fry, lrg	740	39	14	2630	77	15	7	24
Coney Island Fry, ex lrg	1360	67	24	5030	154	30	12	45
Nacho Fry, reg	510	27	9	2570	53	5	3	12
Nacho Fry, lrg	650	35	11	3520	67	7	3	15
Nacho Fry, ex lrg	1190	59	19	6810	132	13	6	28
King Fry, reg	630	39	14	1970	52	5	3	20
King Fry, lrg	880	55	21	2790	66	7	4	31
King Fry, ex lrg	1500	87	33	4980	130	13	7	52
Potato Skins	390	26	12	1070	24	2	4	17

Kids

Kids Nuggets	165	9	2	403	10	1	NP	11
Grilled Cheese w/ Fry	530	28	8	1290	57	6	2	15
Chicken Slider w/ Fry	570	25	7	1560	60	6	5	23
Steak Slider w/ Fry	580	28	8	1530	60	6	5	24
Kids Great Fry	270	13	2	680	36	4	0	4

Dressing/Condiment

Mayonnaise, Dijon, 1 oz	110	11	2	420	3	0	0	0
Mayonnaise, Regular, 1 oz	200	22	3	200	0	0	0	0
Ranch Dressing, 1 oz	170	18	3	160	1	0	1	1
Thousand Island Dressing, 1 oz	130	12	2	280	4	0	3	0
BBQ Sauce, 1 oz	50	0	0	320	11	0	7	0
Buffalo Sauce, 1 oz	10	0	0	855	2	0	0	0
Teriyaki Sauce, 1 oz	25	0	0	960	3	0	3	2

Description & Serving	Cal	Fat	Sfat	Sod	Carb	Fiber	Sugar	Prot
Tzatziki Sauce, 1 oz	50	4	4	80	2	0	1	0
Marinara Dipping Sauce, 3 oz	15	0	0	260	3	0	1	1
Oil, 0.3 oz	60	7	1.5	0	0	0	0	0
Beverage								
Great Steak Lemonade, 12 oz	180	0	0	0	48	0	45	0
Orange Juice, 12 oz	118	0	0	31	30	0	30	0

Harvey's

Description & Serving	Cal	Fat	Sfat	Sod	Carb	Fiber	Sugar	Prot
Breakfast								
Breakfast Club	400	19	8	750	36	2	4	21
Breakfast Club Deluxe	530	28	11	1030	39	2	4	30
Bacon	40	3.5	1	160	0	0	0	3
Extra Egg	90	6	1.5	70	0	0	0	12
Homefries	300	19	2.5	530	29	3	0	3
White Toast	180	2	0	320	35	1	2	6
Whole Wheat Toast	170	2	0.2	320	32	3	2	7
Sandwich/Entrée/Salad								
Original Hamburger	380	16	7	980	37	2	3	20
Original Cheeseburger	460	23	11	1130	39	2	3	25
Original Bacon Cheeseburger	500	26	12	1290	39	2	3	28
Original Patty by Itself	200	14	6	630	4	1	0	13
Angus Burger	560	26	10	1090	47	3	4	35
Angus Burger w/ Cheese	640	32	14	1240	49	3	4	41
Angus Burger w/ Cheese & Bacon	690	35	15	1390	49	3	4	43
Angus Patty	320	23	10	620	4	1	0	26
Hot Dog w/ Bun	300	13	4.5	850	32	2	2	13
Hot Dog by Itself	140	11	4.5	520	3	0	0	7
Grilled Chicken	290	5	1.5	810	28	4	5	34
Grilled Chicken BLT	340	8	2.5	970	30	5	7	38
Grilled Chicken by Itself	140	2.5	1	530	1	1	0	28
Veggie Burger	290	10	1.5	580	33	6	5	18
Veggie Burger by Itself	130	7	1	300	6	3	0	12
Chicken Strips, 3	320	15	1.5	780	27	2	0	20
Warm Grilled Chicken Salad	170	3	1	550	9	4	4	30
Warm Grilled Chicken BLT Salad	230	7	2.5	760	9	4	4	33
Kids								
Hamburger Meal	810	40	43	1710	124	5	45	23
Cheeseburger Meal	890	49	60	1860	125	5	45	28
Hot Dog Meal	730	34	28	1580	118	5	44	16
Chicken Strip Meal, 3 pc	760	37	12	1510	113	5	42	23
Fries	240	10	0.5	710	37	3	0	3
Side								
Fries, reg	320	13	1	950	49	4	0	4
Fries, lrg	410	16	1	1190	61	5	1	4
Onion Rings, reg	270	15	1.5	790	33	2	3	3
Onion Rings, lrg	550	29	2.5	1580	65	4	5	6

Description & Serving	Cal	Fat	Sfat	Sod	Carb	Fiber	Sugar	Prot
Frings	520	24	2	1510	69	5	3	6
Side Garden Salad	40	0.2	0	20	8	3	4	2
Poutine	840	43	15	2210	87	8	1	25
Gravy	30	0.5	0	580	6	0	0	1

Dressing/Condiment/Topping

Description & Serving	Cal	Fat	Sfat	Sod	Carb	Fiber	Sugar	Prot
Honey Mustard Dipping Sauce, 43 g	160	18	2	250	13	0	12	1
Barbecue Dipping Sauce, 43 g	90	0	0	715	21	1	19	1
Sweet N' Sour Dipping Sauce, 43 g	80	1	0	190	17	0	16	0.1
Plum Sauce, 43 g	80	0	0	430	21	0	16	0
Creamy Garlic Peppercorn Ranch Dressing, 28 ml	108	11	2	215	2	0	1	0.2
Creamy Caesar Dressing, 28 ml	100	11	2	216	0.8	0	0	0
Lite Italian Dressing, 28 ml	66	7	1	287	2	0	1	0
Asian Sesame Dressing, 28 ml	60	2.5	0.3	264	9	0	9	0
Balsamic Vinaigrette Dressing, 28 ml	78	7	1	306	3	0	3	0
Ketchup, 8 ml	10	0	0	65	2	0	2	0.1
Mustard, 7 ml	5	0	0	75	0	0	0	0.3
Relish, 20 g	20	0	0	105	5	0	4	0.1
Light Mayonnaise, 15 g	45	8	0	140	1	0	0	0
Barbecue Sauce, 28 g	50	0	0	390	12	0	10	0.3
Frank's Redhot Sauce, 8 ml	2	0	0	270	0	0	0	0.1
Real Canadian Cheddar Cheese Slice	80	9	0.2	150	1	0	0	5
Bacon	15	2	0	50	0	0	0	1
Pickles, 2 slices	5	0	0	150	0	0	0	0.1
Lettuce	4	0	0	3	1	0	1	0.3
Tomato, 2 slices	10	0	0	3	2	1	1	0.4
Onions	10	0	0	2	5	0	2	1
Hot Peppers	0	0	0	115	1	1	1	0.2

Dessert

Description & Serving	Cal	Fat	Sfat	Sod	Carb	Fiber	Sugar	Prot
Chocolate Milkshake, 14 oz	730	33	21	520	91	5	78	17

Hungry Howie's

Small Pizza, 1 slice

Description & Serving	Cal	Fat	Sfat	Sod	Carb	Fiber	Sugar	Prot
Cheese Only Pizza	161	3.6	2.5	370	19.9	9.6	NP	0.8
Pepperoni Topping Only	20	1.8	0.6	68	0	0	NP	0.8
Ham Topping Only	6	0.3	0.3	70	0	0	NP	1.3
Mushroom Topping Only	2	0	0	0	0.4	0.1	NP	0.1
Onions Topping Only	1	0	0	0	0.3	0.1	NP	0
Green Peppers Topping Only	1	0	0	0	0.3	0.1	NP	0
Beef Topping Only	21	1.3	0.3	66	0.3	0.1	NP	0.9
Sausage Topping Only	20	1.2	0.1	86	0.3	0	NP	1
Bacon Topping Only	23	0.1	0	0	0.4	0	NP	4
Black Olives Topping Only	5	0.1	0	33	0.4	0.1	NP	0
Green Olives Topping Only	5	0.1	0	33	0.4	0.1	NP	0
Banana Peppers Topping Only	5	0	0	120	0.4	0	NP	0
Pineapple Topping Only	4	0	0	0	1	0.6	NP	0
Anchovies Topping Only	34	2.7	0.5	652	0	0	NP	5.4

Description & Serving	Cal	Fat	SFat	Sod	Carb	Fiber	Sugar	Prot
Medium Pizza, 1 slice								
Cheese Only Pizza	191	5.7	NP	437	23.2	0.9	NP	11
Pepperoni Topping Only	22	2	NP	75	0	0	NP	1
Ham Topping Only	7	0.4	NP	81	0	0	NP	1.4
Mushroom Topping Only	2	0	NP	0	0.4	0.1	NP	0.1
Onions Topping Only	2	0.6	NP	0.6	0.4	0.2	NP	0.6
Green Peppers Topping Only	2	0.6	NP	0.6	0.4	0.1	NP	0.6
Beef Topping Only	30	2.1	NP	96	0.4	0.1	NP	1.5
Sausage Topping Only	27	1.7	NP	121	0.4	0.1	NP	1.7
Bacon Topping Only	32	0.5	NP	0.6	0.4	0	NP	6.1
Black Olives Topping Only	7	0.1	NP	47	0.4	0.1	NP	0
Green Olives Topping Only	7	0.1	NP	47	0.4	0.1	NP	0.6
Banana Peppers Topping Only	6	0	NP	162	1.1	0	NP	0.2
Pineapple Topping Only	5	0.6	NP	0.6	1.5	0.6	NP	0.6
Anchovies Topping Only	44	2.5	NP	736	0	0	NP	7.2
Large Pizza, 1 slice								
Cheese Only Pizza	208	4.9	3.1	464	25.3	1.1	NP	12.2
Pepperoni Topping Only	22	2	0.8	76	0	0	NP	1
Ham Topping Only	7	0.4	0.4	78	0	0	NP	1.3
Mushroom Topping Only	2	0	0	0	0.5	0.1	NP	0.2
Onions Topping Only	3	0.9	0.9	0.9	0.5	0.4	NP	0.9
Green Peppers Topping Only	2	0	0	0	0.5	0.1	NP	0.1
Beef Topping Only	29	2	0.6	92	0.4	0.1	NP	1.4
Sausage Topping Only	26	1.7	0.2	116	0.4	0.1	NP	1.7
Bacon Topping Only	42	0.5	0.2	1.2	0.7	0	NP	7.6
Black Olives Topping Only	10	0.4	0	59	0.6	0.2	NP	0
Green Olives Topping Only	10	0.4	0	59	0.6	0.2	NP	0
Banana Peppers Topping Only	8	0.1	0	183	1.4	0	NP	0.3
Pineapple Topping Only	5	0.6	0.6	0.6	1.4	0.6	NP	0.6
Anchovies Topping Only	55	3.1	0.7	920	0	0	NP	9
X-Large Pizza, 1 slice								
Cheese Only Pizza	395	9.3	5.9	882	41.9	2.1	NP	23.2
Pepperoni Topping Only	26	2.4	1	91	0	0	NP	1.2
Ham Topping Only	8	0.5	0.5	94	0	0	NP	1.6
Mushroom Topping Only	3	0	0	0	0.6	0.1	NP	0.3
Onions Topping Only	3	1	1	1	0.6	0.4	NP	1
Green Peppers Topping Only	2	0	0	0	0.6	0.1	NP	0.1
Beef Topping Only	37	2.5	0.7	117	0.8	0.1	NP	1.8
Sausage Topping Only	33	2.1	0.2	147	0.5	0.1	NP	2.1
Bacon Topping Only	52	0.6	0.2	1.5	0.9	0	NP	9.5
Black Olives Topping Only	11	0.5	0	74	0.7	0.2	NP	0
Green Olives Topping Only	11	0.5	0	74	0.7	0.2	NP	0
Banana Peppers Topping Only	12	0.1	0	274	2.1	0	NP	0.4
Pineapple Topping Only	6	0.7	0.7	0.7	1.7	0.7	NP	0.7
Anchovies Topping Only	88	5	1.1	1472	0	0	NP	14.4

Description & Serving	Cal	Fat	Sfat	Sod	Carb	Fiber	Sugar	Prot
Medium Thin Crust Pizza, 1 slice								
Cheese Only Pizza	111	5	2.8	256	9.6	0.4	NP	7
Pepperoni Topping Only	22	2	0.7	75	0	0	NP	1
Ham Topping Only	7	0.4	0.4	81	0	0	NP	1.4
Mushroom Topping Only	2	0	0	0	0.4	0.1	NP	0.1
Onions Topping Only	2	0.6	0.6	0.6	0.4	0.2	NP	0.6
Green Peppers Topping Only	2	0.6	0.6	0.6	0.4	0.1	NP	0.6
Beef Topping Only	30	2.1	0.6	96	0.4	0.1	NP	1.5
Sausage Topping Only	27	1.7	0.2	121	0.4	0.1	NP	1.7
Bacon Topping Only	32	0.5	0.4	0.6	0.4	0	NP	6.1
Black Olives Topping Only	7	0.1	0	47	0.4	0.1	NP	0
Green Olives Topping Only	7	0.1	0.6	47	0.4	0.1	NP	0.6
Banana Peppers Topping Only	6	0	0	162	1.1	0	NP	0.2
Pineapple Topping Only	5	0.6	0.6	0.6	1.5	0.6	NP	0.6
Anchovies Topping Only	44	2.5	0.6	736	0	0	NP	7.2
Large Thin Crust Pizza, 1 slice								
Cheese Only Pizza	124	5.6	3.2	323	10.6	0.6	NP	8
Pepperoni Topping Only	22	2	0.8	76	0	0	NP	1
Ham Topping Only	7	0.4	0.4	78	0	0	NP	1.3
Mushroom Topping Only	2	0	0	0	0.5	0.1	NP	0.2
Onions Topping Only	3	0.9	0.9	0.9	0.5	0.4	NP	0.9
Green Peppers Topping Only	2	0	0	0	0.5	0.1	NP	0.1
Beef Topping Only	29	2	0.6	92	0.4	0.1	NP	1.4
Sausage Topping Only	26	1.7	0.2	116	0.4	0.1	NP	1.7
Bacon Topping Only	42	0.5	0.2	1.2	0.7	0	NP	7.6
Black Olives Topping Only	10	0.4	0	59	0.6	0.2	NP	0
Green Olives Topping Only	10	0.4	0	59	0.6	0.2	NP	0
Banana Peppers Topping Only	8	0.1	0	183	1.4	0	NP	0.3
Pineapple Topping Only	5	0.6	0.6	0.6	1.4	0.6	NP	0.6
Anchovies Topping Only	55	3.1	0.7	920	0	0	NP	9
Sandwich, 1/2 Sub								
Pizza Sub	689	33.9	14.3	1722	66.7	2.7	NP	29.7
Pizza Special Sub	606	24.2	10.6	1584	68.1	3	NP	29.4
Turkey Sub	466	12.9	6	1108	63	1.8	NP	25
Turkey Club Sub	556	15.2	7.7	1065	63.2	1.8	NP	41.8
Deluxe Italian Sub	506	18.4	8.4	1005	61.2	1.8	NP	24.3
Vegetarian Sub	530	20.5	10.7	895	64.4	2.7	NP	22
Steak & Cheese Sub	491	14.6	6.7	914	63.7	2	NP	26.5
Ham & Cheese Sub	475	14.5	6.8	1020	60.9	1.8	NP	25.7
Side, 1/4 of Bread								
Howie Bread	300	8.7	1.9	239	46	1	NP	9.4
Three Cheeser Bread	370	13.7	4.9	384	47.1	1	NP	14.7
Cajun Bread	300	8.7	1.9	239	46	1	NP	9.4
Cinnamon Bread	313	8.7	1.9	239	59	1.2	NP	9.4
Chicken								
Howie Wings, 5	180	13	3.5	760	0	0	NP	14
Chicken Tenders, 2	140	4.5	0.5	460	11	0	NP	13

Description & Serving	Cal	Fat	Sfat	Sod	Carb	Fiber	Sugar	Prot
Salad								
Large Garden Salad, 1/4 portion	17	0.3	0	9	2.9	1.5	NP	1
Large Greek Salad, 1/4 portion	109	6.7	4.3	501	7.1	1.8	NP	5.6
Large Chef Salad, 1/4 portion	99	6	3	341	3.6	1.6	NP	8.1
Large Antipasto Salad, 1/4 portion	101	6.7	3.4	477	2.8	1.4	NP	7.8
Small Garden Salad, 1/2 portion	20	0.2	0	10	3.4	1.7	NP	1.1
Small Greek Salad, 1/2 portion	126	7.4	5	581	8.2	2.1	NP	6.5
Small Chef Salad, 1/2 portion	114	6.7	3.5	396	4.2	1.9	NP	9.4
Small Antipasto Salad, 1/2 portion	115	7.3	3.9	554	3.2	1.6	NP	9
Dressing/Condiment								
Blue Cheese, 1 oz	150	16	3	300	1	0	NP	1
Creamy Italian, 1 oz	120	12	2	210	2	0	NP	0
Fat Free Italian, 1.5 oz	25	0	0	390	5	0	NP	0
Fat Free Ranch, 1.5 oz	45	0	0	540	10	1	NP	0
French Style, 1 oz	30	0	0	170	7	0	NP	0
Greek, 1 oz	110	11	2	70	2	0	NP	0
Italian, 1 oz	80	8	1	560	2	0	NP	0
Ranch, 1 oz	180	19	3	250	1	0	NP	0
Thousand Island, 1 oz	140	14	2	240	4	0	NP	0
Dipping Sauce, 3 oz	45	9	3	0	0	1	NP	380
Ranch Dressing, 1 oz	175	1	0	3	3	0	NP	250
Blue Cheese Dressing, 1 oz	152	1	1	3	20	0	NP	300

In-N-Out Burger

	Cal	Fat	Sfat	Sod	Carb	Fiber	Sugar	Prot
Sandwich								
Hamburger w/ Onion	390	19	5	650	39	3	10	16
Cheeseburger w/ Onion	480	27	10	1000	39	3	10	22
Double-Double w/ Onion	670	41	18	1440	39	3	10	37
With Ketchup & Mustard rather than Spread								
Hamburger w/ Onion	310	10	4	730	41	3	10	16
Cheeseburger w/ Onion	400	18	9	1080	41	3	10	22
Double-Double w/ Onion	590	32	17	1520	41	3	10	37
With Lettuce Wrap rather than Bun								
Hamburger w/ Onion Protein Style	240	17	4	370	11	3	7	13
Cheeseburger w/ Onion Protein Style	330	25	9	720	11	3	7	18
Double-Double w/ Onion Protein Style	520	39	17	1160	11	3	7	33
Side								
French Fries	400	18	5	245	54	2	0	7
Beverage/Dessert								
Lemonade, 16 oz	180	0	0	20	40	0	38	0
Chocolate Shake, 15 oz	690	36	24	350	83	0	62	9
Vanilla Shake, 15 oz	680	37	25	390	78	0	57	9
Strawberry Shake, 15 oz	690	33	22	280	91	0	75	9

Description & Serving	Cal	Fat	Sfat	Sod	Carb	Fiber	Sugar	Prot
Jack in the Box								
Breakfast								
Bacon Breakfast Jack	300	14	5	730	29	1	4	16
Bacon, Egg & Cheese Biscuit	440	26	11	1030	37	2	2	16
Biscuit & Gravy	450	28	12	1320	39	2	2	9
Breakfast Jack	290	12	4.5	760	29	1	4	17
Denver Breakfast Bowl	720	53	18	1310	37	5	2	25
Extreme Sausage Sandwich	670	48	17	1300	31	2	5	29
Hash Brown Sticks, 5 pc	230	16	4	330	20	2	0	2
Hearty Breakfast Bowl	780	60	20	1350	34	4	1	26
Homestyle Chicken Biscuit	520	26	10	1230	52	2	1	20
Meaty Breakfast Burrito w/o salsa	610	36	14	1360	39	5	2	32
Original French Toast Sticks, 4 pc	470	23	5	450	58	4	14	7
Sausage Breakfast Jack	450	28	10	840	29	1	4	20
Sausage Croissant	580	39	13	770	37	2	5	21
Sausage, Egg & Cheese Biscuit	590	40	16	1140	38	2	2	20
Sourdough Breakfast Sandwich	420	24	8	980	31	2	3	20
Steak & Egg Burrito w/o salsa	790	48	15	1320	52	6	2	37
Supreme Croissant	450	25	9	860	36	1	5	20
Ultimate Breakfast Sandwich	570	27	10	1700	49	2	8	34
Burger								
Bacon Ultimate Cheeseburger	980	67	27	1880	52	2	11	43
Big Cheeseburger	650	40	15	1170	50	2	9	24
Hamburger	280	12	4.5	540	29	1	5	14
Hamburger w/ cheese	320	15	7	730	30	1	5	16
Hamburger Deluxe	340	18	6	550	31	2	6	14
Hamburger Deluxe w/ cheese	430	25	10	920	33	2	7	19
Jumbo Jack	580	33	11	920	51	2	10	20
Jumbo Jack w/o bun	230	19	9	270	2	1	2	12
Jumbo Jack w/o sauce	470	23	10	790	47	2	8	20
Jumbo Jack w/ cheese	670	40	15	1290	53	2	11	24
Junior Bacon Cheeseburger	400	23	8	800	30	1	6	18
Sirloin Cheeseburger	950	60	19	1920	61	4	10	41
Sirloin Cheeseburger w/ bacon	1010	65	20	2270	62	4	11	46
Sirloin Swiss & Grilled Onions Burger	930	59	18	1880	60	4	10	42
Sirloin Swiss & Grilled Onions Burger w/ bacon	990	64	20	2230	61	4	10	47
Sourdough Jack	680	46	17	1200	41	2	6	26
Sourdough Steak Melt	650	40	14	1500	34	3	4	37
Ultimate Cheeseburger	920	63	26	1530	52	2	11	38
Sandwich								
Chicken Sandwich	400	21	4.5	740	38	2	4	15
Chicken Sandwich w/ bacon	440	24	6	970	38	2	4	19
Homestyle Ranch Chicken Club	720	33	9	1860	74	3	9	33
Jack's Spicy Chicken	550	24	5	1050	59	4	8	24
Jack's Spicy Chicken w/ cheese	630	30	9	1360	61	4	8	29
Sourdough Grilled Chicken Club	530	28	7	1440	34	3	5	36
Sourdough Grilled Chicken Club w/o bun	230	10	4	1020	5	1	3	30

Description & Serving	Cal	Fat	Sfat	Sod	Carb	Fiber	Sugar	Prot
Salad								
Asian Chicken Salad w/ Crispy Chicken w/o dressing & croutons	340	13	3	660	38	8	14	21
Asian Chicken Salad w/ Grilled Chicken w/o dressing & croutons	180	1.5	0	380	22	6	15	22
Chicken Club Salad w/ Crispy Chicken w/o dressing & croutons	480	27	10	1050	28	6	5	33
Chicken Club Salad w/ Grilled Chicken w/o dressing & croutons	320	16	7	780	12	4	5	34
Southwest Chicken Salad w/ Crispy Chicken w/o dressing & croutons	470	23	8	1100	44	9	6	30
Southwest Chicken Salad w/ Grilled Chicken w/o dressing & croutons	310	12	5	820	28	7	6	31
Entrée								
Crispy Chicken Breast Strips, 4 pc	500	25	6	1260	36	3	1	35
Chicken Fajita Pita made w/ whole grain & no salsa	320	11	5	1110	33	4	3	24
Chicken Teriyaki Bowl	580	5	1	1460	106	4	35	26
Grilled Chicken Strips w/o sauce, 4 pc	180	2	0.5	700	3	0	2	37
Fish & Chips, sml	630	35	8	1290	61	5	1	19
Steak Teriyaki Bowl	650	10	3	1740	106	4	35	30
Regular Beef Taco	160	8	3	270	15	2	3	5
Kids								
Applesauce, 1 cup	100	0	0	0	25	1	23	0
Cheeseburger	280	12	4.5	540	29	1	5	14
Crispy Chicken Strips, 2 pc	250	12	3	630	18	2	1	17
Grilled Cheese Sandwich	330	18	6	730	31	2	3	11
Grilled Chicken Strips, 2 pc	250	12	3	630	18	2	1	17
Hamburger w/ cheese	320	15	7	730	30	1	5	16
Natural Cut Fries, kids size	210	11	2.5	380	25	3	0	3
Snack/Side								
Sampler Trio	740	38	15	1720	72	7	6	26
Bacon Cheddar Potato Wedges	760	52	16	960	53	4	2	21
Egg Roll	130	6	2	310	15	2	1	5
Fruit Cup	50	0	0	10	14	1	11	1
Mozzarella Cheese Sticks, 3 pc	240	14	6	510	20	1	1	10
Natural Cut Fries, sml	290	15	3.5	540	35	4	1	4
Natural Cut Fries, med	460	24	6	850	55	6	1	6
Natural Cut Fries, lrg	620	32	7	1150	75	8	1	9
Onion Rings, 8 pc	500	30	6	420	51	3	3	6
Pita Snack, Crispy Chicken	390	19	4.5	780	39	3	2	17
Pita Snack, Grilled Chicken	310	13	3	640	31	3	2	17
Pita Snack, Fish	380	19	4.5	720	39	3	2	13
Pita Snack, Steak	350	16	4.5	640	31	3	2	19
Seasoned Curly Fries, sml	280	15	3	600	30	3	1	4
Seasoned Curly Fries, med	420	24	5	920	46	5	1	6
Seasoned Curly Fries, lrg	570	32	7	1260	63	7	1	8

Description & Serving	Cal	Fat	Sfat	Sod	Carb	Fiber	Sugar	Prot
Side Salad w/o dressing & croutons	50	3	1.5	60	5	2	1	3
Stuffed Jalapenos, 3 pc	230	13	6	690	22	2	2	7

Topping

Description & Serving	Cal	Fat	Sfat	Sod	Carb	Fiber	Sugar	Prot
American Cheese, 1 slice	45	3.5	2	180	1	0	0	2
Gourmet Seasoned Croutons	100	5	1	230	11	0	1	2
Real Swiss Cheese, 1 slice	70	6	3.5	80	0	NP	0	5
Red Onion Rings	5	0	0	0	1	0	1	0
Roasted Slivered Almonds	110	9	0.5	5	4	2	1	4
Short Sliced Onions, Grilled	10	0	0	250	1	0	1	0
Spicy Corn Sticks	130	5	1	150	20	<1	0	2
Swiss-Style Cheese, 1 slice	40	3	2	150	1	0	0	2
Wonton Strips	110	6	1.5	45	13	2	1	2

Dressing/Condiment

Description & Serving	Cal	Fat	Sfat	Sod	Carb	Fiber	Sugar	Prot
Asian Sesame Dressing, 57 g	190	14	2	630	16	0	10	1
Bacon Ranch Dressing, 57 g	260	26	4	700	3	0	2	2
Barbecue Dipping Sauce, 28 g	45	0	0	330	11	0	4	0
Buttermilk House Dipping Sauce, 25 g	130	13	2	210	3	0	0	0
Chipotle Sauce, 20 g	110	12	2	230	1	0	1	0
Creamy Southwest Dressing, 57 g	220	22	3.5	850	3	0	1	1
Fire Roasted Salsa, 21 g	5	0	0	105	1	0	1	0
Grape Jelly, 1 packet	35	0	0	10	9	0	9	0
Honey Mustard Dipping Sauce, 28 g	60	2	0	220	11	0	9	0
Ketchup, 1 packet	10	0	0	105	2	0	2	0
Ketchup Substitute, 19 g	20	0	0	220	5	0	5	0
Lite Ranch Dressing, 57 g	150	15	2.5	560	3	0	2	1
Log Cabin Syrup, 1 packet	190	0	0	35	49	0	18	0
Low Fat Balsamic Dressing, 57 g	35	1.5	0	480	5	0	3	0
Mayonnaise, 1 packet	80	9	1.5	40	0	0	0	0
Mayo-Onion Sauce, .5 oz	90	10	1.5	85	1	0	0	0
Mustard, 1 packet	5	0	0	50	1	0	0	0
Mustard Substitute, 10 g	5	0	0	115	1	0	0	0
Peppercorn Mayo, 1 oz	190	20	3.5	250	1	0	0	0
Ranch Dressing, 57 g	310	33	5	470	3	0	2	1
Smoky Cheddar Mayo, 1 oz	210	22	3.5	220	1	0	1	1
Sour Cream, 1 packet	60	5	3	25	2	<1	1	1
Soy Sauce, 1 packet	5	0	0	480	1	0	0	1
Strawberry Jelly, 1 packet	35	0	0	5	9	0	8	0
Sweet & Sour Dipping Sauce, 28 g	45	0	0	160	11	0	6	0
Taco Sauce, 1 packet	0	0	0	80	0	0	0	0
Tartar Sauce, 43 g	210	22	3.5	370	2	0	1	0
Teriyaki Dipping Sauce, 28 g	60	1	0	530	11	0	10	1
Vinegar, 1 packet	0	0	0	20	0	0	0	0
Zesty Marinara Sauce, 25 g	15	0	0	200	4	0	2	0

Beverage

Description & Serving	Cal	Fat	Sfat	Sod	Carb	Fiber	Sugar	Prot
Mango Smoothie, 16 oz	290	0	0	75	72	0	57	2
Pomegranate-Berry Smoothie, 16 oz	280	0	0	70	69	0	53	2
Strawberry Banana Smoothie, 16 oz	290	0	0	70	73	1	57	2
Strawberry Smoothie, 16 oz	280	0	0	70	68	1	52	2

Description & Serving	Cal	Fat	Sfat	Sod	Carb	Fiber	Sugar	Prot
Dessert								
Cheesecake	310	16	9	220	34	0	23	7
Chocolate Ice Cream Shake, 16 oz	750	36	24	280	95	1	84	12
Chocolate Overload Cake	300	7	1.5	350	57	2	34	4
Mini Churros, 5 pc	320	17	5	270	39	2	11	3
Oreo Cookie Ice Cream Shake, 16 oz	760	40	26	360	87	1	68	12
Strawberry Ice Cream Shake, 16 oz	730	35	24	240	90	0	76	11
Vanilla Ice Cream Shake, 16 oz	650	35	24	230	70	0	59	11

Jamba Juice

Smoothie

Description & Serving	Cal	Fat	Sfat	Sod	Carb	Fiber	Sugar	Prot
Mega Mango, Sixteen (16 oz)	230	0.5	0	5	57	4	50	2
Strawberry Whirl, Sixteen (16 oz)	220	0	0	20	54	4	46	1
Peach Perfection, Sixteen (16 oz)	210	0	0	20	53	4	42	1
Pomegranate Paradise, Sixteen (16 oz)	240	0.5	0	25	60	4	53	1
Berry Fulfilling Jamba Light, Sixteen (16 oz)	150	0.5	0	200	32	4	24	6
Mango Mantra Jamba Light, Sixteen (16 oz)	150	0.5	0	190	31	2	27	6
Strawberry Nirvana Jamba Light, Sixteen (16 oz)	150	0	0	200	31	3	27	5
Strawberry Energizer, Sixteen (16 oz)	280	1	0	20	67	5	58	2
Protein Berry Workout w/ Whey, Sixteen (16 oz)	280	0	0	115	52	3	42	17
Acai Super-Antioxidant, Sixteen (16 oz)	260	4	1	45	53	3	45	4
Protein Berry Workout w/ Soy Protein, Sixteen (16 oz)	270	1	0	170	51	3	42	15
Coldbuster, Sixteen (16 oz)	240	1.5	0.5	20	56	3	49	3
Blackberry Bliss, Sixteen (16 oz)	230	1	0	25	55	4	49	1
Pomegranate Pick-Me-Up, Sixteen (16 oz)	260	1	0	35	61	3	53	2
Aloha Pineapple, Sixteen (16 oz)	290	1	0	50	67	3	63	5
Caribbean Passion, Sixteen (16 oz)	250	1	0	35	57	2	51	2
Mango-a-go-go, Sixteen (16 oz)	280	1	0	35	65	2	59	2
Peach Pleasure, Sixteen (16 oz)	260	1	0.5	35	61	3	51	2
Banana Berry, Sixteen (16 oz)	270	1	0	60	64	3	57	3
Razzmatazz, Sixteen (16 oz)	270	1	0.5	40	63	3	51	2
Strawberry Surf Rider, Sixteen (16 oz)	300	1	0	5	72	2	64	2
Strawberries Wild, Sixteen (16 oz)	250	0	0	95	60	2	52	3
Orange Dream Machine, Sixteen (16 oz)	310	1	0.5	150	66	0	59	7
Peanut Butter MOO'D, Sixteen (16 oz)	470	10	2.5	310	82	3	71	13
Chocolate MOO'D, Sixteen (16 oz)	430	4	2	270	86	2	77	11
Matcha Green Tea Blast, Sixteen (16 oz)	290	0	0	160	62	1	55	8

Juice/Tea Infusion

Description & Serving	Cal	Fat	Sfat	Sod	Carb	Fiber	Sugar	Prot
Carrot Juice, Sixteen (16 oz)	130	0.5	0	230	30	0	26	4
Orange Juice, Sixteen (16 oz)	220	1	0	0	52	<1	42	3
Prickly Pear Tea Infusion, Sixteen (16 oz)	150	0	0	20	38	1	33	1
Pomegranate Tea Infusion, Sixteen (16 oz)	160	0	0	20	40	<1	36	1
Passion Fruit Tea Infusion, Sixteen (16 oz)	150	0	0	20	37	<1	32	1

Shot

Description & Serving	Cal	Fat	Sfat	Sod	Carb	Fiber	Sugar	Prot
Matcha Energy Shot - Orange Juice, Single (4 oz)	60	0	0	0	13	<1	10	1
Matcha Energy Shot - Orange Juice, Double (4 oz)	60	0	0	0	13	1	10	1

Description & Serving	Cal	Fat	Sfat	Sod	Carb	Fiber	Sugar	Prot
Matcha Energy Shot - Soymilk, Single (4 oz)	70	0	0	45	14	0	12	3
Matcha Energy Shot - Soymilk, Double (4 oz)	70	0	0	45	14	<1	12	4
Wheatgrass Detox Shot, 1 oz	5	0	NP	0	1	0	<1	<1
Wheatgrass Detox Shot, 2 oz	15	0	NP	10	2	0	<1	1

Boost

Heart Happy Boost	NP	NP	NP	NP	NP	NP	NP	NP
3G Charger Super Boost	5	0	NP	NP	2	2	NP	NP
Flax & Fiber Boost	30	1.5	NP	NP	7	7	NP	1
Calcium Boost	NP	NP	NP	NP	NP	NP	NP	NP
Daily Vitamin Boost	NP	NP	NP	NP	NP	NP	NP	NP
Whey Protein Super Boost	45	0	NP	20	NP	1	NP	10
Weight Burner Super Boost	30	3	0	NP	NP	NP	NP	NP
Antioxidant Power Super Boost	NP	NP	NP	NP	NP	NP	NP	NP
Soy Protein Boost	30	NP	NP	NP	NP	NP	NP	8
Energy Boost	NP	NP	NP	NP	NP	NP	NP	NP
Immunity Boost	NP	NP	NP	NP	NP	NP	NP	NP

Ideal Meals

Acai Topper, Sixteen (16 oz)	490	10	1.5	40	96	11	57	9
Mango Peach Topper, Sixteen (16 oz)	500	9	1.5	110	95	9	60	13
Berry Topper, Sixteen (16 oz)	480	9	1.5	110	91	9	55	13
Chunky Strawberry Topper, Sixteen (16 oz)	570	17	2.5	180	92	10	54	16

Breakfast

Plain Oatmeal w/ Brown Sugar	220	3.5	1	20	44	5	12	8
Fresh Banana Oatmeal	280	4	1	20	57	6	19	9
Blueberry & Blackberry Oatmeal	290	3.5	1	30	58	6	24	8
Apple Cinnamon Oatmeal	290	4	1	25	60	5	25	8

Sandwich/Wrap

Gobble'licious w/ dijonnaise	570	28	5	1410	49	2	7	28
Gobble'licious w/o dijonnaise	420	14	3.5	1310	47	2	6	28
Tomo Artichoko Flatbread	310	11	3	580	44	3	4	11
Smokehouse Chicken Flatbread	300	8	3	520	41	6	4	15
MediterraneYUM Flatbread	250	8	2.5	620	37	3	4	10
Four Cheesy Flatbread	330	13	7	700	35	2	3	17
Greens & Grain Wrap w/ sauce	640	14	1.5	650	108	9	12	19
Greens & Grain Wrap w/o sauce	600	14	1.5	630	99	9	4	19
Greek Goodness Wrap w/ sauce	550	26	4	1280	70	2	10	15
Greek Goodness Wrap w/o sauce	440	16	3.5	1090	62	2	4	15
Chimichurri Chicken Wrap w/ sauce	560	25	2.5	770	67	3	5	22
Chimichurri Chicken Wrap w/o sauce	410	9	1	710	66	2	5	22
Asian Style Chicken Wrap w/ sauce	430	7	0	600	72	5	13	19
Asian Style Chicken Wrap w/o sauce	400	7	0	590	63	5	5	19

Salad

Couscous & Produce w/ dressing	480	19	1	180	72	9	34	11
Couscous & Produce w/o dressing	360	10	0.5	15	61	9	25	11
Caesar the Day! w/ dressing	330	22	4.5	720	15	3	2	16
Caesar the Day! w/o dressing	180	8	3	280	12	3	2	13

Description & Serving	Cal	Fat	Sfat	Sod	Carb	Fiber	Sugar	Prot
Snack								
Cheddar Tomato Twist	240	4.5	1.5	430	41	2	3	8
Blueberry Oatcake	280	9	1	220	46	6	17	6
Zucchini Walnut Loaf	270	9	1.5	250	43	4	26	5
Reduced-Fat Cranberry Orange Loaf	310	9	2	200	52	4	31	6
Reduced-Fat Blueberry Lemon Loaf	290	8	2	220	53	2	30	2
Sourdough Parmesan Pretzel	410	10	2	640	67	3	4	14
Apple Cinnamon Pretzel	380	4	0	250	76	4	14	11
Dessert								
Omega-3 Chocolate Brownie Cookie	150	3.5	1	15	30	2	24	3
Omega-3 Oatmeal Cookie	150	6	1.5	85	26	3	15	2

Jersey Mike's Subs

Description & Serving	Cal	Fat	Sfat	Sod	Carb	Fiber	Sugar	Prot
Cold Sub								
BLT In a Tub w/o vinegar, oil, or mayo	280	21	9	790	8	2	5	14
BLT Wheat Mini Sub w/o vinegar, oil, or mayo	350	16	7	920	36	3	6	16
BLT White Mini Sub w/o vinegar, oil, or mayo	360	16	6	890	39	2	5	15
Jersey Shore Favorite In a Tub w/o vinegar, oil, or mayo	270	14	7	1060	12	2	5	26
Jersey Shore Favorite Wheat Mini Sub w/o vinegar, oil, or mayo	310	9	4.5	800	38	3	6	20
Jersey Shore Favorite White Mini Sub w/o vinegar, oil, or mayonnaise	330	10	4.5	780	41	2	5	19
American Classic In a Tub w/o vinegar, oil, or mayo	270	14	7	1310	11	2	5	26
American Classic Wheat Mini Sub w/o vinegar, oil, or mayo	320	10	5	1130	37	3	6	23
American Classic White Mini Sub w/o vinegar, oil, or mayo	340	10	5	1110	40	2	5	21
#4 In a Tub w/o vinegar, oil, or mayo	270	14	6	810	13	2	5	25
#4 Wheat Mini w/o vinegar, oil, or mayo	310	9	4.5	740	38	3	6	20
#4 White Mini w/o vinegar, oil, or mayo	330	10	4	720	41	2	5	19
Super Sub In a Tub w/o vinegar, oil, or mayo	290	14	7	1150	13	2	5	29
Super Sub Wheat Mini Sub w/o vinegar, oil, or mayo	340	10	5	1080	39	3	6	25
Super Sub White Mini Sub w/o vinegar, oil, or mayo	360	11	4.5	1060	42	2	5	24
Roast Beef & Provolone In a Tub w/o vinegar, oil, or mayo	430	20	9	190	9	2	5	52
Roast Beef & Provolone Wheat Mini Sub w/o vinegar, oil, or mayo	420	14	6	500	36	3	6	38
Roast Beef & Provolone White Mini Sub w/o vinegar, oil, or mayo	440	14	6	480	39	2	5	37
Turkey Breast & Provolone In a Tub w/o vinegar, oil, or mayo	250	11	6	930	9	2	5	30
Turkey Breast & Provolone Wheat Mini Sub v w/o inegar, oil, or mayo	310	8	4	920	36	3	6	25

Description & Serving	Cal	Fat	Sfat	Sod	Carb	Fiber	Sugar	Prot
Turkey Breast & Provolone White Mini Sub w/o vinegar, oil, or mayo	330	9	4	900	39	2	5	23
Club Sub w/ Mayonnaise In a Tub w/o vinegar & oil	600	47	14	1610	11	2	5	32
Club Sub w/ Mayonnaise Wheat Mini Sub w/o vinegar& oil	490	27	8	1320	37	3	6	27
Club Sub w/ Mayonnaise White Mini Sub w/o vinegar & oil	510	27	8	1300	40	2	5	26
Club Supreme w/ Mayonnaise In a Tub w/o vinegar & oil	650	47	13	910	11	2	5	45
Club Supreme w/ Mayonnaise Wheat Mini Sub w/o vinegar & oil	530	27	8	970	37	3	6	36
Club Supreme w/ Mayonnaise White Mini Sub w/o vinegar & oil	550	28	8	950	40	2	5	35
Albacore Tuna In a Tub w/o vinegar, oil, or mayo	620	55	8	680	12	3	5	21
Albacore Tuna Wheat Mini Sub w/o vinegar, oil, or mayo	530	34	6	790	38	4	6	20
Albacore Tuna White Mini Sub w/o vinegar, oil, or mayo	540	35	5	770	41	3	5	19
#11 In a Tub w/o vinegar, oil, or mayo	340	21	9	1420	11	2	5	27
#11 Wheat Mini w/o vinegar, oil, or mayo	320	11	5	920	37	3	6	19
#11 White Mini w/o vinegar, oil, or mayo	340	12	5	900	40	2	5	18
#12 In a Tub w/o vinegar, oil, or mayo	460	23	10	320	9	2	5	54
#12 Wheat Mini w/o vinegar, oil, or mayo	450	17	7	630	36	3	6	40
#12 White Mini w/o vinegar, oil, or mayo	470	17	7	610	39	2	5	38
Original Italian In a Tub w/o vinegar, oil, or mayo	390	22	10	1600	14	2	5	34
Original Italian Wheat Mini w/o vinegar, oil, or mayo	410	16	7	1340	40	3	6	29
Original Italian White Mini w/o vinegar, oil, or mayo	430	16	7	1320	43	2	5	28
Veggie In a Tub w/o vinegar, oil, or mayo	460	32	19	290	14	3	7	31
Veggie Wheat Mini w/o vinegar, oil, or mayo	400	18	10	530	38	4	7	23
Veggie White Mini w/o vinegar, oil, or mayo	410	18	10	510	41	3	6	22

Hot Sub

Description & Serving	Cal	Fat	Sfat	Sod	Carb	Fiber	Sugar	Prot
Meatball & Cheese Wheat Regular	850	50	21	1880	64	6	11	39
Meatball & Cheese White Regular	870	50	21	1850	68	5	10	37
Chicken Philly Wheat Regular	590	23	13	1660	57	4	11	39
Chicken Philly White Regular	610	24	13	1630	62	3	10	37
Steak Philly Wheat Regular	580	22	11	1640	56	4	10	41
Steak Philly White Regular	600	22	11	1600	60	3	9	39
Chipotle Steak Wheat Regular	860	53	16	2110	58	4	10	42
Chipotle Steak White Regular	890	54	16	2080	63	3	9	40
Chipotle Chicken Wheat Regular	870	54	19	2130	60	4	11	40
Chipotle Chicken White Regular	900	55	18	2100	64	3	10	39
Grilled Chicken Wheat Regular	630	31	5	1220	52	4	7	34
Grilled Chicken White Regular	650	32	5	1190	57	3	6	32
Chicken Parmesan Wheat Regular	610	20	7	1520	69	5	7	37
Chicken Parmesan White Regular	630	21	7	1490	73	4	6	35
BBQ Beef Wheat Regular	670	14	5	1450	75	4	22	59

Description & Serving	Cal	Fat	Sfat	Sod	Carb	Fiber	Sugar	Prot
BBQ Beef White Regular	700	15	5	1420	80	3	20	57
Pastrami & Swiss Wheat Regular	540	16	8	2590	52	3	7	45
Pastrami & Swiss White Regular	570	16	8	2560	57	2	6	43
Reuben Wheat Regular	660	25	9	2610	64	5	13	41
Reuben White Regular	690	26	9	2580	69	3	11	40
Big Kahuna Steak Wheat Regular	630	26	14	2000	57	5	11	43
Big Kahuna Steak White Regular	660	27	14	1960	62	3	10	42
Big Kahuna Chicken Wheat Regular	640	27	16	2020	58	5	12	42
Big Kahuna Chicken White Regular	670	28	16	1990	63	3	11	40
Chipotle Turkey Wheat Regular	820	48	14	2070	59	6	9	44
Chipotle Turkey White Regular	850	49	14	2040	63	4	8	42
Sausage Wheat Regular	560	25	8	1620	58	5	11	26
Sausage White Regular	580	25	7	1590	62	4	10	24
Teriyaki Chicken Cheese Steak Wheat Regular	640	23	13	3830	66	4	19	42
Teriyaki Chicken Cheese Steak White Regular	660	24	13	3800	71	3	18	41
Buffalo Chicken Cheese Steak Wheat Regular	900	53	19	4000	65	5	16	43
Buffalo Chicken Cheese Steak White Regular	920	54	19	3970	70	4	14	41
California Cheese Steak Wheat Regular	830	49	15	1850	57	5	11	42
California Cheese Steak White Regular	860	50	15	1820	62	4	10	40
California Cheese Steak Chicken Wheat Regular	850	51	18	1870	59	5	13	40
California Cheese Steak Chicken White Regular	870	51	17	1840	63	4	12	38

Wrap

Description & Serving	Cal	Fat	Sfat	Sod	Carb	Fiber	Sugar	Prot
BLT Flour Tortilla Wrap w/o vinegar, oil, or mayo	590	29	12	1460	60	7	6	23
BLT Reduced Carb Wrap w/o vinegar, oil, or mayo	550	28	12	1650	50	31	5	26
BLT Spinach Wrap w/o vinegar, oil, or mayo	590	29	12	1630	60	5	8	23
BLT Tomato Wrap w/o vinegar, oil, or mayo	590	29	12	1610	59	5	11	23
BLT Wheat Wrap w/o vinegar, oil, or mayo	580	29	12	1530	58	8	5	23
Jersey Shore Favorite Flour Tortilla Wrap w/o vinegar, oil, or mayo	580	22	10	1730	64	7	6	35
Jersey Shore Favorite Reduced Carb Wrap w/o vinegar, oil, or mayo	540	21	10	1920	54	31	5	38
Jersey Shore Favorite Spinach Wrap w/o vinegar, oil, or mayo	580	22	10	1900	64	5	8	35
Jersey Shore Favorite Tomato Wrap w/o vinegar, oil, or mayo	580	22	10	1880	63	5	11	35
Jersey Shore Favorite Wheat Wrap w/o vinegar, oil, or mayo	570	22	10	1800	62	8	5	34
American Classic Flour Tortilla Wrap w/o vinegar, oil, or mayo	580	22	10	1980	63	7	6	35
American Classic Reduced Carb Wrap w/o vinegar, oil, or mayo	540	21	10	2170	53	31	5	38
American Classic Spinach Wrap w/o vinegar, oil, or mayo	580	22	10	2150	63	5	8	35
American Classic Tomato Wrap w/o vinegar, oil, or mayo	580	22	10	2130	62	5	11	35
American Classic Wheat Wrap w/o vinegar, oil, or mayo	570	22	10	2050	61	8	5	34
#4 Flour Tortilla Wrap w/o vinegar, oil, or mayo	580	22	9	1480	65	7	6	34

Description & Serving	Cal	Fat	Sfat	Sod	Carb	Fiber	Sugar	Prot
#4 Reduced Carb Wrap w/o vinegar, oil, or mayo	540	21	9	1670	55	31	5	37
#4 Spinach Wrap w/o vinegar, oil, or mayo	580	22	9	1650	65	5	8	34
#4 Tomato Wrap w/o vinegar, oil, or mayo	580	22	9	1630	64	5	11	34
#4 Wheat Wrap w/o vinegar, oil, or mayo	570	22	9	1550	63	8	5	33
Super Sub Flour Tortilla Wrap w/o vinegar, oil, or mayo	600	22	10	1820	65	7	6	38
Super Sub Reduced Carb Wrap w/o vinegar, oil, or mayo	560	21	10	2010	55	31	5	41
Super Sub Spinach Wrap w/o vinegar, oil, or mayo	600	22	10	1990	65	5	8	38
Super Sub Tomato Wrap w/o vinegar, oil, or mayo	600	22	10	1970	64	5	11	38
Super Sub Wheat Wrap w/o vinegar, oil, or mayo	590	22	10	1890	63	8	5	37
Roast Beef & Provolone Flour Tortilla Wrap w/o vinegar, oil, or mayo	740	28	12	860	61	7	6	61
Roast Beef & Provolone Reduced Carb Wrap w/o vinegar, oil, or mayo	700	27	12	1050	51	31	5	64
Roast Beef & Provolone Spinach Wrap w/o vinegar, oil, or mayo	740	28	12	1030	61	5	8	61
Roast Beef & Provolone Tomato Wrap w/o vinegar, oil, or mayo	740	28	12	1010	60	5	11	61
Roast Beef & Provolone Wheat Wrap w/o vinegar, oil, or mayo	730	28	12	930	59	8	5	60
Turkey Breast & Provolone Flour Tortilla Wrap w/o vinegar, oil, or mayo	560	19	8	1600	61	7	6	39
Turkey Breast & Provolone Reduced Carb Wrap w/o vinegar, oil, or mayo	520	18	8	1790	51	31	5	42
Turkey Breast & Provolone Spinach Wrap w/o vinegar, oil, or mayo	560	19	9	1770	61	5	8	39
Turkey Breast & Provolone Tomato Wrap w/o vinegar, oil, or mayo	560	19	9	1750	60	5	11	39
Turkey Breast & Provolone Wheat Wrap w/o vinegar, oil, or mayo	550	19	8	1670	59	8	5	38
Club Sub w/ Mayonnaise Flour Tortilla Wrap w/o vinegar & oil	910	55	16	2280	63	7	6	41
Club Sub w/ Mayonnaise Reduced Carb Wrap w/o vinegar & oil	870	54	16	2470	53	31	5	44
Club Sub w/ Mayonnaise Spinach Wrap w/o vinegar & oil	910	55	17	2450	63	5	8	41
Club Sub w/ Mayonnaise Tomato Wrap w/o vinegar & oil	910	55	17	2430	62	5	11	41
Club Sub w/ Mayonnaise Wheat Wrap w/o vinegar & oil	900	55	16	2350	61	8	5	40
Club Supreme w/ Mayonnaise Flour Tortilla Wrap w/o vinegar & oil	960	55	16	1580	63	7	6	54
Club Supreme w/ Mayonnaise Reduced Carb Wrap w/o vinegar & oil	920	54	16	1770	53	31	5	57
Club Supreme w/ Mayonnaise Spinach Wrap w/o vinegar & oil	960	55	16	1750	63	5	8	54
Club Supreme w/ Mayonnaise Tomato Wrap w/o vinegar & oil	960	55	16	1730	62	5	11	54

Description & Serving	Cal	Fat	Sfat	Sod	Carb	Fiber	Sugar	Prot
Club Supreme w/ Mayonnaise Wheat Wrap w/o vinegar & oil	950	55	16	1650	61	8	5	53
Albacore Tuna Flour Tortilla Wrap w/o vinegar, oil, or mayo	930	63	11	1350	64	8	6	30
Albacore Tuna Reduced Carb Wrap w/o vinegar, oil, or mayo	890	62	11	1540	54	32	5	33
Albacore Tuna Spinach Wrap w/o vinegar, oil, or mayo	930	63	11	1520	64	6	8	30
Albacore Tuna Tomato Wrap w/o vinegar, oil, or mayo	930	63	11	1500	63	6	11	30
Albacore Tuna Wheat Wrap w/o vinegar, oil, or mayo	920	63	11	1420	62	9	5	29
#11 Flour Tortilla Wrap w/o vinegar, oil, or mayo	650	29	12	2090	63	7	6	36
#11 Reduced Carb Wrap w/o vinegar, oil, or mayo	610	28	12	2280	53	31	5	39
#11 Spinach Wrap w/o vinegar, oil, or mayo	650	29	12	2260	63	5	8	36
#11 Tomato Wrap w/o vinegar, oil, or mayo	650	29	12	2240	62	5	11	36
#11 Wheat Wrap w/o vinegar, oil, or mayo	640	29	12	2160	61	8	5	35
#12 Flour Tortilla Wrap w/o vinegar, oil, or mayo	770	31	13	990	61	7	6	63
#12 Reduced Carb Wrap w/o vinegar, oil, or mayo	730	30	13	1180	51	31	5	66
#12 Spinach Wrap w/o vinegar, oil, or mayo	770	31	13	1160	61	5	8	63
#12 Tomato Wrap w/o vinegar, oil, or mayo	770	31	13	1140	60	5	11	63
#12 Wheat Wrap w/o vinegar, oil, or mayo	760	31	13	1060	59	8	5	62
Original Italian Flour Tortilla Wrap w/o vinegar, oil, or mayo	700	30	12	2270	66	7	6	43
Original Italian Reduced Carb Wrap w/o vinegar, oil, or mayo	660	29	12	2460	56	31	5	46
Original Italian Spinach Wrap w/o vinegar, oil, or mayo	700	30	13	2440	66	5	8	43
Original Italian Tomato Wrap w/o vinegar, oil, or mayo	700	30	13	2420	65	5	11	43
Original Italian Wheat Wrap w/o vinegar, oil, or mayo	690	30	12	2340	64	8	5	42
Veggie Flour Tortilla Wrap w/o vinegar, oil, or mayo	770	40	22	960	66	8	8	40
Veggie Reduced Carb Wrap w/o vinegar, oil, or mayo	730	39	22	1150	56	32	7	43
Veggie Spinach Wrap w/o vinegar, oil, or mayo	770	40	22	1130	66	6	10	40
Veggie Tomato Wrap w/o vinegar, oil, or mayo	770	40	22	1110	65	6	13	40
Veggie Wheat Wrap w/o vinegar, oil, or mayo	760	40	22	1030	64	9	7	39
Meatball & Cheese Flour Tortilla Wrap	910	55	23	1960	69	8	8	37
Meatball & Cheese Reduced Carb Wrap	870	54	23	2150	59	32	7	40
Meatball & Cheese Spinach Wrap	910	55	23	2130	69	6	10	37
Meatball & Cheese Tomato Wrap	910	55	23	2110	68	6	13	37
Meatball & Cheese Wheat Wrap	900	55	23	2030	67	9	7	36
Chicken Philly Flour Tortilla Wrap	650	28	15	1750	62	6	8	37
Chicken Philly Reduced Carb Wrap	610	27	15	1940	52	30	7	40
Chicken Philly Spinach Wrap	650	28	16	1920	62	4	10	37
Chicken Philly Tomato Wrap	650	28	16	1900	61	4	13	37
Chicken Philly Wheat Wrap	640	28	15	1820	60	7	7	36

Description & Serving	Cal	Fat	Sfat	Sod	Carb	Fiber	Sugar	Prot
Steak Philly Flour Tortilla Wrap	640	27	13	1720	61	6	7	39
Steak Philly Reduced Carb Wrap	600	26	13	1910	51	30	6	42
Steak Philly Spinach Wrap	640	27	13	1890	61	4	9	39
Steak Philly Tomato Wrap	640	27	13	1870	60	4	12	39
Steak Philly Wheat Wrap	630	27	13	1790	59	7	6	38
Chipotle Steak Flour Tortilla Wrap	920	58	18	2190	64	6	6	40
Chipotle Steak Reduced Carb Wrap	880	57	18	2380	54	30	5	43
Chipotle Steak Spinach Wrap	920	58	19	2360	64	4	8	40
Chipotle Steak Tomato Wrap	920	58	19	2340	63	4	11	40
Chipotle Steak Wheat Wrap	910	58	18	2260	62	7	5	39
Chipotle Chicken Philly Flour Tortilla Wrap	940	60	20	2220	65	6	8	38
Chipotle Chicken Philly Reduced Carb Wrap	900	59	20	2410	55	30	7	41
Chipotle Chicken Philly Spinach Wrap	940	60	21	2390	65	4	10	38
Chipotle Chicken Philly Tomato Wrap	940	60	21	2370	64	4	13	38
Chipotle Chicken Philly Wheat Wrap	930	60	20	2290	63	7	7	37
Grilled Chicken Flour Tortilla Wrap	690	37	7	1300	58	6	3	32
Grilled Chicken Reduced Carb Wrap	650	36	7	1490	48	30	2	35
Grilled Chicken Spinach Wrap	690	37	8	1470	58	4	5	32
Grilled Chicken Tomato Wrap	690	37	8	1450	57	4	8	32
Grilled Chicken Wheat Wrap	680	37	7	1370	56	7	2	31
Chicken Parmesan Flour Tortilla Wrap	670	25	9	1610	74	7	4	35
Chicken Parmesan Reduced Carb Wrap	630	24	9	1800	64	31	3	38
Chicken Parmesan Spinach Wrap	670	25	9	1780	74	5	6	35
Chicken Parmesan Tomato Wrap	670	25	9	1760	73	5	9	35
Chicken Parmesan Wheat Wrap	660	25	9	1680	72	8	3	34
BBQ Beef Flour Tortilla Wrap	740	20	7	1540	80	6	18	57
BBQ Beef Reduced Carb Wrap	700	19	7	1730	70	30	17	60
BBQ Beef Spinach Wrap	740	20	7	1710	80	4	20	57
BBQ Beef Tomato Wrap	740	20	7	1690	79	4	23	57
BBQ Beef Wheat Wrap	730	20	7	1610	78	7	17	56
Pastrami & Swiss Flour Tortilla Wrap	610	21	9	2680	58	5	4	43
Pastrami & Swiss Reduced Carb Wrap	570	20	9	2870	48	29	3	46
Pastrami & Swiss Spinach Wrap	610	21	10	2850	58	3	6	43
Pastrami & Swiss Tomato Wrap	610	21	10	2830	57	3	9	43
Pastrami & Swiss Wheat Wrap	600	21	9	2750	56	6	3	42
Reuben Flour Tortilla Wrap	720	31	11	2700	70	7	9	39
Reuben Reduced Carb Wrap	680	30	11	2890	60	31	8	42
Reuben Spinach Wrap	720	31	11	2870	70	5	11	39
Reuben Tomato Wrap	720	31	11	2850	69	5	14	39
Reuben Wheat Wrap	710	31	11	2770	68	8	8	38
Big Kahuna Flour Tortilla Wrap	690	31	16	2080	62	6	7	41
Big Kahuna Reduced Carb Wrap	650	30	16	2270	52	30	6	44
Big Kahuna Spinach Wrap	690	31	16	2250	62	4	9	41
Big Kahuna Tomato Wrap	690	31	16	2230	61	4	12	41
Big Kahuna Wheat Wrap	680	31	16	2150	60	7	6	40
Big Kahuna Chicken Flour Tortilla Wrap	710	33	18	2110	64	6	9	40
Big Kahuna Chicken Reduced Carb Wrap	670	32	18	2300	54	30	8	43
Big Kahuna Chicken Spinach Wrap	710	33	18	2280	64	4	11	40
Big Kahuna Chicken Tomato Wrap	710	33	18	2260	63	4	14	40

Description & Serving	Cal	Fat	Sfat	Sod	Carb	Fiber	Sugar	Prot
Big Kahuna Chicken Wheat Wrap	700	33	18	2180	62	7	8	39
Chipotle Turkey Flour Tortilla Wrap	890	54	16	2160	64	7	6	42
Chipotle Turkey Reduced Carb Wrap	850	53	16	2350	54	31	5	45
Chipotle Turkey Spinach Wrap	890	54	17	2330	64	5	8	42
Chipotle Turkey Tomato Wrap	890	54	17	2310	63	5	11	42
Chipotle Turkey Wheat Wrap	880	54	16	2230	62	8	5	41
Sausage Flour Tortilla Wrap	620	30	9	1710	63	7	8	24
Sausage Reduced Carb Wrap	580	29	9	1900	53	31	7	27
Sausage Spinach Wrap	620	30	10	1880	63	5	10	24
Sausage Tomato Wrap	620	30	10	1860	62	5	13	24
Sausage Wheat Wrap	610	30	9	1780	61	8	7	23
Teriyaki Chicken Cheese Steak Flour Tortilla Wrap	700	28	15	3920	71	6	15	40
Teriyaki Chicken Cheese Steak Reduced Carb Wrap	660	27	15	4110	61	30	14	43
Teriyaki Chicken Cheese Steak Spinach Wrap	700	28	16	4090	71	4	17	40
Teriyaki Chicken Cheese Steak Tomato Wrap	700	28	16	4070	70	4	20	40
Teriyaki Chicken Cheese Steak Wheat Wrap	690	28	15	3990	69	7	14	39
Buffalo Chicken Cheese Steak Flour Tortilla Wrap	960	59	21	4090	70	7	12	41
Buffalo Chicken Cheese Steak Reduced Carb Wrap	920	58	21	4280	60	31	11	44
Buffalo Chicken Cheese Steak Spinach Wrap	960	59	21	4260	70	5	14	41
Buffalo Chicken Cheese Steak Tomato Wrap	960	59	21	4240	69	5	17	41
Buffalo Chicken Cheese Steak Wheat Wrap	950	59	21	4160	68	8	11	40
California Cheese Steak Flour Tortilla Wrap	890	55	17	1940	63	7	8	40
California Cheese Steak Reduced Carb Wrap	870	55	19	2150	54	31	8	41
California Cheese Steak Spinach Wrap	890	55	18	2110	63	5	10	40
California Cheese Steak Tomato Wrap	890	55	18	2090	62	5	13	40
California Cheese Steak Wheat Wrap	880	55	17	2010	61	8	7	39
California Cheese Steak Chicken Flour Tortilla Wrap	910	56	19	1960	64	7	9	38
California Cheese Steak Chicken Reduced Carb Wrap	870	55	19	2150	54	31	8	41
California Cheese Steak Chicken Spinach Wrap	910	56	20	2130	64	5	11	38
California Cheese Steak Chicken Tomato Wrap	910	56	20	2110	63	5	14	38
California Cheese Steak Chicken Wheat Wrap	900	56	19	2030	62	8	8	37
Grilled Veggie Wrap	910	57	22	1480	69	8	10	36
Chicken Caesar Wrap	580	23	5	1470	58	6	4	33
Buffalo Chicken Wrap	740	37	14	2990	62	6	6	40
Baja Chicken Wrap	610	23	11	2640	63	8	7	40
Grilled Ham & Cheese Wrap	740	41	13	1980	63	5	11	29
Grilled Roast Beef & Cheese Wrap	830	45	14	1170	65	5	12	42
Turkey w/ Honey Mustard Sauce Wrap	540	20	4	1700	63	7	10	30

Salad

Tossed Salad	50	0.5	0	20	11	5	7	3
Chef Salad	240	10	5	960	12	5	7	25
Grilled Chicken Caesar Salad	510	35	9	1480	11	2	5	34
Tuna Salad	690	60	9	740	15	5	7	24

Soup

Beef Steak & Black Bean Soup, cup	140	2	0	990	21	9	3	10
Boston Clam Chowder, cup	130	6	2	1030	15	0	0	5
Broccoli Cheese w/ Florets Soup, cup	140	9	5	1100	8	0	2	4

Description & Serving	Cal	Fat	Sfat	Sod	Carb	Fiber	Sugar	Prot
Cape Cod Clam Chowder, cup	140	6	2	1110	17	0	1	4
Chicken Gumbo, cup	100	4.5	1.5	1020	11	1	2	4
Chicken Noodle Soup, cup	90	3.5	1	910	11	0	0	4
Chicken Pot Pie, cup	230	14	5	1240	20	1	3	7
Chicken Tortilla Soup, cup	140	3	1	1010	22	5	2	8
Cream of Broccoli Soup, cup	90	6	3	1220	9	1	3	3
Cream of Potato Soup, cup	180	8	5	810	17	1	0	2
Creamy Tomato Bisque, cup	90	4	1	1130	11	1	5	2
French Onion Soup, cup	80	1	0	940	15	3	3	3
Italian Style Wedding Soup, cup	120	5	2.5	1000	13	1	1	5
Lumberjack Mixed Vegetable Soup, cup	120	4.5	2	1320	16	5	4	2
Maryland Style Crab Soup, cup	70	0.5	0	980	12	2	4	4
Masterpiece Broccoli Cheese w/ Florets Soup, cup	190	10	4.5	1190	16	1	8	7
Masterpiece Chicken & Dumplings Soup, cup	250	18	7	1040	16	0	4	7
Minestrone Soup, cup	70	3	0.5	1540	8	0	6	3
Our Old Fashioned Chicken Noodle Soup, cup	90	2	0.5	1240	11	0	1	7
Potato w/ Bacon Soup, cup	130	5	1.5	1080	18	1	2	4
Spicy Chili w/ Beans, cup	240	8	3.5	1130	25	7	5	16
Split Pea w/ Ham Soup, cup	150	1.5	0.5	1050	25	3	4	9
Timberline Chili w/ Beans, cup	280	9	3.5	680	31	7	9	18
Tomato Florentine, cup	90	1	0	1060	17	1	6	3
Vegetable Beef & Barley Soup, cup	90	3	1	1040	11	2	1	5
Vegetarian Vegetable Soup, cup	80	0.5	0	850	18	4	4	2
Wild & Brown Rice w/ Chicken Soup, cup	310	15	4.5	910	17	1	1	26
Wisconsin Cheese Soup, cup	220	16	4.5	1200	16	0	8	5

Dressing/Condiment/Topping

Description & Serving	Cal	Fat	Sfat	Sod	Carb	Fiber	Sugar	Prot
Mayonnaise Mini, 18 g	130	14	2	100	1	0	0	0
Vinegar Mini, 15 g	5	0	0	0	0	0	0	0
Oil Mini, 15 g	130	15	2	0	0	0	0	0
Sprinklings (Mayo, Vinegar, & Oil) Mini, 48 g	260	29	4	100	1	0	0	0
Mustard Mini, 7 g	0	0	0	90	0	0	0	0
Blue Cheese Dressing, 2 tbsp	120	12	2.5	320	2	0	2	1
Caesar Dressing, 2 tbsp	150	15	2.5	390	2	0	1	2
Chipotle Mayo Dressing, 2 tbsp	180	20	3	150	0	0	0	0
Golden Italian Dressing, 2 tbsp	110	11	1.5	290	3	0	2	0
Italian Light Dressing, 2 tbsp	80	9	1.5	370	0	0	0	0
Italian Fat Free Dressing, 2 tbsp	10	0	0	290	3	0	2	0
Ranch Dressing, 2 tbsp	120	12	2	240	2	0	1	0
Russian Dressing, 2 tbsp	160	16	2.5	200	4	0	4	0
Lettuce Mini	5	0	0	0	1	1	1	0
Onions Mini	5	0	0	0	1	0	1	0
Tomatoes Mini	10	0	0	0	2	1	1	0
Dill Pickle Mini	0	0	0	140	0	0	0	0
Banana Peppers Mini	0	0	0	120	0	0	0	0
Jalapeño Peppers Mini	0	0	0	140	0	0	0	0

Dessert

Description & Serving	Cal	Fat	Sfat	Sod	Carb	Fiber	Sugar	Prot
Chocolate Brownie (David's)	440	20	6	240	60	1	39	5
Chocolate Chip Cookie	200	11	4	150	24	<1	16	2

Description & Serving	Cal	Fat	Sfat	Sod	Carb	Fiber	Sugar	Prot
Chocolate Chip w/ Candy Pieces Cookie	200	11	4	160	24	<1	15	2
Chocolate Chip Walnut Cookie	210	12	3.5	150	23	<1	14	2
Chocolate Chocolate Chip Cookie	180	7	2.5	110	26	1	18	2
Chocolate Chunk Cookie	200	11	4	140	24	0	15	2
Oatmeal Raisin Cookie	180	7	1.5	115	26	1	16	2
Peanut Butter Cookie	200	12	2.5	210	21	<1	14	4
Peanut Butter Cookie (David's)	210	14	4	250	17	1	9	5
Peanut Butter Chocolate Chip Cookie	210	11	3.5	180	23	1	16	3
Sugar Cookie	180	8	3	240	26	0	13	2
Sugar Cookie (David's)	170	8	4.5	240	23	0	11	2
White Chip Macadamia Nut (David's)	190	10	4.5	100	24	1	16	2

Jet's Pizza

Small Pizza

Crispy Crust, 1 slice

	Cal	Fat	Sfat	Sod	Carb	Fiber	Sugar	Prot
Crispy Crust Pizza	164	8	3	320	14	1	1	9

Round, 1 slice

	Cal	Fat	Sfat	Sod	Carb	Fiber	Sugar	Prot
All Meaty Pizza	275	10	4	542	29	2	2	16
BBQ Chicken Pizza	234	5	2	501	33	1	3	15
BLT Pizza	286	14	3	391	28	1	1	13
Cheese & Pepperoni Pizza	236	7	4	412	29	2	1	13
Cheese Pizza	223	6	3	347	29	2	1	13
Cheese, Pepperoni & Ham Pizza	249	8	4	523	29	2	1	15
Cheese, Pepperoni, Ham & Mushroom Pizza	226	6	3	427	29	2	1	13
Cheese, Pepperoni, Ham, Mushroom, Onion & Green Pepper Pizza	223	6	3	400	30	2	1	12
Chicken Parmesan Pizza	233	6	3	455	30	2	2	15
Grilled Chicken Pizza	222	6	3	453	31	2	3	14
Hawaiian Pizza	223	6	2	404	30	2	2	13
Jet 10 Pizza	257	9	3	503	30	2	2	14
Super Special Pizza	223	6	3	400	30	2	2	12
Veggie Pizza	214	5	2	350	31	2	3	11

Square, 1 slice

	Cal	Fat	Sfat	Sod	Carb	Fiber	Sugar	Prot
All Meaty Pizza	334	16	5	595	29	2	2	17
BBQ Chicken Pizza	281	11	3	467	33	1	3	14
BLT Pizza	326	19	4	391	28	1	1	13
Cheese & Pepperoni Pizza	288	13	5	441	29	2	2	14
Cheese Pizza	276	11	4	375	29	2	2	15
Cheese, Pepperoni & Ham Pizza	307	13	5	573	30	2	2	16
Cheese, Pepperoni, Ham & Mushroom Pizza	278	12	4	455	29	2	2	14
Cheese, Pepperoni, Ham, Mushroom, Onion & Green Pepper Pizza	275	11	4	429	30	2	2	14
Chicken Parmesan Pizza	272	10	3	455	30	2	2	15
Grilled Chicken Pizza	272	9	3	746	33	2	4	14
Hawaiian Pizza	276	11	3	433	30	2	2	14
Jet 10 Pizza	320	14	4	815	33	2	3	16
Super Special Pizza	275	11	4	429	30	2	2	14
Veggie Pizza	309	15	4	379	32	2	3	13

Description & Serving	Cal	Fat	Sfat	Sod	Carb	Fiber	Sugar	Prot
Medium Round Pizza, 1 slice								
All Meaty Pizza	276	11	4	554	28	2	2	16
BBQ Chicken Pizza	252	7	2	525	32	1	4	15
BLT Pizza	296	16	4	414	26	1	1	14
Cheese & Pepperoni Pizza	229	7	4	407	28	2	2	13
Cheese Pizza	289	8	4	459	37	2	2	17
Cheese, Pepperoni & Ham Pizza	243	8	4	523	28	2	2	15
Cheese, Pepperoni, Ham & Mushroom Pizza	228	7	3	455	28	2	2	13
Cheese, Pepperoni, Ham, Mushroom, Onion & Green Pepper Pizza	223	6	3	409	29	2	2	13
Chicken Parmesan Pizza	238	6	3	495	28	2	2	16
Grilled Chicken Pizza	227	7	4	519	30	2	3	15
Hawaiian Pizza	229	7	3	442	29	2	3	13
Jet 10 Pizza	257	9	4	523	29	2	2	15
Super Special Pizza	229	7	3	434	29	2	2	13
Veggie Pizza	215	5	2	369	30	2	3	12
Large Pizza								
8 Corner, 1 slice								
All Meaty Pizza	405	19	6	495	35	2	2	22
Grilled Chicken Pizza	368	15	5	1057	39	2	4	18
Super Special Pizza	330	13	5	514	36	2	2	16
Veggie Pizza	315	12	4	422	38	3	3	15
Crispy Crust, 1 slice								
Crispy Crust Pizza	158	8	4	394	10	1	2	10
Round, 1 slice								
All Meaty Pizza	312	12	5	631	32	2	2	19
BBQ Chicken Pizza	275	6	3	643	36	1	4	16
BLT Pizza	325	17	4	451	30	1	1	15
Cheese & Pepperoni Pizza	260	8	4	458	31	2	2	15
Cheese Pizza	248	7	3	401	32	2	2	15
Cheese, Pepperoni & Ham Pizza	276	9	4	591	32	2	2	17
Cheese, Pepperoni, Ham & Mushroom Pizza	251	7	3	491	32	2	2	15
Cheese, Pepperoni, Ham, Mushroom, Onion & Green Pepper Pizza	249	7	3	458	33	2	2	14
Chicken Parmesan Pizza	267	7	3	554	32	2	2	18
Grilled Chicken Pizza	252	8	4	581	33	2	3	16
Hawaiian Pizza	255	7	3	489	32	2	3	15
Jet 10 Pizza	292	10	4	596	33	2	2	17
Super Special Pizza	249	7	3	458	33	2	2	14
Veggie Pizza	238	6	3	407	34	2	3	13
Square, 1 slice								
All Meaty Pizza	373	18	6	662	31	2	2	20
BBQ Chicken Pizza	320	12	3	641	35	1	4	18
BLT Pizza	370	22	5	449	29	1	1	15
Cheese & Pepperoni Pizza	321	15	5	490	31	2	2	16
Cheese Pizza	303	13	5	413	31	2	2	16
Cheese, Pepperoni & Ham Pizza	337	15	6	623	31	2	2	18

Description & Serving	Cal	Fat	Sfat	Sod	Carb	Fiber	Sugar	Prot
Cheese, Pepperoni, Ham & Mushroom Pizza	311	13	5	523	31	2	2	16
Cheese, Pepperoni, Ham, Mushroom, Onion & Green Pepper Pizza	309	13	5	489	32	2	2	16
Chicken Parmesan Pizza	312	12	4	551	32	2	3	18
Grilled Chicken Pizza	297	14	5	578	33	2	3	16
Hawaiian Pizza	316	14	4	521	32	2	3	16
Jet 10 Pizza	345	16	5	613	32	2	2	17
Super Special Pizza	309	13	5	489	32	2	2	16
Veggie Pizza	304	13	4	441	34	2	3	14

Extra Large Square Pizza, 1 slice

	Cal	Fat	Sfat	Sod	Carb	Fiber	Sugar	Prot
All Meaty Pizza	369	18	6	647	31	2	2	20
BBQ Chicken Pizza	217	12	3	616	35	1	4	17
BLT Pizza	364	22	5	432	29	1	1	15
Cheese & Pepperoni Pizza	314	14	5	475	31	2	2	16
Cheese Pizza	295	12	NP	396	31	2	2	15
Cheese, Pepperoni & Ham Pizza	331	15	5	608	31	2	2	18
Cheese, Pepperoni, Ham & Mushroom Pizza	315	14	5	528	31	2	2	17
Cheese, Pepperoni, Ham, Mushroom, Onion & Green Pepper Pizza	313	13	5	493	32	2	2	16
Chicken Parmesan Pizza	306	12	4	528	31	2	3	17
Grilled Chicken Pizza	295	14	5	571	33	2	3	16
Hawaiian Pizza	317	14	4	518	32	2	3	17
Jet 10 Pizza	360	17	6	643	32	2	2	19
Super Special Pizza	364	19	5	493	32	2	2	16
Veggie Pizza	301	12	4	438	33	2	3	15

Salad, no dressing, 1 serving

	Cal	Fat	Sfat	Sod	Carb	Fiber	Sugar	Prot
Caesar Salad	110	5	2	294	11	2	3	8
Greek Salad	116	9	4	676	9	2	4	7
Garden Salad	106	6	3	230	9	3	4	5
Antipasto Salad	191	12	5	739	7	2	3	15
Chicken Caesar Salad	144	6	2	507	11	2	4	13
Additional Chicken on any Salad	34	1	0	213	0	0	1	6

Sandwich

	Cal	Fat	Sfat	Sod	Carb	Fiber	Sugar	Prot
Bold Fold	354	13	6	698	38	2	3	21
Italian Sub w/ Dressing	868	54	15	2475	56	1	3	41
Italian Sub w/o Dressing	632	28	12	2105	56	1	3	41
Tuna Sub w/o Dressing	1443	106	21	2088	55	1	4	81
Steak & Cheese Sub w/ Dressing	776	45	12	1586	56	1	5	39
Steak & Cheese Sub w/o Dressing	541	19	9	1216	55	1	5	39
Ham & Cheese Sub w/ Dressing	835	48	13	2596	57	1	3	46
Ham & Cheese Sub w/o Dressing	599	21	10	2225	56	1	3	46
Veggie Sub w/ Dressing	743	45	11	1460	66	4	8	25
Veggie Sub w/o Dressing	508	18	8	1089	66	4	8	25
Grilled Chicken Sub w/ Dressing	837	47	11	2267	55	1	6	50
Grilled Chicken Sub w/o Dressing	601	20	7	1896	54	1	6	50
Meatball Sub	832	40	17	2020	75	6	13	46
Chicken Parmesan Sub	696	18	7	2243	73	6	16	57

Description & Serving	Cal	Fat	Sfat	Sod	Carb	Fiber	Sugar	Prot
Pizza Sub	713	25	11	2004	78	7	15	44
Steak & Cheese Deli Boat	1235	30	13	2013	164	7	6	78
Italian Deli Boat	1430	48	20	3750	164	7	4	83
Tuna Deli Boat	2670	161	32	3544	163	7	5	159
Ham & Cheese Deli Boat	1570	44	20	4187	167	7	9	119
Veggie Deli Boat	1166	30	12	1833	176	11	9	53
Classic Chicken Deli Boat	1257	30	11	2651	161	7	7	82
Jet Boat	1284	35	16	2116	173	9	9	68
Meatball Boat	1567	60	25	2792	175	9	9	85
Chicken Parmesan Boat	1387	32	13	3017	173	9	12	98

Side

	Cal	Fat	Sfat	Sod	Carb	Fiber	Sugar	Prot
Wings, 1 lb	979	67	21	1907	0	0	0	93
Breaded, Skinless Chicken, 3	160	6	1	520	10	1	0	15
Jet Bread	167	6	2	259	20	1	0	8
Triple Cheese Turbo Stix	129	6	2	177	14	0	0	6
Cinnamon Stix	195	6	1	146	31	1	8	5

Dressing/Condiment/Topping

	Cal	Fat	Sfat	Sod	Carb	Fiber	Sugar	Prot
BBQ Sauce, 113 g	245	0	0	797	61	0	31	0
Italian Dressing, 111 g	461	52	7	725	1	0	0	0
Greek Dressing, 113 g	454	45	8	265	11	0	8	0
Ranch Dressing, 110 g	395	41	6	869	3	0	3	9
Creamy Caesar Dressing, 43 g	210	23	4	420	2	0	2	1
Pizza Sauce, 113 g	66	0	0	255	13	4	8	2

Jimmy John's

Sandwich

	Cal	Fat	Sfat	Sod	Carb	Fiber	Sugar	Prot
#1 Pepe 8" Sub	617.3	30.77	8.03	1262.28	50.12	0.89	NP	27.87
#2 Big John 8" Sub	533.3	23.97	4	1014.28	48.57	0.89	NP	25.97
#3 Totally Tuna 8" Sub	648.35	30.83	4	1592.07	54.13	2.82	NP	32.89
#4 Turkey Tom 8" Sub	514.9	21.83	3	1094.23	50.27	1.28	NP	24.4
#5 Vito 8" Sub	600.14	28.37	8.8	1376.82	51.7	1.21	NP	29.98
#6 Vegetarian 8" Sub	578.35	30.11	7.63	873.07	52.53	1.62	NP	19.29
J.J.B.L.T. 8" Sub	634.3	35.17	9	1329.28	48.57	0.89	NP	25.37
#7 Gourmet Smoked Ham Club	775.3	32.37	8.6	1877.28	68.77	0.89	NP	41.47
#8 Billy Club	799.5	34.07	9.03	1958.28	68.22	1.09	NP	47
#9 Italian Night Club	951.14	50.97	12.33	2165.82	70.35	1.21	NP	43.58
#10 Hunter's Club	807.3	34.77	9.5	1781.28	66.67	0.89	NP	51.67
#11 Country Club	768.3	31.33	8.03	1908.28	68.82	0.89	NP	44.37
#12 Beach Club	729.35	30.67	7.63	1519.07	71.23	1.62	NP	25.79
#13 Gourmet Veggie Club	773.35	38.11	12.13	1235.07	70.63	1.62	NP	30.39
#14 Bootlegger Club	684.3	24.53	4	1660.28	67.27	0.89	NP	42.47
#15 Club Tuna	843.35	38.83	8.5	1954.07	72.23	2.82	NP	43.99
#16 Club Lulu	755.3	33.33	8	1855.28	67.27	0.89	NP	39.57
#17 Ultimate Porker	763.3	39.27	8.53	1751.28	67.22	5.89	NP	36.87
Slim 1 Ham & Cheese	508	9.6	5.03	1244	65.55	0	NP	31.3
Slim 2 Roast Beef	424	2.8	1	996	64	0	NP	29.4

Description & Serving	Cal	Fat	Sfat	Sod	Carb	Fiber	Sugar	Prot
Slim 3 Tuna Salad	722	30.5	4	1746	67.8	1.2	NP	35.4
Slim 4 Turkey Breast	401	0.56	0	1075	65.1	0	NP	27.2
Slim 5 Salami, Capicola, Cheese	599	19.8	8.8	1450	65.58	0	NP	33.2
Slim 6 Double Provolone	545	16	9	991	65	0	NP	28.8
The J.J. Gargantuan Sub	984.3	54.33	13.33	2892.28	52.3	0.89	NP	66.27

Lettuce Wrap

	Cal	Fat	Sfat	Sod	Carb	Fiber	Sugar	Prot
Hunter's Club Unwich	470.1	34.88	9.5	1195.68	3.92	1.73	NP	37.47
The J.J. Gargantuan Unwich	742.1	54.44	13.33	2468.68	7.15	1.73	NP	56.17

Side

	Cal	Fat	Sfat	Sod	Carb	Fiber	Sugar	Prot
Regular Chips	160	8	2	80	18	0	NP	2
BBQ Jimmy Chips	160	9	2	90	17	0	NP	2
Jalapeno Chips	150	7	1.5	290	18	0.5	NP	2
Sea Salt & Vinegar Chips	140	8	1.5	280	16	0	NP	2
Skinny Chips	130	5	1	105	19	2	NP	2
Pickle, Spear	5.5	0	0	579	1.1	1.1	NP	0.3
Pickle, Whole	22	0	0	2314	4.4	4.4	NP	1.1

Dessert

	Cal	Fat	Sfat	Sod	Carb	Fiber	Sugar	Prot
Chocolate Chunk Cookie	420.73	17.76	10.6	427.07	62.35	1.37	NP	5.14
Raisin Oatmeal Cookie	420.85	15.77	8.71	470.86	65.05	3.94	NP	6.99

Johnny Rockets

Breakfast

	Cal	Fat	Sfat	Sod	Carb	Fiber	Sugar	Prot
Pancakes, 1	130	1.5	0	350	26	NP	NP	NP
French Toast, 1 slice	150	3.5	1	260	23	NP	NP	NP
Plain Omlette	220	17	5	250	<1	NP	NP	NP
Breakfast Sausage, 2 links	180	16	6	300	<1	NP	NP	NP
Bacon, 4 slices	180	14	5	840	1	NP	NP	NP
Diced Ham, 1 oz	50	2.5	0.5	330	<1	NP	NP	NP
Country Potatoes	380	17	2	600	50	NP	NP	NP
Eggs - Scrambled, 1	90	6	2	90	1	NP	NP	NP
Eggs - Over Easy, 1	90	7	2	85	0	NP	NP	NP
Eggs - Over Hard, 1	90	6	2	95	2	NP	NP	NP
Eggs - Sunny Side Up, 1	90	7	2	85	1	NP	NP	NP

Appetizer

	Cal	Fat	Sfat	Sod	Carb	Fiber	Sugar	Prot
Onion Rings	790	36	6	2010	80	NP	NP	NP
Half Rings & Half Fries	680	31	5	1080	88	NP	NP	NP
American Fries	550	22	4	50	78	NP	NP	NP
Cheese Fries	780	44	17	460	72	NP	NP	NP
Chili Bowl	872	73	17	1629	24	NP	NP	NP
Chili Fries	1010	62	21	1020	85	NP	NP	NP
Rocket Wings	640	36	7	2600	26	NP	NP	NP
Side Salad	100	5	3	105	7	NP	NP	NP
Side Caesar Salad	189	16	3	388	9	NP	NP	NP
Sliders (traditional), 3	750	42	12	1170	63	NP	NP	NP

Description & Serving	Cal	Fat	Sfat	Sod	Carb	Fiber	Sugar	Prot
Mini Hot Dogs, 3	690	36	14	2040	66	NP	NP	NP
Mini Chili Dogs, 3	1470	105	48	3600	78	NP	NP	NP

Salad

Chicken Club Salad w/ grilled breast	480	26	14	1260	8	NP	NP	NP
Chicken Club Salad w/ chicken tenders	620	37	15	1740	27	NP	NP	NP
Grilled Chicken Caesar Salad	343	31	5	687	13	NP	NP	NP
Caesar Salad	481	35	6	1052	15	NP	NP	NP
Garden Salad	240	14	8	360	12	NP	NP	NP
Scoop Egg Salad	470	42	8	550	2	NP	NP	NP
Scoop Tuna Salad	420	31	6	570	0	NP	NP	NP

Burger/Hot Dog

The Original Hamburger	820	53	14	1270	52	NP	NP	NP
#12 Hamburger	900	59	18	1370	55	NP	NP	NP
Patty Melt	690	37	17	1090	49	NP	NP	NP
St. Louis Hamburger	991	56	20	1491	53	NP	NP	NP
Route 66 Hamburger	920	60	18	1010	55	NP	NP	NP
Bacon Cheddar Single Burger	860	53	18	1220	42	NP	NP	NP
Bacon Cheddar Double Burger	1400	92	37	1850	57	NP	NP	NP
Rocket Single Burger	710	44	15	770	45	NP	NP	NP
Rocket Double Burger	1020	63	25	1020	52	NP	NP	NP
Streamliner Hamburger	410	8	2	1120	57	NP	NP	NP
Chili Cheese Hamburger	850	50	21	1090	53	NP	NP	NP
Smoke House Single Burger	950	55	19	1720	68	NP	NP	NP
Smoke House Double Burger	1359	80	28	2511	99	NP	NP	NP
Hot Dog	370	20	8	1220	34	NP	NP	NP
Chili Dog	810	55	25	1960	48	NP	NP	NP

Sandwich/Chicken Tenders

Grilled Chicken Breast	560	25	5	1080	47	NP	NP	NP
Chicken Club Sandwich	930	51	10	1860	58	NP	NP	NP
Tuna Melt	900	62	17	1448	40	NP	NP	NP
Tuna Salad Sandwich	800	50	8	1010	41	NP	NP	NP
Philly Cheese Steak	715	46	21	1085	58	NP	NP	NP
Egg Salad Sandwich	870	64	12	1100	46	NP	NP	NP
Grilled Cheese	540	29	14	1600	48	NP	NP	NP
Bacon, Lettuce & Tomato	510	31	7	1040	40	NP	NP	NP
Chicken Tenders	610	33	5	2300	39	NP	NP	NP

Kids

Hamburger	370	19	7	430	32	NP	NP	NP
Mini Hamburgers, 2	400	17	6	570	40	NP	NP	NP
Peanut Butter & Jelly	490	19	4	540	66	NP	NP	NP
Hot Dog	450	26	10	1280	39	NP	NP	NP
Mini Hot Dogs, 2	460	24	9	1360	44	NP	NP	NP
Grilled Cheese	440	20	10	1230	48	NP	NP	NP
Chicken Tenders	350	17	3	1360	24	NP	NP	NP
Iced Tea, 12 oz	3	0	0	6	0	NP	NP	NP
Lemonade, 12 oz	102	0	0	84	29	NP	NP	NP

Description & Serving	Cal	Fat	Sfat	Sod	Carb	Fiber	Sugar	Prot
Vanilla Shake, 12 oz	620	32	19	160	74	NP	NP	NP
Chocolate Shake, 12 oz	660	37	22	135	72	NP	NP	NP
Strawberry Shake, 12 oz	600	35	21	160	62	NP	NP	NP

Dressing/Condiment

Ancho Chipotle, 0.75 oz	80	6	3	214	5	NP	NP	NP
Dijonnaise, 1 oz	150	16	2	240	1	NP	NP	NP
Gourmet Blue Cheese, 0.75 oz	150	16	3	230	1	NP	NP	NP
Pepper Relish Mayo, 1.5 oz	187	18	3	217	7	NP	NP	NP

Substitution/Topping

Boca Patty, 1	100	2	0	450	8	NP	NP	NP
Turkey Patty, 1	170	10	3	120	0	NP	NP	NP
Wheat Bun, 1	250	4	1	370	48	NP	NP	NP
Grilled Onions, 1 oz	48	6	1	0	3	NP	NP	NP
Cheddar Cheese, 1 slice	90	7	5	125	0	NP	NP	NP
American Cheese, 1 slice	70	6	4	310	0	NP	NP	NP
Swiss Cheese, 1 slice	62	5	3	35	0	NP	NP	NP
Pepper Jack Cheese, 1 slice	80	6	4	130	1	NP	NP	NP
Chili, 3 oz	155	12	5	313	5	NP	NP	NP
Grilled Mushrooms, 1 oz	33	3	1	0	1	NP	NP	NP
Grilled Peppers & Onions, 1 oz	20	1	0	10	3	NP	NP	NP

Dessert

Chocolate Original Shake, 16 oz	890	44	27	160	102	NP	NP	NP
Strawberry Original Shake, 16 oz	750	44	27	130	77	NP	NP	NP
Vanilla Original Shake, 16 oz	840	44	26	160	100	NP	NP	NP
Oreo Cookies & Cream Deluxe Shake, 16 oz	820	50	29	280	79	NP	NP	NP
Butterfinger Deluxe Shake, 16 oz	1020	65	31	310	85	NP	NP	NP
Strawberry-Banana Deluxe Shake, 16 oz	970	54	31	220	106	NP	NP	NP
Mocha Fudge Deluxe Shake, 16 oz	810	47	29	110	82	NP	NP	NP
Chocolate Peanut Butter Deluxe Shake, 16 oz	890	50	31	190	96	NP	NP	NP
Big Apple Deluxe Shake, 16 oz	890	54	30	350	89	NP	NP	NP
Super Sundae	1110	74	46	266	120	NP	NP	NP
Apple Pie	800	33	14	640	119	NP	NP	NP
a la mode	250	16	10	40	25	NP	NP	NP
Single Scoop	410	26	16	65	40	NP	NP	NP
The Perfect Brownie	750	42	10	220	94	NP	NP	NP
The Perfect Brownie Sundae	1464	91	39	382	176	NP	NP	NP

Beverage/Add-On

Iced Tea, 20 oz	5	0	0	10	0	NP	NP	NP
Lemonade, 20 oz	170	0	0	140	49	NP	NP	NP
Coffee, 12 oz	10	0	0	10	2	NP	NP	NP
Hot Tea, 12 oz	0	0	0	0	0	NP	NP	NP
Hot Chocolate, 12 oz	140	5	3	210	25	NP	NP	NP
Cherry Flavor Shot	22	0	0	0	2	NP	NP	NP
Chocolate Flavor Shot	60	0	0	10	13	NP	NP	NP
Vanilla Flavor Shot	21	0	0	0	5	NP	NP	NP
Lemon Flavor Shot	0	0	0	0	1	NP	NP	NP

Description & Serving	Cal	Fat	Sfat	Sod	Carb	Fiber	Sugar	Prot
Kentucky Fried Chicken								
Sandwich/Wrap								
KFC Snacker w/ Oven Roasted Strip	270	12	3	560	28	2	5	15
KFC Snacker w/ Oven Roasted Strip & w/o Sauce	230	7	2	500	27	2	4	15
KFC Snacker w/ Crispy Strip	300	14	3	470	28	2	4	15
KFC Snacker w/ Crispy Strip & w/o Sauce	250	9	2.5	410	27	2	4	15
KFC Snacker w/ Oven Roasted Strip, Buffalo	240	7	2	670	29	2	4	15
KFC Snacker w/ Crispy Strip, Buffalo	260	9	2.5	580	30	2	4	15
KFC Snacker, Fish	320	14	3	640	31	2	5	16
KFC Snacker, Fish w/o Sauce	290	12	2.5	550	29	1	4	16
KFC Snacker, w/ Oven Roasted Strip, Ultimate Cheese	260	9	3	650	29	2	5	15
KFC Snacker w/ Crispy Strip, Ultimate Cheese	280	11	3	560	29	2	4	16
KFC Snacker, Honey BBQ	210	3	1	470	32	2	12	13
Honey BBQ Sandwich	310	4	1	810	42	1	19	23
Double Crunch Sandwich w/ Oven Roasted Strip	470	23	6	1020	35	2	6	27
Double Crunch Sandwich w/ Oven Roasted Strip & w/o Sauce	360	12	4	870	33	2	4	27
Double Crunch Sandwich w/ Crispy Strip	510	27	6	840	36	1	5	27
Double Crunch Sandwich w/ Crispy Strip & w/o Sauce	410	16	4.5	690	34	1	4	27
Crispy Twister w/ Oven Roasted Strip	540	26	7	1430	48	4	6	28
Crispy Twister w/ Oven Roasted Strip & w/o Sauce	440	15	5	1280	47	3	4	28
Crispy Twister w/ Crispy Strip	580	30	7	1250	49	3	5	28
Crispy Twister w/ Crispy Strip & w/o Sauce	480	20	6	1100	48	2	4	28
Tender Roast Twister	440	18	4	1120	42	2	5	29
Tender Roast Twister w/o Sauce	340	7	2.5	980	41	2	4	29
Tender Roast Sandwich	400	15	3	810	29	1	6	34
Tender Roast Sandwich w/o Sauce	300	4	1.5	660	28	0	4	34
Oven Roasted Filet Sandwich	480	23	4	1230	38	2	6	25
Oven Roasted Filet Sandwich w/o Sauce	370	12	2.5	1080	36	2	5	25
Toasted Wrap w/ Oven Roasted Strip	340	18	6	820	27	2	3	17
Toasted Wrap w/ Oven Roasted Strip & w/o Sauce	270	11	5	730	26	2	2	17
Toasted Wrap w/ Crispy Strip	360	20	6	730	27	2	2	17
Toasted Wrap w/ Crispy Strip & w/o Sauce	300	14	5	640	27	1	1	17
Toasted Wrap w/ Tender Roast Filet	310	14	5	740	24	1	2	22
Toasted Wrap w/ Tender Roast Filet & w/o Sauce	250	8	3.5	650	24	1	2	22
Chicken								
Pieces								
Oven Roasted Chicken - Whole Wing	110	7	1.5	310	3	0	0	9
Oven Roasted Chicken - Breast	370	21	5	1050	7	0	0	38
Oven Roasted Chicken - Breast w/o skin or breading	140	2	0	510	1	0	0	29
Oven Roasted Chicken - Drumstick	110	7	1.5	290	2	0	0	10
Oven Roasted Chicken - Thigh	260	19	5	670	6	0	0	16
Extra Crispy Chicken - Whole Wing	150	10	2	320	6	1	0	11
Extra Crispy Chicken - Breast	490	31	7	1080	17	0	0	38
Extra Crispy Chicken - Drumstick	150	9	2	360	6	0	0	11

Description & Serving	Cal	Fat	Sfat	Sod	Carb	Fiber	Sugar	Prot
Extra Crispy Chicken - Thigh	370	27	6	840	12	0	0	18
Hot & Spicy Chicken - Whole Wing	160	8	2.5	460	10	1	0	12
Hot & Spicy Chicken - Breast	470	28	6	1310	15	4	0	38
Hot & Spicy Chicken - Drumstick	160	10	2	400	5	1	0	12
Hot & Spicy Chicken - Thigh	380	28	6	810	11	2	1	22
Grilled Chicken - Whole Wing	80	4	1	160	0	0	0	10
Grilled Chicken - Breast	180	4	1	440	0	0	0	35
Grilled Chicken - Drumstick	70	4	1	200	0	0	0	10
Grilled Chicken - Thigh	140	9	2.5	320	0	0	0	15
Strips & Popcorn								
Oven Roasted Chicken Strips, 2	200	10	3.5	660	7	1	1	31
Crispy Chicken Strips, 2	250	15	4	480	8	1	0	22
Popcorn Chicken, Kids	290	19	3.5	850	16	2	0	16
Popcorn Chicken, Individual	400	26	4.5	1160	22	3	0	21
Popcorn Chicken, lrg	550	35	6	1600	30	3	0	29
Popcorn Chicken Snack Box	660	38	7	1900	55	5	0	25
Wings								
Hot Wings Snack Box	470	27	6	1190	41	4	0	16
Fiery Buffalo Hot Wings Snack Box	500	27	6	1580	46	4	0	16
HBBQ Hot Wings Snack Box	520	27	6	1530	53	4	7	16
Boneless HBBQ Wings, 1	80	3.5	0.5	340	7	1	2	5
Boneless Fiery Buffalo Wings, 1	80	3.5	0.5	390	6	1	0	5
HBBQ Wings, 1	80	5	1	170	5	1	2	4
Fiery Buffalo Wings, 1	80	5	1	230	4	1	0	4
Hot Wings, 1	70	5	1	150	3	0	0	4
HBBQ Hot Wings, 1	90	5	1	260	7	0	2	4
Fiery Buffalo Hot Wings, 1	80	5	1	280	5	1	0	4
Other Chicken Entrées								
Chicken Pot Pie	690	40	31	1760	57	3	14	27
KFC Kentucky Nuggets, 1	45	3	0.5	135	2	0	0	3
KFC Gizzards	200	11	2	800	15	1	0	11
KFC Livers	180	10	2	620	11	0	0	11
Country Fried Steak w/o Gravy	360	24	8	1040	19	2	0	16
Country Fried Steak w/ Gravy	390	26	8	1200	23	2	0	16
Side								
KFC Famous Bowls - Rice & Gravy	790	28	7	2690	106	5	4	29
KFC Famous Bowls - Mashed Potato w/ Gravy	700	32	8	2260	77	6	3	26
Snack Bowl	320	15	4.5	990	34	3	1	12
Green Beans	25	0	0	380	5	2	1	1
Seasoned Rice	140	0.5	0	560	31	1	1	3
Mashed Potatoes w/ Gravy	130	4.5	1	550	20	1	0	2
Mashed Potatoes w/o Gravy	100	3	0.5	350	16	1	0	2
Macaroni & Cheese	180	9	3	880	20	2	4	6
Potato Wedges	260	13	2.5	740	33	3	0	4
Corn on the Cob, 3"	70	0.5	0	0	16	2	3	2
Corn on the Cob, 5.5"	140	1	0	5	33	4	5	5
BBQ Baked Beans	200	1.5	0	680	39	9	18	8

Description & Serving	Cal	Fat	Sfat	Sod	Carb	Fiber	Sugar	Prot
Potato Salad	200	10	2	540	24	3	5	2
Cole Slaw	180	10	1.5	270	22	3	18	1
Biscuit	180	8	6	530	23	1	2	4
Sweet Kernel Corn	110	0.5	0	0	23	2	4	4
KFC Mean Greens	30	0	0	400	4	2	1	3
Macaroni Salad	180	9	2	400	20	1	6	3
Three Bean Salad	70	0	0	170	14	3	7	3
KFC Red Beans w/ Sausage & Rice	160	2.5	0.5	340	26	4	0	24
KFC Cornbread Muffin	210	9	1.5	240	28	1	11	3
Chicken Little	190	10	2	390	20	1	3	6
Jalapeno Peppers, 1	20	1.5	0	480	1	1	0	0

Salad, w/o dressing

Description & Serving	Cal	Fat	Sfat	Sod	Carb	Fiber	Sugar	Prot
Roasted Chicken Caesar Salad	190	6	3	530	5	2	3	29
Oven Roasted Chicken Caesar Salad	280	14	6	840	11	4	3	28
Crispy Chicken Caesar Salad	320	19	6	660	12	3	3	28
Caesar Side Salad	35	2	1	90	2	1	1	3
Roasted Chicken BLT Salad	200	7	2	720	7	3	5	30
Oven Roasted Chicken BLT Salad	300	15	5	1020	13	4	5	29
Crispy Chicken BLT Salad	340	19	5	840	14	3	4	30
House Side Salad	15	0	0	10	2	1	2	1

Dressing/Condiment

Description & Serving	Cal	Fat	Sfat	Sod	Carb	Fiber	Sugar	Prot
Fiery Buffalo Dipping Sauce	25	0	0	530	6	0	1	0
Garlic Parmesan Dipping Sauce	130	13	2.5	220	2	0	1	0
Sweet & Sour Dipping Sauce	45	0	0	95	12	0	10	0
Honey Mustard Dipping Sauce	120	10	1.5	110	6	0	5	0
Creamy Ranch Dipping Sauce	140	15	2.5	230	1	0	1	0
HBBQ Dipping Sauce	40	0	0	310	9	0	8	0
Heinz Buttermilk Ranch Dressing	160	17	2	220	1	0	1	0
Hidden Valley The Original Ranch Fat Free Dressing	35	0	0	410	8	0	2	1
Marzetti Light Italian Dressing	10	0.5	0	510	2	0	1	0
KFC Creamy Parmesan Caesar Dressing	260	26	5	540	4	0	2	2
Parmesan Garlic Croutons Pouch	70	3	0	140	8	1	1	2

Dessert

Description & Serving	Cal	Fat	Sfat	Sod	Carb	Fiber	Sugar	Prot
Apple Turnover	260	13	3	170	35	1	14	2
Café Valley Bakery Chocolate Chip Cake	280	9	3.5	160	47	1	21	3
Lil' Bucket Lemon Crème Parfait Cup	390	14	8	220	60	0	47	7
Lil' Bucket Chocolate Crème Parfait Cup	280	14	9	220	37	1	22	2
Lil' Bucket Strawberry Shortcake Parfait Cup	230	8	4	220	39	1	20	2
Strawberry Cream Cheese Pie Slice	270	15	10	220	31	0	22	3
Pecan Pie Slice	410	21	6	220	52	1	22	4
Lemon Meringue Pie Slice	250	7	3.5	210	42	0	33	4
Dutch Apple Pie Slice	320	14	6	300	47	1	24	2
Cookie Dough Pie Slice	240	12	7	190	31	1	21	3
Sara Lee Sweet Potato Pie Slice	340	16	7	330	46	0	25	5
Sara Lee Apple Pie Slice	310	13	5	290	48	1	24	2
Sara Lee Pecan Pie Slice	450	22	8	460	61	1	22	5
Sweet Life Sugar Cookie	160	7	3	125	22	0	11	2
Sweet Life Oatmeal Raisin Cookie	150	6	2.5	130	23	1	13	2
Sweet Life Chocolate Chip Cookie	170	8	4	90	23	1	15	2

Description & Serving	Cal	Fat	Sfat	Sod	Carb	Fiber	Sugar	Prot
Krispy Kreme								
Doughnut								
Original Glazed	200	12	5	95	22	<1	11	2
Chocolate Iced Glazed	250	12	5	100	33	<1	21	3
Chocolate Iced Glazed w/ Sprinkles	270	12	5	100	38	<1	24	3
Chocolate Iced Kreme Filled	350	20	10	140	39	<1	23	3
Chocolate Iced Custard Filled	300	17	8	150	35	<1	19	3
Glazed Lemon Filled	290	16	8	135	35	<1	17	3
Powdered Strawberry Filled	290	16	8	135	33	<1	13	3
Powdered Cake	290	14	6	320	37	<1	19	3
Glazed Raspberry Filled	300	16	8	125	36	<1	20	3
Cinnamon Apple Filled	290	16	8	150	32	<1	14	3
New York Cheesecake	340	20	10	200	34	<1	17	4
Caramel Kreme Crunch	380	19	9	170	49	<1	30	4
Glazed Chocolate Cake	260	13	6	320	33	2	18	3
Traditional Cake	230	13	6	315	25	<1	9	3
Glazed Kreme Filled	340	20	10	140	39	<1	23	3
Glazed Cinnamon	210	12	6	100	24	<1	12	2
Cinnamon Bun	260	16	8	125	28	<1	13	3
Cinnamon Twist	240	15	7	130	23	<1	7	3
Maple Iced Glazed	240	12	6	100	32	<1	20	2
Glazed Sour Cream	300	13	7	250	43	<1	28	2
Sugar	200	12	6	90	21	0	10	2
Chocolate Iced Cake	280	14	6	320	36	<1	20	3
Chocolate Glazed Cruller	290	15	7	240	37	<1	25	2
Glazed Pumpkin Spice Cake	300	14	7	250	42	<1	27	2
Dulche De Leche	300	18	9	160	31	<1	14	3
Apple Fritter	380	20	10	220	47	2	24	4
Original Glazed Doughnut Holes, 4	200	11	5	90	25	<1	15	2
Glazed Blueberry Doughnut Holes, 4	220	12	5	280	27	<1	9	3
Glazed Cake Doughnut Holes, 4	210	10	4	240	29	<1	17	2
Glazed Chocolate Cake Doughnut Holes, 4	210	10	4	240	29	<1	17	2
Glazed Pumpkin Spice Doughnut Holes, 4	210	11	4	230	28	<1	17	2
Beverage								
Very Berry Chiller, 12 oz	170	0	0	10	43	0	43	0
Orange You Glad Chiller, 12 oz	180	0	0	10	43	0	43	0
Berries & Kreme Chiller, 12 oz	620	28	24	220	92	<1	71	3
Oranges & Kreme Chiller, 12 oz	630	28	24	220	92	<1	71	3
Lemon Sherbert Chiller, 12 oz	630	28	24	220	95	<1	71	3
Mocha Dream Chiller, 12 oz	670	28	24	320	105	1	58	3
Lotta Latte Chiller, 12 oz	670	28	24	380	49	<1	60	4
Chocolate, Chocolate Chiller, 12 oz	670	29	24	320	104	2	62	4
Krystal								
Breakfast								
4Carb Scrambler (Bacon)	370	29	10	830	4	1	0	24
4Carb Scrambler (Sausage)	600	51	18	1040	3	2	1	32

Description & Serving	Cal	Fat	Sfat	Sod	Carb	Fiber	Sugar	Prot
Scrambler	440	26	11	840	33	3	<1	20
Country Breakfast	660	42	14	1450	46	8	3	24
Kryspers	190	13	5	340	17	2	0	1
Chik Biscuit	360	15	3	1030	40	0	2	13
Biscuit & Gravy	280	14	3	710	34	0	2	5
Bacon Egg Cheese Biscuit	390	23	7	1090	33	0	2	11
Sausage Biscuit	480	33	10	980	33	0	2	12
Plain Biscuit	270	13	3	660	33	0	2	5
Krystal Sunriser	240	14	5	460	14	2	1	12

Buger/Sandwich/Hot Dog

	Cal	Fat	Sfat	Sod	Carb	Fiber	Sugar	Prot
Krystal Burger	160	7	3	260	17	1	1	7
Cheese Krystal Burger	180	9	4	430	17	2	1	9
Bacon Cheese Krystal Burger	190	10	4.5	430	16	2	2	10
DBL Cheese Krystal Burger	310	16	7	800	26	<1	2	16
Double Krystal Burger	260	13	6	550	24	2	2	13
BA Burger	470	27	8	760	39	2	6	22
BA Burger w/ Cheese	530	32	11	1020	40	2	6	25
BA Double Bacon Cheese	800	53	20	1600	41	2	6	44
Krystal Chik	240	11	3.5	640	24	2	1	11
Corn Pup	260	19	8	480	19	1	5	5
Chili Cheese Pup	210	12	5	510	17	2	2	9
Plain Pup	170	9	3.5	500	15	1	NP	6

Side

	Cal	Fat	Sfat	Sod	Carb	Fiber	Sugar	Prot
Krystal Chili	200	7	3.5	1130	22	7	2	13
Chili Cheese Fries	540	28	13	800	59	6	1	13
Regular Fries	470	20	8	90	53	7	0	4
Chik'n Bites	310	19	8	790	16	1	0	17
Chik'n Bites Salad	290	20	11	490	12	4	1	20

Dessert/Beverage

	Cal	Fat	Sfat	Sod	Carb	Fiber	Sugar	Prot
Lemon Icebox Pie	260	9	2	180	41	2	37	5
Fried Apple Turnover	220	10	3.5	300	31	2	7	3
Green Apple Freeze	230	0	0	10	57	0	57	0
Blueberry Freeze	230	0	0	10	58	0	58	0
Cherry Freeze	230	0	0	10	58	0	58	0
Orange Freeze	220	0	0	10	54	0	54	0
Pomegranate Freeze	230	0	0	10	57	0	56	0
Grape Freeze	230	0	0	10	57	0	57	0

Little Caesars

Pizza

Slice (1/8 of pizza)

	Cal	Fat	Sfat	Sod	Carb	Fiber	Sugar	Prot
14" Round Hot-N-Ready Just Cheese Pizza	240	9	4.5	410	30	1	3	12
14" Round Hot-N-Ready Pepperoni Pizza	280	11	5	520	30	1	3	14
Deep Dish Pepperoni Pizza	360	16	6	610	38	1	4	16
Deep Dish Just Cheese Pizza	320	13	5	490	38	1	3	14
Ultimate Supreme Pizza	310	14	6	640	31	2	3	15

Description & Serving	Cal	Fat	Sfat	Sod	Carb	Fiber	Sugar	Prot
3 Meat Treat Pizza	350	18	8	730	30	1	3	17
Hula Hawaiian Pineapple & Ham Pizza	270	9	4.5	600	33	1	6	15
Hula Hawaiian Pineapple & Canadian Bacon Pizza	280	9	4.5	640	34	1	6	15
Vegetarian Pizza	270	10	4.5	530	32	2	4	13
Pan, 1 slice								
Baby Pan!Pan! Cheese & Pepperoni Pizza	360	18	7	610	33	1	3	16
Baby Pan!Pan! Just Cheese Pizza	320	15	6	500	33	1	3	14
Chicken								
Oven Roasted Caesar Wings, 1	50	3.5	1	150	0	0	0	4
Mild Caesar Wings, 1	60	4	1	290	1	0	0	4
Hot Caesar Wings, 1	60	4.5	1	430	1	0	0	4
Barbecue Caesar Wings, 1	70	4	1	220	3	0	2	4
Side								
Crazy Bread, 1 stick	100	3	0.5	150	15	1	1	3
Little Caesars Italian Cheese Bread, 1 pc	130	7	2.5	230	13	0	1	6
Little Caesars Pepperoni Cheese Bread, 1 pc	150	8	3	280	13	0	1	7
Churros	150	4	0.5	95	25	1	10	2
Condiment								
Crazy Sauce	45	0	0	260	10	1	8	2
Dulce De Leche Churro Sauce	90	2.5	0.5	90	16	0	13	0
Chocolate Churro Sauce	90	3	1	60	16	0	13	0
Cheezy Dip	210	21	4	450	3	0	2	1
Ranch Dip	250	26	4	380	3	0	2	0
Buffalo Ranch Dip	230	24	3.5	520	3	0	2	0
Chipotle Dip	220	24	3.5	560	2	0	0	0
Buttery Garlic Dip	380	42	9	420	0	0	0	0
Buffalo Dip	140	14	2	940	4	0	2	0

Lone Star Steakhouse

Appetizer								
Amarillo Cheese Fries	2640.71	NP	38.29	16887.52	356.01	15.3	NP	68.77
Bavarian Loaf	150	NP	0.91	264	28.5	1.8	NP	NP
Chicken Tenders	1093.82	NP	12.12	1769.76	91	7.06	NP	35.33
Chicken Tenders, buffalo style	1197.43	NP	15.6	4172.17	92.32	6.95	NP	37.18
Lone Star Skins	1310.52	NP	21.75	1542.12	134.38	8.41	NP	53.23
Lone Star Wings, mild	953.65	NP	8.19	841.56	15.25	2.77	NP	83.35
Spinach Artichoke Dip	491.49	NP	24.12	1534.83	13.98	3.25	NP	18.53
Texas Rose	1258.28	NP	36.98	2704.19	108.39	6.62	NP	19.51
Yeast Rolls	366.33	NP	5.6	NP	72.49	2.31	NP	10.13
Salad								
Caesar Salad w/ Grilled Chicken	479.25	NP	5.21	2876.93	19.34	5.22	NP	46.18
Chicken Caesar Salad	479.25	NP	5.21	2876.93	19.34	5.22	NP	46.18
Classic Dinner Salad	130.63	NP	9.88	381.9	15.59	3.35	NP	12.96
Cobb Salad	684.65	NP	12.96	3357.3	22.68	5.84	NP	67.02
Dinner Caesar Salad	142.54	NP	2.42	344.62	8.32	3.04	NP	4.08
Dinner Salad	130.63	NP	9.88	381.9	15.59	3.35	NP	12.96

Description & Serving	Cal	Fat	Sfat	Sod	Carb	Fiber	Sugar	Prot
El Paso Salad	351.12	NP	11.38	1087.45	25.1	6.88	NP	23.99
Side Caesar Salad	142.54	NP	2.42	344.62	8.32	3.04	NP	4.08
Signature Lettuce Wedge	396.57	NP	14.38	818.4	9.81	0.35	NP	13.7
Steakhouse Salad	708.19	NP	22.41	1328.28	1.74	5.64	NP	55.76
Soup/Chili								
Chicken Pot Pie Soup, cup (4 oz)	18.97	NP	0.45	289.51	4.68	0.59	NP	3.44
Steak Soup, cup (4 oz)	26.17	NP	0.94	112.41	4.36	0.44	NP	9.59
Chili, cup (4 oz)	138.04	NP	2.63	350.63	5.39	1.53	NP	12.2
Burger/Sandwich								
Alamo Burger	937.17	NP	12.01	1807.07	77.69	2.94	NP	54.61
Bacon Bleu Burger	821.14	NP	16.52	1641.32	50.6	3.33	NP	67.78
Bubba Burger	1086.67	NP	22.99	4268.22	66.93	3.35	NP	72.61
Cajun Burger	695.65	NP	10.19	1769.41	48.06	2.55	NP	60.26
Lone Star Burger	639.96	NP	10.19	1169.12	47.77	2.5	NP	60.22
Lone Star Cheeseburger	893.96	NP	20.18	2089.12	49.77	2.5	NP	70.22
Swiss & Mushroom Burger	843.65	NP	16.62	1348.85	52.52	2.56	NP	69.19
Willie Burger	1006.99	NP	22.38	1698.23	48.26	2.5	NP	72.39
Lone Star Chicken Sandwich	1047.08	NP	4.02	4431.15	135.03	8.45	NP	49.92
Mesquite Grilled Chicken Sandwich	212.13	NP	0.81	897.72	27.36	1.71	NP	10.11
Steak Sandwich	638.49	NP	5.01	2967.72	54.84	3.13	NP	55.19
Entrée								
Chicken								
Chicken Tenders	516.42	NP	7.3	1241.13	38.51	3.96	NP	30.64
Grilled Chicken Breast	169.15	NP	0.34	1335.21	0	0.1	NP	32.68
Combination								
Garlic Lover's Medallions & Shrimp	370.74	NP	6.43	2242.57	0	0	NP	68.56
Superstar Combo	646.09	NP	8.53	8021.68	5.25	1.17	NP	89.87
Texas Trio	1205.61	NP	18.64	8386.36	63.83	1.53	NP	107.97
Pork								
Baby Back Ribs (half rack)	486	NP	16.2	126	0	0	NP	29.4
Baby Back Ribs (full rack)	972	NP	32.4	252	0	0	NP	58.8
Grilled Pork Chop	317.47	NP	4.65	3044.4	0	0	NP	42.61
Seafood								
Fried Shrimp, 5 pc (in Steak Combo)	251.89	NP	1.82	299.83	26.31	0.33	NP	7.25
Fried Shrimp Dinner	865.68	NP	5.46	1859.49	96.94	0.99	NP	21.76
Grilled Lobster Tail (in Steak Combo)	83.92	NP	0	213.14	7.65	0	NP	12.3
Grilled Shrimp, 5 pc (in Steak Combo)	44.2	NP	0.19	1455.99	0.58	0.28	NP	9.45
Mesquite-Grilled Shrimp Dinner	230.84	NP	1.42	3665.71	17.23	1.41	NP	21.27
Sweet Bourbon Salmon	309.88	NP	4.87	538.9	0	0	NP	36.48
Steak								
Cajun Ribeye	816.52	NP	20.36	703.07	5.47	0	NP	80.75
Chopped Steak	712.27	NP	6.23	364.02	0	0	NP	61.76
Five Star Filet, 6 oz	332.9	NP	6.83	241.54	1.84	0	NP	41.92
Lunch Cut Steak	389.91	NP	7.19	1554.86	0.61	0.23	NP	36.46
New York Strip	524.74	NP	15.55	617.49	0	0	NP	68.87
Texas Ribeye	710.2	NP	14.59	1339.19	5.58	0.15	NP	83.27

Description & Serving	Cal	Fat	Sfat	Sod	Carb	Fiber	Sugar	Prot
Side								
1/2 Mushrooms & 1/2 Onions	138.34	NP	1.02	504.83	15.49	2.04	NP	3.79
Baked Potato, plain	226.2	NP	0.06	32.65	50	5.36	NP	6.13
Garlic Mashed Potatoes	130	NP	2.5	430	19	2	NP	3
Jumbo Baked Sweet Potato, plain	332.09	NP	0.13	132.84	76.42	12.18	NP	7.42
Sauteed Mushrooms	140.38	NP	1.29	419.22	10.79	0.21	NP	4.5
Sauteed Onions	85.68	NP	0.4	400.23	14.23	3.01	NP	1.73
Steak Fries, 8 oz	610.07	NP	2.66	351.92	86.39	5.33	NP	8.5
Steamed Mixed Vegetables	189.57	NP	2.66	989.26	14.38	6.53	NP	5.33
Sweet Potato, plain	332.09	NP	0.13	132.84	76.42	12.18	NP	7.42
Texas Rice	101.94	NP	0.74	580.39	14	0.46	NP	2.07

LongHorn Steakhouse

Description & Serving	Cal	Fat	Sfat	Sod	Carb	Fiber	Sugar	Prot
Appetizer								
Wild West Shrimp	760	49	13	4180	43	NP	NP	NP
Texas Tonion	1130	68	12	2320	116	NP	NP	NP
Western Cheese Fries	1730	96	35	4940	138	NP	NP	NP
LongHorn Shrimp & Lobster Dip w/ Chips	1030	53	17	2080	92	NP	NP	NP
Crispy Chicken Trio	730	39	9	1590	32	NP	NP	NP
Boneless Buffalo Wings	990	63	11	5160	40	NP	NP	NP
Firecracker Chicken Wraps	640	36	13	2330	52	NP	NP	NP
Salad/Soup/Burger								
Grilled Chicken & Strawberry Salad w/ Raspberry Vinaigrette	960	58	10.5	860	56	NP	NP	NP
Strawberry Pecan Salad w/ Raspberry Vinaigrette	380	26	4.5	245	28	NP	NP	NP
7-Pepper Sirloin Salad	670	36	12	1500	32	NP	NP	NP
Sonoma Chicken Salad w/ Vinaigrette	720	39	11	1770	19	NP	NP	NP
Southern Fried Chicken Salad	1100	68	12	1740	63	NP	NP	NP
Mixed Greens Salad w/ Salmon	490	24	9	600	28	NP	NP	NP
Caesar Salad w/ Salmon	730	50	10	1040	29	NP	NP	NP
Authentic Ranch House Chili, cup	255	13	6	730	15	NP	NP	NP
Authentic Ranch House Chili, bowl	360	18	8	1020	20	NP	NP	NP
Shrimp & Lobster Chowder, cup	170	7	3	595	21	NP	NP	NP
Shrimp & Lobster Chowder, bowl	250	10	5	870	31	NP	NP	NP
French Onion Soup, cup	215	14	6	1220	13	NP	NP	NP
French Onion Soup, bowl	320	21	9	1820	20	NP	NP	NP
Cheeseburger	840	47	20	1180	53	NP	NP	NP
Entrée								
Steak								
Flo's Filet, 7 oz	420	28	8.5	330	0	NP	NP	NP
Flo's Filet, 9 oz	505	32	10	350	0	NP	NP	NP
LongHorn Porterhouse	1290	83	35	1180	0	NP	NP	NP
Outlaw Ribeye, 18 oz	1070	79	33	1640	0	NP	NP	NP
Fontina & Wild Mushroom Stuffed Filet	490	27	13	1130	8	NP	NP	NP
Portabella Peppercorn Filet	563	36	10	600	0	NP	NP	NP
Big Sky Bleu Filet, 7 oz	610	43	16	987	4	NP	NP	NP

Description & Serving	Cal	Fat	Sfat	Sod	Carb	Fiber	Sugar	Prot
Big Sky Bleu Filet, 9 oz	695	47	18	1000	4	NP	NP	NP
Fire-Grilled T-Bone	830	57	21.9	1710	1	NP	NP	NP
Renegade Top Sirloin, 8 oz	430	25	7	600	0	NP	NP	NP
Renegade Top Sirloin, 12 oz	580	30	9	870	0	NP	NP	NP
New York Strip/Kansas City Strip, 11 oz	780	55	19.5	650	0	NP	NP	NP
New York Strip/Kansas City Strip, 14 oz	957	66	23.5	816	0	NP	NP	NP
Ribeye, 12 oz	910	69	25	1260	0	NP	NP	NP
Sirloin & Shrimp Scampi	510	30	7	1650	2	NP	NP	NP
Eye of Prime Rib w/ Au Jus, 12 oz	660	42	19	570	0	NP	NP	NP
Eye of Prime Rib w/ Au Jus, 16 oz	924	59	27	798	0	NP	NP	NP
Eye of Prime Rib w/ French Onion Au Jus, 12 oz	880	58	22	1700	18	NP	NP	NP
Eye of Prime Rib w/ French Onion Au Jus, 16 oz	1144	75	30	1928	18	NP	NP	NP
Eye of Prime Rib w/ Roasted Garlic Cream Sauce, 12 oz	780	50	22	1380	9	NP	NP	NP
Eye of Prime Rib w/ Roasted Garlic Cream Sauce, 16 oz	1044	67	30	1608	9	NP	NP	NP
Chop Steak	1220	80	22	5040	66	NP	NP	NP
LongHorn Churrasco Steak w/ Plantains	1070	72	26	1090	40	NP	NP	NP
LongHorn Steak Tips	630	39	14.5	920	10	NP	NP	NP
Ribs/Pork								
Half-Rack of Spiced Rum Ribs	570	36	12	640	12	NP	NP	NP
Full-Rack of Spiced Rum Ribs	1140	72	24	1270	24	NP	NP	NP
Spiced Rum BBQ Ribs & Sirloin	990	61	19	1240	12	NP	NP	NP
Spiced Rum BBQ Ribs & Filet	1030	66	20	1140	12	NP	NP	NP
Half-Rack of Vidalia Onion BBQ Ribs	660	44	15	830	18	NP	NP	NP
Full-Rack of Vidalia Onion BBQ Ribs	1320	87	29	1650	35	NP	NP	NP
Vidalia Onion BBQ Ribs & Filet	1120	74	23	1330	18	NP	NP	NP
Vidalia Onion BBQ Ribs & Sirloin	1080	69	22	1430	18	NP	NP	NP
Baby Back Ribs - Full-Rack	1140	74	25	1710	15	NP	NP	NP
Baby Back Ribs - Half-Rack	550	37	13	1140	13	NP	NP	NP
Half-Rack of Ribs	550	37	13	570	2	NP	NP	NP
Cowboy Pork Chop	400	14	5	1600	1	NP	NP	NP
Chicken								
Rocky Top Chicken	870	39	19	3150	34	NP	NP	NP
Chicken Tenders	730	37	7	1460	34	NP	NP	NP
Sierra Chicken	410	12	3	1240	2	NP	NP	NP
Parmesan Crusted Chicken	1080	69	25	2440	16	NP	NP	NP
Honey Mustard Chicken Sandwich	700	28	9	1320	54	NP	NP	NP
Seafood								
Shrimp & Crab Gratin	300	14	8	1190	6	NP	NP	NP
Shrimp Scampi	200	9	5	1050	2	NP	NP	NP
Grilled Shrimp	45	0.5	0	560	1	NP	NP	NP
LongHorn Salmon, 7 oz	290	13	2.5	300	3	NP	NP	NP
LongHorn Salmon, 10 oz	410	19	4	430	4	NP	NP	NP
Golden Fried Shrimp	880	48	9	3180	71	NP	NP	NP
Redrock Grilled Shrimp	130	1.5	0.5	1690	2	NP	NP	NP

Description & Serving	Cal	Fat	Sfat	Sod	Carb	Fiber	Sugar	Prot
Combination								
Flo's Filet & Shrimp & Crab Gratin	720	42	16.5	1520	6	NP	NP	NP
Flo's Filet & Lobster Tail	580	39	19	1200	2	NP	NP	NP
Flo's Filet & LongHorn Salmon	700	41	11.5	697	6	NP	NP	NP
Side								
Baked Potato - Plain	260	0	0	0	55	NP	NP	NP
Add Bacon	50	3.5	1	0	1	NP	NP	NP
Add Butter	100	11	7	95	1	NP	NP	NP
Add Cheese	45	3.5	2	80	1	NP	NP	NP
Add Sour Cream	40	3.5	2	30	2	NP	NP	NP
Mashed Potatoes	270	14	7	620	30	NP	NP	NP
Seasoned French Fries	290	13	2.5	370	38	NP	NP	NP
Sweet Potato - Plain	240	1	0	0	50	NP	NP	NP
Add Butter	100	11	7	95	1	NP	NP	NP
Add Cinnamon Sugar	30	0	0	0	7	NP	NP	NP
Freshly Baked Bread (loaf)	510	5	1	590	96	NP	NP	NP
Add Butter	100	11	7	95	1	NP	NP	NP
Seasoned Rice Pilaf	200	0.5	0	1600	43	NP	NP	NP
Caesar Side Salad w/ Caesar Dressing	350	27	6	550	18	NP	NP	NP
Mixed Greens Side Salad	110	4.5	2	200	12	NP	NP	NP
Jalapeno Cole Slaw	310	26	4	670	16	NP	NP	NP
Fresh Seasonal Vegetables	90	4	1	350	9	NP	NP	NP
Fresh Steamed Asparagus	80	4.5	1	55	5	NP	NP	NP
Brandied Cinnamon Apples	230	0	0	170	58	NP	NP	NP
Grilled Onions	90	4	0.5	750	11	NP	NP	NP
Sauteed Mushrooms	90	5	1	530	5	NP	NP	NP
Sauteed Mushrooms & Onions	90	4.5	1	640	8	NP	NP	NP
Dressing/Condiment								
Avocado-Lime Dipping Sauce, 1 oz	108	11	2	240	2	NP	NP	NP
Bleu Cheese Dipping Sauce, 1 oz	100	9.5	2.5	310	2	NP	NP	NP
Honey Pepper Glaze Dipping Sauce, 1 oz	50	0.5	0	240	11	NP	NP	NP
Tangy Tonion Dipping Sauce, 1 oz	150	15	2.5	250	4	NP	NP	NP
Ranch Dipping Sauce, 1 oz	130	13.5	2	230	2	NP	NP	NP
Honey Mustard Dipping Sauce, 1 oz	175	17	2.5	175	5	NP	NP	NP
Garlic Butter for Grilled Shrimp,1 oz	170	18	9.5	200	1.5	NP	NP	NP
BBQ Sauce, 1 oz	30	0.5	0	380	7	NP	NP	NP
Bordelaise Sauce,1 oz	60	3	0.5	660	5	NP	NP	NP
Horseradish Sauce, 1 oz	70	6	3.4	220	4	NP	NP	NP
Lemon Butter Sauce, 1 oz	130	14	2.5	60	0	NP	NP	NP
Ranch, 1 oz	200	20	3.5	340	3	NP	NP	NP
Fat-Free Ranch, 1 oz	30	0	0	310	8	NP	NP	NP
Balsamic Vinaigrette, 1 oz	134	14	2	290	2	NP	NP	NP
Thousand Island,1 oz	140	14	2	150	3	NP	NP	NP
Chipotle Ranch, 1 oz	142	14	2	530	4	NP	NP	NP
Bleu Cheese, 1 oz	148	16	3	320	1	NP	NP	NP
Caesar, 1 oz	140	15	2	430	1	NP	NP	NP
Italian, 1 oz	64	6	1	450	3	NP	NP	NP

Description & Serving	Cal	Fat	Sfat	Sod	Carb	Fiber	Sugar	Prot
Honey Mustard, 1 oz	170	17	2.5	520	5	NP	NP	NP
Oil & Vinegar, 1 oz	120	12	1.5	360	2	NP	NP	NP
Bacon Honey Mustard, 1 oz	320	31	5.3	360	8	NP	NP	NP

Long John Silver's

Entrée

	Cal	Fat	Sfat	Sod	Carb	Fiber	Sugar	Prot
Battered Fish, 1 pc	260	16	4	790	17	0	0	12
Battered Shrimp, 3 pc	130	9	2.5	480	8	0	0	5
Popcorn Shrimp, 1 snack box	270	16	4	570	23	1	1	9
Baked Cod, 1 pc	120	4.5	1	240	1	0	0	22
Alaskan Flounder, 1 pc	250	11	2.5	910	26	2	0	12
Buttered Lobster Bites, 1 snack box	230	9	3	520	24	2	0	13
Breaded Clam Strips, 1 snack box	320	19	4.5	1190	29	2	1	9
Grilled Pacific Salmon, 2 filets	150	5	1	440	2	0	1	24
Grilled Tilapia, 1 filet	110	2.5	1	250	1	0	1	22
Shrimp Scampi, 8 pc	110	5	1	610	1	0	0	16
Lobster Stuffed Crab Cake, 1 cake	170	9	2	390	16	1	0	6
Baja Fish Taco	350	22	5	840	29	1	1	9
Freshside Grille Smart Choice Salmon, 1 plate	280	7	2	1010	27	3	5	27
Freshside Grille Smart Choice Tilapia, 1 plate	250	4.5	2	820	27	3	4	25
Freshside Grille Smart Choice Shrimp Scampi, 1 plate	250	7	2	1180	27	3	4	19
Salmon Bowl w/o sauce, 1 bowl	380	8	2	1270	47	4	5	29
Salmon Bowl w/ sauce, 1 bowl	460	8	2.5	1660	65	4	22	30
Shrimp Bowl w/o sauce, 1 bowl	300	4	1.5	1200	46	4	4	20
Shrimp Bowl w/ sauce, 1 bowl	380	4.5	1.5	1580	64	4	21	21
Chicken Plank, 1 pc	140	8	2	480	9	0	0	8

Sandwich

	Cal	Fat	Sfat	Sod	Carb	Fiber	Sugar	Prot
Fish Sandwich	470	23	5	1210	48	3	4	18
Ultimate Fish Sandwich	530	28	8	1400	49	3	4	21
Chicken Sandwich	360	15	3.5	900	10	3	4	14

Side

	Cal	Fat	Sfat	Sod	Carb	Fiber	Sugar	Prot
Fries, Platter portion (3 oz)	230	10	2.5	350	34	3	0	3
Fries, Basket Combo portion (4 oz)	310	14	3.5	460	45	4	0	3
Hushpuppy	60	2.5	0.5	200	9	1	1	1
Cole Slaw, 4 oz	200	15	2.5	340	15	3	10	1
Corn Cobbette w/o butter oil	90	3	0.5	0	14	3	6	3
Corn Cobbette w/ butter oil	150	10	2	30	14	3	6	3
Crumblies, 1 oz	170	12	2.5	410	14	1	0	1
Breadstick	170	3.5	1	290	29	1	2	6
Vegetable Medley, 4 oz	50	2	0.5	360	8	3	3	1
Rice, 5 oz	180	1	0.5	470	37	2	1	4
Broccoli Cheese Soup, 1 bowl	220	18	8	650	8	1	2	5

Dressing/Condiment

	Cal	Fat	Sfat	Sod	Carb	Fiber	Sugar	Prot
Cocktail Sauce, 1 oz	25	0	0	250	6	0	5	0
Tartar Sauce, 1 oz	100	9	1.5	250	4	0	3	0
Malt Vinegar, 0.5 oz	0	0	0	35	0	0	0	0

Description & Serving	Cal	Fat	Sfat	Sod	Carb	Fiber	Sugar	Prot
Ginger Teriyaki Sauce, 1 packet	80	0	0	380	18	0	17	1
Ketchup, 1 packet	10	0	0	100	2	0	2	0

Dessert

Chocolate Cream Pie, 1 slice	310	22	14	170	24	1	18	5
Pineapple Cream Pie, 1 slice	290	13	7	210	39	1	26	4
Pecan Pie, 1 slice	370	15	3	190	55	2	20	4

MaggieMoo's Ice Cream and Treatery

Ice Cream/Sorbet

Udderly Cream Ice Cream, half cup	180	11	8	40	18	0	16	3
NSA Ice Cream, half cup	110	3.5	3.5	20	28	0	0	0
Low Fat/Lactose Free Ice Cream, half cup	90	3	2	100	15	0	12	0
Fat Free Sorbet, half cup	120	0	0	0	30	0	29	0

Smoothie

Triple Berry Pomegranate Zoomer, 16 oz	400	1	0	5	101	13	86	1
Raspberry Pomegranate Zoomer, 16 oz	410	0.5	0	5	99	12	84	1
Creamy Mango Zoomer, 16 oz	400	2.5	1.5	75	95	0	85	1
Strawberry Banana Zoomer, 16 oz	430	13	7	390	82	3	62	2
Peach Orange-Blossom Zoomer, 16 oz	350	9	6	310	65	2	52	2
Pineapple Coconut-Colada Zoomer, 16 oz	560	28	22	330	80	6	63	2
Mocha Coffee Zoomer, 16 oz	550	16	9	480	103	1	73	2
Caramel Coffee Zoomer, 16 oz	450	14	9	490	80	0	64	1
Iced Cream Coffee Zoomer, 16 oz	380	14	8	440	66	0	54	1

Marble Slab Creamery

Ice Cream, 99 g

Amaretto Ice Cream	229	14	9	0	23	0	15	3
Amaretto Reduced Fat Ice Cream	210	10	7	0	24	0	24	3
Apple N Spice Ice Cream	224	12	8	7	26	0	19	3
Banana Ice Cream	202	11	7	0	22	1	15	3
Banana Rum Ice Cream	211	12	8	8	23	0	15	3
Birthday Cake Ice Cream	236	14	9	25	25	0	16	3
Blackberry Ice Cream	230	14	9	5	24	0	16	3
Black Walnut Ice Cream	227	14	9	1	24	0	16	3
Blueberry Ice Cream	216	12	8	3	24	0	17	3
Bubblegum Ice Cream	224	13	9	0	23	0	15	3
Butter Pecan Ice Cream	228	12	8	33	26	0	19	3
Butter Pecan Reduced Fat Ice Cream	230	12	8	33	26	0	19	3
Caramel Ice Cream	228	13	9	0	24	0	17	3
Cheesecake Ice Cream	228	13	8	0	26	0	17	3
Cheesecake Reduced Fat Ice Cream	211	10	6	0	27	0	25	3
Chocolate Amaretto Ice Cream	229	13	8	1	25	1	17	3
Chocolate Mint Ice Cream	229	13	8	1	25	1	17	3
Chocolate Peanut Butter Ice Cream	261	17	9	87	25	1	20	5
Chocolate Rum Ice Cream	230	13	8	10	25	1	17	3
Chocolate Swiss Ice Cream	229	13	8	1	26	1	18	3

Description & Serving	Cal	Fat	Sfat	Sod	Carb	Fiber	Sugar	Prot
Chocolate Swiss Reduced Fat Ice Cream	213	10	6	1	27	1	26	3
Cinnamon Ice Cream	229	14	9	0	23	1	15	3
Coconut Ice Cream	230	14	9	0	23	0	15	3
Coffee Ice Cream	227	14	10	0	23	0	15	3
Cookie Dough Ice Cream	234	12	8	9	29	0	23	3
Dark Chocolate Ice Cream	235	13	9	18	26	1	18	4
Egg Nog Ice Cream	237	12	8	1	29	0	19	3
French Vanilla Ice Cream	236	13	8	5	26	0	18	3
Fudge Ice Cream	243	13	8	15	29	0	21	3
Honey Ice Cream	232	13	9	0	25	0	18	3
Lemon Custard Ice Cream	240	13	8	3	27	0	20	3
Mango Ice Cream	228	14	9	0	23	0	15	3
Maple Ice Cream	230	13	9	0	24	0	16	3
Mocha Ice Cream	228	13	8	1	25	1	17	3
Peach Ice Cream	219	12	8	3	24	0	16	3
Peanut Butter Ice Cream	263	17	9	42	23	1	15	5
Peanut Butter Banana Ice Cream	243	15	9	30	23	1	15	4
Peppermint Ice Cream	239	13	9	0	26	0	18	3
Pina Colada Ice Cream	214	12	8	0	22	0	15	3
Pistachio Ice Cream	258	16	9	0	25	1	17	4
Praline Ice Cream	244	12	8	49	31	0	20	3
Pumpkin Ice Cream	201	11	7	29	23	1	16	3
Rum Ice Cream	231	13	9	17	23	0	16	3
Strawberry Ice Cream	207	12	8	1	22	0	15	3
Strawberry Reduced Fat Ice Cream	191	9	6	1	23	0	23	3
Sweet Cream Ice Cream	229	14	9	0	23	0	15	3
Vanilla Ice Cream	229	13	9	0	22	0	15	3
Vanilla Reduced Fat Ice Cream	211	10	7	0	24	0	24	3
Vanilla Bean Ice Cream	230	13	9	1	23	0	15	3
Vanilla Cinnamon Ice Cream	230	13	9	0	23	0	15	3

Ice Cream Creations, small

Description & Serving	Cal	Fat	Sfat	Sod	Carb	Fiber	Sugar	Prot
S'More	409	19	11	91	57	2	37	5
Cookies N' Cream	363	19	10	150	42	1	26	4
Snickerdoodle	342	17	10	69	41	0	28	4
Rocky Road	440	26	12	21	48	3	34	6
Rainbownanza	312	17	11	10	36	0	27	4
Peanut Butter Crunch	373	21	12	67	43	2	32	6
Almond Joy	384	24	14	59	36	5	23	7
Smooth Mint Masterpiece	414	22	15	35	48	0	29	5
White Chocolate Raspberry Swirl	273	21	10	85	40	3	26	7
Strawberries 'N' Cream	238	14	9	0	25	1	17	3
Red, White & Blue	242	14	9	0	26	1	17	3
Cherries Jubilee	299	16	10	71	36	1	20	4
Bear Necessities	341	14	9	12	51	0	32	3
Birthday Bonanza	305	14	9	31	42	0	28	3
Raspberry Cheesecake	297	14	9	71	38	1	21	4
Blue Cheese	239	13	9	0	29	1	24	4
Chocolate Delight Cheesecake	405	21	13	23	52	1	31	5

Description & Serving	Cal	Fat	Sfat	Sod	Carb	Fiber	Sugar	Prot
Butter Than Nuttin'	420	32	10	33	30	2	20	6
Southern Pecan Pie	371	23	10	71	38	1	25	4
Coffee Bar	375	21	12	81	40	1	31	4
Caramel Nut Latte'	360	19	10	150	43	1	26	4
Trail Mix	461	29	12	12	42	3	28	8
Bananas Foster	287	14	9	38	35	0	23	4
Candylicious	452	25	15	80	50	1	40	5
The Bart	360	19	12	65	43	1	28	5
Willy Wonka	347	18	12	32	44	3	32	5
Pineapple Mixed Up Cake	312	15	9	96	40	1	23	4
Tipsy Sailor	382	25	12	2	35	3	24	7
Cherry Amaretto Cake	300	16	10	70	36	1	20	4
Chocolate Covered Strawberries	255	13	9	13	31	1	22	3
Blueberry Pie	286	14	8	73	37	1	22	4
Berry Bash	223	12	8	2	26	2	17	3
Blackberry Crumble	341	17	10	9	42	2	27	5
Ultimate Cookie Dough	405	18	11	52	56	0	35	4
Swiss Cocoa Buttercup	416	22	13	71	51	2	39	6
Caramel Peanut Butter Crisp	410	21	13	70	52	1	35	5

Ice Cream Cake, per serving

	Cal	Fat	Sfat	Sod	Carb	Fiber	Sugar	Prot
Birthday Cake Ice Cream Cake	460	24	17	100	58	0	45	4
Caramel Peanut Butter Crisp Ice Cream Cake	520	28	20	95	63	1	45	5
Cookie Dough Drizzle Ice Cream Cake	510	27	17	100	63	1	44	5
Smooth Mint Masterpiece Ice Cream Cake	490	28	20	40	55	0	33	5
Sweet Cream & Strawberries Ice Cream Cake	370	22	15	20	40	0	29	4
Swiss Cocoa Buttercup Ice Cream Cake	540	31	20	110	60	2	47	7
Turtle Ice Cream Cake	590	37	15	95	60	3	40	7
Vanilla & Oreo Ice Cream Cake	470	26	17	130	54	1	37	5

Marco's Pizza

Small Pizza, 1 slice

	Cal	Fat	Sfat	Sod	Carb	Fiber	Sugar	Prot
Cheese Pizza	200	6	3.5	370	23	1	2	11
Pepperoni Pizza	210	8	4	440	23	1	2	10
White Cheesy Pizza	170	7	3.5	360	17	1	1	9
Deluxe Uno Pizza	200	9	4.5	360	18	1	2	10
Meat Supremo Pizza	210	10	4.5	430	18	1	2	11
Chicken Fresco Pizza	180	7	3.5	480	19	1	2	11
Hawaiian Chicken Pizza	180	6	3	430	18	1	2	10
Garden Pizza	160	5	3	360	19	1	2	8

Medium Pizza, 1 slice

	Cal	Fat	Sfat	Sod	Carb	Fiber	Sugar	Prot
Cheese Pizza	210	6	3.5	390	24	1	2	11
Pepperoni Pizza	230	9	4.5	470	24	1	2	11
White Cheesy Pizza	260	11	5	550	24	1	2	13
Deluxe Uno Pizza	280	12	6	520	26	1	2	15
Meat Supremo Pizza	300	15	7	640	25	1	2	15
Chicken Fresco Pizza	260	10	5	670	26	1	3	15

Description & Serving	Cal	Fat	Sfat	Sod	Carb	Fiber	Sugar	Prot
Hawaiian Chicken Pizza	260	10	5	620	26	1	3	15
Garden Pizza	230	8	4.5	530	26	2	3	12
Large Pizza, 1 slice								
Cheese Pizza	280	8	5	510	33	2	3	14
White Cheesy Pizza	340	15	7	730	33	2	2	17
Deluxe Uno Pizza	380	16	8	700	35	2	3	20
Meat Supremo Pizza	430	21	10	900	34	2	3	23
Chicken Fresco Pizza	350	13	7	900	35	2	4	20
Hawaiian Chicken Pizza	380	15	8	890	35	2	4	22
Garden Pizza	310	10	6	740	36	2	4	16
Pepperoni Pizza	310	11	6	640	33	2	3	15
Extra Large Pizza, 1 slice								
Cheese Pizza	240	7	4	440	29	1	3	12
Pepperoni Pizza	270	10	5	550	29	1	2	13
White Cheesy Pizza	300	13	6	630	29	1	2	15
Deluxe Uno Pizza	330	14	7	600	31	2	3	17
Meat Supremo Pizza	350	17	8	710	29	1	2	18
Chicken Fresco Pizza	300	11	6	770	31	2	3	17
Hawaiian Chicken Pizza	300	11	5	720	31	1	4	17
Garden Pizza	270	9	5	620	31	2	3	14
Deep Pan Pizza, 1 slice								
Deep Pan Pepperoni Pizza	330	12	6	650	36	2	3	16
Deep Pan Cheese Pizza	290	8	5	530	36	2	3	15
Chicken								
BBQ Chicken Wings	71	4.3	1.2	174	2.8	0	2.5	5.3
Hot & Spicy Chicken Wings	60	4.3	1.2	167	0	0	0	5.3
Naked Chicken Wings	60	4.3	1.2	130	0	0	0	5.3
BBQ Chicken Tumblers	67	2.3	0.5	164	7.4	0	2.5	4
Hot & Spicy Chicken Tumblers	57	2.3	0.5	157	4.7	0	0	4
Naked Chicken Tumblers	57	2.3	0.5	120	4.7	0	0	4
Sandwich								
Italian Sub	430	22.5	9.5	1175	34.5	1.5	2.5	23.5
Steak & Cheese Sub	380	14.5	7	605	32.5	1	1.5	29
Ham & Cheese Sub	400	21	9	865	33	1	1.5	21
Chicken Club Sub	385	15.5	7	1150	33.5	1.5	2	27.5
Veggie Sub	355	16	8.5	1135	39	2.5	2	15.5
Side/Salad								
Cheezybread	80	1.5	1	105	11	0	1	3
Cinnasquares	60	1.5	0	60	9	0	5	1
Italian Salad	230	17	9	930	11	3	3	12
Chicken Ranch Salad	240	13	6	1220	10	3	2	22

Maui Wowi Hawaiian

Smoothie, 12 oz

Description & Serving	Cal	Fat	Sfat	Sod	Carb	Fiber	Sugar	Prot
Strawberry Banana Smoothie	240	0	0	35	57	<1	47	2
Passion Papaya Smoothie	220	0	0.6	50	54	<1	38	2

Description & Serving	Cal	Fat	Sfat	Sod	Carb	Fiber	Sugar	Prot
Mango Orange Banana Smoothie	240	0	0.6	35	57	<1	43	3
Banana Banana Smoothie	210	0	0.6	55	50	2	36	2
Pina Colada Smoothie w/o a fresh banana	240	0	2.5	70	57	0	46	3
Kiwi Lemon-Lime Smoothie w/o a fresh banana	180	0	0	35	42	0	34	3
Black Raspberry Smoothie	240	0	0	40	59	0	46	2
Lemon Wave Smoothie	415	0.3	0.1	1.2	108	0.4	108	0.4

Mazzio's Italian Eatery

Appetizer

	Cal	Fat	Sfat	Sod	Carb	Fiber	Sugar	Prot
Toasted Ravioli w/o Sauce	118	5.1	1.8	212.1	13.3	0.7	0.3	5.2
Mozzarella Sticks w/o Sauce	181	12.1	4.5	368.7	10	NP	NP	8.5
Cheese Dippers w/o Sauce	405	17.5	4.9	638.8	47.3	1.8	2.2	12.9
Garlic Cheese Toast w/o Sauce	205	13.4	3.7	419.3	15.6	1	1.1	6.2
Garlic Toast w/o Sauce	160	10	2	280	15	1	1	3
Breadsticks w/o Sauce	150	3	0.7	352.9	26	0.9	1.35	5
Artichoke Spin Dip w/ Bread	245	16.4	5.6	475.1	17.8	2.4	1.1	6.2
Meat Nachos - Sausage w/ Jalapenos	505	36.9	18.6	970.6	19.59	1.8	0.2	23.3
Meat Nachos - Chicken w/ Jalapenos	448	30.3	16.3	866.3	19.6	1.5	0.2	24.1
Meat Nachos - Beef w/ Jalapenos	484	34.3	18.2	918.7	19.8	2.1	0.1	24.5
Cheese Nachos w/ Jalapenos	423	29.9	16.2	695.3	18.7	1.48	NP	19.7
Dippin' Tostitos Chips	284	14.2	2	243	36.5	2	0	4.1
Cinnamon Sticks w/o Sauce	626	36.1	5.7	559	70.3	1.8	36.5	5.3
Wings of Fire w/o Dippin' Sauce, 10 pc	161	10.9	2.7	411.9	0.6	0	0	15.1
Roasted & BBQ Tossed Wings, 10 pc	191	11.9	3.1	36.7	6.9	0	6.5	13.5
Boneless Dippin' Chicken, 10 pc	122	5.7	1	326.9	6.8	0.28	0	10.1
Rib Dippers (3/4 lb), tossed w/ BBQ	458	32.4	13.4	862.3	13.2	0	12	28.3
Pepperoni Calzone Ring	260	9.6	3.7	555.3	32.7	1.2	1.5	9.6
Ham Bacon & Cheddar Calzone Ring	244	7.5	3.4	519.8	32.2	1.2	1.6	10.9
Four Meat/Four Cheese Calzone Ring	274	10.6	3.9	603.1	33.1	1.4	1.6	10.5
Pepperoni Quesapizza	332	16.1	6.1	668.9	32	1.2	0.8	13.4
Chicken Quesapizza	317	13.1	4.7	707	32.8	1.2	1.1	16.1

Sandwich

	Cal	Fat	Sfat	Sod	Carb	Fiber	Sugar	Prot
Tuscan Smash on Hoagie	986	36	9.3	2723.4	117	5.4	8	45.6
Tuscan Smash on Wheatberry	645	33.7	8.59	2223.9	45.1	1.3	4.3	33.4
Turkey & Swiss on Hoagie	1059	40.4	12.3	2750.2	117.5	5.4	8.1	52.9
Turkey & Swiss on Wheatberry	718	38.1	11.6	2250.8	45.6	1.3	4.4	40.8
Mazzio's Sub on Hoagie	1109	51.7	15.6	3290.3	116.6	5.1	8.4	48.7
Mazzio's Sub on Wheatberry	768	49.4	14.9	2790.8	44.7	1	4.7	36.6
Ham & Cheddar on Hoagie	1088	49.5	14	3260.4	118.7	5.1	8.9	48.6
Ham & Cheddar on Wheatberry	747	47.2	13.3	2761	46.8	1	5.2	36.4
Chicken, Bacon & Swiss on Hoagie	1362	72.4	18.5	2391.2	120.2	5.6	7.4	60.1
Chicken, Bacon & Swiss on Wheatberry	1022	70.1	17.8	1891.7	48.3	1.5	3.7	48

Pizza

Medium Thin Crust, 1 slice

	Cal	Fat	Sfat	Sod	Carb	Fiber	Sugar	Prot
Cheese Pizza	182	8.7	3.7	484.4	18.4	1.2	1.3	8.7
Canadian Bacon Pizza	179	7.8	3.2	571.8	18.3	1.2	1.5	9.8
Chicken Pizza	187	7.6	3	592.3	19	1.2	1.6	11.7

Description & Serving	Cal	Fat	Sfat	Sod	Carb	Fiber	Sugar	Prot
Hamburger (Beef) Pizza	208	10.5	4.4	588.8	18.9	1.7	1.4	10.9
Pepperoni Pizza	202	10.7	4.3	554.2	18.1	1.8	1.3	8.9
Sausage Pizza	224	12.4	4.7	627.8	18.8	1.4	1.5	10.1
Combo Pizza	231	12.7	5	752.6	19.4	1.6	1.8	9.8
4 Meat Pizza	253	14.9	5.8	728.8	18.8	1.5	1.5	11.6
Lucky 7 Pizza	203	10.1	4.1	642.6	19.7	1.6	2.1	8.7
Greek Pizza	263	17	5.2	607.6	18.5	0.8	0.6	12
California Alfredo Pizza	233	12.9	6	568	18.5	0.9	1.1	12.2
Mexican Pizza	263	13.9	5.7	776.3	23	2.6	2	12
Chicken Club Pizza	205	9.1	3.5	653.6	19.1	1.3	1.8	12.7
Veggie Pizza	180	8.1	3.4	617	19.4	1.6	1.8	7.6
Mazzio's "Works" Pizza	255	14.6	5.7	859.1	19.7	1.7	1.9	11.3
Cheesebuster Pizza	197	9.1	4	513.5	18.5	1.1	1.5	9.8
Meatbuster Pizza	234	13.3	5.1	667.7	18.7	1.5	1.5	10.5
Supremebuster Pizza	206	10.7	4.1	572.2	18.9	1.5	1.6	8.9
Medium Original Crust, 1 slice								
Cheese Pizza	234	8.5	3.6	522.2	30.1	1.6	2	10.3
Canadian Bacon Pizza	231	7.5	3.1	609.6	30.1	1.6	2.2	11.4
Chicken Pizza	239	7.3	2.9	630.1	30.7	1.6	2.2	13.2
Hamburger (Beef) Pizza	260	10.2	4.3	626.6	30.7	2.1	2.1	12.5
Pepperoni Pizza	254	10.4	4.3	592	29.9	1.6	2	10.5
Sausage Pizza	276	12.1	4.7	665.6	30.5	1.8	2.2	11.6
Combo Pizza	283	12.4	5	790.4	31.2	2	2.5	11.4
4 Meat Pizza	305	14.6	5.8	766.7	30.6	1.9	2.2	13.1
Lucky 7 Pizza	255	9.8	4.1	680.4	31.5	2	2.8	10.2
Greek Pizza	315	16.7	5.1	645.4	30.3	1.2	1.3	13.6
California Alfredo Pizza	285	12.6	6	605.9	30	1.3	1.8	13.8
Mexican Pizza	314	13.7	5.7	814.1	34.7	3	2.6	13.5
Chicken Club Pizza	257	8.8	3.5	691.4	30.9	1.7	2.5	14.2
Veggie Pizza	232	7.8	3.3	654.8	31.1	2	2.5	9.2
Mazzio's "Works" Pizza	307	14.3	5.7	896.9	31.4	2.1	2.6	12.9
Cheesebuster Pizza	249	8.9	4	551.4	30.2	1.5	2.2	11.3
Meatbuster Pizza	286	13	5.1	705.5	30.5	1.9	2.2	12.1
Supremebuster Pizza	257	10.4	4.1	610	30.7	1.9	2.3	10.4
Medium Deep Pan, 1 slice								
Cheese Pizza	332	15.3	4.6	658.2	37.6	2	2.5	11.4
Canadian Bacon Pizza	330	14.3	4.1	745.5	37.6	1.9	2.7	12.5
Chicken Pizza	339	14.1	3.9	766.1	38.2	2	2.8	14.4
Hamburger (Beef) Pizza	359	17	5.3	762.6	38.2	2.4	2.6	13.6
Pepperoni Pizza	352	17.2	5.3	728	37.4	1.9	2.5	11.6
Sausage Pizza	374	18.9	5.6	801.6	38	2.2	2.7	12.7
Combo Pizza	381	19.2	6	926.4	38.7	2.3	3	12.5
4 Meat Pizza	403	21.4	6.7	902.6	38.1	2.2	2.7	14.2
Lucky 7 Pizza	353	16.6	5.1	816.4	39	2.3	3.3	11.3
Greek Pizza	414	23.5	6.1	781.4	37.8	1.6	1.8	14.7
California Alfredo Pizza	383	19.4	6.9	741.8	37.5	1.6	2.3	14.9
Mexican Pizza	413	20.5	6.6	950.1	42.2	3.3	3.2	14.7
Chicken Club Pizza	356	15.6	4.5	827.4	38.4	2	3	15.4
Veggie Pizza	331	14.6	4.3	790.8	38.6	2.3	3	10.3

Description & Serving	Cal	Fat	Sfat	Sod	Carb	Fiber	Sugar	Prot
Mazzio's "Works" Pizza	406	21.1	6.6	1032.9	39	2.4	3.1	14
Cheesebuster Pizza	348	15.7	5	687.3	37.7	1.8	2.7	12.5
Meatbuster Pizza	385	19.8	6.1	841.5	38	2.2	2.7	13.2
Supremebuster Pizza	356	17.2	5.1	746	38.2	2.2	2.9	11.5

Pasta

Description & Serving	Cal	Fat	Sfat	Sod	Carb	Fiber	Sugar	Prot
Chicken Parmesan	947	27.4	7	2478.2	134.8	8.9	20.2	64.6
Lasagna Red & White	984	61.6	33.5	3003.6	64.3	5.4	11.9	45.8
Lasagna w/ Alfredo	1264	93.7	54.5	2581.1	55.2	2.7	4.4	53.1
Lasagna w/ Meat Sauce	949	51.9	21.7	3018.1	63.9	7.6	8.8	57.1
Lasagna w/ Marinara	704	29.5	12.5	3426.1	73.4	8	19.5	38.5
Greek Pasta	1456	94.2	18.5	2582.4	107.3	5.8	8.3	40.8
Chicken Spinach Artichoke Pasta	1005	38.1	20	1631.1	112.9	10.1	7.8	48.6
Fettuccine Alfredo	1061	56.4	33.2	1054.7	106.5	4.2	8.5	33
Chicken-Fried Chicken Alfredo	1290	69.2	35.4	1591.8	120.1	4.7	8.8	70
Spaghetti w/ Marinara	641	8.2	1.7	1688.5	120.2	8.2	19.9	22.1
Spaghetti w/ Meat Sauce	825	25	8.6	1382.4	113.1	7.9	11.8	36
Spaghetti w/ Meatballs (4) & Marinara	972	33.5	12.4	2337.7	126.4	9.6	20.6	41.5
Spaghetti w/ Meatballs (4) & Meat Sauce	1156	50.4	19.3	2031.7	119.3	9.3	12.6	55.4

Side

Description & Serving	Cal	Fat	Sfat	Sod	Carb	Fiber	Sugar	Prot
Greek Bread, 1	623	30.7	10.3	2074.4	60.8	3.2	3.4	28.2
Deli Bread, 1	480	20.1	6.9	1637	60	3.3	3.3	17.7
Hawaiian Bread, 1	449	13.1	5.8	1410.7	62.4	3.1	5.8	22.8
Southwestern Chicken Bread, 1	532	20.3	6.9	1599.7	61.3	3.2	4.1	27.9
Pepperoni Bread, 1	495	21.1	8.9	1474	58.3	3	2.5	21.7
Garlic Toast, 1 pc	160	10	2	280	15	1	1	3
Kosher Pickle Spear	5	0	0	300	1	0	0	0
Fries w/ Sandwich	558	28.8	5.6	1621	67.3	6.7	0	6.3
Full Order of Fries	279	14.4	2.8	810.4	33.6	3.3	0	3.1
Cheese Fries	432	25.6	8.3	1306.7	35.4	3.4	0.3	14.4

Sauce/Condiment

Description & Serving	Cal	Fat	Sfat	Sod	Carb	Fiber	Sugar	Prot
Marinara, 2 oz	29	0.8	0.1	295.5	4.6	0.8	2.6	0.8
Picante, 2 oz	20	0	0	700	4	0.5	4	0
Buffalo, 2 oz	19	0	0	1436.4	3.78	0	0	0
BBQ, 2 oz	140	0	0	580	34	0	32	0
Honey Mustard, 2 oz	260	22	3	420	14	0	12	0
Vanilla, 2 oz	181	0	0	0	45.4	0.1	42	0
Chocolate, 2 oz	178	1.4	0.6	0	42.6	0.7	38.7	0
Cool Ranch, 2 oz	372	39.4	6.7	694.3	1.9	0.1	1.3	0.9
Southwestern Ranch, 2 oz	321	33.6	5.7	707	2.4	0.2	1.8	0.8
Blue Cheese, 2 oz	302	32.1	6.6	585.9	1.9	0	1.9	1.9
Ketchup, 2 oz	50	0	0	600.4	13.3	0	13.3	0

McAlister's Deli

Sandwich/Wrap

Description & Serving	Cal	Fat	Sfat	Sod	Carb	Fiber	Sugar	Prot
BLT	911	64	10	1523	61	2	3	24
French Dip	433	15	8	1315	43	2	3	36

Description & Serving	Cal	Fat	Sfat	Sod	Carb	Fiber	Sugar	Prot
Greek Chicken Pita	591	27	8	1771	49	4	7	31
Grilled Chicken Club	997	56	16	2017	79	7	8	50
Ham Melt	687	33	10	3354	46	4	6	51
McAlister's Club	1029	56	16	3143	79	7	10	54
Memphian	552	23	6	2473	47	4	6	40
Muffuletta Sandwich	649	48	0	2285	25	1	2	26
New Yorker	465	13	6	2427	49	4	5	42
Orange Cranberry Club	976	39	39	3021	102	5	42	53
Reuben	679	34	9	4052	66	4	12	42
Roast Beef Melt	563	27	8	1649	26	4	4	38
Submarine	730	36	11	3977	49	3	7	53
The Big Nasty	753	18	10	2761	90	6	10	67
The Veggie	527	12	6	1945	82	16	29	21
Turkey Melt	563	25	7	2095	48	4	6	36
Basil Parmesan Chicken Panini	683	21	8	2132	81	9	15	43
Havarti Chicken Panini	656	17	9	1686	88	3	26	36
Horseradish Roast Beef & Cheddar Panini	796	43	14	1511	73	2	11	33
Sicilian Cheese Panini	587	19	11	1201	71	4	8	30
Smokey Pepper Jack Turkey Panini	690	32	10	1810	78	2	19	28
Chipotle Chicken Wrap	444	11	2	1313	57	8	4	27
Grill Chicken Caesar Wrap	591	27	8	1771	49	4	7	31

Build-Your-Own-Deli-Sandwich

Description & Serving	Cal	Fat	Sfat	Sod	Carb	Fiber	Sugar	Prot
Chicken Breast, 4 oz	130	4	1	790	3	0	0	21
Chicken Salad, 4 oz	338	26	4	477	6	0	2	20
Corned Beef, 4 oz	101	2	1	1235	2	0	2	20
Hickory Smoked Ham, 4 oz	126	5	2	1431	1	0	1	18
Meatloaf, 5 oz	335	23	9	512	9	2	2	24
Pastrami, 4 oz	122	3	2	1357	2	0	2	20
Roast Beef, 4 oz	101	2	1	850	2	0	0	20
Salami, 4 oz	405	36	12	1903	0	0	0	24
Smoked Turkey, 4 oz	101	0	0	1296	4	0	2	18
Croissant	360	21	13	470	37	1	6	7
Harvest Wheat Bread, 2 slices	367	5	1	652	69	4	12	12
Pita Bread, 1 whole	240	5	1	510	41	2	2	7
Rye Bread, 2 slices	241	3	0	703	46	4	2	10
Sliced Wheat, 2 slices	200	3	0	360	36	4	4	8
Sourdough Bread, 2 slices	298	3	0	557	60	2	2	12
Wheat Hoagie, 1 whole	195	2	0	420	40	3	3	9
Wheat Wrap, 1 whole	295	8	2	773	48	6	1	9
White Hoagie, 1 whole	195	2	0	465	40	2	3	8
American Cheese	52	4	3	224	1	0	1	3
Cheddar Cheese	88	7	4	144	1	1	1	6
Havarti Cheese	59	5	3	106	0	0	0	3
Pepper Jack Cheese	53	5	3	127	0	0	0	3
Provolone Cheese	81	6	4	198	0	0	0	6
Swiss Cheese	80	6	4	46	0	0	0	6

Salad

Description & Serving	Cal	Fat	Sfat	Sod	Carb	Fiber	Sugar	Prot
Basil Parmesan Chicken Salad	503	31	9	1724	25	3	22	30
Caesar Salad w/ Grilled Chicken	700	51	12	1891	24	2	4	35

Description & Serving	Cal	Fat	Sfat	Sod	Carb	Fiber	Sugar	Prot
Caesar Salad	599	49	11	1395	23	2	3	17
Greek Chicken Salad	485	31	8	1549	19	3	8	27
Greek Salad	347	30	8	1053	18	3	7	9
Grilled Chicken Salad	374	19	9	1322	16	2	4	35
McAlister's Chef	254	12	6	1242	14	2	5	22
Sweet Chipotle Chicken Salad	425	11	2	1242	58	4	28	22
Taco Salad	593	32	13	1102	47	6	11	27

Soup/Chili

Asiago Cheese Bisque, 8 oz	240	17	9	720	17	0	1	5
Broccoli Cheddar Soup, 8 oz	213	15	9	947	13	0	4	8
Cheddar Potato Soup, 8 oz	213	13	8	773	19	1	0	5
Cheesy Chicken Tortilla Soup, 8 oz	150	6	3	1470	13	0	4	10
Chicken & Dumplings Soup, 8 oz	270	10	3	1199	25	1	1	21
Chicken & Sausage Gumbo, 8 oz	150	5	2	1040	17	2	3	8
Chicken Chili, 8 oz	150	3	0	490	20	4	4	20
Chicken Noodle Soup, 8 oz	110	2	0	1280	15	1	1	8
Chili w/ Meat, 8 oz	390	22	5	1070	18	17	2	23
Clam Chowder, 8 oz	200	11	6	960	19	0	4	8
Country Potato Soup, 8 oz	173	8	4	760	23	0	4	4
Country Vegetable Soup, 8 oz	93	1	0	973	17	3	4	3
French Onion Soup, 8 oz	80	1	1	144	11	1	5	1
Golden Lentil Soup, 8 oz	213	3	2	831	35	9	4	12
Southwest Roasted Corn Soup, 8 oz	120	4	1	900	20	4	3	3
Vegetarian Chili, 8 oz	133	1	0	987	28	15	4	8
Minestrone Soup, 9 oz	220	10	2	690	24	4	2	8
Bread Bowl for 12 oz Soup or Chili	140	1	0	310	28	1	1	5

Entrée

Beef

Meatloaf Platter	680	46	18	1050	19	4	4	48
Pot Roast Classic	398	19	7	1384	24	3	2	34

Nachos

Chili Nacho	448	25	6	642	44	3	2	13
Chili Nacho w/ Veggie Chili	397	20	5	636	47	6	1	10
Nacho Basket	433	25	10	986	42	2	4	12

Pizza

Basil Parmesan Pizza	385	23	8	1242	15	4	2	17
Mediterranean Feta Pizza	392	20	12	1050	31	4	4	22
Simply Cheese Pizza	314	15	8	808	30	4	4	15

Spud

Bacon Spud	320	14	8	430	34	3	1	15
Cheese Spud	509	18	11	370	69	6	2	22
Grilled Chicken Spud	558	12	7	870	70	6	7	41
Justaspud	298	0	0	18	68	5	3	8
Pot Roast Spud	538	11	5	1048	72	6	3	40
Spud Max	759	31	16	1883	34	6	4	43
Spud Ole	694	28	13	871	77	7	3	32

Description & Serving	Cal	Fat	Sfat	Sod	Carb	Fiber	Sugar	Prot
Spud Ole w/ Veggie Chili	591	18	11	860	83	13	4	26
Veggie Spud	585	19	6	907	77	6	5	25

Side

Applesauce, 4 oz	100	0	0	0	24	1	22	0
Fruit Salad, 5 oz	81	0	0	13	11	1	18	1
Macaroni & Cheese, 6 oz	302	16	5	714	28	1	6	11
Mashed Potatoes, 7 oz	254	13	3	584	32	3	2	3
Potato Salad, 5 oz	261	17	2	472	24	1	5	2

Kids

Cheese Pita Pizza, 7 oz	463	20	20	866	47	4	6	23
Ham & Cheese, 7 oz	385	13	5	1951	38	4	6	28
Kid's Nacho, 5 oz	573	32	11	1108	61	3	4	14
Kid's Garden Salad, 4 oz	89	5	3	154	7	1	2	5
Mac & Cheese, 6 oz	302	16	5	714	28	1	6	11
Mac's Dog, 3 oz	248	11	4	550	25	1	4	9
PB&J, 7 oz	687	31	5	626	85	8	43	22
Toasted Cheese, 4 oz	346	16	7	987	38	4	6	16
Turkey & Cheese, 5 oz	324	9	4	1321	39	4	6	21

Dressing/Condiment

Blue Cheese Dressing, 3 oz	397	43	6	822	3	0	3	3
Caesar Dressing, 3 oz	539	57	9	1163	3	0	0	3
Chipotle Peach Dressing, 3 oz	170	0	0	567	40	0	34	0
Greek Dressing, 3 oz	255	26	4	709	6	0	3	0
Lite Ranch Dressing, 3 oz	283	28	4	822	3	0	3	3
McAlister's Honey Mustard Dressing, 3 oz	319	27	4	451	24	0	24	0
Olive Oil & Balsamic Vinaigrette, 3 oz	170	17	3	652	9	0	6	0
Ranch Dressing, 3 oz	283	31	4	822	3	0	3	0
Thousand Island Dressing, 3 oz	340	31	4	850	14	0	11	0
Fat-Free Chipotle Peach, 2 tbsp	60	0	0	200	14	0	12	0
Horseradish Sauce, 2 tbsp	132	12	2	265	6	0	5	0
McAlister's Honey Mustard Dressing, 1 oz	106	9	1	151	8	0	8	0
Orange Cranberry Sauce, 2 tbsp	130	0	0	110	31	0	31	0
Au Jus, 4 oz	8	0	0	567	0	0	0	0
Comeback Gravy, 4 oz	11	1	0	26	1	0	0	0

McDonald's

Breakfast

Egg McMuffin	300	12	5	820	30	2	3	18
Sausage McMuffin	370	22	8	850	29	2	2	14
Sausage McMuffin w/ Egg	450	27	10	920	30	2	2	21
English Muffin	160	3	0.5	280	27	2	2	5
Bacon, Egg & Cheese Biscuit, reg	420	23	12	1160	37	2	3	15
Bacon, Egg & Cheese Biscuit, lrg	480	27	12	1270	43	3	4	15
Sausage Biscuit w/ Egg, reg	510	33	14	1170	36	2	2	18
Sausage Biscuit w/ Egg, lrg	570	37	15	1280	42	3	3	18
Sausage Biscuit, reg	430	27	12	1080	34	2	2	11

Description & Serving	Cal	Fat	Sfat	Sod	Carb	Fiber	Sugar	Prot
Sausage Biscuit, lrg	480	31	13	1190	39	3	3	11
Southern Style Chicken Biscuit, reg	410	20	8	1180	41	2	3	17
Southern Style Chicken Biscuit, lrg	470	24	9	1290	46	3	4	17
Biscuit, reg	260	12	7	740	33	2	2	5
Biscuit, lrg	320	16	8	850	39	3	3	5
Bacon, Egg & Cheese McGriddles	420	18	8	1110	48	2	15	15
Sausage, Egg & Cheese McGriddles	560	32	12	1360	48	2	15	20
Sausage McGriddles	420	22	8	1030	44	2	15	11
Big Breakfast, reg	740	48	17	1560	51	3	3	28
Big Breakfast, lrg	800	52	18	1680	56	4	3	28
Deluxe Breakfast, reg	1090	56	19	2150	111	6	17	36
Deluxe Breakfast, lrg	1150	60	20	2260	116	7	17	36
Sausage Burrito	300	16	7	830	26	1	2	12
McSkillet Burrito w/ Sausage	610	36	14	1390	44	3	4	27
McSkillet Burrito w/ Steak	570	30	12	1470	44	3	4	32
Sausage Patty	170	15	5	340	1	0	0	7
Scrambled Eggs, 2	170	11	4	180	1	0	0	15
Hash Brown	150	9	1.5	310	15	2	0	1
Hotcakes	350	9	2	590	60	3	14	8
Hotcakes & Sausage	520	24	7	930	61	3	14	15
Hotcake Syrup, 60 g	180	0	0	20	45	0	32	0
Whipped Margarine, 6 g	40	4.5	1.5	55	0	0	0	0
Grape Jam, 0.5 oz	35	0	0	0	9	0	9	0
Strawberry Preserves, 0.5 oz	35	0	0	0	9	0	0	0

Burger/Sandwich

Description & Serving	Cal	Fat	Sfat	Sod	Carb	Fiber	Sugar	Prot
Hamburger	250	9	3.5	520	31	2	6	12
Cheeseburger	300	12	6	750	33	2	6	15
Double Cheeseburger	440	23	11	1150	34	2	7	25
McDouble	390	19	8	920	33	2	7	22
Quarter Pounder	410	19	7	730	37	2	8	24
Quarter Pounder w/ Cheese	510	26	12	1190	40	3	9	29
Double Quarter Pounder w/ Cheese	740	42	19	1380	40	3	9	48
Big Mac	540	29	10	1040	45	3	9	25
Big N' Tasty	460	24	8	720	37	3	8	24
Big N' Tasty w/ Cheese	510	28	11	960	38	3	8	27
Angus Bacon & Cheese	790	39	17	2070	63	4	13	45
Angus Deluxe	750	39	16	1700	61	4	10	40
Angus Mushroom & Swiss	770	40	17	1170	59	4	8	44
Filet-O-Fish	380	18	3.5	640	38	2	5	15
McChicken	360	16	3	830	40	2	5	14
McRib	500	26	10	980	44	3	11	22
Premium Grilled Chicken Classic Sandwich	420	10	2	1190	51	3	11	32
Premium Crispy Chicken Classic Sandwich	530	20	3.5	1150	59	3	12	28
Premium Grilled Chicken Club Sandwich	530	17	6	1410	52	4	12	39
Premium Crispy Chicken Club Sandwich	630	28	7	1360	60	4	13	35
Premium Grilled Chicken Ranch BLT Sandwich	470	12	3	1440	54	3	12	36
Premium Crispy Chicken Ranch BLT Sandwich	580	23	4.5	1400	62	3	13	31
Southern Style Crispy Chicken Sandwich	400	17	3	1030	39	1	6	24

Description & Serving	Cal	Fat	Sfat	Sod	Carb	Fiber	Sugar	Prot
Wrap								
Ranch Snack Wrap (Crispy)	340	17	4.5	810	33	1	2	14
Ranch Snack Wrap (Grilled)	270	10	4	830	26	1	2	18
Honey Mustard Snack Wrap (Crispy)	330	16	4.5	780	34	1	4	14
Honey Mustard Snack Wrap (Grilled)	260	9	3.5	800	27	1	4	18
Chipotle BBQ Snack Wrap (Crispy)	330	15	4.5	810	35	1	4	14
Chipotle BBQ Snack Wrap (Grilled)	260	9	3.5	830	28	1	5	18
Chicken								
Chicken McNuggets, 4 pc	190	12	2	400	11	0	0	10
Chicken McNuggets, 6 pc	280	17	3	600	16	0	0	14
Chicken McNuggets, 10 pc	460	29	5	1000	27	0	0	24
Chicken Selects Premiun Breast Strips, 3	400	24	3.5	1010	23	0	0	23
Chicken Selects Premiun Breast Strips, 5	660	40	6	1680	39	0	0	38
French Fries								
French Fries, sml	230	11	1.5	160	29	3	0	3
French Fries, med	380	19	2.5	270	48	5	0	4
French Fries, lrg	500	25	3.5	350	63	6	0	6
Salad								
Premium Southwest Salad w/ Grilled Chicken	320	9	3	960	30	6	11	30
Premium Southwest Salad w/ Crispy Chicken	430	20	4	920	38	6	12	26
Premium Southwest Salad (w/o chicken)	140	4.5	2	150	20	6	6	6
Premium Bacon Ranch Salad w/ Grilled Chicken	260	9	4	1010	12	3	5	33
Premium Bacon Ranch Salad w/ Crispy Chicken	370	20	6	970	20	3	6	29
Premium Bacon Ranch Salad (w/o chicken)	140	7	3.5	300	10	3	4	9
Premium Caesar Salad w/ Grilled Chicken	220	6	3	890	12	3	5	30
Premium Caesar Salad w/ Crispy Chicken	330	17	4.5	840	20	3	6	26
Premium Caesar Salad (w/o chicken)	90	4	2.5	180	9	3	4	7
Side Salad	20	0	0	10	4	1	2	1
Snack Size Fruit & Walnut Salad	210	8	1.5	60	31	2	25	4
Dressing/Condiment/Topping								
Butter Garlic Croutons	60	1.5	0	140	10	1	0	2
Newman's Own Southwest Dressing, 1.5 oz	100	6	1	340	11	0	3	1
Newman's Own Creamy Caesar Dressing, 2 oz	190	18	3.5	500	4	0	2	2
Newman's Own Low Fat Balsamic Vinaigrette, 1.5 oz	40	3	0	730	4	0	3	0
Newman's Own Low Fat Family Recipe Italian Dressing, 1.5 oz	60	2.5	0	730	8	0	1	1
Newman's Own Ranch Dressing, 2 oz	170	15	2.5	530	9	0	4	1
Spicy Buffalo Sauce, 43 g	70	7	1	960	1	2	0	0
Creamy Ranch Sauce, 43 g	200	22	3.5	320	2	0	1	0
Tangy Honey Mustard Sauce, 43 g	70	2.5	0	170	13	0	9	1
Southwestern Chipotle Barbeque Sauce, 43 g	70	0	0	260	18	1	13	0
Ketchup, 10 g	15	0	0	110	3	0	2	0
Barbeque Sauce, 28 g	50	0	0	260	12	0	10	0
Honey, 14 g	50	0	0	0	12	0	11	0
Hot Mustard Sauce, 28 g	60	2.5	0	250	9	2	6	1
Sweet 'N Sour Sauce, 28 g	50	0	0	150	12	0	10	0

Description & Serving	Cal	Fat	Sfat	Sod	Carb	Fiber	Sugar	Prot
Dessert								
Fruit 'n Yogurt Parfait	160	2	1	85	31	1	21	4
Fruit 'n Yogurt Parfait w/o granola	130	2	1	55	25	0	19	4
Apple Dippers	35	0	0	0	8	0	6	0
Vanilla Reduced Fat Ice Cream Cone	150	3.5	2	60	24	0	18	4
Kiddie Cone	45	1	0.5	20	8	0	6	1
Strawberry Sundae	280	6	4	95	49	1	45	6
Hot Caramel Sundae	340	8	5	160	60	1	44	7
Hot Fudge Sundae	330	10	7	180	54	2	48	8
Peanuts for Sundae	45	3.5	0.5	0	2	1	0	2
Low Fat Caramel Dip, 0.8 oz	70	0.5	0	35	15	0	9	0
McFlurry w/ M&M's Candies, 12 oz	620	20	12	190	96	1	85	14
McFlurry w/ Oreo Cookies, 12 oz	550	17	9	250	88	1	73	13
Chocolate Triple Thick Shake, 12 oz	440	10	6	290	76	1	63	10
Strawberry Triple Thick Shake, 12 oz	420	10	6	130	73	0	63	10
Vanilla Triple Thick Shake, 12 oz	420	10	6	140	72	0	54	9
Baked Hot Apple Pie	250	13	7	170	32	4	13	2
Cinnamon Melts	460	19	9	370	66	3	32	6
McDonaldland Cookies	260	8	2.5	300	43	1	13	4
Chocolate Chip Cookie	160	8	3.5	90	21	1	15	2
Oatlmeal Raisin Cookie	150	6	2.5	135	22	1	13	2
Sugar Cookie	160	7	3	120	21	0	11	2
Beverage								
Iced Coffee & Tea								
Iced Coffee - Caramel, med (11.5 oz)	190	8	5	115	27	0	27	2
Iced Coffee - Hazelnut, med (11.5 oz)	190	8	5	60	29	0	29	2
Iced Coffee - Regular, med (11.5 oz)	200	8	5	60	30	0	30	2
Iced Coffee - Vanilla, med (11.5 oz)	190	8	5	60	29	0	28	2
Iced Coffee w/ Sugar Free Vanilla Syrup, med (11.5 oz)	90	8	5	100	11	0	2	2
Sweet Tea, child (12 oz)	90	0	0	5	23	0	23	0
Sweet Tea, sml (16 oz)	120	0	0	10	30	0	30	0
Nonfat Coffee & Tea								
Nonfat Cappuccino, sml (12 oz)	60	0	0	85	9	0	9	6
Nonfat Latte, sml (12 oz)	90	0	0	115	13	0	13	9
Nonfat Caramel Cappuccino, sml (12 oz)	150	0	0	120	33	0	32	5
Nonfat Caramel Latte, sml (12 oz)	170	0	0	150	36	0	36	7
Nonfat Hazelnut Cappuccino, sml (12 oz)	150	0	0	70	34	0	34	5
Nonfat Hazelnut Latte, sml (12 oz)	180	0	0	95	37	0	37	7
Nonfat Vanilla Cappuccino, sml (12 oz)	150	0	0	70	34	0	34	5
Nonfat Vanilla Latte, sml (12 oz)	180	0	0	95	37	0	37	7
Nonfat Cappuccino w/ Sugar Free Vanilla Syrup, sml (12 oz)	50	0	0	100	15	0	8	5
Nonfat Latte w/ Sugar Free Vanilla Syrup, sml (12 oz)	80	0	0	130	18	0	11	7
Mocha w/ Nonfat Milk, sml (12 oz)	240	5	3	130	41	0	34	7
Hot Chocolate w/ Nonfat Milk, sml (12 oz)	250	5	3	140	14	0	37	8
Iced Nonfat Latte, sml (12 oz)	50	0	0	70	2	0	7	5

Description & Serving	Cal	Fat	Sfat	Sod	Carb	Fiber	Sugar	Prot
Iced Nonfat Caramel Latte, sml (12 oz)	140	0	0	105	30	0	30	3
Iced Nonfat Hazelnut Latte, sml (12 oz)	140	0	0	50	32	0	32	3
Iced Nonfat Vanilla Latte, sml (12 oz)	140	0	0	50	31	0	31	3
Iced Nonfat Latte w/ Sugar Free Vanilla Syrup, sml (12 oz)	40	0	0	85	13	0	5	4
Iced Mocha w/ Nonfat Milk, med (16 oz)	270	8	4.5	140	43	0	35	7
Whole Milk Coffee & Tea								
Cappuccino, sml (12 oz)	120	7	4	85	9	0	9	6
Latte, sml (12 oz)	150	8	4.5	105	11	0	11	8
Caramel Cappuccino, sml (12 oz)	200	5	3	125	32	0	32	5
Caramel Latte, sml (12 oz)	230	7	4	140	35	0	35	7
Hazelnut Cappuccino, sml (12 oz)	200	5	3	70	34	0	34	5
Hazelnut Latte, sml (12 oz)	230	7	4	90	36	0	36	7
Vanilla Cappuccino, sml (12 oz)	200	5	3	70	34	0	34	5
Vanilla Latte, sml (12 oz)	230	7	4	90	36	0	36	7
Cappuccino w/ Sugar Free Vanilla Syrup, sml (12 oz)	100	5	3	105	15	0	7	5
Latte w/ Sugar Free Vanilla Syrup, sml (12 oz)	130	7	4	125	17	0	10	7
Mocha, sml (12 oz)	280	11	6	125	40	0	33	6
Hot Chocolate, sml (12 oz)	300	12	7	135	41	0	35	8
Iced Latte, sml (12 oz)	80	4.5	2.5	65	6	0	6	4
Iced Caramel Latte, sml (12 oz)	160	3	1.5	100	29	0	29	3
Iced Hazelnut Latte, sml (12 oz)	160	3	1.5	45	31	0	31	3
Iced Vanilla Latte, sml (12 oz)	160	3	1.5	45	31	0	31	3
Iced Latte w/ Sugar Free Vanilla Syrup, sml (12 oz)	60	3	2	80	12	0	4	3
Iced Mocha, med (16 oz)	310	13	8	140	42	0	35	7

Moe's Southwest Grill

Burrito

Homewrecker	890	33	15	2645	93	18	8	46
Triple Lindy w/ Sour Cream	845	31	15	225	88	16	5	46
Triple Lindy w/ Guacamole	795	26	9.5	2630	90	18	5	45
Joey Bag of Donuts	755	24	9.5	2210	86	16	3	44
Art Vandalay	740	27	13.5	2135	90	18	8	25
Homewrecker Streaker	580	24	12	1815	44	17	7	38
Triple Lindy Streaker w/ Sour Cream	535	22	12	1395	39	15	4	38
Triple Lindy Streaker w/ Guacamole	485	17	6.5	1800	41	14	4	37
Joey Bag of Donuts Streaker	445	15	6.5	1380	37	15	2	36
Art Vandalay Streaker	430	18	10.5	1305	41	17	7	17

Fajita

Fat Sam	1220	52	21.5	3145	88	8	14	67
Alfredo Garcia	990	44	16	2710	82	6	10	65

Nacho

Billy Barou	1490	87	30	3085	117	23	8	55
Ruprict	1340	81	28.5	2575	114	23	8	34
Nacho Bar	1530	88	30	2760	130	27	9	58

Description & Serving	Cal	Fat	Sfat	Sod	Carb	Fiber	Sugar	Prot
Quesadilla								
John Coctosan	765	37	19	1835	56	16	5	48
Instant Friend	605	31	17.5	1135	51	16	3	27
Super Kingpin	510	31	17.5	1085	35	1	5	21
Taco								
Overachiever Hardshell Taco	315	15	6.5	780	23	10	3	19
Unanimous Decision Hardshell Taco	240	12	5.5	525	21	10	3	9
The Funk Meister Hardshell Taco	250	11	4	560	20	9	2	18
Overachiever Soft Taco	345	14	7	1020	29	10	4	21
Unanimous Decision Soft Taco	270	11	6	765	27	10	4	11
The Funk Meister Soft Taco	280	10	4.5	800	26	9	3	20
Taco Bar	620	28	11	1460	47	17	4	44
Salad								
Close Talker	1030	68	15	2130	67	18	9	41
Personal Trainer	880	62	13.5	1620	64	18	9	20
Close Talker Streaker	680	45	10.5	1610	34	16	8	36
Personal Trainer Streaker	530	39	9	1100	31	16	8	15
Salad Bar	910	46	13	2250	70	24	7	56
Salad Bar (Streaker)	560	24	8	1740	37	22	6	51
Side								
Chips	375	20	4	65	43	3	0	5
Rice	120	0	0	450	25	1	1	3
Beans	220	1.5	0	470	37	28	0	14
Baja Chicken Enchilada Soup	180	11	4.5	860	13	2	4	9
Kids								
Moo Moo Mr. Cow	395	14	5.5	1170	47	6	2	22
Power Wagon (Hardshell)	135	8	3.5	345	2	0	1	14
Power Wagon (Soft)	225	10	4.5	585	16	1	2	17
Mini Masterpiece	330	19	11.5	715	24	0	4	12
Dressing/Condiment/Topping								
Chipotle Ranch, 2 tbsp	160	18	2.5	160	2	0	1	1
Southwest Vinagrette, 2 tbsp	120	13	1	170	1	0	0	0
Queso, 2 oz	130	11	7	390	3	0	2	6
Guacamole, 2 oz	25	1	0	310	3	1	1	0
Pico de Gallo, 2 oz	10	0	0	150	2	1	1	0
Sour Cream, 2 oz	90	7	5.5	15	2	0	2	2
El Guapo Salsa, 2 oz	15	0	0	230	3	1	1	1
Kaiser Salsa, 2 oz	20	0	0	360	4	1	1	1
Tomatillo Salsa, 2 oz	15	0	0	250	3	2	1	0
Rock & Roll Salsa, 2 oz	25	1	0	320	4	1	0	1
Hard Rock Salsa, 2 oz	20	1	0	290	3	1	0	1
Grilled Peppers, 4 oz	25	1	0	35	3	1	1	1
Grilled Onions, 4 oz	70	3	0.5	90	9	4	6	1
Grilled Mushrooms, 4 oz	60	3.5	0.5	115	5	2	2	3

Description & Serving	Cal	Fat	Sfat	Sod	Carb	Fiber	Sugar	Prot
Dessert								
Chocolate Chunk Cookie	170	8	4	130	23	1	13	2
White Chocolate Macadamia Cookie	180	9	4	125	22	1	14	2
Oatmeal Raisin Cookie	160	6	2.5	115	23	1	12	2

Mr. Sub

Description & Serving	Cal	Fat	Sfat	Sod	Carb	Fiber	Sugar	Prot
Sandwich								
Assorted Cold Cuts Sub	290	9	3	1000	38	2	5	16
Italian Salami Sub	280	10	3.5	730	35	2	5	14
Maple Baked Ham Sub	250	4	1	970	40	2	5	15
White Albacore Tuna Sub	280	8	1	510	37	2	5	18
Meatball Sub	360	15	6	710	38	1	3	20
Roast Beef Sub	280	8	2.5	1430	35	1	3	21
Pizza Supremo Sub	270	10	3.5	730	34	1	3	14
Veggie Sub	180	2	0.5	260	34	2	4	7
BLT Sub	260	8	2.5	540	34	2	4	12
Grilled Chicken Sub	260	5	1.5	560	38	2	6	20
Breaded Chicken Sub	370	13	2	740	46	2	4	20
Montreal Style Corned Beef Sub	280	7	2.5	1200	34	1	3	21
Santa Fe Spicy Chicken Sub	370	13	2	740	46	2	4	20
Seafood w/ Crab Sub	300	10	1	750	43	2	8	11
Smoked Turkey Breast Sub	230	3.5	1	700	36	2	4	14
Louisiana Chicken Sub	290	8	2	820	35	1	3	19
Philly Style Steak Sub w/o Cheese	260	5	2	580	34	1	4	18
Philly Style Steak Sub w/ Cheese	300	8	3.5	780	36	1	5	21
Great Canadian Club Sub	300	8	2.5	1120	38	2	5	19
BBQ Rib Sub	360	17	5	640	34	1	3	20
Specialty Sandwich/Wrap								
Buffalo Chicken Panini Grilled Sub	260	5	1.5	560	38	8	6	20
Classic Reuben Panini Grilled Sub	290	7	2.5	1400	35	8	3	21
Ultimate Club Panini Grilled Sub w/o Cheddar	320	9	3	1340	38	8	5	31
Ultimate Cheddar Club Panini Grilled Sub w/ Cheese	440	18	9	1530	38	8	5	27
Tuna Melt Panini Grilled Sub	340	10	5	590	34	4	4	29
Louisiana Chicken Wrap	430	15	3	1470	48	20	0	25
Roast Beef Wrap	440	14	3	2280	49	20	1	28
Albacore Tuna Wrap	460	16	1	1100	52	24	4	25
Smoked Turkey Breast Wrap	360	9	1	1320	51	24	2	19
Seafood w/ Crab Wrap	470	19	1.5	1460	61	20	7	15
Veggie Wrap	310	8	0.5	730	49	24	1	10
Salad								
Garden Salad	35	0.5	0	10	6	8	3	3
Classic Caesar Salad	70	4.5	1.5	200	2	4	1	5
Grilled Chicken Caesar Salad	160	7	2	500	6	4	4	18
Seafood w/ Crab Salad	150	8	0.5	500	15	8	8	6
Maple Baked Ham Salad	85	1.5	0.5	550	10	8	4	8
Mediterranean Greek Salad	70	3	0.5	125	8	12	4	3

Description & Serving	Cal	Fat	Sfat	Sod	Carb	Fiber	Sugar	Prot
Smoked Turkey Breast Salad	80	2	0.3	460	8	8	4	9
Albacore Tuna Salad	140	6	0.4	260	8	8	5	13

Chili/Soup

Description & Serving	Cal	Fat	Sfat	Sod	Carb	Fiber	Sugar	Prot
Chili w/ Beef	198	1	0	1110	34	40	6	13
Hearty Chili w/ Beef	231	2	1	1590	36	44	8	18
Cream of Broccoli Soup	170	10	4.5	990	16	8	5	3
Creamy Tomato & Roasted Red Pepper Soup	110	2.5	1	950	19	8	9	4
Chicken w/ Rice Soup	90	2	0.5	930	15	4	1	3
Garden Vegetable Soup	60	0	0	890	13	4	2	2
Minestrone Soup	80	0	0	830	17	8	3	4
Italian Wedding Soup	140	3.5	1	970	24	4	2	4
Cream of Mushroom Soup	170	10	4.5	1080	16	4	5	4
Cream of Potato & Leek Soup	190	9	4.5	1040	23	8	4	4
Chicken Noodle Soup	110	2.5	0.5	1080	17	4	1	4
Cream of Tomato Soup	150	6	2	950	20	8	8	4
Vegetable Beef & Barley Soup	90	1	0	820	18	8	1	3
Pasta Fagioli Soup	150	1.5	0	970	28	24	5	7
Mediterranean Chicken Soup	110	3.5	1	800	15	4	3	4

Dessert

Description & Serving	Cal	Fat	Sfat	Sod	Carb	Fiber	Sugar	Prot
Double Chocolate Chip Cookie	160	8	5	135	23	1	15	2
Milk Chocolate Chunk Cookie	170	8	4	140	23	0	14	2
Triple Chocolate Chip Cookie	170	8	3.5	115	23	0	14	2
Carnival Cookie	160	7	3.5	140	24	0	15	2
Oatmeal Raisin Cookie	150	7	4	130	23	2	13	2

Bread

Description & Serving	Cal	Fat	Sfat	Sod	Carb	Fiber	Sugar	Prot
White Reduced Salt Sub Bun, sml	170	2	0.5	260	32	4	3	7
Whole Wheat Reduced Salt Sub Bun, sml	170	2	0.5	200	32	8	3	7
Multigrain Reduced Salt Sub Bun, sml	170	2	0.5	195	32	8	3	7
Mozza-Cheddar Reduced Salt Sub Bun, sml	200	4	1.5	290	33	4	3	9
Greek Seasoning Reduced Salt Sub Bun, sml	200	3.5	1	440	35	4	3	7
Whole Wheat Tortilla	180	4.5	0	450	30	13	0	6
Regular Tortilla	200	4.5	0.5	460	32	5	0	6
Cheese Tortilla	190	4.5	0.5	510	31	5	0	5
Sun Dried Tortilla	190	4.5	0.5	470	32	5	0	5

Topping

Description & Serving	Cal	Fat	Sfat	Sod	Carb	Fiber	Sugar	Prot
Bacon, 2 strips	50	4	1.5	190	0	0	0	3
Iceberg Lettuce	15	0	0	10	3	1	2	1
Tomatoes, 3 wheels	20	0	0	5	4	1	3	1
Red Onions	4	0	0	0	1	0	0	0.1
Green Pepper	2	0	0	0	1	0	0	0.1
Dill Pickles, 3 slices	1	0	0	110	0	0	0	0
Green Olives	10	0.5	0.1	160	1	0	0	0.1
Cucumbers, 3 slices	2	0	0	0	0	0	0	0.1
Jalapeño Peppers	2	0	0	160	0	0	0	0
Banana Peppers	2	0	0	110	0	0	0	0.1
Sliced Mushrooms	3	0	0	100	1	0	0	0.2
Croutons, 14 g	60	1.5	0.2	230	10	0	0	1

Description & Serving	Cal	Fat	Sfat	Sod	Carb	Fiber	Sugar	Prot
Process Slice Cheese for most sml subs	40	3	2	200	2	0	1	3
Process Slice Cheese for sml Pizza subs	80	6	3.5	390	3	0	2	5
Cheddar Cheese for sml Ultimate Cheddar Club Sub	120	9	6	190	0	0	0	6
Cheddar/Mozzarella Cheese Shred for wraps	50	3.5	2	85	1	0	1	4
Cheddar/Mozzarella Cheese Shred for most salads	75	5	4	130	1	0	1	6
Parmesan for Caesar salads	60	4	2.5	100	1	0	1	4
Feta Cheese for Greek Salad	85	7	4.5	360	1	0	1	5

Dressing/Condiment

Description & Serving	Cal	Fat	Sfat	Sod	Carb	Fiber	Sugar	Prot
Secret Sauce, 10 g	40	4	0.3	25	0	0	0	0
Light Mayo, 10 g	40	3.5	0.3	85	2	0	1	0.1
Buttermilk Ranch, 10 g	40	4	0.3	85	0.5	0	0.5	0.2
Honey Mustard, 10 g	20	0.1	0	65	5	0	4	0.1
Hot Sauce, 10 g	3	0.1	0	330	0	0	0	0.4
Pizza Sauce, 10 g	5	0	0	80	2	0	1	0.1
Louisiana Chicken Sauce, 10g	10	0	0	140	2	0	1	0.1
BBQ Sauce, 30 g	45	0	0	310	11	0	10	0.4
Meatball Sauce, 30 g	20	0	0	230	4	0	3	0.3
Mustard, 10 g	5	0.3	0	115	1	0	0	0.4
Caesar Dressing, 1 pouch	200	21	2.5	340	2	0	1	1
Greek Feta Dressing, 1 pouch	170	17	2	230	4	0	2	0.5
Ranch Dressing, 1 pouch	190	20	2	300	2	0	2	0.5
Lite Italian Dressing, 1 pouch	80	9	1	340	1	0	1	0
French Dressing, 1 pouch	130	13	1.5	410	5	0	4	0.1

Mrs. Fields

Cookie, 1 per serving

Description & Serving	Cal	Fat	Sfat	Sod	Carb	Fiber	Sugar	Prot
Oatmeal Peanut Butter Scotchy Cookie	300	16	7	220	34	2	22	5
Butter Toffee Cookie	280	13	4	190	37	1	21	3
Chewy Fudge Cookie	280	14	8	65	37	2	25	3
Chocolate Lovers Cookie	280	13	8	170	39	1	26	3
Cinnamon Sugar Cookie	270	12	6	160	39	1	20	3
Debra's Special (Oatmeal Raisin Walnut) Cookie	270	12	5	210	38	2	23	3
M&M Milk Chocolate Chip Cookie	320	15	8	190	43	1	29	3
M&M Sugar Butter Cookie	290	13	7	170	41	1	24	3
Milk Chocolate Chip Cookie	280	13	7	180	39	1	26	3
Milk Chocolate Macadamia Nut Cookie	300	16	7	160	36	1	24	3
Milk Chocolate Walnut Cookie	290	15	7	170	37	1	25	3
Peanut Butter Cookie	290	15	6	240	33	1	18	5
Peanut Butter Milk Chocolate Chip Cookie	320	17	6	260	36	2	20	6
Semi Sweet Chocolate Chip Cookie	280	13	7	170	39	1	25	3
Semi Sweet Walnut Cookie	290	15	7	160	38	2	24	3
Sugar Butter Cookie	260	11	6	160	37	1	20	3
White Chocolate Macadamia Cookie	310	16	8	170	36	0	25	3
Frosted Sugar Butter Cookie	360	17	7	170	49	1	32	3

Description & Serving	Cal	Fat	Sfat	Sod	Carb	Fiber	Sugar	Prot
Nibblers, 3 per serving								
Cinnamon Sugar Nibblers	160	7	4	95	24	0	12	2
M&M Nibblers	170	7	4	85	23	0	10	2
Milk Chocolate Chip Nibblers	170	8	5	105	23	1	15	2
Milk Chocolate Walnut Nibblers	170	9	4	100	22	1	14	2
Oatmeal Raisin Walnut Nibblers	160	7	3	125	23	1	13	2
Peanut Butter Nibblers	170	9	4	140	20	1	11	3
Semi Sweet Chocolate Chip Nibblers	170	8	5	100	23	1	15	2
Sugar Butter Nibblers	170	7	4	105	23	0	12	2
White Chunk Macadamia Nibblers	180	10	5	100	22	0	15	2
Other Desserts								
Double Fudge Brownie	490	26	15	180	65	3	51	5
Frosted Fudge Brownie	500	24	12	200	70	2	58	4
Peanut Butter Dream Bar Brownie	640	39	19	300	70	4	59	9
Pecan Fudge Brownie	430	25	12	150	51	2	39	5
Rocky Mountain Mogul Brownie	640	37	18	170	77	4	59	7
Walnut Fudge Brownie	430	24	12	150	51	2	39	5
Big Cookie Cake - 16 servings	470	22	10	260	66	2	46	4
Cookie Cake Slice	680	31	16	400	95	3	64	6
Cookie Card	500	23	11	270	71	2	51	4
Heart Cookie Cake	420	20	9	230	60	2	43	3
Little Sweethearts	500	23	11	270	71	2	51	4
Cranberry White Chunk	270	12	5	200	39	1	24	3
Frosted Lemon Cookie	370	15	7	160	56	0	37	3
Pumpkin Harvest	260	14	7	330	31	1	18	3
Hand-Dipped Chewy Fudge	430	22	15	95	58	2	46	4
Hand-Dipped Peanut Butter	440	24	11	260	51	2	35	7
SWO Cookie Sandwich	810	40	18	360	111	3	82	5
MWO Cookie Sandwich	820	40	18	370	110	2	83	6
Chewy Fudge Cookie Cup	460	24	11	80	60	2	48	3
Disney Cookie Cup	340	16	6	170	47	1	34	2
Peanut Butter Cookie Cup	470	25	8	260	56	1	40	5
Semi Sweet Cookie Cup	460	23	10	180	62	1	48	3
Peanut Butter Mini Cookie Cup	70	4	2	50	8	0	5	1
Semi Sweet Mini Cookie Cup	70	3.5	2	35	9	0	7	1
Blueberry Muffin	370	16	5	510	49	1	28	5
Chocolate Chip Muffin	430	21	8	500	56	2	33	5
Raspberry Muffin	370	16	5	510	50	2	27	5
Blueberry Mini Muffin	80	4	1	115	11	0	6	1
Chocolate Chip Mini Muffin	100	5	2	120	13	0	8	1
Raspberry Mini Muffin	80	4	1	115	11	0	6	1
Desserts w/o Trans Fats								
Frosted Fudge Brownie	500	24	14	210	70	2	57	4
Big Cookie Cake - 16 servings	460	22	11	260	66	2	46	4
Cookie Cake Slice	650	30	16	390	92	3	62	5
Cookie Card	500	23	12	270	71	2	51	4
Heart Cookie Cake	420	20	10	230	60	2	43	3

Description & Serving	Cal	Fat	Sfat	Sod	Carb	Fiber	Sugar	Prot
Little Sweethearts Cookie Cake	500	23	12	270	71	2	51	4
SWO Cookie Sandwich	810	40	20	360	111	3	82	5
MWO Cookie Sandwich	830	41	20	380	110	2	84	6
Chewy Fudge Cookie Cup	450	24	12	80	60	2	47	3
Disney Cookie Cup	360	17	8	170	50	1	37	2
Peanut Butter Cookie Cup	470	25	10	260	56	1	40	5
Semi Sweet Cookie Cup	70	3.5	1.5	35	9	0	7	1
Mini Peanut Butter Cookie Cup	70	4	1.5	50	8	0	5	1
Mini Semi Sweet Cookie Cup	460	23	11	180	62	1	48	3

Beverage

Cappuccino Smoothie	620	20	13	140	106	0	106	6
Lemon Smoothie	710	18	11	110	123	6	117	11
Mango Smoothie	660	20	13	95	116	0	113	6
Mocha Smoothie	620	20	13	140	106	0	106	6
Peach Smoothie	650	20	13	110	117	0	115	6
Peach Smoothie, nondairy	480	0	0	20	130	0	127	0
Pina-Colada Smoothie	690	38	28	310	78	0	76	6
Raspberry Smoothie	650	20	13	95	117	0	112	6
Raspberry Smoothie, nondairy	480	0	0	0	130	0	123	0
Strawberry Banana Smoothie	650	20	13	95	115	0	108	6
Strawberry Banana Smoothie, nondairy	480	0	0	0	128	0	117	0
Cookies & Cream Chiller	1210	65	40	560	137	3	109	18

Nathan's Famous

Hot Dog

Nathan's Famous Beef Hot Dog	296.9	18.21	6.88	692.07	23.98	0.75	4	10.88
Nathan's Famous Beef Chili Dog	400	23	6	1000	33	2	5	16
Nathan's Famous Beef Cheese Dog	340	21	8	970	27	1	5	11
Hot Dog Nuggets	350.14	28.01	6	400.24	20.01	0	5	5
Corn Dogs on a Stick	380	21	5	730	39	1	13	7

Burger/Sandwich/Wrap

Super Cheeseburger	986.64	71.77	23.01	1348.62	46.91	2.79	10.61	35.16
5 oz Burger w/ Cheese	704.64	43.42	16.31	1070.54	44.54	2.2	10.28	32.61
Bacon Cheeseburger	782.73	50.11	19.66	1364.19	44.77	2.2	10.28	36.4
Double Burger w/ Cheese	1178.32	83.84	32.11	1298.79	44.98	2.2	10.28	57.08
Philly Cheese Steak	849.16	44.57	20.53	1554.15	70.21	2.4	1.21	43.96
Philly Cheese Steak Supreme	878.93	44.52	20.47	1625.15	75.52	3.3	2.57	46.39
Chicken Cheese Steak	600.78	19.16	9.06	1719.26	69.54	3.36	2.57	39.5
Original Krispy Chicken Sandwich	660	37	5	1180	57	4	9	26
Krispy Chicken Chipotle Club	750	36	10	1630	72	4	19	63
Krispy Homestyle Chicken Sandwich	720	45	6	1720	54	4	3	25
Grilled Chicken Sandwich	553.84	31.9	5.06	1157.53	39.93	2.59	3.34	27.39
Grilled Chicken Club Sandwich	598.84	35.2	6.36	1304.19	39.93	2.59	3.34	59.39
Grilled Chicken Caesar Wrap	700	34	11	1340	60	1	2	38
Grilled Chicken Santa Fe Wrap	750	39	13	1160	62	1	3	68

Salad

Garden Salad	100	3	0	110	15	5	4	4
Krispy Chicken Salad	290	10	1.5	850	31	5	4	52

Description & Serving	Cal	Fat	Sfat	Sod	Carb	Fiber	Sugar	Prot
Caesar Salad	410	31	8	970	16	4	3	15
Chicken Caesar Salad	530	35	8	1650	17	4	3	34

Soup

Manhattan Clam Chowder	270	4.5	0	2730	48	6	9	9
Chicken Noodle Soup	190	5	1.5	1560	27	3	7	10
New England Clam Chowder	250	4.5	3	1590	42	3	7	10

Entrée

Chicken

Chicken Tender Order, 3 ea	525.93	39	5.56	900	24	3	7.5	21
Chicken Tender Platter	1245.01	90.1	13.86	1352.18	80.27	9.52	31.03	26
Grilled Chicken Breast Platter	839.35	55.61	8.8	1133.69	58.28	6.52	23.52	24.15
Chicken Wing Order w/ Bleu Cheese, 5 ea	670	55	11	650	12	0	0	27
Chicken Wing Order w/ Bleu Cheese & Fries, 10 ea	1680	130	25	1360	59	4	4	57

Seafood

Fish & Chips Platter	1536.26	94.85	15.5	2742.87	163.01	10.57	40.73	34.78
Seafood Sampler	2080	111	18	3990	214	17	52	48
Fish Sandwich	435.28	18.31	3.21	714.78	49.77	2.72	7.24	18.18
Breaded Clam Order	470	27	4	470	40	6	4	18
Breaded Clam & Chips	933.93	61.09	8.75	525.28	75.01	9.69	7.69	21.69
Shrimp & Chips	1510	76	12	3510	176	11	45	25
Shrimp Boat	3710	176	25	8680	454	24	66	69

Side

French Fries, med	440	29	4.5	55	36	4	4	4
Cheese French Fries, med	490	34	7	460	41	4	5	4
French Fries, lrg	610	41	6	80	50	5	5	5
Cheese French Fries, lrg	680	46	9	620	56	5	7	6
French Fries, super	940	63	10	125	78	8	8	8
Cheese French Fries, super	1070	73	14	1070	89	8	11	10
Onion Rings, reg	543.76	44.55	6.25	579.89	36.24	1.45	4.35	2.9
Onion Rings, lrg	785.43	64.35	9.03	837.61	52.35	2.09	6.28	4.19
Mozzarella Sticks	385.93	27.63	8.16	940.5	20.25	0.9	6.3	13.5
Southwest Munchers	70	3.5	1.5	170	6	1	0	2
Cole Slaw	180	12	2.5	280	15	2	14	1
Hush Puppies	520	16	2	1960	84	4	16	10
Corn on the Cob	140	1.5	0	20	34	2	8	5

Dressing/Condiment

Nathan's Mustard, 1 tsp	0	0	0	40	0	0	4	0
Ketchup, 1 tbsp	15	0	0	190	4	0	4	0
Relish, 9 g	10	0	0	65	3	0	2	0
Mayonnaise, 1 tbsp	110	12	2	70	0	0	0	0
Honey Mustard Dipping Sauce, 1 oz	174	18	3	136	3	0	2	0
Barbeque Sauce, 1 oz	45	0	0	281	11	1	6	0
Tartar Sauce, 2 tbsp	100	8	1.5	240	5	0	4	0
1000 Island Dressing, 1 oz	220	21	3	350	6	0	6	0
Tzatzki Sauce, 2 tbsp	50	5	3.5	125	2	0	1	1
Garlic Sauce, 2 tbsp	60	5	1	420	4	1	2	0
Wing Sauce, 2 tbsp	30	8	1	230	0	0	0	0

Description & Serving	Cal	Fat	Sfat	Sod	Carb	Fiber	Sugar	Prot
Topping								
Aged Cheddar Cheese Sauce, 2.12 oz	100	8	2	720	6	0	1	1
Chili w/ Beans, 2 oz	80	4.75	2.25	382.5	4.75	1.5	0.5	4.75
Sauerkraut, 2 oz	13	0	0	600	2.5	1.5	0.5	0.5
Dessert								
Apple Pie	310	19	4	310	33	0	9	3
Beverage								
Nathan's Old Fashioned Lemonade, 16 oz	170	0	0	0	42	0	42	0
Nathan's Old Fashioned Orangeade, 16 oz	160	0	0	20	40	0	40	0

Noble Roman's

Description & Serving	Cal	Fat	Sfat	Sod	Carb	Fiber	Sugar	Prot
Pizza								
7" Cheese Pizza	623	22	10	1638	81	4	7	26
7" Pepperoni Pizza	721	34	14	1998	81	4	7	31
7" Sausage Pizza	881	45	18	2217	82	4	7	35
7" Works Pizza	822	39	18	2255	85	5	9	37
14" Cheese Pizza, whole	2232	80	36	5769	294	12	26	92
14" Cheese Pizza, 1 slice	223	8	4	577	29	1	3	9
14" Pepperoni Pizza, whole	2500	105	46	6759	294	12	26	104
14" Pepperoni Pizza, 1 slice	250	10	5	676	29	1	3	10
14" Sausage Pizza, whole	3091	157	62	7702	298	12	26	121
14" Sausage Pizza, 1 slice	309	16	6	770	30	1	3	12
14" Works Pizza, whole	3289	165	70	8748	317	17	33	144
14" Works Pizza, 1 slice	329	16	7	875	32	2	3	14
Wings								
Hot-N-Spicy Wings, 6	360	28	7	519	3	0	0	27
Bar-B-Que Wings, 6	360	22	6	1028	15	0	10	24
Pasta & Sandwich								
Lasagna	600	32	13	1150	56	6	7	27
Fettuccini	530	16	10	1260	78	2	6	22
Spaghetti	490	13	4	1150	72	3	12	20
Pizza Stuffer	420	18	6	1040	48	4	5	19
Baked Ham & Cheese Sandwich	787	54	20	2541	43	2	4	35
Baked Italian Roast Beef Sandwich	750	49	17	2636	37	2	4	41
Baked Stromboli Sandwich	1012	72	28	2985	50	5	9	44
Side								
Breadsticks w/ Cheese, 3	410	113	4	1050	59	3	4	16
Breadsticks w/ Tomato, 3	335	6	0	740	60	3	7	13
Breakfast								
Sausage, Egg & Cheese Biscuit Sandwich	589	40	15	1438	35	26	4	23
Bacon, Egg & Cheese Biscuit Sandwich	455	27	10	1272	35	1	4	14
Sausage Biscuit Sandwich	440	28	10	1020	34	26	4	14
Biscuits & Gravy	720	36	11	2800	84	2	12	16
Cinnamon Round	750	24	3	1073	126	3	31	12

Description & Serving	Cal	Fat	Sfat	Sod	Carb	Fiber	Sugar	Prot
Old Country Buffet								

Breakfast

Description & Serving	Cal	Fat	Sfat	Sod	Carb	Fiber	Sugar	Prot
Cinnamon Bread, 1 slice	160	2.5	0.5	140	32	1	13	3
Cinnamon Roll, 1	140	5	1	115	23	<1	10	2
Cinnamon Sugared Donut Holes, 1 pc	50	3	0.5	75	5	0	2	<1
French Toast, 1 slice	220	9	2	270	29	1	12	8
French Toast Stick	110	7	1	130	12	0	2	2
Glazed Donut	140	8	2	115	15	0	6	2
1 Pancake	130	5	1	280	19	<1	6	2
1 Waffle	120	3	0.5	420	19	<1	5	3
Denver Scrambled Eggs, 1 spoon	140	11	3	230	1	0	0	9
Egg, Poached	70	5	1.5	150	0	0	0	6
Eggs Benedict	260	16	4	780	16	1	2	14
Breakfast Quiche, 1 spoon	200	13	4	400	12	0	4	9
Scrambled Eggs, 1 spoon	120	10	2.5	100	0	0	0	7
Bacon, 1 slice	30	2.5	1	145	0	0	0	2
Sausage Link, 1	90	8	3	210	0	4	0	4
Grits, 4 oz	60	0	0	125	13	0	0	1
Oatmeal, 4 oz	60	1.5	0	110	12	2	0	2
Cheesy Hashbrowns, 1 spoon	140	9	5	320	10	6	1	6
Hash Browns, 1 spoon	100	6	1	170	11	2	0	2

Salad

Description & Serving	Cal	Fat	Sfat	Sod	Carb	Fiber	Sugar	Prot
Ambrosia Salad, 1 spoon	160	9	8	50	23	1	19	0
BLT Salad, 1 spoon	120	12	2	180	2	<1	2	2
Broccoli Apple Salad, 1 spoon	160	11	2	150	13	2	9	4
Bruschetta Tomato Salad, 1 spoon	90	7	1.5	180	4	1	3	3
Caesar Salad, 1 spoon	70	6	1	110	4	1	1	1
California Coleslaw, 1 spoon	100	0	0	85	24	1	22	1
Carrot & Raisin Salad, 1 spoon	140	9	1.5	115	17	2	13	1
Chicken Pasta Salad, 1 spoon	240	18	3.5	320	13	<1	1	6
Creamy Pea Salad, 1 spoon	180	15	4.5	220	10	3	4	6
Cucumber Tomato Salad, 1 spoon	30	1	0	360	4	<1	3	<1
Dilled Potato Salad, 1 spoon	110	8	2	240	10	1	1	1
Flavored Gelatin, 1 spoon	40	0	0	30	10	0	10	<1
Gelatin Whip, 1 spoon	80	3	2.5	55	13	0	11	<1
Greek Salad, 1 spoon	120	8	2	210	10	1	4	3
Macaroni Vegetable Salad, 1 spoon	240	16	3	330	21	1	4	5
Oriental Pasta, 1 spoon	150	8	1	330	14	2	2	8
Potato Salad, 1 spoon	110	6	1	260	13	1	4	2
Raisin Fluff, 1 spoon	120	4	2.5	125	21	<1	10	1
Seafood Salad, 1 spoon	310	26	3.5	500	15	1	3	4
Seven Layer Salad, 1 spoon	190	17	4.5	250	4	1	2	5
Sicilian Pasta Salad, 1 spoon	140	7	1.5	430	16	1	2	4
Spring Mix, 1 cup	5	0	0	5	1	1	0	<1
Strawberry-Banana Salad, 1 spoon	80	0.5	0	0	20	2	13	1
Strawberry-Peach-Banana Salad, 1 spoon	70	0	0	170	18	1	14	<1
Strawberry Whip, 1 spoon	230	18	11	140	17	0	11	1
Tarragon Potato Salad, 1 spoon	120	7	1.5	155	13	1	1	1

Description & Serving	Cal	Fat	Sfat	Sod	Carb	Fiber	Sugar	Prot
Three Bean Salad, 1 spoon	90	4.5	0.5	480	12	3	0	2
Tossed Green Salad, 1 cup	5	0	0	5	1	1	0	<1
Waldorf Salad, 1 spoon	110	7	1	40	12	1	10	2
Whipped Pineapple-Banana Salad, 1 spoon	120	2	1.5	65	25	<1	21	1
Strawberry Walnut Salad, 1 spoon	80	7	0.5	5	6	2	3	2

Soup

Chicken Noodle Soup, 4 oz	80	2	0.5	300	8	<1	1	6
Chicken Rice Soup, 4 oz	60	1.5	0.5	300	5	<1	1	6
Chili Bean Soup, 4 oz	80	3.5	1.5	340	9	3	2	7
Corn Chowder, 4 oz	130	8	6	250	14	1	2	1
Cream of Broccoli Soup, 4 oz	80	6	3.5	170	6	1	1	1
Navy Bean Soup w/ Ham, 4 oz	50	0.5	0	350	9	2	2	4
New England Clam Chowder, 4 oz	150	11	8	440	12	<1	1	2
Potato Cheese Soup, 4 oz	120	9	5	260	9	1	<1	3

Sandwich/Hot Dog

Grilled Cheese Sandwich, 1	310	18	7	830	28	1	3	10
Hamburger Patty, 1	200	14	5	55	0	0	0	19
Turkey Hot Dog, 1	130	11	3.5	570	2	0	1	6
Mini Corn Dogs, 1 pc	45	2.5	0.5	120	5	0	1	1

Entrée

Beef

BBQ Beef Ribs, 1 serving	300	23	9	350	7	0	6	17
Beef & Broccoli, 1 spoon	190	15	4	160	7	1	4	7
BBQ Carved Beef Brisket, 3 oz	210	11	4	630	2	0	1	25
Carved Roast Beef, 3 oz	230	15	7	55	0	0	0	23
Taco Meat, Beef, 2 oz	100	5	2	310	3	0	1	11

Chicken/Turkey

Buffalo Chicken Tender, 1	80	5	0.5	350	5	0	0	4
Chicken & Dumplings, 1 spoon	170	6	1	530	17	<1	3	11
Chicken Cacciatore, 1 spoon	220	11	3	320	3	<1	1	26
Chicken Fajitas, 1 spoon	150	12	2.5	830	3	1	1	9
Hand Breaded Fried Chicken Breast, 1	280	12	3	240	3	1	0	40
Hand Breaded Fried Chicken Drumstick, 1	130	8	2	115	1	0	0	12
Hand Breaded Fried Chicken Thigh, 1	250	16	4	220	3	<1	0	23
Hand Breaded Fried Chicken Wing, 1	70	3	1	60	1	0	0	10
Roasted Jerk Chicken Breast, 1	280	13	3.5	450	0	0	0	40
Roasted Jerk Chicken Drumstick, 1	140	9	2.5	330	0	0	0	13
Roasted Jerk Chicken Thigh, 1	250	17	4.5	520	0	0	0	25
Roasted Jerk Chicken Wing, 1	80	4	1	240	0	0	0	10
Rotisserie Style Chicken Breast, 1	270	12	3.5	330	1	0	0	40
Rotisserie Style Chicken Drumstick, 1	130	9	2.5	160	<1	0	0	13
Rotisserie Style Chicken Thigh, 1	250	17	4.5	250	<1	0	0	25
Chicken Strip, 1	70	3.5	0.5	210	5	0	0	4
Teriyaki Chicken, 1 pc	60	2.5	0.5	350	3	0	3	6
Traditional Baked Chicken Breast, 1	270	12	3.5	270	<1	0	0	40
Traditional Baked Chicken Drumstick, 1	130	9	2.5	160	<1	0	0	13
Traditional Baked Chicken Thigh, 1	240	16	4.5	200	<1	0	0	24

Description & Serving	Cal	Fat	Sfat	Sod	Carb	Fiber	Sugar	Prot
Chinese Chicken Livers, 1 spoon	200	12	2	340	17	1	3	8
Country BBQ Chicken Breast, 1	300	12	3	320	6	1	3	40
Country BBQ Chicken Drumstick, 1	150	8	2	140	5	0	2	13
Country BBQ Chicken Thigh, 1	260	16	4	280	6	<1	3	23
Country BBQ Chicken Wing, 1	80	3	1	100	3	0	1	10
Honey BBQ Chicken, 1 spoon	200	9	2.5	480	9	0	8	21
Hot Wings-Drummies, 1	50	3.5	0.5	160	0	0	0	6
Hot Wings-Wing, 1	70	4	1	180	0	0	0	9
Orange Chicken, 1 spoon	240	9	2	510	32	1	14	8
Carved Roast Turkey, 3 oz	170	8	2.5	60	0	0	0	24

Pasta/Pizza

Description & Serving	Cal	Fat	Sfat	Sod	Carb	Fiber	Sugar	Prot
Chicken Alfredo, 1 spoon	220	12	5	260	16	1	2	11
Italian Sausage Penne, 1 spoon	180	9	3	430	20	1	6	6
Macaroni & Cheese, 1 spoon	120	2.5	1	530	19	<1	1	4
Baked Mostaciolli, 1 spoon	100	3	1.5	260	13	1	3	7
Pasta Margherita, 1 spoon	150	7	2.5	300	18	1	4	5
Pasta Primavera, 1 spoon	180	10	4	230	17	2	2	4
Shrimp Alfredo, 1 spoon	200	10	4	280	14	<1	1	14
Spaghetti, 1 spoon	130	2.5	0.5	90	23	4	1	4
Cheese Pizza, 1 pc	150	4	2	350	22	1	2	8

Pork

Description & Serving	Cal	Fat	Sfat	Sod	Carb	Fiber	Sugar	Prot
BBQ Smoked Sausage, 1 spoon	140	10	4	380	9	<1	7	4
Carved Ham, 3 oz	140	9	3	970	0	0	0	13
Smoked Sausage & Sauerkraut (Sauerkraut only), 1 spoon	5	0	0	110	1	0	0	0
Smoked Sausage & Sauerkraut (Sausage only), 1 link	190	17	8	460	2	0	0	7

Seafood

Description & Serving	Cal	Fat	Sfat	Sod	Carb	Fiber	Sugar	Prot
Buttercrumb Baked Fish, 1 pc	190	10	2.5	280	3	0	0	23
Butterfly Shrimp, 1	35	1.5	0	70	4	0	0	1
Breaded Catfish, 1 pc	120	7	1.5	170	7	<1	0	6
Carved Salmon Filet, 3 oz	190	11	2	390	0	0	0	19
Clam Strip, 1	15	1	0	45	2	0	0	1
Fish Patties, 1 pc	180	9	1.5	510	17	<1	0	8
Fried Fish, 1 pc	90	4.5	1	210	10	<1	0	3
Fried Shrimp, 6	200	10	2	420	22	<1	1	7

Steak

Description & Serving	Cal	Fat	Sfat	Sod	Carb	Fiber	Sugar	Prot
Country Fried Steak, 1 pc	210	13	4	630	15	<1	0	9
Salisbury Steak, 1 pc	150	9	3.5	300	8	1	1	9

Side

Description & Serving	Cal	Fat	Sfat	Sod	Carb	Fiber	Sugar	Prot
Biscuit, 1	130	6	1.5	340	16	<1	1	3
Garlic Cheese Biscuit, 1	290	19	5	850	24	1	4	6
Breadstick, 1	120	4.5	1	170	16	<1	<1	3
Cornbread, 1 pc	140	5	1	280	22	<1	10	3
Dinner Rolls, White, 1	130	5	1	120	18	<1	4	3
Dinner Rolls, White-Pull-A-Part, 1	130	5	1	120	18	<1	4	3
Dinner Rolls, White-Parkerhouse, 1	230	7	1.5	220	36	1	8	6

Description & Serving	Cal	Fat	Sfat	Sod	Carb	Fiber	Sugar	Prot
English Muffin, half	60	0.5	0	200	13	<1	<1	2
Taco Shell, 1	50	2.5	0.5	45	7	<1	0	<1
Flour Tortilla, 1	120	3	0.5	240	20	1	<1	3
Cantaloupe, 1 spoon	25	0	0	10	6	<1	7	<1
Grapes, 1 spoon	60	0	0	0	15	<1	12	<1
Honeydew, 1 spoon	30	0	0	15	8	<1	7	<1
Pineapple, 1 spoon	35	0	0	0	10	1	7	0
Strawberries, 1 spoon	25	0	0	0	6	1	4	<1
Watermelon, 1 spoon	25	0	0	0	6	0	5	<1
Spanish Rice, 1 spoon	140	7	3.5	370	9	<1	2	9
White Rice, 1 spoon	100	0	0	5	23	2	0	2
Fried Rice w/ Ham, 1 spoon	130	6	1.5	720	14	<1	1	5
Vegetable Lo Mein, 1 spoon	90	2	0.5	410	16	2	4	3
Marinated Vegetables, 1 spoon	50	3.5	0.5	150	5	2	3	2
Pickled Beets, 1 spoon	60	0	0	110	18	2	16	<1
Stewed Prunes, 1 spoon	100	0	0	0	27	2	19	<1
BBQ Baked Beans, 1 spoon	170	4	1.5	890	33	5	19	5
Bread Dressing, 1 spoon	150	6	1	440	21	1	2	4
German Boiled Cabbage, 1 spoon	40	2.5	1	230	4	1	2	3
Green Cabbage, 1 spoon	70	5	1	500	6	2	4	2
Steamed Carrots, 1 spoon	40	2.5	0.5	65	7	3	4	<1
Chesapeake Corn, 1 spoon	80	3	0.5	360	13	2	3	2
Corn on the Cob, 1 pc	80	2.5	0.5	20	13	2	2	2
Steamed Corn, 1 spoon	90	2.5	0.5	210	17	2	2	3
Green Bean Casserole, 1 spoon	100	7	2	400	9	1	2	2
Green Beans, 1 spoon	15	0	0	340	3	1	1	<1
Green Beans El Greco, 1 spoon	20	0	0	150	6	2	3	1
Joe's Cracked Pepper Green Beans, 1 spoon	70	4.5	1.5	210	6	2	2	3
Montreal Vegetable Medley, 1 spoon	50	4.5	0.5	160	3	1	2	1
Breaded Okra, 1 spoon	220	12	1	590	28	3	2	3
Pinto Beans w/ Bacon, 1 spoon	70	2	1	380	13	4	0	4
Baked Potatoes, 1 ea	180	0	0	10	31	4	1	4
Baked Sweet Potatoes, 1 ea	160	0	0	5	47	3	9	3
Cowboy Potatoes, 1 spoon	180	9	1.5	640	23	3	1	3
Red Potatoes, 1 spoon	90	2	0.5	15	18	2	1	2
Red Beans w/ Ham, 1 spoon	90	1	0	440	18	8	1	8
Spinach Marie, 1 spoon	190	14	5	480	8	7	1	7
Winter Squash, 1 spoon	150	9	2	10	18	1	9	1
Turnip or Collard Greens w/ Bacon, 1 spoon	40	2.5	1	310	3	2	1	2
Candied Yams, 1 spoon	140	1.5	0	45	33	1	15	1
Sauteed Zucchini, 1 spoon	50	4	0.5	60	4	1	2	1

Dressing/Condiment

Description & Serving	Cal	Fat	Sfat	Sod	Carb	Fiber	Sugar	Prot
Bleu Cheese Dressing, 30 g	170	18	3	130	1	0	1	1
Creamy Italian Dressing, 29 g	110	11	1.5	450	3	0	2	0
Fat Free French Dressing, 30 g	35	0	0	210	8	<1	6	0
French Dressing, 33 g	150	12	2	230	12	0	12	0
Italian Dressing, 32 g	120	11	1.5	420	5	0	3	0
Low Fat Italian Dressing, 30 g	25	2	0	420	2	0	2	0
Ranch Dressing, 30 g	140	15	2.5	240	2	0	<1	0

Description & Serving	Cal	Fat	Sfat	Sod	Carb	Fiber	Sugar	Prot
Reduced Fat Ranch Dressing, 30 g	60	5	0	280	5	0	1	0
Fat Free Creamy Italian Dressing, 30 g	15	0	0	330	3	<1	1	0
Au Jus, 2 oz	0	0	0	120	0	0	0	0
Beef Gravy, 2 oz	25	1.5	0	230	2	0	0	0
Blueberry Syrup, 2 oz	250	0	0	80	63	0	61	0
Chicken Gravy, 2 oz	60	2	0	340	8	0	1	<1
Cocktail Sauce, 1 ladle	30	0	0	330	8	0	6	0
Country Gravy, 2 oz	40	2	1	190	5	0	1	<1
Cranberry Sauce, 1 ladle	45	0	0	10	12	0	12	0
Creamy Cheese Sauce, 2 oz	45	1.5	0.5	510	7	0	1	1
Hollandaise Sauce, 2 oz	140	13	3	260	5	0	2	1
Horseradish Sauce, 1 ladle	60	5	3	90	2	0	<1	1
Hot Sauce, 1 tsp	0	0	0	125	0	0	0	0
Jelly, packet	40	0	0	0	10	0	7	0
Ketchup, 1 tbsp	15	0	0	190	4	0	4	0
Maple Syrup, 2 oz	180	0	0	40	47	0	46	0
Margarine, melted	410	45	9	440	0	0	0	0
Margarine, packet	35	4	1	40	0	0	0	0
Marinara Sauce, 2 oz	50	1.5	0.5	300	7	0	6	1
Mayonnaise, 1 tbsp	100	11	1.5	85	0	0	0	0
Meat Sauce, 4 oz	80	3.5	1.5	400	4	<1	4	8
Mustard, 1 tbsp	10	0.5	0	170	1	<1	0	<1
Peanut Butter, 1 tbsp	100	8	1.5	80	3	1	1	4
Salsa, 1 ladle	10	0	0	150	2	0	0	0
Sour Cream, 1 spoon	25	2.5	1.5	5	<1	0	0	0
Soy Sauce, 1 tsp	2	0	0	340	<1	0	0	0
Tabasco Sauce, 1 tsp	0	0	0	125	0	0	0	0
Tartar Sauce, 1 ladle	150	14	2	220	4	0	3	0
Turkey Gravy, 2 oz	20	0.5	0	160	4	0	0	0

Topping

Description & Serving	Cal	Fat	Sfat	Sod	Carb	Fiber	Sugar	Prot
Croutons, 7	35	1	0	90	4	0	0	<1
Chow Mein Noodles, 1 spoon	35	1.5	0	50	4	<1	0	1
Shredded Cheddar Cheese, 1 spoon	40	3.5	2	60	0	0	0	3
Grated Parmesan Cheese, 1 spoon	30	2	1	110	0	0	0	3
Feta Cheese, 1 spoon	110	9	6	450	2	0	2	6
Imitation Shredded Cheese, 1 spoon	25	1.5	1	135	1	0	0	0
Imitation Bacon Bits, 1 spoon	30	1	0	125	2	<1	0	3
Real Bacon Bits, 1 spoon	25	1.5	0.5	220	0	0	0	3
Eggs, hard cooked & diced, 1 spoon	20	1.5	0.5	20	0	0	0	2
Black Olives, sliced, 1 spoon	15	1.5	0	130	1	<1	0	0
Cherry Peppers, 1 spoon	4	0	0	60	1	0	<1	0
Crushed Red Pepper, 1 tsp	10	0.5	0	0	1	<1	0	0
Diced Onions, 1 spoon	5	0	0	0	2	0	0	0
Jalapeño Peppers, 1 spoon	2	0	0	0	<1	0	0	0
Pepperoncini Peppers, 1 spoon	2	0	0	170	<1	0	0	0
Sauteed Green Peppers, 1 spoon	25	1.5	0.5	30	4	<1	2	<1
Sauteed Mushrooms, 1 spoon	45	3.5	0.5	20	2	<1	1	1
Sauteed Onions, 1 spoon	30	1	0	25	5	<1	2	<1
Sliced Pickles, 1 spoon	2	0	0	140	<1	0	0	0

Description & Serving	Cal	Fat	Sfat	Sod	Carb	Fiber	Sugar	Prot
Sliced/Diced Tomatoes, 1 spoon	2	0	0	0	<1	0	0	0
Sweet Pickle Relish, 1 tbsp	25	0	0	140	6	0	3	0
Julienne Carrots, 1 spoon	5	5	0	5	1	0	0	0
Cherry Tomatoes, 1	5	0	0	0	1	0	0	0
Sliced Cucumbers, 1 slice	2	0	0	0	<1	0	0	0
Sliced Mushrooms, 1 spoon	2	0	0	0	<1	0	0	0
Peas, 1 spoon	10	0	0	10	2	1	1	1
Red Onion, sliced, 1 ring	2	0	0	0	<1	0	0	0

Dessert

Description & Serving	Cal	Fat	Sfat	Sod	Carb	Fiber	Sugar	Prot
Apple Crisp, 1 spoon	150	2.5	0.5	75	32	1	27	0
Apple Reduced Sugar Pie, 1 pc	230	13	3	160	28	2	10	3
Apple Spice Cake, 1 pc	180	7	1	210	26	0	18	3
Apple Struedel Bites, 1 pc	80	5	1.5	35	7	0	2	2
Banana Nut Cake, 1 pc	270	12	2.5	190	37	<1	27	2
Bread Pudding, 1 spoon	190	8	3.5	170	27	<1	15	3
Butterscotch Brownie	170	9	2	210	20	0	14	2
Carrot Cake, 1 pc	240	12	2.5	220	29	<1	22	2
Cherry Cobbler, 1 spoon	200	9	2	100	31	1	7	1
Cherry Reduced Sugar Pie, 1 pc	170	10	7	330	18	0	2	2
Chocolate Cake, 1 pc	180	8	1.5	210	25	0	9	3
Chocolate Chip Cookie	130	7	2	110	16	1	9	1
Chocolate Chip Cookie Pizza, 1 slice	160	8	3	130	21	1	12	1
Chocolate Cream Pie, 1 slice	180	9	4.5	120	24	<1	15	2
Chocolate Cream Pie-Reduced Sugar, 1 slice	190	12	9	260	19	<1	1	2
Chocolate Decadence Cake, 1 pc	220	10	4	250	30	0	14	4
Chocolate Pudding, 1 spoon	120	4.5	1	100	19	<1	14	1
Chocolate Reduced Sugar/Calorie Pudding, 1 spoon	70	1	0.5	360	12	<1	4	4
Chocolate Soft Serve, 4 oz	120	3	2.5	70	21	<1	15	2
Coconut Cream Pie, 1 slice	160	5	3	125	27	1	20	2
Donut Hole	50	3	0.5	75	5	0	2	<1
Fudge Brownie	100	3	1	75	18	<1	14	1
Fudge, 1 pc	40	1.5	0.5	10	7	0	6	0
Glazed Donut	140	8	2	115	15	0	6	2
Hot Fudge Sundae Cake, 1 spoon	160	3	1	250	33	1	24	2
Ice Cream Cone	15	0	0	15	2	0	<1	0
Lemon Cream Pie, 1 slice	170	4	1.5	130	32	<1	26	3
Lemon Reduced Sugar Pie, 1 pc	170	10	7	330	18	0	2	2
Lime Reduced Sugar Pie, 1 pc	170	10	7	330	18	0	2	2
Nonfat NutraSweet Vanilla Soft Serve Frozen Yogurt, 4 oz	80	0	0	80	16	0	6	4
Nonfat Strawberry Soft Serve Frozen Yogurt, 4 oz	90	0	0	55	22	0	9	3
Nonfat Vanilla Soft Serve Frozen Yogurt, 4 oz	100	0	0	55	21	0	12	3
Oatmeal Raisin Cookie	120	5	1.5	100	16	1	8	1
Orange Reduced Sugar Pie, 1 pc	170	10	7	330	18	0	2	2
Peach Cobbler, 1 spoon	210	8	2	95	33	1	10	1
Peanut Butter Cookie	120	6	1.5	150	14	1	8	2
Plain Cheesecake, 1 pc	230	12	6	280	28	0	22	3
Raspberry Reduced Sugar Pie, 1 pc	170	10	7	330	18	0	2	2
Snickerdoodle Cookie	120	5	1	55	17	0	10	1

Description & Serving	Cal	Fat	Sfat	Sod	Carb	Fiber	Sugar	Prot
Strawberry Reduced Sugar Pie, 1 pc	170	10	7	330	18	0	2	2
Sugar Free Ranger Cookie	90	5	2	100	10	<1	0	1
Turtle Brownie	70	2	0.5	70	12	<1	8	1
Vanilla Pudding, 1 spoon	130	5	1	120	19	0	15	1
Vanilla Reduced Sugar/Calorie Pudding, 1 spoon	40	1	0.5	65	5	0	4	3
Vanilla Soft Serve, 4 oz	130	5	3.5	65	19	0	12	2

Dessert Topping

Description & Serving	Cal	Fat	Sfat	Sod	Carb	Fiber	Sugar	Prot
Butterfinger Pieces, 1 spoon	70	2.5	1.5	35	11	0	8	1
Butterscotch Topping, 1 pump	230	1	0.5	180	56	0	55	0
Chocolate Chips, 1 spoon	90	5	4	0	10	0	9	0
Chocolate Syrup, 1 pump	80	0	0	30	21	0	16	0
FunE Chips, 1 spoon	80	3	2	0	12	0	11	0
Gummy Bears, 9 pc	60	0	0	10	15	0	14	1
Honey Nut Topping, 1 spoon	170	12	2	125	9	2	5	5
Hot Fudge Topping, 1 pump	120	3	0.5	85	24	<1	18	1
Hydrox Cookies, crushed, 1 spoon	35	1.5	0	20	6	0	3	0
Malted Milk Balls, ground, 1 spoon	70	3	2.5	40	11	0	9	0
Nestle Crunch Pieces, 1 spoon	80	4	2.5	20	10	0	8	<1
Non-Dairy Whipped Topping, 1 spoon	60	5	4.5	20	3	0	3	0
Rainbow Sprinkles, 1 spoon	70	2	1.5	0	13	0	11	0
Strawberry Topping, 1 pump	70	0	0	10	18	0	17	0

Olive Garden

Appetizer

Description & Serving	Cal	Fat	Sfat	Sod	Carb	Fiber	Sugar	Prot
Alfredo Dipping Sauce	380	35	22	510	9	1	NP	NP
Breadstick (w/ garlic-butter spread)	150	2.5	0.5	350	28	2	NP	NP
Bruschetta	620	13	2.5	1760	100	10	NP	NP
Calamari	890	54	5	2330	64	2	NP	NP
Caprese Flatbread	600	33	10.5	1520	46	5	NP	NP
Chicken & Gnocchi, 1 serving	250	8	3	1180	29	2	NP	NP
Chicken Alfredo Pizza	1180	40	17	3330	144	11	NP	NP
Marinara Sauce	70	2.5	0.42	550	10	3	NP	NP
Parmesan-Peppercorn Sauce	300	30	5	340	6	1	NP	NP
Tomato Sauce (part of Sampler Italiano)	45	1.5	0.28	270	6	1	NP	NP
Calamari (part of Sampler Italiano)	440	27	2.5	1170	32	0	NP	NP
Chicken Fingers (part of Sampler Italiano)	330	16	1.5	940	23	0	NP	NP
Fried Mozzarella (part of Sampler Italiano)	370	22	9	800	26	2	NP	NP
Fried Zucchini (part of Sampler Italiano)	370	20	1.5	630	42	4	NP	NP
Stuffed Mushrooms (part of Sampler Italiano)	410	28	8	990	20	3	NP	NP
Toasted Beef & Pork Ravioli (part of Sampler Italiano)	360	16	2.5	780	39	2	NP	NP
Grilled Chicken Caesar	850	64	13	1880	14	4	NP	NP
Grilled Chicken Flatbread	760	44	14.5	1500	46	5	NP	NP
Hot Artichoke-Spinach Dip	660	32	15	1450	68	6	NP	NP
Lasagna Fritta	1030	63	24	1780	77	9	NP	NP
Mussels di Napoli	180	8	4	1800	13	0	NP	NP
Sicilian Scampi	500	22	10	1850	43	7	NP	NP
Smoked Mozzarella Fonduta	940	48	28	1940	72	7	NP	NP
Stuffed Mushrooms	410	28	8	990	20	3	NP	NP

Description & Serving	Cal	Fat	Sfat	Sod	Carb	Fiber	Sugar	Prot
Pizza								
Create Your Own Pizza (w/ cheese & sauce only)	910	28	12	2970	129	8	NP	NP
Bell Peppers (pizza topping)	10	0	0	0	2	1	NP	NP
Black Olives (pizza topping)	45	4	0.5	350	3	1	NP	NP
Italian Sausage (pizza topping)	140	11	4	360	1	0	NP	NP
Mushrooms (pizza topping)	5	0	0	0	1	0	NP	NP
Onions (pizza topping)	15	0	0	0	4	1	NP	NP
Pepperoni (pizza topping)	120	11	4.5	460	1	0	NP	NP
Roma Tomatoes (pizza topping)	10	0	0	0	2	1	NP	NP
Salad & Soup								
Garden-Fresh Salad, 1 serving w/ dressing	350	27	4.5	1990	22	3	NP	NP
Garden-Fresh Salad, 1 serving w/o dressing	120	3.5	0.5	550	17	3	NP	NP
Minestrone, 1 serving	100	1.5	0	1090	19	3	NP	NP
Pasta e Fagioli, 1 serving	130	2.5	1	730	19	6	NP	NP
Zuppa Toscana, 1 serving	170	4	2	950	23	2	NP	NP
Lunch Portion								
Pasta								
Braised Beef & Tortelloni	740	41	17	1280	60	5	NP	NP
Capellini Pomodoro	480	11	2	970	78	11	NP	NP
Cheese Ravioli w/ Marinara Sauce	530	18	9	1160	64	6	NP	NP
Cheese Ravioli w/ Meat Sauce	610	22	12	1210	65	8	NP	NP
Chicken Parmigiana	570	18	5	1720	66	18	NP	NP
Eggplant Parmigiana	620	26	8	1540	70	11	NP	NP
Fettuccine Alfredo	800	48	30	810	69	4	NP	NP
Five Cheese Ziti al Forno	770	32	17	1450	89	5	NP	NP
Lasagna Classico	580	32	18	1930	35	7	NP	NP
Linguine alla Marinara	310	4	1	670	55	5	NP	NP
Manicotti Formaggio	680	33	18	2100	58	7	NP	NP
Ravioli di Portobello	450	19	11	970	53	8	NP	NP
Spaghetti & Italian Sausage	830	44	16	1920	61	9	NP	NP
Spaghetti & Meatballs	820	40	16	1600	65	6	NP	NP
Spaghetti w/ Meat Sauce	550	21	8	1040	59	6	NP	NP
Chicken & Seafood								
Chicken & Gnocchi Veronese	710	42	20	2040	50	3	NP	NP
Chicken Alfredo	910	52	31	1150	71	4	NP	NP
Chicken Scampi	720	34	14	1370	69	17	NP	NP
Grilled Chicken Spiedini	460	13	2.5	1180	26	7	NP	NP
Grilled Shrimp Caprese	820	39	17	2800	81	0	NP	NP
Seafood Alfredo	670	36	21	1320	59	5	NP	NP
Shrimp Primavera	510	9	1.5	1130	79	12	NP	NP
Venetian Apricot Chicken	280	3	1	1180	32	8	NP	NP
Entrée (Dinner Portion)								
Pasta								
Braised Beef & Tortelloni	1020	53	22	2060	82	10	NP	NP
Capellini Pomodoro	840	17	3	1250	141	19	NP	NP
Cheese Ravioli w/ Marinara Sauce	660	22	11	1440	84	7	NP	NP
Cheese Ravioli w/ Meat Sauce	790	28	14	1510	88	12	NP	NP
Chicken Parmigiana	1090	49	18	3380	79	27	NP	NP
Eggplant Parmigiana	850	35	10	1900	98	19	NP	NP

Description & Serving	Cal	Fat	Sfat	Sod	Carb	Fiber	Sugar	Prot
Fettuccine Alfredo	1220	75	47	1350	99	5	NP	NP
Five Cheese Ziti al Forno	1050	48	26	2370	112	9	NP	NP
Lasagna Classico	850	47	25	2830	39	19	NP	NP
Linguine alla Marinara	430	6	1	900	76	9	NP	NP
Manicotti Formaggio	940	46	25	2530	81	8	NP	NP
Ravioli di Portobello	670	30	17	1400	74	15	NP	NP
Spaghetti & Italian Sausage	1270	68	24	3100	98	15	NP	NP
Spaghetti & Meatballs	1110	50	20	2180	103	9	NP	NP
Spaghetti w/ Meat Sauce	710	22	8	1340	94	9	NP	NP
Tour of Italy	1450	74	33	3830	97	10	NP	NP
Chicken & Seafood								
Chicken & Gnocchi Veronese	1030	58	26	2580	72	8	NP	NP
Chicken & Shrimp Carbonara	1440	88	38	3000	80	9	NP	NP
Chicken Alfredo	1430	82	48	2030	103	5	NP	NP
Chicken Marsala	770	37	5	1800	59	16	NP	NP
Chicken Scampi	1020	53	22	1880	84	17	NP	NP
Garlic-Herb Chicken con Broccoli	960	41	18	2180	90	12	NP	NP
Grilled Shrimp Caprese	900	41	17	3490	82	0	NP	NP
Herb-Grilled Salmon	510	26	6	760	5	6	NP	NP
Parmesan Crusted Tilapia	590	25	10	910	42	6	NP	NP
Seafood Alfredo	1020	52	31	2430	88	9	NP	NP
Seafood Portofino	800	33	14	1880	85	16	NP	NP
Shrimp & Asparagus Risotto	620	30	17	2530	44	19	NP	NP
Shrimp Primavera	730	12	2	1620	110	14	NP	NP
Stuffed Chicken Marsala	800	36	16	2830	40	6	NP	NP
Venetian Apricot Chicken	380	4	1.5	1420	32	8	NP	NP
Beef & Pork								
Chianti Braised Short Ribs	1060	58	26	2970	71	17	NP	NP
Mixed Grill	770	24	5	1980	48	13	NP	NP
Pork Milanese	1510	87	37	3100	118	11	NP	NP
Steak Gorgonzola-Alfredo	1310	73	41	2190	82	9	NP	NP
Steak Toscano	880	43	14	1700	45	12	NP	NP
Kids								
Cheese Pizza	470	14	6	1170	66	4	NP	NP
Cheese Ravioli w/ Tomato Sauce	300	8	4	440	43	4	NP	NP
Chicken Fingers	330	16	1.5	940	23	0	NP	NP
Children's Grilled Chicken	210	5.5	0.7	505	12	0	NP	NP
Broccoli	25	0	0	10	3	2	NP	NP
Fries	400	21	2	880	47	4	NP	NP
Fettuccine Alfredo	800	48	30	810	69	4	NP	NP
Grilled Chicken w/ Pasta & Broccoli	310	5	1	680	33	6	NP	NP
Macaroni & Cheese	340	6	2.5	1000	58	3	NP	NP
Spaghetti & Tomato Sauce	250	3	0.5	370	45	4	NP	NP
Chocolate Milkshake	520	22	14	230	72	7	NP	NP
Strawberry Milkshake	500	24	15	160	62	10	NP	NP
Sundae	180	9	6	21	45	0	NP	NP
Vanilla Milkshake	530	23	14	170	73	16	NP	NP
Dessert								
Black Tie Mousse Cake	760	48	27	270	73	8	NP	NP
Chocolate Gelato	620	25	20	150	89	6	NP	NP

Description & Serving	Cal	Fat	Sfat	Sod	Carb	Fiber	Sugar	Prot
Lemon Cream Cake	620	35	16	430	69	2	NP	NP
Tiramisu	510	32	19	75	48	2	NP	NP
Torta di Chocolate	800	51	29	125	75	4	NP	NP
White Chocolate Raspberry Cheesecake	890	62	36	490	70	6	NP	NP
Zeppoli	920	35	3.5	590	131	4	NP	NP
Chocolate Sauce	210	2.5	1.5	75	44	2	NP	NP

Beverage

Description & Serving	Cal	Fat	Sfat	Sod	Carb	Fiber	Sugar	Prot
Bellini Peach-Raspberry Iced Tea	70	0	0	0	16	NP	NP	NP
Berry Sangria	230	0	0	15	35	NP	NP	NP
Bianco Wine (White)	146	0	0	20	8	NP	NP	NP
Caffè la Toscana Coffee	0	0	0	5	0	NP	NP	NP
Caffè Latte	130	4	2	85	15	NP	NP	NP
Caffè Mocha	180	4	2.5	80	31	NP	NP	NP
Cappuccino	150	8	4	65	14	NP	NP	NP
Caramel Hazelnut Macchiato	220	4.5	2.5	40	43	NP	NP	NP
Chocolate Almond Amore	600	21	13	135	82	NP	NP	NP
Chocolate Martini	260	3.5	2	50	36	NP	NP	NP
Cream Sodas	200	6	4	50	36	NP	NP	NP
Frozen Cappuccino	320	10	6	60	53	NP	NP	NP
Frozen Tiramisu	410	14	8	95	54	NP	NP	NP
Italian Margarita	240	0	0	10	32	NP	NP	NP
Italian Sodas	120	0	0	5	30	NP	NP	NP
Lavazza Espresso	0	0	0	25	0	NP	NP	NP
Lime-Mint Fresco	230	0	0	45	29	NP	NP	NP
Limoncello Lemonade	260	0	0	5	42	NP	NP	NP
Mango Daiquiri	240	0	0	10	43	NP	NP	NP
Mango Martini	180	0	0	0	31	NP	NP	NP
Peach Bellini	170	0	0	0	33	NP	NP	NP
Peach Daiquiri	270	0	0	10	50	NP	NP	NP
Peach Fresco	200	1	0	10	22	NP	NP	NP
Peach Sangria	250	0	0	50	40	NP	NP	NP
Pomegranate Margarita Martini	290	0	0	5	44	NP	NP	NP
Raspberry Lemonade	110	0	0	15	29	NP	NP	NP
Rosato Wine (Blush)	146	0	0	20	8	NP	NP	NP
Rosso Wine (Red)	146	0	0	20	8	NP	NP	NP
Sicilian Citrus Fresco	210	0	0	10	25	NP	NP	NP
Sicilian Splash	100	0	0	15	25	NP	NP	NP
Sour Apple Martini	210	0	0	0	22	NP	NP	NP
Sparkling Wine	126	0	0	20	8	NP	NP	NP
Strawberry Bellini	220	0	0	0	46	NP	NP	NP
Strawberry Daiquiri	250	0	0	15	47	NP	NP	NP
Strawberry Fresco	230	0	0	5	31	NP	NP	NP
Strawberry Frozen Margarita	340	0	0	25	66	NP	NP	NP
Strawberry-Limoncello Martini	300	0	0	15	42	NP	NP	NP
Strawberry-Mango Frozen Margarita	350	0	0	20	68	NP	NP	NP
Strawberry Siciliano	360	10	6	50	46	NP	NP	NP
Tropical Sangria	220	0	0	10	32	NP	NP	NP
Venetian Sunset	190	0	0	10	38	NP	NP	NP
Wild Berry Bellini	160	0	0	10	31	NP	NP	NP
Wild Berry Daiquiri	270	0	0	5	50	NP	NP	NP
Wild Berry Frozen Margarita	290	0	0	20	55	NP	NP	NP

Description & Serving	Cal	Fat	Sfat	Sod	Carb	Fiber	Sugar	Prot

On The Border

Appetizer

Description & Serving	Cal	Fat	Sfat	Sod	Carb	Fiber	Sugar	Prot
Border Sampler, 1 serving	2090	141	50	5230	99	11	NP	101
Guacamole Live! w/o chips, 1 serving	570	50	10	3490	34	31	NP	11
Chicken Empanadas w/ Chile con Queso, 5 ea	1150	82	30	1970	71	3	NP	34
Beef Empanadas w/ Chile con Queso, 5 ea	1210	86	31	1950	72	5	NP	39
Firecracker Stuffed Jalapenos w/ Chile con Queso, 1 serving	1950	134	36	6540	123	3	NP	67
Chicken Flautas w/ Chile con Queso, 4 ea	1190	83	20	2860	57	6	NP	50
Grande Fajita Nachos - Mesquite-Grilled Chicken, 1 serving	1580	84	38	5220	88	16	NP	112
Grande Fajita Nachos - Mesquite-Grilled Steak, 1 serving	1670	101	46	3920	86	16	NP	92
Chicken Fajita Quesadillas, 1 serving	1250	83	31	2910	59	5	NP	62
Beef Fajita Quesadillas, 1 serving	1290	91	36	2260	58	5	NP	53
OTB Dip Trio w/o chips, 1 serving	470	36	14	1610	22	5	NP	17
Chile con Queso w/o chips, 1 bowl	390	30	19	1870	13	1	NP	26
Chile con Queso w/o chips, 1 cup	250	18	12	1170	8	1	NP	16
Chile con Queso Carne Style w/o chips, 1 bowl	480	35	21	2360	16	2	NP	32
Chile con Queso Carne Style w/o chips, 1 cup	330	24	14	1540	10	2	NP	22
Queso Blanco w/o chips, 1 bowl	620	48	31	2510	8	1	NP	33
Queso Blanco w/o chips, 1 cup	390	30	19	1560	5	0	NP	21
Queso Blanco Carne Style w/o chips, 1 bowl	710	53	33	3000	10	2	NP	40
Queso Blanco Carne Style w/o chips, 1 cup	470	35	21	1930	7	1	NP	27
Ultimate Loaded Queso w/o chips, 1 serving	780	52	27	2790	36	11	NP	45
Guacamole w/o chips, 1 serving	170	14	3	500	11	9	NP	4
Fajita Chicken Con Queso w/ tortillas, 1 serving	1520	90	47	4120	74	4	NP	102
Chips & Salsa, 1 basket	430	22	3.5	440	52	5	NP	5
Chipotle Chicken Rolls, 1 serving	770	27	14	1570	95	4	NP	27

Salad

Description & Serving	Cal	Fat	Sfat	Sod	Carb	Fiber	Sugar	Prot
Sizzling Fajita Salad - Chicken, no dressing	740	47	21	2210	26	7	NP	53
Sizzling Fajita Salad - Steak, no dressing	860	61	28	2120	26	11	NP	47
Grande Taco Salad w/ Spicy Chicken, no dressing	1260	84	28	2270	82	11	NP	44
Grande Taco Salad w/ Seasoned Ground Beef, no dressing	1390	95	33	2250	83	14	NP	53
Mexican Chopped Chicken Salad w/ Smoked Jalapeno Vinaigrette	720	39	7	2640	42	12	NP	46
Citrus Chipotle Chicken Salad w/ Mango Citrus Vinaigrette	290	3.5	2	840	42	11	NP	25
Chicken Fiesta Salad w/ Chipotle Honey Mustard	1070	72	22	2700	57	6	NP	58
Create Your Own Combo - Side House Salad w/o dressing	210	12	3.5	260	20	4	NP	6
Create Your Own Combo - Side Mexican Chopped Salad w/ Smoked Jalapeno Vinaigrette	230	15	3.5	470	19	6	NP	6

Soup

Description & Serving	Cal	Fat	Sfat	Sod	Carb	Fiber	Sugar	Prot
Chicken Tortilla Soup, bowl	490	25	8	2060	51	5	NP	19
Chicken Tortilla Soup, cup	320	18	7	1010	26	4	NP	14

Description & Serving	Cal	Fat	Sfat	Sod	Carb	Fiber	Sugar	Prot
Lunch								
Lunch Taco Salad w/ Seasoned Ground Beef, no dressing	950	67	22	1520	57	9	NP	32
Lunch Taco Salad w/ Spicy Chicken, no dressing	870	60	19	1540	56	7	NP	27
Lunch Fajita Nachos - Chicken	1090	59	27	3470	60	12	NP	75
Lunch Fajita Nachos - Beef	1150	70	32	2610	60	12	NP	62
Border's Best Chicken Lunch Fajitas w/ rice & w/o beans, tortillas, & condiments	480	16	2.5	1850	47	2	NP	32
Border's Best Steak Lunch Fajitas w/ rice & w/o beans, tortillas, & condiments	600	30	9	1760	47	5	NP	25
Lunch Chimichanga - Ground Beef w/o Sauce	1060	62	18	1860	93	4	NP	32
Lunch Chimichanga - Spicy Chicken w/o Sauce	920	48	14	1870	92	2	NP	26
Lunch Beef Burrito w/o Sauce	770	26	10	1580	91	2	NP	40
Lunch Chicken Burrito w/o Sauce	680	23	9	1870	92	2	NP	26
Entrée								
Beef								
Classic Beef Burrito w/ rice & w/o beans & sauce	1020	38	17	2030	106	2	NP	59
Big Beef Bordurrito w/ rice & side salad (no dressing) & w/o beans	2050	110	27	3840	171	13	NP	63
Little Bordurrito - Beef w/o dressing	1200	72	17	2020	90	8	NP	33
Classic Chimichanga Beef w/ rice & w/o beans & sauce	1410	87	27	2450	108	5	NP	47
Tres Enchiladas Dinner - Cheese & Onion w/ Chile Con Carne, w/ rice & w/o beans	1360	73	33	3460	130	7	NP	52
Tres Enchiladas Dinner - Beef w/ Chile Con Carne, w/ rice & w/o beans	1150	49	15	3030	130	10	NP	48
Grilled Enchilada - Smoky Beef Brisket w/ rice & w/o beans	1050	48	19	3140	103	3	NP	45
Create Your Own Combo - Beef Enchilada w/ Chile Con Carne	210	11	3.5	570	18	2	NP	10
Create Your Own Combo - Cheese & Onion Enchilada w/ Chile Con Carne	260	17	8	680	18	2	NP	11
Create Your Own Combo - Beef Empanadas w/ Chile con Queso	540	39	15	1040	30	2	NP	19
Beef Fajita Quesadillas	1290	91	36	2260	58	5	NP	53
Create Your Own Combo - Crispy Beef Taco	320	19	7	600	19	4	NP	18
Create Your Own Combo - Soft Beef Taco	340	18	8	890	24	3	NP	20
Taco Melt - Beef (Crispy) w/ rice & w/o beans	920	50	18	1830	81	6	NP	35
Taco Melt - Beef (Soft) w/ rice & w/o beans	1060	49	19	2700	111	7	NP	41
Brisket Tacos w/ Jalapeno BBQ Sauce, w/ rice & w/o beans	1360	55	20	4700	154	6	NP	58
Brisket Tacos	1030	38	14	3560	127	4	NP	41
Chicken (make H3)								
Classic Chicken Burrito w/ rice & w/o beans & sauce	900	33	15	2460	108	3	NP	38
Three Sauce Fajita Chicken Burrito w/ rice & w/o beans	1360	55	17	5050	122	4	NP	81
Big Chicken Bordurrito w/ rice & side salad (no dressing) & w/o beans	1970	93	8	5140	172	13	NP	83

Description & Serving	Cal	Fat	Sfat	Sod	Carb	Fiber	Sugar	Prot
Little Bordurrito - Chicken w/o dressing	1160	63	12	2670	91	8	NP	42
Classic Chimichanga Chicken w/ rice & w/o beans & sauce	1270	76	22	2460	108	3	NP	38
Tres Enchiladas Dinner - Chicken w/ Sour Cream Sauce, w/ rice & w/o beans	1180	65	13	2630	122	5	NP	27
Enchilada Suizas w/ rice & w/o beans	1090	56	16	2950	115	5	NP	32
Grilled Enchilada - Pepper Jack Chicken w/ rice & w/o beans	1210	52	16	3560	108	4	NP	56
Create Your Own Combo - Chicken Enchilada w/ Sour Cream Sauce	220	15	3	480	16	1	NP	5
Create Your Own Combo - Chicken Empanadas w/ Chile con Queso	510	37	15	1050	30	1	NP	17
Create Your Own Combo - Chicken Flautas w/ Chile con Queso	330	23	8	990	15	1	NP	16
Tender Mesquite-Grilled Chicken Fajita w/o rice, beans, tortillas, & condiments	360	18	3	1040	4	0	NP	36
Monterey Ranch Chicken Fajita w/ rice & w/o beans, tortillas, & condiments	1040	54	19	3570	69	1	NP	68
Chipotle Chicken Fajita w/ rice & w/o beans, tortillas, & condiments	940	42	11	3230	73	2	NP	55
Chicken Fajita Quesadillas	1250	83	31	2910	59	5	NP	62
Chicken Quesadilla Combo (quesadilla only)	610	38	14	1550	28	1	NP	35
Create Your Own Combo - Crispy Chicken Taco	240	12	4	620	19	2	NP	12
Create Your Own Combo - Soft Chicken Taco	250	11	4.5	910	24	2	NP	14
Taco Melt - Chicken (Crispy) w/ rice & w/o beans	790	39	13	1850	80	4	NP	26
Taco Melt - Chicken (Soft) w/ rice & w/o beans	930	38	15	2730	110	4	NP	32
Southwest Chicken Tacos w/ Creamy Red Chile Sauce, w/ rice & w/o beans	1530	88	21	3350	130	5	NP	55
Spicy Buffalo Chicken Tacos w/ Creamy Red Chile Sauce, w/ rice & w/o beans	1350	74	15	3880	115	4	NP	49
Grilled Fajita Chicken Tacos w/ black beans & grilled veggies	570	9	2	1910	78	18	NP	54
Fajita Chicken Tacos w/ black beans & veggies	570	9	2	1650	78	18	NP	54
Honey Chipotle Chicken	870	26	5	2450	117	3	NP	47
Chicken Salsa Fresca	520	9	3	2410	60	12	NP	50
Spice Crusted Chicken	850	25	5	2110	114	3	NP	47
Pork								
Savoy Pulled Pork (Carnitas) Fajita w/o rice, beans, tortillas, & condiments	820	68	14	1440	2	2	NP	34
Create Your Own Combo - Pork Tamale w/ Chile Con Carne	290	20	7	960	14	3	NP	13
Seafood								
Seasoned, Sauteed Shrimp Fajita w/o rice, beans, tortillas, & condiments	480	34	6	920	2	0	NP	26
Dos XX Fish Tacos w/ Creamy Red Chile Sauce, w/ rice & w/o beans	2350	152	31	4060	173	5	NP	58
Grilled Mahi Mahi Tacos	1050	55	12	2170	96	7	NP	39
Pico Shrimp Tacos w/ black beans & grilled veggies	490	5	1	1650	78	17	NP	34
Bacon-Wrapped Shrimp & Steak Medallions	1530	89	24	2090	99	2	NP	66

Description & Serving	Cal	Fat	Sfat	Sod	Carb	Fiber	Sugar	Prot
Mahi Mahi	950	33	5	1810	102	4	NP	54
Jalapeno-BBQ Salmon	590	21	6	1120	45	24	NP	54
Grilled Mahi Mahi w/ Creamy Red Chile Sauce, w/ rice & w/o beans	1220	61	13	3080	118	7	NP	45
Steak								
Three Sauce Fajita Steak Burrito w/ rice & w/o beans	1450	72	25	3760	121	4	NP	61
Ranchiladas w/ rice & w/o beans	1430	79	35	3750	114	10	NP	67
Mesquite-Grilled Steak Fajita w/o rice, beans, tortillas, & condiments	520	38	12	920	4	4	NP	26
Smothered Steak Fajita w/ rice & w/o beans, tortillas, & condiments	1160	65	27	2910	74	7	NP	57
The Ultimate Fajita w/ rice & w/o beans, tortillas, & condiments	1440	99	23	3710	79	7	NP	52
Steak Quesadilla Combo (quesadilla only)	630	44	17	1120	27	1	NP	28
Loaded Carne Asada Tacos w/ Creamy Red Chile Sauce, w/ rice & w/o beans	1610	92	19	2250	113	4	NP	56
Vegetarian								
Grilled Enchilada - Avocado w/ Red Chile Pesto, w/ rice & w/o beans	1120	57	19	2140	109	11	NP	32
Create Your Own Combo - Cheese Chile Relleno w/ Ranchero Sauce	680	57	5	1190	28	6	NP	31
Grilled Vegetables Fajita w/o rice, beans, tortillas, & condiments	280	14	1	380	20	4	NP	4
Side								
Black Beans w/ cheese	180	7	2	690	20	6	NP	8
Refried Beans w/ cheese	210	8	3.5	710	23	7	NP	10
Homemade Flour Tortillas, 3 ea w/ fajita order	360	11	3	900	57	3	NP	9
Mexican Rice	290	4	1	680	56	0	NP	6
Vegetables - Grilled	70	0	0	20	16	3	NP	2
Vegetables - House	170	14	2.5	250	11	2	NP	2
Classic Veggies (for all fajitas)	100	5	1	660	11	3	NP	2
Baja Blend Veggies (for all fajitas)	200	15	2.5	680	15	3	NP	3
El Diablo Veggies (for all fajitas)	50	2	0	15	8	1	NP	1
Kids								
Mexican Dinner - Crispy Beef Taco	320	19	7	600	19	4	NP	18
Mexican Dinner - Crispy Chicken Taco	240	12	4	620	19	2	NP	12
Mexican Dinner - Soft Beef Taco	340	18	8	890	24	3	NP	20
Mexican Dinner - Soft Chicken Taco	250	11	4.5	910	24	2	NP	14
Mexican Dinner - Cheese Enchiladas	410	29	15	1180	20	2	NP	20
Nachos - Bean & Cheese	780	43	23	1570	59	11	NP	41
Nachos - Cheese	550	36	20	770	31	3	NP	32
Corn Dog	280	17	3.5	650	25	2	NP	5
Cheese Quesadilla	850	66	26	1250	36	1	NP	33
Grilled Chicken Sandwich	330	18	4	790	25	1	NP	22
Grilled Chicken	90	2.5	1	520	2	0	NP	18
Chicken Tenders	540	36	6	1640	44	2	NP	25

Description & Serving	Cal	Fat	Sfat	Sod	Carb	Fiber	Sugar	Prot
Hamburger	440	31	10	310	23	1	NP	17
Cheeseburger	550	40	15	490	24	1	NP	24
Black Beans w/ cheese	180	7	2	690	20	6	NP	8
Refried Beans w/ cheese	210	8	3.5	710	23	7	NP	10
House Salad, no dressing	10	0	0	5	2	1	NP	1
French Fries	370	32	5	480	19	2	NP	2
Mexican Rice	290	4	1	680	56	0	NP	6
Vegetables - House, kids size	170	14	2.5	250	11	2	NP	2
Sundae w/ chocolate syrup	360	18	14	95	51	1	NP	3
Sundae w/ strawberry puree	390	18	14	60	58	0	NP	3

Dressing/Condiment

Description & Serving	Cal	Fat	Sfat	Sod	Carb	Fiber	Sugar	Prot
Chipotle Honey Mustard	310	29	4.5	370	11	0	NP	0
Ranch	230	23	4	440	2	0	NP	2
Fat Free Mango Citrus Vinaigrette	45	0	0	20	11	0	NP	0
Smoked Jalapeno Vinaigrette	230	23	4	760	8	0	NP	0
Mixed Cheese	110	9	5	180	1	0	NP	7
Guacamole	40	3.5	0.5	125	3	2	NP	1
Pico de Gallo	15	0.5	0	55	1	0	NP	0
Sour Cream	60	4.5	3.5	45	2	0	NP	1
Tequila Lime Chile Sauce	170	14	2.5	670	6	2	NP	1
Chipotle Honey Sauce	230	4	1.5	1020	48	0	NP	0
Habanero Fire Sauce	120	9	0	1740	9	3	NP	0
Side Chile Con Carne for Chimi/Burrito	100	5	2	550	7	1	NP	5
Side Queso for Chimi/Burrito	150	11	7	700	5	0	NP	10
Side Ranchero Sauce for Chimi/Burrito	60	3	0	420	8	1	NP	1
Side Sour Cream Sauce for Chimi/Burrito	200	20	4.5	350	4	0	NP	1

Dessert

Description & Serving	Cal	Fat	Sfat	Sod	Carb	Fiber	Sugar	Prot
Border Brownie Sundae w/ vanilla ice cream	1300	70	35	230	160	6	NP	15
OTB Sweet Sampler	2500	124	34	2540	313	11	NP	32
Sopapillas	1350	44	7	1090	235	12	NP	12
Chocolate Turtle Empanadas	1200	72	27	440	136	4	NP	10
Kaluha Ice Cream Pie	820	42	16	380	99	4	NP	9
Sizzling Apple Crisp	1120	45	22	470	177	6	NP	10
Dulce De Leche Cheesecake	1270	105	44	990	125	3	NP	13

Orange Julius

Fruit Drink

Description & Serving	Cal	Fat	Sfat	Sod	Carb	Fiber	Sugar	Prot
Bananarilla, 16 oz	320	7	6	70	65	5	44	3
Blackberry, 16 oz	280	7	6	64	55	4	37	2
Lemon Julius, 16 oz	220	0	0	20	58	0	55	0
Mango Julius, 16 oz	150	0.5	0	20	38	1	36	1
Orange Julius, 16 oz	130	0.5	0	20	33	0	30	1
Orange Passion Julius, 16 oz	150	0	0	25	37	0	36	0
Peach Julius, 16 oz	140	0	0	20	34	1	32	1
Pina Colada, 16 oz	260	7	6	75	52	2	41	2
Pineapple Julius, 16 oz	120	0	0	25	31	1	29	0

Description & Serving	Cal	Fat	Sfat	Sod	Carb	Fiber	Sugar	Prot
Pomegranate Julius, 16 oz	160	0.5	0	25	40	1	39	1
Raspberry, 16 oz	300	7	6	70	59	3	48	2
Raspberry Julius, 16 oz	200	1	0	20	51	3	49	1
Strawberry Banana, 16 oz	300	7	6	65	60	4	44	3
Strawberry Julius, 16 oz	170	0	0	20	44	1	42	0
Strawberry Lemonade Julius, 16 oz	200	0	0	20	54	1	51	1
Tripleberry, 16 oz	310	7	6	65	63	4	49	2
Tropical, 16 oz	350	7	6	70	71	4	49	3

Smoothie

Description & Serving	Cal	Fat	Sfat	Sod	Carb	Fiber	Sugar	Prot
3-Berry Blast Smoothie, 20 oz	460	0	0	150	108	6	89	8
Berry Banana Squeeze Smoothie, 20 oz	270	0	0	10	70	4	59	1
Berry Lemon Lively Smoothie, 20 oz	420	0	0	150	99	5	80	8
Blackberry Storm Smoothie, 20 oz	680	15	13	290	128	6	90	12
Blackberry Toner Smoothie, 20 oz	410	0	0	150	94	4	71	8
Blueberrathon Smoothie, 20 oz	350	0.5	0	15	87	6	67	2
Blueberry Blast Smoothie, 20 oz	380	0	0	160	90	3	75	8
Cocoa Latte Swirl Smoothie, 20 oz	960	23	19	870	156	5	119	34
Mango Passion Smoothie, 20 oz	370	0	0	170	86	1	75	7
Orange Swirl Smoothie, 20 oz	540	12	10	150	103	3	77	4
Peaches & Cream Smoothie, 20 oz	360	0	0	170	83	2	69	8
Pomegranate & Berries Smoothie, 20 oz	400	0	0	150	92	3	81	7
Raspberry Crème Smoothie, 20 oz	650	15	13	290	118	5	87	12
Raspberry Crush Smoothie, 20 oz	390	1	0	5	98	9	80	2
Strawberry Sensation Smoothie, 20 oz	430	0	0	160	100	2	88	7
Strawberry Xtreme Smoothie, 20 oz	390	0	0	160	89	2	74	8
Tart 'N' Berry Smoothie, 20 oz	410	2.5	1	55	99	7	84	2
Tropical Tango Smoothie, 20 oz	380	0	0	120	92	3	75	1
Tropi-Colada Smoothie, 20 oz	530	10	9	260	99	3	75	11
Wild Blue Twist Smoothie, 20 oz	420	0	0	160	100	4	81	8
Strawberry Delight Light Smoothie, 20 oz	250	0	0	75	60	3	47	2
Berry-Pom Twilight Light Smoothie, 20 oz	230	0	0	70	55	5	39	3
Tropical Sunlight Light Smoothie, 20 oz	220	0	0	85	55	3	44	2

Coffee Drink

Description & Serving	Cal	Fat	Sfat	Sod	Carb	Fiber	Sugar	Prot
Cool Cappuccino, 16 oz	300	10	9	250	45	2	33	8
Cool Mocha, 16 oz	400	13	10	360	62	3	46	9

Supplement/Add-In

Description & Serving	Cal	Fat	Sfat	Sod	Carb	Fiber	Sugar	Prot
Heart Health Boost, 4 g	15	0	0	0	3	0	0	0
Joint Care Boost, 6 g	20	0	0	135	5	0	0	0
Fiber Plus Boost, 6 g	5	0	0	60	4	4	0	0
Protein Boost, 19 g	90	3	0.5	115	8	1	3	6
Banana, 1 whole	110	0	0	0	29	3	15	1

Pita

Description & Serving	Cal	Fat	Sfat	Sod	Carb	Fiber	Sugar	Prot
Santa Fe Grilled Chicken Pita	470	22	6	930	47	7	2	21
Chicken Caesar Pita	470	23	3.5	1010	45	6	1	19
Turkey Club Pita	460	23	6	1240	46	6	1	21
Garden Veggie Pita	460	26	13	810	49	7	5	14
Chicken Fajita Pita	380	1	4	1190	49	7	3	21
Steak Fajita Pita	400	14	5	1210	51	6	3	23

Description & Serving	Cal	Fat	Sfat	Sod	Carb	Fiber	Sugar	Prot
Hot Dog								
Relish Dog	420	27	11	1240	28	1	7	15
Chili Melt Dog	470	33	14	1250	25	1	3	20
Chili Slaw Dog	470	31	12	1280	28	2	3	17
Cheese Dog	460	31	14	1220	24	1	3	18
Chicago Dog	430	27	11	2120	29	3	6	16
Pepperoni Cheese Dog	460	31	13	1250	26	2	3	18
Sauerkraut Dog	410	27	11	1320	24	2	3	15
Reuben Dog	520	36	16	1450	24	2	3	23
Bacon Cheese Dog	490	33	14	1380	24	1	3	22
Southwest Chili Dog	500	34	15	1370	27	2	4	21
Triple Cheese Dog	540	38	17	1340	24	1	3	25
Snack								
Nachos, small	280	15	3.5	600	36	2	0	4
Salted Pretzel	160	1	0	920	34	1	1	5

Panago

Description & Serving	Cal	Fat	Sfat	Sod	Carb	Fiber	Sugar	Prot
Pizza, 1 slice								
Grilled Veggie & Goat Cheese Thin Pizza	180	6	2.5	270	19	1	2	8
Grilled Veggie & Goat Cheese Hand-Tossed Pizza	220	6	3	270	29	2	2	9
Grilled Veggie & Goat Cheese Multigrain Pizza	210	6	3	290	25	2	2	9
Grilled Veggie & Goat Cheese Multigrain Thin Pizza	170	6	2.5	280	17	1	2	8
Garden Veggie Thin Pizza	170	6	2.5	240	21	2	4	9
Garden Veggie Hand-Tossed Pizza	210	6	2.5	250	29	2	4	11
Garden Veggie Multigrain Pizza	200	6	2.5	270	28	3	4	11
Garden Veggie Multigrain Thin Pizza	160	6	2.5	250	20	2	4	9
Quattro Formaggio Thin Pizza	140	4.5	2.5	180	18	1	1	8
Quattro Formaggio Hand-Tossed Pizza	190	5	2.5	180	26	1	1	9
Quattro Formaggio Multigrain Pizza	180	5	2.5	200	24	2	2	9
Quattro Formaggio Multigrain Thin Pizza	140	5	2.5	190	17	1	2	7
Veggie Pepperoni Thin Pizza	160	5	2.5	280	19	1	2	11
Veggie Pepperoni Hand-Tossed Pizza	200	5	2.5	290	27	2	2	12
Veggie Pepperoni Multigrain Pizza	200	5	2.5	310	25	2	2	12
Veggie Pepperoni Multigrain Thin Pizza	160	5	2.5	300	18	2	2	11
Primo Vegetarian Thin Pizza	180	8	2.5	190	20	1	1	8
Primo Vegetarian Hand-Tossed Pizza	220	9	2.5	200	28	2	1	10
Primo Vegetarian Multigrain Pizza	220	9	2.5	220	26	2	2	9
Primo Vegetarian Multigrain Thin Pizza	180	8	2.5	210	18	2	1	8
Veggie Mediterranean Thin Pizza	180	10	3.5	300	19	2	2	7
Veggie Mediterranean Hand-Tossed Pizza	220	12	3.5	300	28	2	2	7
Veggie Mediterranean Multigrain Pizza	210	12	3.5	320	26	3	2	7
Veggie Meditterranean Multigrain Thin Pizza	170	10	3.5	310	18	2	2	7
Chorizo & Goat Cheese Thin Pizza	200	9	3.5	270	17	1	1	7
Chorizo & Goat Cheese Hand-Tossed Pizza	240	10	3.5	280	26	1	1	8
Chorizo & Goat Cheese Multigrain Pizza	230	10	3.5	300	24	2	1	8
Chorizo & Goat Cheese Multigrain Thin Pizza	190	9	3.5	280	16	1	1	7
Genoa Classic Thin Pizza	200	8	3.5	360	18	1	1	8

Description & Serving	Cal	Fat	Sfat	Sod	Carb	Fiber	Sugar	Prot
Genoa Classic Hand-Tossed Pizza	240	10	3.5	370	27	1	1	8
Genoa Classic Multigrain Pizza	240	10	3.5	390	25	2	2	8
Genoa Classic Multigrain Thin Pizza	200	8	3.5	370	17	1	1	8
Italia Classic Thin Pizza	180	10	3	420	19	1	2	7
Italia Classic Hand-Tossed Pizza	220	12	3	420	27	2	2	7
Italia Classic Multigrain Pizza	210	12	3	440	25	2	2	7
Italia Classic Multigrain Thin Pizza	170	10	3	430	18	2	2	7
Meatball Thin Pizza	200	12	4.5	330	19	2	2	9
Meatball Hand-Tossed Pizza	250	13	4.5	330	28	2	2	10
Meatball Multigrain Pizza	240	13	4.5	350	26	2	2	10
Meatball Multigrain Thin Pizza	200	12	4.5	340	18	2	2	9
Sicilian Sausage Thin Pizza	200	11	4	350	19	1	2	9
Sicilian Sausage Hand-Tossed Pizza	250	12	4	360	27	2	2	10
Sicilian Sausage Multigrain Pizza	240	12	4	380	26	2	2	10
Sicilian Sausage Multigrain Thin Pizza	200	11	4	360	18	2	2	9
The Mediterranean Thin Pizza	200	12	4	270	19	2	2	8
The Mediterranean Hand-Tossed Pizza	240	14	4.5	280	28	2	2	8
The Mediterranean Multigrain Pizza	230	13	4.5	300	26	3	2	8
The Mediterranean Multigrain Thin Pizza	190	12	4.5	280	18	2	2	8
Panago Classic Thin Pizza	180	10	3	350	19	2	2	7
Panago Classic Hand-Tossed Pizza	220	12	3	350	28	2	2	7
Panago Classic Multigrain Pizza	210	12	3	370	26	2	2	7
Panago Classic Multigrain Thin Pizza	170	10	3	360	18	2	2	7
Tropical Hawaiian Thin Pizza	200	12	3.5	410	22	1	5	8
Tropical Hawaiian Hand-Tossed Pizza	250	13	3.5	420	30	1	5	8
Tropical Hawaiian Multigrain Pizza	240	13	3.5	440	29	2	5	8
Tropical Hawaiian Multigrain Thin Pizza	200	12	3.5	430	21	1	5	8
Primo Shrimp Thin Pizza	140	3	1.5	200	22	1	5	7
Primo Shrimp Hand-Tossed Pizza	180	3	1.5	210	30	2	5	9
Primo Shrimp Multigrain Pizza	180	3.5	1.5	230	29	2	5	9
Primo Shrimp Multigrain Thin Pizza	140	3	1.5	220	21	2	5	7
Pesto Shrimp Thin Pizza	210	10	3	300	19	1	1	11
Pesto Shrimp Hand-Tossed Pizza	250	10	3	300	27	2	1	13
Pesto Shrimp Multigrain Pizza	240	10	3.5	320	25	2	1	13
Pesto Shrimp Multigrain Thin Pizza	200	10	3	310	18	2	1	11
Shrimp Club Thin Pizza	200	10	2.5	290	17	1	1	9
Shrimp Club Hand-Tossed Pizza	240	13	3.5	370	27	1	1	13
Shrimp Club Multigrain Pizza	260	13	3.5	390	25	2	2	13
Shrimp Club Multigrain Thin Pizza	190	11	3.5	300	17	1	2	9
Simple Pepperoni Thin Pizza	170	6	3	280	18	1	1	10
Simple Pepperoni Hand-Tossed Pizza	210	7	3	290	26	1	1	11
Simple Pepperoni Multigrain Pizza	200	7	3	310	25	2	2	11
Simple Pepperoni Multigrain Thin Pizza	160	6	3	290	17	1	2	10
Simple Cheese Thin Pizza	150	4.5	2.5	200	18	1	1	9
Simple Cheese Hand-Tossed Pizza	190	5	2.5	290	26	1	1	10
Simple Cheese Multigrain Pizza	180	5	2.5	230	24	2	2	10
Simple Cheese Multigrain Thin Pizza	140	4.5	2.5	220	17	1	2	9
Simple Ham & Pineapple Thin Pizza	160	5	2.5	300	20	1	3	10
Simple Ham & Pineapple Hand-Tossed Pizza	210	5	2.5	310	28	2	3	11
Simple Ham & Pineapple Multigrain Pizza	200	5	2.5	330	26	2	4	11
Simple Ham & Pineapple Multigrain Thin Pizza	160	5	2.5	310	19	2	3	10

Description & Serving	Cal	Fat	Sfat	Sod	Carb	Fiber	Sugar	Prot
Side								
Rosemary Garlic Torizoné Breadsticks	110	1	0	340	22	1	2	4
Cinnamon Torizoné Breadsticks	140	3.5	2	290	23	1	6	3
Formaggio Shaker	40	2.5	1	190	1	0	0	3
Italiano Shaker	15	0	0	440	3	1	0	1
Chili Shaker	0	0	0	0	2	0	0	1
Wings, 10 packs								
Hot Buffalo Wings	280	19	4	1070	4	0	2	20
Tikka Masala Wings	310	21	4.5	920	4	0	2	22
Mediterranean Wings	280	19	4	830	4	0	2	20
Honey Mustard Wings	280	20	4	960	4	0	3	20
Salad								
Antipasto Salad	250	13	5	780	16	10	8	8
Chicken Caesar Salad	260	9	3	780	17	2	2	28
Chicken Garden Salad	250	7	3	830	18	4	6	35
Mediterranean Salad	190	10	5	410	18	11	8	9
Caesar Salad	150	7	2	370	16	2	2	7
Garden Salad	160	7	3	290	18	4	6	8
Shrimp Caesar Salad	195	7	2	820	16	2	2	16
Shrimp Garden Salad	205	7	3	740	18	4	6	17
Dressing/Condiment								
Jalapeno Ranch Dip, 38 g	160	17	2	290	1	0	1	0
Frank's Original Red Hot Dip, 42 g	10	0	0	1250	1	1	2	0
Italian Garlic Ranch, 35 g	150	16	1	210	1	0	1	1
Cheezy Cheddar, 32 g	150	16	2	200	1	0	1	1
BBQ, 43 g	60	0	0	450	14	1	10	0
Italian Tomato, 43 g	45	1.5	0	510	9	2	2	2
Chipotle Cilantro, 33 g	160	17	0	200	2	0	0	0
Classic Caesar, 28 g	130	14	1	190	2	0	1	0
Balsamic Vinaigrette, 28 g	50	4.5	0	90	3	0	3	0
Blue Cheese, 28 g	100	10	2	130	1	0	1	1
Cheezy Formaggio Cucina Dip, 250 ml	120	14	1	270	1	0	1	0
Creamy Ranch Jalapeno Cucina Dip, 250 ml	120	13	1	210	1	0	1	0
Italiano Garlic Cucina Dip, 250 ml	140	15	1	180	2	0	1	1

Panda Express

Description & Serving	Cal	Fat	Sfat	Sod	Carb	Fiber	Sugar	Prot
Entrée								
Mixed Vegetables	100	6	1	220	7	3	2	3
Black Pepper Chicken	200	11	2.5	740	11	2	4	14
Broccoli Chicken	180	9	2	630	11	3	2	13
Kung Pao Chicken	300	20	4	900	13	2	4	20
Mandarin Chicken	310	16	4	740	8	0	8	34
Mushroom Chicken	180	10	2	720	10	2	4	14
Orange Chicken	400	20	3.5	640	42	0	18	15
Pineapple Chicken	230	10	2	710	21	2	16	13
Potato Chicken	220	11	2	760	18	3	4	11
String Bean Chicken	190	9	2	660	13	3	5	12

Description & Serving	Cal	Fat	Sfat	Sod	Carb	Fiber	Sugar	Prot
Sweet & Sour Chicken	400	17	3	370	46	1	23	15
Pineapple Chicken Breast	230	12	2	560	19	1	14	11
String Bean Chicken Breast	200	12	2	550	12	2	5	10
Thai Cashew Chicken Breast	330	22	3.5	630	17	2	5	15
Beijing Beef	660	41	7	860	52	4	22	24
Broccoli Beef	150	6	1.5	720	12	3	2	11
Mongolian Beef	200	9	2	830	16	3	6	15
BBQ Pork	360	19	8	1310	13	1	12	34
Sweet & Sour Pork	400	23	4.5	360	36	2	15	13
Crispy Shrimp, 6	260	13	2.5	810	26	1	2	9
Kung Pao Shrimp	230	14	2.5	850	13	2	4	13
Tangy Shrimp	140	4.5	1	660	16	1	13	8
Side								
Chow Mein	400	12	2	1060	61	8	10	12
Fried Rice	570	18	4	900	85	8	0	16
Steamed Rice	420	0	0	0	93	0	0	8
Eggplant & Tofu	310	24	3	680	19	3	13	7
Mixed Vegetables	190	13	2	440	14	5	4	5
Chicken Egg Roll, 1	200	12	4	390	16	2	2	8
Chicken Potsticker, 3	220	11	2.5	280	23	1	2	7
Cream Cheese Rangoon, 3	190	8	5	180	24	2	1	5
Veggie Spring Roll, 2	160	7	1	540	22	4	2	4
Egg Flower Soup	90	2	0	810	15	1	4	3
Hot & Sour Soup	90	3.5	0.5	970	12	1	3	4
Fortune Cookie, 1	32	0	0	8	7	0	3	1
Condiment								
Mandarin Sauce	160	0	0	340	40	0	40	0
Potsticker Sauce	45	0	0	1030	10	0	8	1
Sweet & Sour Sauce	80	0	0	180	21	0	21	0

Panera Bread

Breakfast

	Cal	Fat	Sfat	Sod	Carb	Fiber	Sugar	Prot
Asiago Cheese Bagel	330	6	3.5	570	55	2	3	13
Blueberry Bagel	330	1.5	0	490	67	2	9	10
Chocolate Chip Bagel	370	6	4	480	69	2	14	10
Cinnamon Crunch Bagel	430	8	5	430	81	3	30	9
Cinnamon Swirl Bagel	320	2.5	1	460	65	3	11	10
Dutch Apple & Raisin Bagel	360	3	1	620	77	2	33	8
Everything Bagel	300	2.5	0	630	59	2	4	10
Plain Bagel	290	1.5	0	450	59	2	3	10
Salt Bagel	290	1.5	0	2790	59	2	3	10
Sesame Bagel	310	3	0	450	59	2	3	10
French Toast Bagel	350	5	2	610	67	2	15	9
Whole Grain Bagel	370	3.5	0	420	70	6	5	13
Cheese Pastry	400	23	14	340	41	1	13	8
Cherry Pastry	450	22	13	340	55	2	24	8

Description & Serving	Cal	Fat	Sfat	Sod	Carb	Fiber	Sugar	Prot
Chocolate Pastry	340	20	12	230	37	2	13	6
Fresh Apple Pastry	380	19	13	320	44	1	17	7
Gooey Butter Pastry	350	19	12	250	39	1	11	7
Pecan Braid Pastry	440	25	11	270	46	2	20	8
Carrot Walnut Muffin	430	19	4	380	61	2	33	8
Chocolate Chip Muffie	270	12	3	140	40	1	23	4
Pumpkin Muffie	250	10	2	200	39	1	22	3
Pumpkin Muffin	530	20	3.5	430	81	2	47	6
Reduced Fat Wild Blueberry Muffin	360	10	2	220	61	1	35	6
Wild Blueberry Muffin	390	15	2.5	290	58	1	34	5
Cinnamon Chip Scone	530	27	16	310	67	2	32	8
Orange Scone	460	20	11	290	65	1	28	8
Wild Blueberry Scone	390	16	11	780	56	2	23	6
French Croissant	290	17	11	220	31	1	3	6
Pastry Ring - Cherry Cheese	220	10	6	150	27	1	13	3
Cinnamon Roll	620	24	14	480	89	3	33	13
Cobblestone Roll	650	13	5	410	123	3	62	12
Pecan Roll	720	38	11	310	88	2	48	11
Four Cheese Baked Egg Souffle	480	31	16	700	34	2	6	16
Spinach & Artichoke Baked Egg Souffle	500	32	18	830	35	2	6	19
Spinach & Bacon Baked Egg Souffle	570	37	20	990	36	2	6	21
Turkey Sausage & Potato Baked Egg Souffle	460	28	15	600	35	2	6	15
Bacon, Egg & Cheese Grilled Breakfast Sandwich	510	24	10	1060	44	2	2	28
Egg & Cheese Grilled Breakfast Sandwich	380	14	6	620	43	2	1	18
Sausage, Egg & Cheese Grilled Breakfast Sandwich	550	30	12	800	44	2	2	15
Strawberry Granola Parfait	310	12	3.5	100	41	4	29	3

Sandwich

Description & Serving	Cal	Fat	Sfat	Sod	Carb	Fiber	Sugar	Prot
Half Chicken Bacon Dijon on Country	470	18	7	1010	48	2	7	29
Half Chicken Bacon Dijon on French	390	18	7	770	32	1	8	27
Half Frontega Chicken on Focaccia	430	20	4.5	1080	40	2	3	23
Half Smokehouse Turkey on Focaccia	430	18	6	1310	41	2	4	26
Half Smokehouse Turkey on Three Cheese	410	15	7	1330	41	2	3	27
Half Tomato & Mozzarella on Ciabatta	390	15	5	650	50	4	5	15
Half Turkey Artichoke on Focaccia	370	13	3.5	1170	44	3	5	20
Half Asiago Roast Beef on Asiago Cheese	360	16	6	640	29	1	2	24
Half Bacon Turkey Bravo on Tomato Basil	420	16	5	1460	43	2	4	25
Half Chicken Caesar on Focaccia	430	19	4	820	41	2	3	22
Half Chicken Caesar on Three Cheese	400	16	5	820	42	2	3	23
Half Chipotle Chicken on Artisan French	530	28	7	1280	43	2	3	27
Half Chipotle Chicken on French	450	28	7	1050	26	2	4	25
Half Italian Combo on Ciabatta	520	23	9	1530	47	2	3	30
Half Chicken Salad on Sesame Semolina	360	13	2.5	970	50	7	5	15
Half Chicken Salad on Whole Grain	320	13	2.5	770	40	9	5	16
Half Mediterranean Veggie on Tomato Basil	310	7	1.5	730	51	5	4	11
Half Sierra Turkey on Focaccia w/ Asiago Cheese	480	27	6	990	40	2	3	19
Half Smoked Ham & Swiss on Rye	350	18	7	940	28	2	4	20
Half Smoked Ham & Swiss on Stone-Milled Rye	390	14	5	1290	41	3	3	24
Half Smoked Turkey Breast on Country	310	9	1.5	1040	40	2	2	17

Description & Serving	Cal	Fat	Sfat	Sod	Carb	Fiber	Sugar	Prot
Half Smoked Turkey Breast on Sourdough	240	9	1.5	840	25	1	2	15
Half Tuna Salad on Honey Wheat	380	23	4.5	570	32	3	6	10

Salad

Full Fresh Fruit Cup, sml	70	0	0	15	19	1	9	1
Half Asian Sesame Chicken Salad	210	10	1.5	450	16	2	3	16
Half Caesar Salad	200	14	4	310	13	2	1	6
Half Classic Café Salad	90	5	1	135	9	2	6	1
Half Fuji Apple Salad	200	14	3	310	16	3	10	4
Half Fuji Apple w/ Chicken Salad	260	15	3	450	17	3	11	16
Half Greek Salad	220	20	4	690	7	3	2	5
Half Grilled Chicken Caesar Salad	250	14	4	500	13	1	1	18
Half Chopped Chicken Cobb Salad	250	18	4	650	4	1	1	18
Half Strawberry Poppyseed Salad	80	3	0	100	13	2	9	2
Half Strawberry Poppyseed w/ Chicken Salad	140	4.5	0	230	14	2	9	13
Half Tomato & Mozzarella Salad	440	24	10	830	42	3	9	18

Soup

Baked Potato Soup, 8 oz (You Pick Two size)	230	14	9	720	21	2	3	5
Baked Potato Soup, 12 oz	370	22	14	1140	33	3	5	8
Broccoli Cheddar Soup, 8 oz (You Pick Two size)	190	10	6	1020	16	5	0	8
Broccoli Cheddar Soup, 12 oz	290	16	9	1540	24	7	0	12
Cream of Chicken & Wild Rice, 8 oz (You Pick Two size)	200	12	6	970	19	1	2	5
Cream of Chicken & Wild Rice, 12 oz	300	17	9	1450	29	1	4	7
Creamy Tomato Soup, 8 oz (You Pick Two size)	210	15	8	770	20	3	10	3
Creamy Tomato Soup, 12 oz	290	20	11	1040	28	3	13	4
Creamy Tomato Soup w/ croutons, 8 oz (You Pick Two size)	300	18	9	580	31	4	10	4
Creamy Tomato Soup w/ croutons, 12 oz	370	23	12	740	39	5	13	4
French Onion Soup w/ cheese & croutons, 8 oz (You Pick Two size)	210	9	4.5	1670	23	2	4	8
French Onion Soup w/ cheese & croutons, 12 oz	250	11	5	2370	30	3	6	10
French Onion Soup w/o cheese & croutons, 8 oz (You Pick Two size)	90	3	1.5	1560	13	1	4	2
French Onion Soup w/o cheese & croutons, 12 oz	130	4.5	2.5	2340	20	2	6	3
Forest Mushroom Soup, 8 oz (You Pick Two size)	170	12	6	770	14	1	2	3
Forest Mushroom Soup, 12 oz	250	18	8	1150	21	2	3	4
Low-Fat Chicken Noodle, 8 oz (You Pick Two size)	100	2	0	1110	16	1	1	6
Low-Fat Chicken Noodle, 12 oz	160	3	0.5	1670	23	2	2	9
Low-Fat Vegetarian Black Bean, 8 oz (You Pick Two size)	90	1	0	870	16	4	4	4
Low-Fat Vegetarian Black Bean, 12 oz	140	1.5	0	1410	26	7	7	6
Low-Fat Vegetarian Garden Vegetable, 8 oz (You Pick Two size)	70	0.5	0	1200	15	4	1	3
Low-Fat Vegetarian Garden Vegetable, 12 oz	120	1	0	1970	24	7	2	4
New England Clam Chowder, 8 oz (You Pick Two size)	300	23	13	790	19	2	0	5
New England Clam Chowder, 12 oz	450	34	20	1190	29	3	0	8

Description & Serving	Cal	Fat	Sfat	Sod	Carb	Fiber	Sugar	Prot
Summer Corn Chowder, 8 oz (You Pick Two size)	260	14	8	730	28	5	7	5
Summer Corn Chowder, 12 oz	170	9	6	490	19	4	4	3

Kids

Panera Kids Deli Sandwich - Roast Beef	320	10	5	790	35	3	3	23
Panera Kids Deli Sandwich - Smoked Ham	300	9	6	1210	34	3	3	21
Panera Kids Deli Sandwich - Smoked Turkey	300	10	5	1160	35	3	4	21
Panera Kids Grilled Cheese Sandwich	300	12	9	890	35	3	4	25
Panera Kids Peanut Butter & Jelly Sandwich	410	17	3	410	56	5	22	23
Panera Kids Organic Yogurt (blueberry, strawberry, orange)	70	1	0.5	40	12	0	11	2

Dessert

Caramel Pecan Brownie	490	25	6	170	64	2	51	5
Very Chocolate Brownie	460	22	5	180	61	2	48	5
Chocolate Chipper Cookie	440	23	14	320	59	2	33	5
Chocolate Duet w/ Walnuts Cookie	450	24	13	330	55	3	36	6
Nutty Chocolate Chipper Cookie	460	27	13	300	54	3	31	5
Oatmeal Raisin Cookie	370	14	8	310	57	2	28	5
Toffee Nut Cookie	460	19	13	330	59	1	29	5
Oatmeal Raisin Cookie, Petite	90	3.5	2	75	14	1	7	1
Shortbread Cookie, Petite	90	5	3	40	9	0	3	1
Chocolate Chipper Cookie, Petite	110	6	3.5	80	15	1	8	1
Chocolate Duet w/ Walnuts Cookie, Petite	110	6	3	80	14	1	9	2
Shortbread Cookie	350	21	12	160	36	1	11	3
Lemon Poppyseed Mini Bundt Cake	460	20	4	440	63	0	33	6
Pineapple Upside-Down Mini Bundt Cake	510	22	10	480	75	3	49	5
Bear Claw	460	24	13	400	54	2	18	9

Bread

Ciabatta Bread, 6.25 oz	460	5	1	760	84	3	3	16
Country Loaf, 2 oz	140	0.5	0	310	27	1	0	5
Country Miche, 2 oz	140	0.5	0	330	28	1	0	5
Focaccia, 2 oz	160	2	0	330	29	1	1	5
Focaccia w/ Asiago Cheese, 2 oz	160	5	1.5	230	23	1	1	5
French Baguette, 2 oz	150	0.5	0	370	30	1	0	5
French Miche, 2 oz	140	0.5	0	360	28	1	0	5
Sesame Semolina Loaf, 2 oz	140	0.5	0	350	29	1	1	4
Sesame Semolina Miche, 2 oz	140	1	0	360	30	1	1	5
Stone-Milled Rye Loaf, 2 oz	140	0.5	0	380	28	2	0	5
Stone-Milled Rye Miche, 2 oz	140	0.5	0	410	27	2	0	5
Three Cheese Demi, 2 oz	140	2	1	300	26	1	1	6
Three Cheese Loaf, 2 oz	140	2	1	300	26	1	1	6
Three Cheese Miche, 2 oz	150	2	1	320	27	1	1	6
Three Seed Demi, 2 oz	160	3.5	0	300	27	2	0	6
Whole Grain Baguette, 2 oz	140	1	0	320	28	3	2	6
Whole Grain Loaf, 2 oz	130	1	0	240	26	3	1	6
Whole Grain Miche, 2 oz	130	1	0	240	25	3	2	5
Asiago Cheese Demi, 2 oz	160	4	2.5	320	22	1	0	7
Asiago Cheese Loaf, 2 oz	160	4	2.5	320	22	1	0	7

Description & Serving	Cal	Fat	Sfat	Sod	Carb	Fiber	Sugar	Prot
Challah Bread, 2 oz	180	2.5	1	290	34	1	6	6
Cinnamon Raisin Loaf, 2 oz	180	3	1.5	135	34	1	11	5
French Baguette, 2 oz	160	2	0	330	31	1	1	6
French Loaf, 2 oz	150	2	0	310	29	1	1	5
French Roll, 2.25 oz	180	2	0	370	35	1	1	6
French XL Loaf, 2 oz	150	2	0	300	29	1	1	5
Honey Wheat Loaf, 2 oz	160	3	1.5	240	30	2	4	5
Sourdough Baguette, 2 oz	160	0.5	0	320	31	1	0	6
Sourdough Loaf, 2 oz	140	0.5	0	290	28	1	0	5
Sourdough Roll, 2.5 oz	200	1	0	400	39	1	0	7
Sourdough Soup Bowl, 8 oz	590	2.5	0	1210	117	4	1	22
Sourdough XL Loaf, 2 oz	140	0.5	0	290	28	1	0	5
Tomato Basil Loaf, 2 oz	140	0.5	0	330	27	1	1	5
White Whole Grain Loaf, 2 oz	140	2.5	1	310	27	2	1	5

Dressing/Condiment

Description & Serving	Cal	Fat	Sfat	Sod	Carb	Fiber	Sugar	Prot
Plain Cream Cheese, 1 oz	100	10	6	110	1	0	1	2
Reduced Fat Hazelnut Cream Cheese, 1 oz	80	6	3.5	110	3	0	3	2
Reduced Fat Honey Walnut Cream Cheese, 1 oz	80	6	3.5	105	4	0	4	2
Reduced Fat Plain Cream Cheese, 1 oz	70	6	4	120	1	0	1	3
Reduced Fat Raspberry Cream Cheese, 1 oz	70	5	3	105	4	1	3	2
Reduced Fat Sun-Dried Tomato Cream Cheese, 1 oz	70	6	3.5	115	2	1	1	3
Reduced Fat Veggie Cream Cheese, 1 oz	60	5	3	110	1	1	1	2
Half Reduced Fat Balsamic Vinaigrette, 0.75 oz	60	5	1	120	4	0	4	0
Half Caesar Dressing, 0.75 oz	80	8	1.5	95	1	0	0	0
Half Cherry Balsamic Vinaigrette, 0.75 oz	70	6	1	135	3	0	3	0
Half Fat-Free Raspberry Dressing, 0.75 oz	15	0	0	45	4	0	3	0
Half FF Reduced-Sugar Poppyseed Dressing, 0.75 oz	5	0	0	80	2	1	0	0
Half Greek Dressing/Herb Vinaigrette, 0.75 oz	110	12	2	190	1	0	0	0
Half Light Buttermilk Ranch, 0.75 oz	40	2	0	170	4	0	1	0
Half Reduced-Sugar Asian Sesame Vinaigrette, 0.75 oz	45	4	0.5	190	3	0	2	0
Half White Balsamic Apple Vinaigrette, 0.75 oz	80	6	1	160	6	0	5	0

Beverage

Description & Serving	Cal	Fat	Sfat	Sod	Carb	Fiber	Sugar	Prot
Frozen Caramel, Grande (16 oz)	580	25	17	170	83	1	70	6
Frozen Lemonade, Grande (16 oz)	90	0	0	10	21	0	21	0
Mango Smoothie, Grande (16 oz)	330	10	7	30	61	3	54	2
Frozen Mocha, Grande (16 oz)	550	25	16	140	78	2	63	7
Strawberry Smoothie, Grande (16 oz)	240	1.5	0.5	190	51	3	39	5
Iced Chai Tea Latte, 16 oz	150	3.5	2	75	25	0	23	6
Iced Green Tea, Grande (16 oz)	90	0	0	10	23	0	23	0
Lemonade, Grande (16 oz)	90	0	0	10	22	0	22	0
Caffe Latte, 8.5 oz	110	4.5	3	95	11	0	11	7
Café Mocha, 11.5 oz	380	17	11	160	48	2	41	11
Cappuccino, 8.5 oz	110	4.5	3	95	11	0	11	7
Caramel Latte, 11.5 oz	410	18	12	190	54	0	49	9
Hot Chai Tea Latte, 10 oz	190	4	2.5	85	31	0	29	7
Hot Chocolate, 11.5 oz	390	17	12	170	49	2	42	11

Description & Serving	Cal	Fat	Sfat	Sod	Carb	Fiber	Sugar	Prot

Papa Gino's

Thin Crust Pizza, small, 1 slice

Description & Serving	Cal	Fat	Sfat	Sod	Carb	Fiber	Sugar	Prot
Cheese Pizza	160	4	2	420	24	1	1	7
BBQ Chicken Pizza	210	5	2.5	640	31	1	1	10
Buffalo Chicken Pizza	180	5	2.5	580	23	1	1	10
Chicken & Roasted Garlic Pizza	210	7	3.5	530	25	1	2	12
Chicken Pepper Pizza	210	7	3.5	490	25	1	2	12
Hawaiian Pizza	180	5	2.5	470	26	1	4	8
Meat Combo Pizza	260	13	5	710	24	1	1	13
Papa Roni Pizza	230	11	5	660	24	1	1	11
Pepperoni Pizza	200	8	3.5	560	24	1	1	9
Super Veggie Pizza	180	5	2.5	480	27	2	3	8
The Works Pizza	210	8	4	540	25	1	2	10

Thin Crust Pizza, large, 1 slice

Description & Serving	Cal	Fat	Sfat	Sod	Carb	Fiber	Sugar	Prot
Cheese Pizza	220	6	3.5	570	31	1	2	10
BBQ Chicken Pizza	270	7	3.5	800	38	1	1	14
Buffalo Chicken Pizza	240	7	3.5	900	31	2	2	14
Chicken & Roasted Garlic Pizza	290	10	5	730	34	2	3	17
Chicken Pepper Pizza	270	9	4.5	690	32	2	3	17
Hawaiian Pizza	240	6	3.5	640	35	1	5	11
Meat Combo Pizza	320	15	7	900	32	1	2	16
Papa Roni Pizza	320	15	7	910	32	1	2	15
Pepperoni Pizza	270	11	5	740	31	1	2	12
Super Veggie Pizza	240	7	3.5	620	35	2	3	11
The Works Pizza	300	12	6	740	33	2	2	14

Large Pizza, 1 slice

Description & Serving	Cal	Fat	Sfat	Sod	Carb	Fiber	Sugar	Prot
Cheese Pizza	330	9	5	860	47	2	2	15
BBQ Chicken Pizza	390	9	4.5	1130	56	2	2	20
Breakfast Bacon/Egg Pizza	560	29	13	1340	46	2	2	31
Breakfast Egg & Cheese Pizza	460	20	9	960	46	2	2	26
Breakfast Sausage Egg & Cheese Pizza	480	22	10	1020	47	2	2	26
Breakfast Veg Egg & Cheese Pizza	450	18	9	940	50	2	4	25
Buffalo Chicken Pizza	350	9	4.5	1260	46	3	2	20
Chicken Pepper Pizza	390	12	6	980	48	2	4	23
Hawaiian Pizza	340	9	4.5	910	52	2	6	16
Meat Combo Pizza	460	20	9	1250	47	2	2	22
Papa Roni Pizza	460	21	10	1270	48	2	3	21
Pepperoni Pizza	380	14	7	1040	47	2	2	17
Super Veggie Pizza	340	9	4.5	880	51	3	4	16
The Works Pizza	420	16	8	1050	49	2	3	20

Extra Large Pizza, 1 slice

Description & Serving	Cal	Fat	Sfat	Sod	Carb	Fiber	Sugar	Prot
Cheese Pizza	230	7	4	630	32	1	2	11
BBQ Chicken Pizza	300	8	4	940	40	1	2	17
Buffalo Chicken Pizza	270	8	4	1030	31	2	2	17
Chicken & Roasted Garlic Pizza	300	10	5	820	35	2	3	20
Chicken Pepper Pizza	290	11	5	850	32	2	3	19

Description & Serving	Cal	Fat	Sfat	Sod	Carb	Fiber	Sugar	Prot
Hawaiian Pizza	250	7	4	720	35	2	5	12
Meat Combo Pizza	430	24	10	1150	33	2	2	21
Papa Roni Pizza	360	18	9	1060	32	1	2	17
Pepperoni Pizza	290	13	6	840	32	1	2	13
Super Veggie Pizza	260	8	4	680	36	3	4	12
The Works Pizza	340	16	7	860	34	2	3	17

Thick Crust Pizza, 1 slice

Description & Serving	Cal	Fat	Sfat	Sod	Carb	Fiber	Sugar	Prot
Cheese Pizza	450	13	7	1260	62	3	2	21
BBQ Chicken Pizza	470	9	5	1430	70	3	1	23
Breakfast Bacon Egg & Cheese Pizza	680	31	14	1640	63	3	1	37
Breakfast Egg & Cheese Pizza	560	20	10	1230	63	3	1	30
Breakfast Sausage Egg & Cheese Pizza	600	25	11	1320	63	3	1	32
Breakfast Veg Egg & Cheese Pizza	570	21	10	1240	67	4	3	31
Buffalo Chicken Pizza	430	10	5	1560	61	4	1	23
Chicken & Roasted Garlic Pizza	480	12	7	1280	65	3	3	27
Chicken Pepper Pizza	470	13	7	1380	63	4	2	26
Hawaiian Pizza	430	9	5	1210	66	3	5	19
Meat Combo Pizza	540	21	10	1550	62	3	1	26
Papa Roni Pizza	540	21	10	1570	62	3	2	25
Pepperoni Pizza	480	15	7	1340	64	3	1	21
Super Veggie Pizza	430	10	5	1180	66	4	3	19
The Works Pizza	500	17	8	1350	64	4	2	23

Rustic Pizza, 1 slice

Description & Serving	Cal	Fat	Sfat	Sod	Carb	Fiber	Sugar	Prot
Cheese Pizza	200	9	4	490	23	1	1	8
BBQ Chicken Pizza	240	9	4	620	28	1	1	11
Buffalo Chicken Pizza	220	9	4	690	23	2	1	11
Chicken & Roasted Garlic Pizza	240	10	4.5	550	25	1	2	12
Chicken Pepper Pizza	230	10	4.5	520	24	2	2	12
Hawaiian Pizza	220	9	4	540	26	1	3	8
Meat Combo Pizza	280	15	7	720	24	1	1	13
Papa Roni Pizza	280	15	7	730	24	1	1	12
Pepperoni Pizza	240	12	5	610	24	1	1	10
Super Veggie Pizza	230	9	4.5	530	26	2	2	9
The Works Pizza	250	13	5	580	24	2	2	10

Topping, per large slice

Description & Serving	Cal	Fat	Sfat	Sod	Carb	Fiber	Sugar	Prot
Bacon	80	7	2.5	250	0	0	0	4
Black Olives	15	1	0	100	1	0	0	0
Broccoli	5	0	0	5	1	1	0	1
Capicola	5	0	0	75	0	0	0	1
Extra Cheese	35	3	2.5	105	0	0	0	2
Green Pepper	0	0	0	0	1	0	0	0
Hamburger	50	4	1.5	80	0	0	0	4
Mushrooms	5	0	0	0	0	0	0	0
Onions	5	0	0	0	1	0	1	0
Sausage	70	6	2	125	0	0	0	3
Sliced Tomato	0	0	0	0	0	0	0	0

Description & Serving	Cal	Fat	Sfat	Sod	Carb	Fiber	Sugar	Prot
Appetizer, small, 2 servings								
Mozzarella Sticks	950	59	21	2350	69	3	2	44
BBQ Chicken Tenders	520	18	3	1520	55	2	0	29
Buffalo Chicken Tenders	450	19	3	1970	36	4	1	29
Cheese Breadsticks	970	39	18	2260	116	4	6	44
Chicken Tenders	430	18	3	1010	36	2	0	29
Buffalo Chicken Wings	930	76	16	4350	33	6	7	29
Honey BBQ Chicken Wings	650	34	7	2560	62	3	17	28
Plain Chicken Wings	480	32	7	1880	24	2	0	26
BBQ Chicken Wings	640	32	7	2820	58	2	0	26
Plain Chicken Wings w/ Honey Mustard	650	36	7	2290	65	4	33	30
Plain Chicken Wings w/ Ranch	720	51	10	2840	30	3	4	28
Spicy BBQ Chicken Wings	580	33	7	3240	41	4	1	26
Teriyaki Chicken Wings	660	32	7	4000	64	3	33	29
Cinnamon Sticks	620	19	8	430	100	4	33	11
French Fries	540	23	4.5	120	80	8	4	8
Salad								
Buffalo Chicken Tender Salad	330	15	2	1010	29	5	4	20
Caesar Side Salad	70	4	1.5	135	6	2	1	4
Garden Side Salad	70	3	0.5	105	10	2	2	2
Caesar Salad	190	10	3.5	380	19	5	3	9
Chicken Bacon Cheddar Salad	530	33	13	1460	22	4	6	39
Chicken Caesar Salad	320	11	4.5	1150	14	5	3	42
Chicken Tender Salad	320	14	2	650	29	4	4	20
Garden Salad	180	8	1.5	300	25	5	5	5
Pasta								
Papa Platter-Penne	990	32	13	1380	135	6	11	40
Papa Platter-Spaghetti	990	32	13	1380	135	10	11	40
Pasta Trio Plate	990	34	17	1270	138	5	12	34
Penne	650	11	1.5	1130	118	3	12	21
Penne Alfredo	900	36	22	560	111	1	3	29
Penne Alfredo Chicken Broccoli	1050	42	25	1070	116	4	3	49
Ravioli	590	24	12	1360	71	3	14	24
Spaghetti	650	11	1.5	1130	118	7	12	21
Spaghetti & Meatballs	890	29	10	1710	123	10	13	34
Spaghetti Alfredo	900	36	22	560	111	5	3	29
Spaghetti Alfredo Chicken Broccoli	1050	42	25	1070	116	7	3	49
Spaghetti Chicken Parmesan	1070	39	12	2850	129	7	15	52
Side								
Single Breadstick	190	8	3.5	440	23	1	1	9
Meatballs, 2	280	21	9	870	9	3	3	14
Penne	330	6	0.5	640	61	2	7	10
Penne Alfredo	450	18	11	280	55	1	1	14
Spaghetti	330	6	0.5	640	61	4	7	10
Spaghetti Alfredo	450	18	11	280	55	3	1	14
Sandwich								
BLT Sub, sml	720	35	13	1740	71	3	4	29
Hot Dog, sml	400	25	7	890	31	2	4	13

Description & Serving	Cal	Fat	Sfat	Sod	Carb	Fiber	Sugar	Prot
Italian Sub, sml	910	48	20	2800	69	3	2	47
Lobster Roll Sub, sml	550	34	5	910	31	2	4	29
Meatball Sub, sml	740	32	14	1830	76	7	4	35
Meatball Parmesan Sub, sml	840	41	19	2150	76	7	4	42
Steak Sub, sml	630	25	9	780	65	2	0	34
Steak & Cheese Sub, sml	720	32	14	1260	68	2	1	39
Super Steak Sub, sml	760	32	14	1210	76	4	5	42
Tuna Sub, sml	740	39	6	1150	67	3	0	30
Turkey Sub, sml	460	4	0.5	1300	72	2	0	33
Turkey Club Sub, sml	630	23	6	1590	70	3	2	37
Basil Chicken Sub Panini	1080	60	17	2990	85	3	2	49
Eggplant Sub Panini	860	40	13	1930	95	7	7	31
Italian Deli Sub Panini	1050	69	21	2410	69	4	4	39
Sausage & Pepper Sub Panini	1150	69	28	2350	75	3	3	58
Kids								
Cheese Slice	310	9	5	810	42	2	2	14
Chicken Tender Meal	510	21	3.5	800	54	4	1	24
Hot Dog Meal	620	35	9	940	64	5	6	17
Penne	330	6	0.5	640	61	2	7	10
Pepperoni Slice	380	16	8	1050	42	2	2	19
Spaghetti & Meatball	460	15	5	950	63	5	7	17
Dressing/Condiment								
Balsamic Dressing, 85 g	180	18	3	700	9	0	6	0
Bleu Cheese Dressing, 30 g	150	15	3	280	2	0	2	1
Caesar Dressing, 85 g	400	44	7	709	2	0	0	2
Fat Free Honey Dijon Dressing, 43 g	60	0	0	400	13	1	8	1
Honey Mustard Dressing, 30 g	150	14	2	210	7	0	6	0
Ranch Dressing, 85 g	280	30	5	830	4	0	2	2
Marinara Dip Sauce, 31 g	20	1	0	180	3	0	2	0
Cinnamon Stick Icing, 71 g	240	1	1	35	57	0	55	0

Papa John's

Small Pizza, 1 slice

	Cal	Fat	Sfat	Sod	Carb	Fiber	Sugar	Prot
BBQ Chicken & Bacon Pizza, Original Crust	220	8	2.5	640	30	1	4	10
Cheese Pizza, Original Crust	180	6	1.5	430	25	1	3	7
Garden Fresh Pizza, Original Crust	190	6	1.5	460	26	2	4	8
Hawaiian BBQ Chicken Pizza, Original Crust	230	8	2.5	640	31	1	6	10
Pepperoni Pizza, Original Crust	210	9	2.5	540	25	1	3	9
Sausage Pizza, Original Crust	220	10	3	540	25	2	3	8
Spicy Italian Pizza, Original Crust	230	7	5	600	26	2	3	9
Spinach Alfredo Pizza, Original Crust	190	7	3	420	24	1	3	8
The Meats Pizza, Original Crust	230	11	3.5	620	25	1	3	10
The Works Pizza, Original Crust	220	7	3.5	600	26	2	4	9
Tuscan Six Cheese Pizza, Original Crust	210	8	3	530	26	1	3	10

Medium Pizza, 1 slice

	Cal	Fat	Sfat	Sod	Carb	Fiber	Sugar	Prot
BBQ Chicken & Bacon Pizza, Original Crust	240	8	2.5	690	32	1	5	11
BBQ Chicken & Bacon Pizza, Pan Crust	430	22	7	940	43	1	5	15

Description & Serving	Cal	Fat	Sfat	Sod	Carb	Fiber	Sugar	Prot
Cheese Pizza, Original Crust	210	8	2.5	510	27	1	3	9
Cheese Pizza, Pan Crust	410	23	7	750	38	1	3	13
Garden Fresh Pizza, Original Crust	200	7	2	490	28	2	4	8
Garden Fresh Pizza, Pan Crust	370	19	6	660	39	2	4	11
Hawaiian BBQ Chicken Pizza, Original Crust	240	8	2.5	690	33	1	6	11
Hawaiian BBQ Chicken Pizza, Pan Crust	440	22	7	940	45	1	7	15
Pepperoni Pizza, Original Crust	220	9	3	580	26	1	3	9
Pepperoni Pizza, Pan Crust	410	24	8	820	37	1	3	13
Sausage Pizza, Original Crust	240	11	3.5	580	26	2	3	9
Sausage Pizza, Pan Crust	420	25	8	790	37	2	3	12
Spicy Italian Pizza, Original Crust	260	8	7	680	27	2	4	11
Spicy Italian Pizza, Pan Crust	470	21	14	950	38	3	4	15
Spinach Alfredo Pizza, Original Crust	210	8	3	450	26	1	3	8
Spinach Alfredo Pizza, Pan Crust	380	22	8	610	35	1	2	11
The Meats Pizza, Original Crust	240	11	3.5	640	26	1	3	11
The Meats Pizza, Pan Crust	440	26	8	890	37	1	3	15
The Works Pizza, Original Crust	230	8	3.5	620	27	2	4	10
The Works Pizza, Pan Crust	420	21	9	860	38	2	4	14
Tuscan Six Cheese Pizza, Original Crust	230	9	3.5	570	27	1	3	11
Tuscan Six Cheese Pizza, Pan Crust	410	23	8	760	37	1	3	15

Large Pizza, 1 slice

	Cal	Fat	Sfat	Sod	Carb	Fiber	Sugar	Prot
BBQ Chicken & Bacon Pizza, Original Crust	340	11	3.5	960	44	2	7	15
BBQ Chicken & Bacon Pizza, Thin Crust	270	13	3.5	750	27	<1	3	12
Cheese Pizza, Original Crust	280	10	3	700	38	2	5	12
Cheese Pizza, Thin Crust	220	12	3	490	21	1	2	9
Garden Fresh Pizza, Original Crust	280	9	2.5	680	39	2	6	11
Garden Fresh Pizza, Thin Crust	210	11	2.5	470	23	2	3	8
Hawaiian BBQ Chicken Pizza, Original Crust	340	11	3.5	960	46	2	8	16
Hawaiian BBQ Chicken Pizza, Thin Crust	290	14	3.5	740	31	1	6	13
Pepperoni Pizza, Original Crust	310	13	4	810	38	2	5	13
Pepperoni Pizza, Thin Crust	250	15	4.5	600	21	1	2	10
Sausage Pizza, Original Crust	330	15	4.5	810	37	3	5	13
Sausage Pizza, Thin Crust	270	16	5	600	21	2	2	9
Spicy Italian Pizza, Original Crust	370	11	10	960	38	4	5	15
Spicy Italian Pizza, Thin Crust	310	13	11	760	22	3	2	12
Spinach Alfredo Pizza, Original Crust	280	11	4.5	630	36	2	4	11
Spinach Alfredo Pizza, Thin Crust	220	13	4.5	410	19	1	1	8
The Meats Pizza, Original Crust	350	16	5	930	38	2	5	15
The Meats Pizza, Thin Crust	280	17	5	720	21	1	2	12
The Works Pizza, Original Crust	330	11	6	890	39	3	5	14
The Works Pizza, Thin Crust	260	13	6	680	22	2	2	11
Tuscan Six Cheese Pizza, Original Crust	320	13	4.5	780	38	2	5	15
Tuscan Six Cheese Pizza, Thin Crust	250	14	5	580	21	1	2	12

Extra Large Pizza, 1 slice

	Cal	Fat	Sfat	Sod	Carb	Fiber	Sugar	Prot
BBQ Chicken & Bacon Pizza, Original Crust	350	12	3.5	1010	47	2	7	16
Cheese Pizza, Original Crust	300	10	3	720	41	2	5	12
Garden Fresh Pizza, Original Crust	290	9	2.5	720	42	3	6	12
Hawaiian BBQ Chicken Pizza, Original Crust	360	12	3.5	1010	49	2	9	16

Description & Serving	Cal	Fat	Sfat	Sod	Carb	Fiber	Sugar	Prot
Pepperoni Pizza, Original Crust	330	13	4	850	40	2	5	13
Sausage Pizza, Original Crust	340	15	4.5	840	40	3	5	13
Spicy Italian Pizza, Original Crust	390	12	11	1020	41	4	5	16
Spinach Alfredo Pizza, Original Crust	310	12	4.5	660	39	2	4	12
The Meats Pizza, Original Crust	370	17	5	980	40	2	5	16
The Works Pizza, Original Crust	350	11	6	940	42	3	6	15
Tuscan Six Cheese Pizza, Original Crust	330	13	4.5	820	41	2	5	15

Breadstick/Appetizer

	Cal	Fat	Sfat	Sod	Carb	Fiber	Sugar	Prot
Breadsticks	290	4.5	0.5	540	53	2	5	9
Cheesesticks	370	16	4.5	830	42	2	4	15
Garlic Parmesan Breadsticks	330	10	1.5	720	54	2	5	10
BBQ Wings	160	10	3	560	4	0	3	14
Buffalo Wings	160	11	3.5	680	1	1	1	14
Honey Chipotle Wings	190	12	3	730	8	0	5	12
Chickenstrips	160	8	2	350	10	0	1	10

Dessert

	Cal	Fat	Sfat	Sod	Carb	Fiber	Sugar	Prot
Applepie	480	10	2	510	89	3	43	9
Cinnapie	560	19	4	560	89	3	39	9
Cinnamon Sweetsticks	570	15	3	750	98	3	33	12
Chocolate Pastry Delights	180	11	6	140	18	1	6	2

Condiment

	Cal	Fat	Sfat	Sod	Carb	Fiber	Sugar	Prot
Barbeque Sauce Dipping Sauce	45	0	0	240	11	0	10	0
Blue Cheese Dipping Sauce	160	16	3.5	250	1	0	1	1
Buffalo Sauce Dipping Sauce	15	0.5	0	1030	2	0	2	0
Cheese Sauce Dipping Sauce	40	3.5	1	160	2	0	0	1
Honey Mustard Dipping Sauce	150	15	2.5	120	5	0	4	0
Pizza Sauce Dipping Sauce	20	1	0	230	3	0	1	0
Ranch Sauce Dipping Sauce	100	10	1.5	260	1	0	1	1
Special Garlic Dipping Sauce	150	17	3	310	0	0	0	0

Papa Murphy's

Pizza

Family Size, 1 Slice

	Cal	Fat	Sfat	Sod	Carb	Fiber	Sugar	Prot
5-Meat Stuffed Pizza	370	16	7	910	39	0	7	18
Big Murphy Stuffed Pizza	370	16	7	890	40	<1	7	17
Chicago Style Stuffed Pizza	370	16	7	850	40	<1	7	17
Chicken & Bacon Stuffed Pizza	370	15	7	820	39	0	6	20
All Meat Original Crust Pizza	360	18	9	900	31	0	6	19
Awesome Foursome Original Crust Pizza	270-320	11-15	6-8	560-800	30-34	<1	6-9	13-16
Barbeque Chicken Original Crust Pizza	340	13	7	720	37	0	10	19
Cheese Original Crust Pizza	270	11	6	560	30	0	6	13
Cowboy Original Crust Pizza	350	18	8	900	32	<1	6	17
Gourmet Chicken Garlic Original Crust Pizza	320	14	7	630	30	0	5	19
Gourmet Classic Italian Original Crust Pizza	350	18	8	790	31	<1	5	17
Gourmet Vegetarian Original Crust Pizza	300	14	7	700	31	1	5	14

Description & Serving	Cal	Fat	Sfat	Sod	Carb	Fiber	Sugar	Prot
Hawaiian Original Crust Pizza	290	11	6	670	33	<1	9	15
Herb Chicken Mediterranean Original Crust Pizza	340	14	7	630	35	3	7	17
Meat Sampler Original Crust Pizza	280-	11-	6-	670-	31-	<1	6	15-
	340	16	8	840	32			17
Murphy's Combo Original Crust Pizza	360	18	9	940	33	<1	6	18
Papa-Roni Original Crust Pizza	350	18	9	810	31	0	6	16
Papa's Favorite Original Crust Pizza	360	18	8	910	33	<1	6	18
Pepperoni Original Crust Pizza	320	15	8	710	31	0	6	15
Perfect Original Crust Pizza	290-	11-	6-	670-	30-	<1	6-	15
	320	15	8	710	34		9	
Rancher Original Crust Pizza	330	16	8	790	31	<1	6	17
Specialty of the House Original Crust Pizza	320	15	7	800	32	<1	6	16
Taco Grande Original Crust Pizza	340	16	7	850	34	2	5	17
Veggie Combo Original Crust Pizza	300	13	6	670	33	<1	6	14
Veggie Mediterranean Original Crust Pizza	310	14	6	610	34	3	7	13
Large Size, 1 slice								
5-Meat Stuffed Pizza	370	16	7	900	38	0	7	18
Big Murphy Stuffed Pizza	360	15	7	870	39	<1	7	17
Chicago Style Stuffed Pizza	370	16	7	840	39	<1	7	17
Chicken & Bacon Stuffed Pizza	360	14	7	790	38	0	6	20
All Meat Original Crust Pizza	320	16	8	790	28	0	5	17
Barbeque Chicken Original Crust Pizza	310	11	6	680	35	0	11	17
Cheese Original Crust Pizza	250	10	6	500	27	0	5	12
Cowboy Original Crust Pizza	320	16	8	810	29	<1	5	16
Gourmet Chicken Garlic Original Crust Pizza	290	13	6	560	27	0	4	17
Gourmet Classic Italian Original Crust Pizza	310	16	7	700	28	<1	4	15
Gourmet Vegitarian Original Crust Pizza	270	12	6	610	28	1	4	13
Hawaiian Original Crust Pizza	270	10	6	600	30	<1	8	13
Herb Chicken Mediterranean Original Crust Pizza	300	13	6	560	31	2	6	15
Murphy's Combo Original Crust Pizza	330	17	8	850	29	<1	6	16
Papa-Roni Original Crust Pizza	300	15	8	690	28	0	5	14
Papa's Favorite Original Crust Pizza	330	17	8	820	29	<1	6	16
Pepperoni Original Crust Pizza	290	14	7	640	27	0	5	13
Perfect Original Crust Pizza	270-	10-	6-	600-	27-	<1	5-	13
	290	14	7	640	30		8	
Rancher Original Crust Pizza	300	14	7	700	28	0	6	16
Specialty of the House Original Crust Pizza	300	14	7	730	29	<1	6	15
Taco Grande Original Crust Pizza	310	14	6	760	30	1	5	16
Veggie Combo Original Crust Pizza	270	11	6	610	30	<1	6	13
Veggie Mediterranean Original Crust Pizza	280	12	6	540	31	2	6	12
All Meat deLITE Thin Crust Pizza	190	11	5	430	13	0	2	11
Barbeque Chicken deLITE Thin Crust Pizza	180	8	4.5	340	17	0	5	12
Cheese deLITE Thin Crust Pizza	140	7	4	230	13	0	2	8
Chicken Bacon Artichoke deLITE Thin Crust Pizza	180	9	4	400	13	<1	1	12
Cowboy deLITE Thin Crust Pizza	190	11	5	460	14	0	2	11
Gourmet Chicken Garlic deLITE Thin Crust Pizza	170	9	4.5	270	13	0	1	11
Gourmet Classic Italian deLITE Thin Crust Pizza	190	10	5	380	14	<1	2	11
Gourmet Vegitarian deLITE Thin Crust Pizza	160	9	4.5	300	12	<1	1	9
Hawaiian deLITE Thin Crust Pizza	160	7	4	290	15	0	4	9

Description & Serving	Cal	Fat	Sfat	Sod	Carb	Fiber	Sugar	Prot
Herb Chicken Mediterranean deLITE Thin Crust Pizza	180	9	4	270	15	2	2	10
Meat deLITE Thin Crust Pizza	190	11	5	400	13	0	2	11
Murphy's Combo deLITE Thin Crust Pizza	200	12	6	490	14	0	2	11
Papa's Favorite deLITE Thin Crust Pizza	200	12	5	460	15	<1	2	11
Pepperoni deLITE Thin Crust Pizza	170	9	5	320	13	0	2	9
Rancher deLITE Thin Crust Pizza	180	10	5	370	14	0	2	10
Specialty of the House deLITE Thin Crust Pizza	180	10	5	400	14	0	2	10
Taco Grande deLITE Thin Crust Pizza	180	10	5	380	16	<1	<1	10
Vegetarian Combo deLITE Thin Crust Pizza	160	8	4	310	15	<1	2	8
Veggie deLITE Thin Crust Pizza	160	9	4	250	13	<1	1	8
Veggie Mediterranean deLITE Thin Crust Pizza	170	9	4	260	15	2	2	8
Medium Size, 1, slice								
All Meat Original Crust Pizza	290	14	7	710	25	0	5	15
Barbeque Chicken Original Crust Pizza	280	10	6	590	30	0	8	16
Cheese Original Crust Pizza	230	9	5	460	25	0	5	11
Cowboy Original Crust Pizza	290	15	7	740	26	0	5	14
Gourmet Chicken Garlic Original Crust Pizza	260	12	6	510	25	0	4	15
Gourmet Classic Italian Original Crust Pizza	280	13	7	640	26	<1	5	14
Gourmet Vegetarian Original Crust Pizza	250	11	6	550	25	<1	4	12
Hawaiian Original Crust Pizza	240	10	5	540	28	0	7	12
Herb Chicken Mediterranean Original Crust Pizza	270	12	5	510	27	2	5	14
Murphy's Combo Original Crust Pizza	300	15	7	780	27	<1	5	15
Papa-Roni Original Crust Pizza	270	14	7	620	25	0	5	13
Papa's Favorite Original Crust Pizza	300	15	7	750	27	<1	5	15
Pepperoni Original Crust Pizza	260	13	6	580	25	0	5	12
Perfect Original Crust Pizza	240-260	10-13	5-6	540-580	25-28	0	5-7	12
Rancher Original Crust Pizza	270	13	6	640	26	0	5	14
Specialty of the House Original Crust Pizza	270	13	6	670	26	0	5	13
Taco Grande Original Crust Pizza	220	10	5	520	23	<1	3	11
Veggie Combo Original Crust Pizza	250	11	5	560	27	<1	6	11
Veggie Mediterranean Original Crust Pizza	260	11	5	490	27	2	5	11
Pasta/Calzone								
Lasagna, 1/8 portion	330	18	9	760	26	2	9	17
Chicken Florentine Calzone, fam size, 1/8 portion	470	20	9	1050	46	1	7	26
Combo Calzone, fam size, 1/8 portion	450	21	11	1030	46	<1	8	21
Italian Calzone, fam size, 1/8 portion	470	21	10	1170	47	<1	8	23
Veggie Calzone, fam size, 1/8 portion	410	17	9	970	46	2	8	19
Chicken Florentine Calzone, lrg size, 1/6 portion	460	19	9	1040	46	1	7	26
Combo Calzone, lrg size, 1/6 portion	450	20	10	1020	45	<1	8	21
Italian Calzone, lrg size, 1/6 portion	450	20	10	1090	46	<1	8	22
Veggie Calzone, lrg size, 1/6 portion	400	16	9	920	46	1	8	18
Side/Salad/Dressing/Condiment								
Cheesy Bread	220	7	3	480	31	0	5	7
Caesar Salad	50	2	1	120	4	2	2	4
Chicken Caesar Salad	140	5	2.5	320	5	3	2	18
Club Salad	140	8	4	480	6	3	2	13

Description & Serving	Cal	Fat	Sfat	Sod	Carb	Fiber	Sugar	Prot
Garden Salad	100	6	3	260	8	3	2	6
Italian Salad	140	10	4	400	7	3	1	7
Buttermilk Ranch Dressing, 15 g	120	13	1	210	2	0	2	0
Caesar Salad Dressing, 15 g	140	14	1	170	2	0	1	1
Low Calorie Italian Salad Dressing, 15 g	10	0.5	0	280	1	0	1	0
Marinara Sauce for Cheesy Bread	10	0	0	60	2	0	1	0
Croutons	90	3.5	0	140	11	0	0	2
Dessert								
Cookie Dough w/ Hershey's Chocolate Chips	120	6	2	115	17	0	10	1
Apple Dessert Pizza	240	4.5	1	340	46	<1	19	4
Cherry Dessert Pizza	240	4.5	1	330	44	<1	16	4
Cinnamon Wheel	250	7	2	410	42	0	13	5
Cream Cheese Frosting	50	3	2	40	4	0	4	0

Pei Wei Asian Diner

Appetizer

	Cal	Fat	Sfat	Sod	Carb	Fiber	Sugar	Prot
Minced Chicken w/ Cool Lettuce Wraps, 1/2 of dish (no rice sticks)	250	4	NP	NP	31	3	15	22
Pei Wei Spring Rolls, 2	90	5	NP	NP	11	1	3	2
Crab Wontons, 4	190	13	NP	NP	9	0	0	8
Crab Wontons, 6	230	16	NP	NP	9	0	0	11
Crispy Potstickers, 4	130	7	NP	NP	10	1	1	6
Crispy Potstickers, 6	150	8	NP	NP	10	1	1	8
Edamame, 1/2 of dish	156	8	NP	NP	12	4	4	14
Hot & Sour Soup, cup	150	9	NP	NP	11	0	0	7
Hot & Sour Soup, bowl	500	28	NP	NP	37	1	1	24

Salad

	Cal	Fat	Sfat	Sod	Carb	Fiber	Sugar	Prot
Asian Chopped Chicken Salad w/ dressing, 1/2 of dish	280	15	NP	NP	13	2	4	24
Asian Chopped Chicken Salad w/o dressing, 1/2 of dish	200	8	NP	NP	10	2	2	23
Pei Wei Spicy Chicken Salad w/ dressing, 1/2 of dish	350	16	NP	NP	28	2	8	22
Pei Wei Spicy Chicken Salad w/o dressing, 1/2 of dish	210	2.5	NP	NP	23	2	3	22
Vietnamese Chicken Salad Rolls, 1/3 of dish	53	3	NP	NP	5	0.5	3	3

Entrée

Beef

	Cal	Fat	Sfat	Sod	Carb	Fiber	Sugar	Prot
Mongolian Beef, 1/2 of dish	420	22	NP	NP	14	1	8	36
Lemon Pepper Beef, 1/2 of dish	550	31	NP	NP	32	2	18	38
Thai Coconut Curry Beef, 1/2 of dish	550	37	NP	NP	20	2	10	36
Pei Wei Spicy Beef, 1/2 of dish	480	26	NP	NP	25	2	8	34
Ginger Broccoli Beef, 1/2 of dish	450	22	NP	NP	19	2	11	37
Mandarin Kung Pao Beef, 1/2 of dish	610	34	NP	NP	31	3	10	40
Orange Peel Beef, 1/2 of dish	660	31	NP	NP	52	3	33	42
Spicy Korean Beef, 1/2 of dish	490	24	NP	NP	26	3	12	41

Description & Serving	Cal	Fat	Sfat	Sod	Carb	Fiber	Sugar	Prot
Chicken								
Thai Dynamite Chicken, 1/2 of dish	390	19	NP	NP	20	2	7	33
Mongolian Chicken, 1/2 of dish	280	9	NP	NP	14	1	8	30
Lemon Pepper Chicken, 1/2 of dish	440	20	NP	NP	34	2	18	31
Thai Coconut Curry Chicken, 1/2 of dish	380	19	NP	NP	23	2	10	30
Pei Wei Spicy Chicken, 1/2 of dish	330	13	NP	NP	25	2	8	28
Ginger Broccoli Chicken, 1/2 of dish	300	9	NP	NP	19	2	11	31
Mandarin Kung Pao Chicken, 1/2 of dish	450	21	NP	NP	28	3	10	34
Orange Peel Chicken, 1/2 of dish	520	18	NP	NP	52	3	33	36
Honey Seared Chicken, 1/2 of dish	420	15	NP	NP	45	1	17	21
Spicy Korean Chicken, 1/2 of dish	350	11	NP	NP	26	3	12	35
Sweet & Sour Chicken, 1/2 of dish	440	13	NP	NP	61	2	30	21
Noodles/Rice								
Chicken Pad Thai, 1/2 of dish	560	20	NP	NP	61	2	19	35
Beef Pad Thai, 1/2 of dish	670	30	NP	NP	63	2	19	40
Vegetables & Tofu Pad Thai, 1/2 of dish	470	17	NP	NP	66	4	21	18
Shrimp Pad Thai, 1/2 of dish	490	17	NP	NP	60	2	19	27
Chicken Dan Dan Noodles, 1/2 of dish	390	7	NP	NP	54	3	9	26
Chicken Lo Mein Noodles, 1/2 of dish	460	11	NP	NP	61	5	9	31
Beef Lo Mein Noodles, 1/2 of dish	570	21	NP	NP	61	5	9	36
Vegetables & Tofu Lo Mein Noodles, 1/2 of dish	400	8	NP	NP	66	7	11	16
Shrimp Lo Mein Noodles, 1/2 of dish	400	8	NP	NP	60	5	9	23
Chicken Thai Blazing Noodles, 1/2 of dish	520	22	NP	NP	55	4	11	24
Beef Thai Blazing Noodles, 1/2 of dish	630	32	NP	NP	55	4	11	28
Vegetables & Tofu Thai Blazing Noodles, 1/2 of dish	430	18	NP	NP	59	6	14	10
Shrimp Thai Blazing Noodles, 1/2 of dish	482	22	NP	NP	55	4	11	16
Chicken Fried Rice Bowl, 1/2 of dish	525	11	NP	NP	68	3	9	32
Beef Fried Rice Bowl, 1/2 of dish	630	21	NP	NP	68	3	9	37
Vegetables & Tofu Fried Rice Bowl, 1/2 of dish	440	7	NP	NP	73	5	12	17
Shrimp Fried Rice Bowl, 1/2 of dish	475	10	NP	NP	67	3	9	24
Chicken Japanese Teriyaki Bowl w/ Brown Rice, 1/2 of dish	460	7	NP	NP	64	4	21	28
Chicken Japanese Teriyaki Bowl w/ White Rice, 1/2 of dish	440	6	NP	NP	60	3	21	28
Beef Japanese Teriyaki Bowl w/ Brown Rice, 1/2 of dish	580	17	NP	NP	66	4	21	33
Beef Japanese Teriyaki Bowl w/ White Rice, 1/2 of dish	560	16	NP	NP	62	3	21	32
Vegetables & Tofu Japanese Teriyaki Bowl w/ Brown Rice, 1/2 of dish	410	6	NP	NP	71	7	24	13
Vegetables & Tofu Japanese Teriyaki Bowl w/ White Rice, 1/2 of dish	390	5	NP	NP	68	5	24	13
Shrimp Japanese Teriyaki Bowl w/ Brown Rice, 1/2 of dish	410	5	NP	NP	64	4	21	20
Shrimp Japanese Teriyaki Bowl w/ White Rice, 1/2 of dish	390	4.5	NP	NP	61	3	21	20

Description & Serving	Cal	Fat	Sfat	Sod	Carb	Fiber	Sugar	Prot
Shrimp								
Thai Dynamite Shrimp, 1/2 of dish	280	16	NP	NP	20	2	8	15
Mongolian Shrimp, 1/2 of dish	210	6	NP	NP	12	1	8	21
Lemon Pepper Shrimp, 1/2 of dish	380	18	NP	NP	34	2	18	22
Thai Coconut Curry Shrimp, 1/2 of dish	300	17	NP	NP	18	2	10	21
Pei Wei Spicy Shrimp, 1/2 of dish	300	11	NP	NP	29	2	8	19
Ginger Broccoli Shrimp, 1/2 of dish	230	7	NP	NP	18	2	11	22
Mandarin Kung Pao Shrimp, 1/2 of dish	400	19	NP	NP	28	3	10	25
Orange Peel Shrimp, 1/2 of dish	460	16	NP	NP	51	3	33	27
Honey Seared Shrimp, 1/2 of dish	370	14	NP	NP	43	0	17	14
Spicy Korean Shrimp, 1/2 of dish	280	9	NP	NP	24	3	12	26
Sweet & Sour Shrimp, 1/2 of dish	390	11	NP	NP	59	2	30	14
Vegetarian								
Thai Dynamite Vegetables & Tofu, 1/2 of dish	220	16	NP	NP	15	3	9	6
Mongolian Vegetables & Tofu, 1/2 of dish	180	6	NP	NP	19	3	11	10
Lemon Pepper Vegetables & Tofu, 1/2 of dish	230	10	NP	NP	29	4	19	10
Thai Coconut Curry Vegetables & Tofu, 1/2 of dish	220	14	NP	NP	19	2	11	8
Pei Wei Spicy Vegetables & Tofu, 1/2 of dish	250	16	NP	NP	21	3	8	6
Ginger Broccoli Vegetables & Tofu, 1/2 of dish	170	3.5	NP	NP	23	4	14	10
Mandarin Kung Pao Vegetables & Tofu, 1/2 of dish	290	15	NP	NP	23	4	10	13
Orange Peel Vegetables & Tofu, 1/2 of dish	330	10	NP	NP	46	4	33	14
Spicy Korean Vegetables & Tofu, 1/2 of dish	240	9	NP	NP	27	4	14	15
Side								
Rice Sticks, 1 cup	130	0	NP	NP	33	0	0	0
Fortune Cookie	30	0	NP	NP	7	0	3	0
Brown Rice, 1/2 of dish	170	1.5	NP	NP	37	3	0	4
White Rice, 1/2 of dish	200	0	NP	NP	44	1	0	4
Fried Rice, 1/2 of dish	260	5	NP	NP	44	2	5	9
Egg Noodles, 1/2 of dish	210	2.5	NP	NP	39	2	0	7
Rice Noodles, 1/2 of dish	130	0	NP	NP	32	0	0	0
Kids								
Kids Wei Teriyaki Chicken	240	5	NP	NP	20	0	18	23
Kids Wei Honey Seared Chicken	290	17	NP	NP	19	0	8	16
Kids Wei Lo Mein Chicken	180	7	NP	NP	7	0	3	20
Brown Rice, 1/2 of dish	100	0.5	NP	NP	20	2	0	2
White Rice, 1/2 of dish	110	0	NP	NP	24	0	0	2
Egg Noodles, 1/2 of dish	210	2.5	NP	NP	39	2	0	7
Rice Noodles, 1/2 of dish	130	0	NP	NP	32	0	0	0
Dressing/Condiment								
Lime Vinaigrette	230	20	NP	NP	13	0	11	0
Sesame Ginger Dressing	170	16	NP	NP	5	0	4	1
Sweet Chile Sauce	140	0	NP	NP	34	2	28	0
Thai Peanut Sauce	168	11	NP	NP	15	1	11	5
Lettuce Wrap Sauce	70	4.5	NP	NP	2	0	1	4
Dessert								
Chocolate Chip Cookie	342	14	NP	NP	53	2	37	5

Description & Serving	Cal	Fat	Sfat	Sod	Carb	Fiber	Sugar	Prot
Penn Station East Coast Subs								
Bread								
Bread, sml, 7"	273	1.66	NP	692.25	54	NP	NP	NP
Wrap, 10"	206.6	5.78	NP	786.13	34	NP	NP	NP
Meat (3 oz per small sub)								
Bacon, 2 slices	55	4	NP	181	0.28	NP	NP	NP
Chicken Salad, 1 oz	66	5	NP	140	3.4	NP	NP	NP
Chicken, 1 oz	47	1	NP	21	0	NP	NP	NP
Corned Beef, 1 oz	73	2	NP	603	1	NP	NP	NP
Ham, 1 oz	33	0.5	NP	290	0	NP	NP	NP
Pepperoni, 1 oz	140	13	NP	470	0	NP	NP	NP
Salami, 1 oz	120	11	NP	500	0	NP	NP	NP
Sausage, 1 oz	90	7	NP	270	0.76	NP	NP	NP
Steak, 1 oz	38	2	NP	16	0	NP	NP	NP
Tuna Salad, 1 oz	60	4	NP	150	3.4	NP	NP	NP
Turkey (white), 1 oz	25	0.25	NP	220	0	NP	NP	NP
Vegetables (portion on small sub)								
Artichokes, 1 oz	8	0	NP	95	1.5	NP	NP	NP
Banana Peppers, grilled, .25 oz	1.25	0	NP	120	0.25	NP	NP	NP
Green Peppers, grilled, .5 oz	4	0.03	NP	0.2	0.91	NP	NP	NP
Lettuce, 1.25 oz	5	0.07	NP	4	0.74	NP	NP	NP
Mushrooms, grilled, .37 oz	3	0.04	NP	0.3	0.49	NP	NP	NP
Pickles, .19 oz	1	0.01	NP	75	0.22	NP	NP	NP
Red Onions, 1.4 oz	17	0.08	NP	0	3.41	NP	NP	NP
Tomato, .8 oz	5	0.07	NP	2	1.06	NP	NP	NP
Yellow Onions, grilled, 1.87 oz	21	0.11	NP	0	4.56	NP	NP	NP
Cheese (portion on small sub)								
American, 1 oz	100	5	NP	510	1	NP	NP	NP
Provolone, 1 oz	100	8	NP	200	0.6	NP	NP	NP
Swiss, 1 oz	100	8	NP	60	0.94	NP	NP	NP
Dressing/Condiment (portion on small sub)								
1,000 Island Dressing, 2 oz	215	20.26	NP	397	8.62	NP	NP	NP
Honey Mustard, 0.5 oz	66	6.14	NP	85	2.36	NP	NP	NP
Mayonnaise, 0.5 oz	101	11.26	NP	81	0.38	NP	NP	NP
Olive Oil & Vinegar, 0.38 oz	96	11	NP	0	0.32	NP	NP	NP
Oregano, 0.009 tbsp	16	1.75	NP	14	0.01	NP	NP	NP
Parmesan Cheese, 0.19 oz	25	1.62	NP	100	0.2	NP	NP	NP
Pizza Sauce, 1.31 oz	18	0.24	NP	80	3.54	NP	NP	NP
Sauerkraut, 4 oz	16	0.16	NP	1096	3.78	NP	NP	NP
Teriyaki, 1 oz	28	0	NP	1153	5.42	NP	NP	NP
P.F. Chang's China Bistro								
Appetizer								
Chang's Chicken Lettuce Wraps	153	7	1	655	15	NP	NP	8
Chang's Vegetarian Lettuce Wraps	135	7	1	535	10	NP	NP	6

Description & Serving	Cal	Fat	Sfat	Sod	Carb	Fiber	Sugar	Prot
Crispy Green Beans	167	14	13	27	8	NP	NP	2
Spring Rolls, 2	313	16	4	542	34	NP	NP	7
Seared Ahi Tuna	44	1	0	335	2	NP	NP	7
Spicy Mustard Sauce, 2 oz	187	18	2	955	5	NP	NP	1
Crab Wontons, 2	169	11	4	304	13	NP	NP	5
Plum Sauce, 2 oz	247	0	0	1863	63	NP	NP	0
Salt & Pepper Calamari	345	21	4	725	36	NP	NP	13
Sichuan Chicken Flatbread	179	8	5	454	12	NP	NP	16
Sichuan Chicken Sauce, 2 oz	335	36	5	556	4	NP	NP	0
Cabbage Slaw	147	14	2	314	4	NP	NP	1
Northern Style Spare Ribs	342	19	2	985	11	NP	NP	31
Dynamite Shrimp	482	42	6	1133	10	NP	NP	19
Chang's Spare Ribs	344	24	7	336	7	NP	NP	26
Pan-Fried Peking Dumplings, 1	93	5	1	215	7	NP	NP	6
Steamed Peking Dumplings, 1	66	3	1	178	6	NP	NP	5
Pan-Fried Shrimp Dumplings, 1	68	2	1	347	8	NP	NP	6
Steamed Shrimp Dumplings, 1	58	0	0	347	8	NP	NP	6
Pan-Fried Vegetable Dumplings, 1	66	2	0	172	11	NP	NP	2
Steamed Vegetable Dumplings, 1	56	0	0	172	11	NP	NP	2
Egg Rolls, 1	174	8	1	673	22	NP	NP	5

Salad

Chicken Chopped Salad w/ Ginger Dressing	940	68	10	2225	33	NP	NP	47
Chang's Wedge Salad	665	60	13	1080	17	NP	NP	12
Chang's Wedge Salad w/ Chicken	865	64	13	1900	19	NP	NP	52
Asian Shrimp Salad	541	31	4	827	33	NP	NP	38

Soup

Wonton Soup	150	7	2	820	10	NP	NP	9
Chang's Noodle Soup	130	4	1	770	16	NP	NP	7
Hot & Sour Soup, cup	80	3	1	1000	9	NP	NP	5
Hot & Sour Soup, bowl	510	19	4	5990	54	NP	NP	28
Egg Drop Soup, cup	70	3	0	1050	10	NP	NP	1
Egg Drop Soup, bowl	400	15	3	6310	58	NP	NP	6

Lunch

Beef

Beef w/ Broccoli, 1 bowl	790	23	5	4085	98	NP	NP	46

Chicken

Sesame Chicken, 1 bowl	1025	25	4	2489	148	NP	NP	49
Almond & Cashew Chicken, 1 bowl	990	37	6	4963	114	NP	NP	48
Moo Goo Gai Pan, 1 bowl	833	24	4	4435	109	NP	NP	41
Crispy Honey Chicken, 1 bowl	1271	50	9	618	150	NP	NP	56

Gluten Free

Shrimp w/ Lobster Sauce, 1 bowl	715	21	4	4745	100	NP	NP	31
Moo Goo Gai Pan, 1 bowl	809	25	4	4437	101	NP	NP	41

Seafood

Shrimp w/ Lobster Sauce, 1 bowl	722	20	4	4745	103	NP	NP	31
Asian Grilled Salmon, 1 bowl	785	35	16	1203	73	NP	NP	43

Description & Serving	Cal	Fat	Sfat	Sod	Carb	Fiber	Sugar	Prot
Steak								
Pepper Steak, 1 bowl	776	23	5	3489	96	NP	NP	42
Vegetarian								
Buddha's Feast Steamed, 1 bowl	574	10	0	1831	102	NP	NP	22
Entrée								
Beef								
Hong Kong Beef w/ Snow Peas	370	20	4	75	24	NP	NP	24
Mongolian Beef	471	25	8	3094	27	NP	NP	33
Wok-Charred Beef	170	6	3	2009	15	NP	NP	15
Beef w/ Broccoli	345	14	3	2159	26	NP	NP	29
Beef a La Sichuan	518	22	5	2196	40	NP	NP	40
Orange Peel Beef	272	12	3	700	21	NP	NP	21
Chicken								
Chang's Spicy Chicken	300	12	2	800	29	NP	NP	18
Sweet & Sour Chicken	276	13	2	280	29	NP	NP	11
Almond & Cashew Chicken	280	12	2	2258	26	NP	NP	16
Dali Chicken	276	13	2	300	24	NP	NP	20
Moo Goo Gai Pan	278	11	2	1880	26	NP	NP	19
Crispy Honey Chicken	336	10	2	125	46	NP	NP	13
Orange Peel Chicken	295	15	2	454	21	NP	NP	21
Philip's Better Lemon Chicken	229	10	2	74	23	NP	NP	14
Mu Shu Chicken	232	12	2	870	13	NP	NP	19
Mu Shu Pancake, 1	90	2	0	30	14	NP	NP	2
Kung Pao Chicken	393	22	3	756	24	NP	NP	27
Sesame Chicken	374	16	2	932	31	NP	NP	27
Ginger Chicken w/ Broccoli	283	13	2	1304	21	NP	NP	22
Chicken w/ Black Bean Sauce	218	12	2	1295	12	NP	NP	17
Ground Chicken & Eggplant	188	6	1	1830	23	NP	NP	10
Mandarin Chicken	360	15	2	1715	29	NP	NP	33
Canton Chicken & Mushrooms	735	4	4	2430	89	NP	NP	47
Duck								
VIP Duck	495	18	5	1431	58	NP	NP	31
Gluten Free								
Chicken Lettuce Wraps	328	6	1	63	53	NP	NP	12
Singapore Street Noodles	285	8	1	203	39	NP	NP	11
P.F. Chang's Chicken Fried Rice	300	10	2	560	38	NP	NP	12
P.F. Chang's Shrimp Fried Rice	300	9	2	580	39	NP	NP	12
Shrimp w/ Lobster Sauce	262	10	2	2638	25	NP	NP	18
Moo Goo Gai Pan	277	11	2	1880	26	NP	NP	19
Ginger Chicken w/ Broccoli	306	14	2	154	23	NP	NP	22
Philip's Better Lemon Chicken	407	17	3	132	40	NP	NP	25
Chang's Spicy Chicken	534	22	4	1437	51	NP	NP	32
Chang's Lemon Scallops	188	3	0	258	20	NP	NP	22
Salmon Steamed w/ Ginger	272	14	2	159	14	NP	NP	22
Cantonese Shrimp	147	6	1	974	10	NP	NP	13
Cantonese Scallops	167	8	1	1006	14	NP	NP	9
Spinach Stir-Fried w/ Garlic, sml	80	4	1	448	8	NP	NP	6

Description & Serving	Cal	Fat	Sfat	Sod	Carb	Fiber	Sugar	Prot
Garlic Snap Peas, sml	100	3	0	162	12	NP	NP	3
Shanghai Cucumbers, sml	63	3	0	1109	5	NP	NP	3
Lamb								
Wok-Seared Lamb	227	13	3	1102	7	NP	NP	20
Chengdu Spiced Lamb	362	18	2	1173	16	NP	NP	33
Noodles/Rice								
Singapore Street Noodles	263	7	1	873	36	NP	NP	12
Beef Lo Mein	483	21	2	1366	68	NP	NP	23
Pork Lo Mein	473	24	4	1723	56	NP	NP	24
Chicken Lo Mein	522	27	4	1581	59	NP	NP	26
Shrimp Lo Mein	436	19	1	1415	65	NP	NP	20
Combo Lo Mein	492	24	3	1465	59	NP	NP	26
Cantonese Chow Fun, Chicken	352	13	2	995	39	NP	NP	17
Cantonese Chow Fun, Beef	338	12	2	1161	39	NP	NP	17
Garlic Noodles	384	5	1	849	72	NP	NP	12
Double Pan-Fried Noodles, Beef	396	18	1	1911	43	NP	NP	15
Double Pan-Fried Noodles, Pork	395	18	1	1865	41	NP	NP	16
Double Pan-Fried Noodles, Chicken	403	19	1	1831	43	NP	NP	14
Double Pan-Fried Noodles, Shrimp	364	17	1	1945	41	NP	NP	12
Double Pan-Fried Noodles, Combo	408	20	2	1918	39	NP	NP	18
Dan Dan Noodles	472	24	1	1752	75	NP	NP	20
P.F. Chang's Beef Fried Rice	384	16	3	1208	44	NP	NP	16
P.F. Chang's Pork Fried Rice	406	20	5	1603	41	NP	NP	14
P.F. Chang's Chicken Fried Rice	383	16	3	1137	41	NP	NP	18
P.F. Chang's Shrimp Fried Rice	343	13	2	1251	41	NP	NP	13
P.F. Chang's Combo Fried Rice	401	18	4	1332	38	NP	NP	21
P.F. Chang's Vegetarian Fried Rice	214	2	1	421	43	NP	NP	6
Pork								
Hunan Pork	350	14	2	2315	29	NP	NP	24
Sweet & Sour Pork	253	9	5	576	33	NP	NP	9
Mu Shu Pork	249	16	5	1541	10	NP	NP	17
Mu Shu Pancake, 1	90	2	0	30	14	NP	NP	2
Seafood								
Asian Grilled Salmon w/ Rice	367	16	7	653	27	NP	NP	28
Lemongrass Prawns w/ Garlic Noodles	608	44	10	1428	58	NP	NP	27
Mahi-Mahi	325	16	4	749	22	NP	NP	23
Oolong Marinated Sea Bass	291	15	4	1695	20	NP	NP	20
Cantonese Scallops	297	14	2	1800	25	NP	NP	17
Kung Pao Scallops	269	12	2	878	16	NP	NP	26
Salt & Pepper Prawns	146	7	1	670	15	NP	NP	8
Chang's Lemon Scallops	188	3	0	257	20	NP	NP	22
Salmon Steamed w/ Ginger	125	14	2	533	9	NP	NP	23
Sichuan from the Sea, Scallops	201	10	2	716	18	NP	NP	11
Sichuan from the Sea, Calamari	366	23	4	365	26	NP	NP	13
Sichuan from the Sea, Shrimp	177	7	1	676	13	NP	NP	16
Hot Fish	305	18	4	1395	18	NP	NP	20
Shanghai Shrimp w/ Garlic Sauce	210	11	2	1125	10	NP	NP	19
Crispy Honey Shrimp	422	14	2	363	58	NP	NP	12

Description & Serving	Cal	Fat	Sfat	Sod	Carb	Fiber	Sugar	Prot
Cantonese Shrimp	262	10	2	1742	18	NP	NP	23
Shrimp w/ Lobster Sauce	273	11	2	2712	27	NP	NP	18
Kung Pao Shrimp	258	12	2	844	16	NP	NP	24
Orange Peel Shrimp	182	7	1	794	15	NP	NP	14
Shrimp w/ Candied Walnuts	412	26	1	754	30	NP	NP	18
Lemon Pepper Shrimp	227	10	2	1225	16	NP	NP	21
Steak								
Asian Marinated New York Strip	186	10	4	288	10	NP	NP	16
Pepper Steak	314	13	3	1864	24	NP	NP	25
Vegetarian								
Buddha's Feast, Steamed	161	3	0	1073	24	NP	NP	12
Buddha's Feast, Stir-Fried	189	5	0	1064	28	NP	NP	12
Stir-Fried Eggplant	96	3	0	438	16	NP	NP	2
Coconut Curry Vegetables	295	21	8	565	16	NP	NP	7
Ma Po Tofu	260	15	5	1144	18	NP	NP	14
Vegetable Chow Fun	391	20	0	640	76	NP	NP	16
Side								
Shanghai Cucumbers, sml	63	3	0	1109	5	NP	NP	3
Garlic Snap Peas, sml	100	3	0	162	12	NP	NP	3
Spinach Stir-Fried w/ Garlic, sml	90	5	0	448	8	NP	NP	6
Spicy Green Beans, sml	96	5	1	13	10	NP	NP	3
Sichuan-Style Asparagus, sml	107	5	1	131	11	NP	NP	3
Asian Slaw, sml	302	29	4	646	8	NP	NP	3
Wok-Seared Mushrooms, sml	251	19	8	949	12	NP	NP	6
Green Tea Noodles, sml	407	18	2	1749	51	NP	NP	9
White Rice Steamed, 1/2 cup	121	0	0	0	27	NP	NP	2
Brown Rice Steamed, 1/2 cup	109	1	0	1	23	NP	NP	2
Kids								
Kid's Chicken w/ Honey	220	6	1	745	28	NP	NP	12
Kid's Chicken w/ Sweet & Sour	180	6	1	860	18	NP	NP	12
Baby Buddha's Feast, Steamed	30	0	0	25	12	NP	NP	2
Baby Buddha's Feast, Stir-Fried	95	5	1	685	11	NP	NP	3
Kid's Fried Rice	187	5	1	503	25	NP	NP	8
Kid's Lo Mein	195	5	1	480	6	NP	NP	6
Dessert								
Banana Spring Rolls	992	45	23	480	145	NP	NP	15
The Great Wall of Chocolate	1440	61	20	1120	231	NP	NP	10
Flourless Chocolate Dome	440	26	8	290	52	NP	NP	7
New York-Style Cheesecake	870	56	35	620	70	NP	NP	16
Mini Carrot Cake	170	7	3	110	25	NP	NP	1
Mini Red Velvet Cake	170	9	3	110	23	NP	NP	2
Mini Great Wall	150	5	2	130	26	NP	NP	1
Mini Strawberry Cheesecake	229	17	9	162	17	NP	NP	3
Mini Apple Pie	127	5	1	127	20	NP	NP	1
Mini Tiramisu	234	17	7	96	17	NP	NP	3
Mini Lemon Dream	190	4	2	30	30	NP	NP	4
Mini S'mores	268	10	3	184	44	NP	NP	2

Description & Serving	Cal	Fat	Sfat	Sod	Carb	Fiber	Sugar	Prot

Pizza Delight

Appetizer

Fire Bread w/ Spinach & Artichoke Dip	814.11	31.95	12.22	2193.95	109.41	10.48	5.23	26.43
Garlic Cheese Fingers	336.4	11.21	5.57	861	44.13	1.75	4.07	15.71
Bruschetta Cheese Fingers	334.49	11.37	3.7	950.63	46.63	2.43	5.64	12.38
Oven-Baked Chicken Wings, 6	380.93	28.29	6.29	923.4	14.58	0	1.62	22.68
French Onion Soup	370.46	16.48	8.22	3044.06	37.42	4.33	10.98	17.96
Fajita Flat'za	442.41	18.46	10.92	1735.51	41.14	1.97	4.41	20.84
Southwest Flat'za	718.61	55.32	13.96	1598.37	34.29	2.28	2.01	21.88

Entrée

Chicken Skillet	285.78	11.47	1.27	862.24	12.76	3.63	5.96	35.77
Seafood Skillet	330.66	21.79	6.83	1280.07	14.34	3.63	5.95	21.76
Quarter Chicken Dinner	973.69	42.61	7.55	2348.37	75.59	3.99	3.64	68.29
BBQ Chicken Skillet	474.52	13.42	5.61	1826.72	57.54	7.52	34.94	42.71
Super Donair Skillet	855.3	53.98	26.8	2706.1	51.24	4.96	30.73	44.58
Sweet & Sour Chicken Skillet	533.94	17.72	8.73	361.53	60.02	4.47	49.98	36.73

Pasta, per portion

Chicken Carbonara	1458.4	79.66	16.7	2357.6	109.29	7.73	10.5	79.89
Chicken Portobello Rosa	1099.93	48.77	8.79	1506.13	98.46	9.74	15.84	66.8
Oven-Baked Lasagna	638.06	27.71	15.05	1549.68	60.96	6.65	2.96	38.82
Chicken Broccoli Penne	700.3	21.61	10.96	1129.34	74.84	6.9	3.35	51.15
Spaghetti w/ Italian Meatballs	629.81	19.27	7.2	1247.78	79.44	5.78	6.29	31.82
Spaghetti Supreme	777.79	30.39	14.3	1611.43	81.16	6.06	7.55	43.72
Pasta Classica	714.92	28.21	8.62	1510.59	73.58	4.35	4.14	41.11
Seafood Pasta	694.52	23.07	12.04	1278.93	80.33	4.62	8.38	41.5
Chickan Tetrazzini	884.35	28.74	11.46	2272.2	93.99	5.74	3.02	62.48
Fettuccine Alfredo w/ Chicken	745.43	31.88	8.81	1465.71	71.93	3.97	2.38	42.1
BBQ Chicken Penne	752.51	26.05	15.32	1113.67	83.06	5.78	7.37	46.87
Chicken & Peppered Bacon Fettuccine	850.07	35.04	16.68	1641.12	82.66	5.47	8.94	55.78
Oven-Baked Lasagna Combo	638.05	27.71	15.05	1550	60.96	6.65	2.98	38.82
Eight Layer Lasagna	287.76	8.92	4.73	696.45	34.73	5.15	1.05	18.56
Portobello Beef Penne	1067.58	48.09	11.85	2208.28	102.83	11.02	14.83	55.18

Donair/Panzerotti

Famous Donair	463.82	15.64	7.05	1480.34	60.42	3.02	15.62	21.08
Super Donair	625.65	28.09	13.51	2051.53	62.12	3.4	16.22	32.61
Classic Panzerotti	420.2	15.74	7	1350.65	49.51	3.75	7.51	22.08
Seafood Panzerotti	376.02	11.28	5.47	1059.85	46.67	1.89	6.69	22.89
Greek Panzerotti	420.76	19.52	7.07	1245.61	46.84	2.7	6.48	16.38
Donair Panzerotti	595.73	24.33	11.27	1841.21	68.62	2.81	23.35	27.24
Regular Classic Panzerotti Combo	420.2	15.74	7	1351	49.51	3.75	7.51	22.08

Pizza

Works Pizza, 1 slice	275.5	10.8	5.1	762.96	30.51	1.75	4.03	15.22
All-Star Meat Pizza, 1 slice	280.18	10.77	5.12	830.74	29.67	1.59	3.65	17.17
Hawaiian Delight Pizza, 1 slice	286.9	11.2	5.95	784.26	31.01	1.38	5.45	17.02
Broadway Classic Pizza, 1 slice	226.28	10.81	5.15	645.92	19.83	1.86	3.78	13.87

Description & Serving	Cal	Fat	Sfat	Sod	Carb	Fiber	Sugar	Prot
Chunky Vegetable Greek Pizza, 1 slice	270.67	11.99	4.95	748.85	30.66	1.59	4.14	11.21
Ultimate Pizza, 1 slice	295.06	12.12	5.57	832.42	30.83	1.9	4.2	16.84
BBQ Chicken Pizza, 1 slice	221.3	5.86	3.38	587.31	29.41	1.28	3.59	13.56
Seafood Pizza, 1 slice	225.18	5.83	3.47	550.71	29.99	1.12	4	13.83
Donair Pizza, 1 slice	267.15	8.99	4.83	687.22	34.59	1.31	8.06	12.85
Chicken & Chunky Vegetable Tetrazzini Pizza	273.93	10.16	5.98	673.83	29.92	1.44	3.34	16.86
Multigrain Thin Crust - Pepperoni	668.47	32.56	14.72	2047.83	64.98	6.84	8.46	33.51
Multigrain Thin Crust - Rustic Italian	694.39	35.23	15.39	1947.04	65.09	6.74	8.77	33.64
Multigrain Thin Crust - BBQ Chicken	624.19	21.02	10.36	2036.12	70.62	7.1	12.02	43.41
Multigrain Thin Crust - Garden Fresh	463.6	14.82	6.32	1120.34	73.52	9.56	14.47	23.97
Multigrain Thin Crust - Spicy Chicken	645.79	22.89	11.24	1855.64	69.64	7.22	11.7	47
Deep Dish Pizza - Works	1468.87	62.41	30.21	4680.93	154.73	9.45	19.21	77.89
Deep Dish Pizza - Gourmet Deli	1345.19	49.39	25.43	4379.08	148.78	6.54	17.13	82.82
Deep Dish Pizza - Vegetarian Delight	1149.81	33.55	19.88	3139.67	162.89	11.24	24.61	57.46

Sandwich/Wrap

	Cal	Fat	Sfat	Sod	Carb	Fiber	Sugar	Prot
Tuscan Chicken Sandwich	1002.54	29.77	7.58	1423	137.25	6.05	12.54	43.95
Italian Club Sandwich	1032.56	33.82	8.34	1451.89	135.52	5.84	11.48	43.94
Tuscan Chicken Panini	619.39	30.77	10.79	1804.86	54.49	4.02	3.91	34.85
BBQ Steak Panini	738.77	35.69	12.56	2394.7	64.02	5.85	8.12	44.88
Sicilian Club Panini	703.81	39.06	13.08	2029.86	55.14	4.19	5.09	38.64
Classic Ham & Cheese Panini	708.77	39.63	13.58	2560.46	53.76	5.4	4.04	37.94
Club Wrap	526.33	32.45	6.52	926	32.71	2.27	1.81	28.31
Caesar Wrap	416.74	24.22	4.02	1097.53	31.69	2.09	0.84	18.3

Salad

	Cal	Fat	Sfat	Sod	Carb	Fiber	Sugar	Prot
Tuscan Chicken Salad	357.64	27.41	3.71	918.77	17.71	2.36	4.46	11.34
BBQ Chicken Chopped Meal Salad	786.39	4.91	1.1	517.82	15.96	3.84	4.61	38.05
Thai Crispy Chicken Chopped Salad	280.81	13.51	2.07	1117.97	29.04	4.25	7.84	12.7
Hot-Top Salad	677.42	40.34	8.83	1653.14	52.2	4.83	29.78	28.9
Mediterranean Chopped Salad	1009.84	78.93	17.06	1956.06	58.2	13.9	5.95	18.99
Famous Caesar Salad	382.94	34.41	7.19	923.78	9.38	2.58	1.93	9.53
Chicken Caesar Salad	542.61	37.96	7.56	1261.67	22.93	3.43	2.58	28.16
Garden Salad	34.49	0.39	0.06	58	7.25	2.85	3.4	2.12
Italian Pasta Salad	331.2	15.43	2.4	580	42.13	3.18	8.1	7.01

Kids

	Cal	Fat	Sfat	Sod	Carb	Fiber	Sugar	Prot
6" Garlic Cheese Fingers & Fries	560.6	21.25	5.54	1589	75.68	3.33	4.22	17.33
6" Kitty Cat Pizza	372.69	11.41	6.16	865	52.39	2.02	10.88	15.87
9" Bad Dog Pizza	763.44	25.81	1291	2007	98.56	4.38	13.7	36.71
Chicken Nuggets & Fries or Salad	439.78	20.67	2.99	1284	47.01	1.7	0.55	15.69
Spaghetti & Meat Sauce	422.14	6.22	1.31	715.88	74.51	5.66	5.55	16.51

Dessert

	Cal	Fat	Sfat	Sod	Carb	Fiber	Sugar	Prot
Red Cherry Temptation	730.03	10.75	6.99	513.22	151.76	4.48	80.89	11.18
Apple Cinnamon Sensation	740.64	8.88	5.88	578.39	159.56	3.58	83.99	10.62
Apple Skillet	477.72	16.18	7.93	337.72	77.96	2.54	49.18	5.96
Brownie Skillet Supreme	705.89	34.01	19.52	263.85	102.46	2.97	74.48	6.15
Chocolate Eruption	737.94	42.48	25.24	491.98	83.5	3.48	57.53	8.48

Description & Serving	Cal	Fat	Sfat	Sod	Carb	Fiber	Sugar	Prot

Pizza Inn

Pizza, per slice

14" Cheese Pizza w/ New York Crust	288.8	13.75	5.22	582	30.6	NP	NP	10.67
14" Pepperoni Pizza w/ New York Crust	339.9	18.27	7.21	771	30.7	NP	NP	13.16
14" Monster Pizza w/ New York Crust	375.6	20.52	7.84	999	32.3	NP	NP	15.44
14" Pork Pizza w/ New York Crust	337.5	17.24	6.65	819	31.6	NP	NP	14.01
14" Beef Pizza w/ New York Crust	351.4	18.55	7.17	815	31.7	NP	NP	14.37

Wrap

Pepperoni Wrap	282.2	12.98	5.08	680	30.4	NP	NP	10.9

Pizza Pizza

Pizza

Small, 1 slice

Bacon Double Cheeseburger Pizza	220	8	3.5	600	27	1	1	10
Big Bacon Bonanza Pizza	230	9	4	570	27	1	1	10
Cheese Pizza	190	5	2.5	450	27	1	1	9
Canadian Eh! Pizza	220	8	3.5	620	27	1	1	10
Classic Super Pizza	200	6	2.5	550	27	1	2	9
Garden Veggie Pizza	180	4.5	2	420	28	2	2	8
New York Pepperoni Pizza	210	8	3.5	580	27	1	1	9
Pepperoni Pizza	200	6	2.5	550	27	1	1	9
Pepperoni & Mushroom Pizza	200	6	2.5	550	27	1	1	9
Spicy BBQ Chicken Pizza	190	4.5	2	500	28	2	2	10
Tropical Hawaiian Pizza	210	7	3	610	28	1	3	10
Bacon Chicken Mushroom Melt Pizza	260	12	3	570	27	1	1	11
Chicken Bruschetta Parm Pizza	190	6	2.5	560	23	1	2	10
Meat Supreme Pizza	280	13	5	860	28	1	1	14
Mediterranean Vegetarian Pizza	190	5	2	500	28	2	2	8
Pesto Amore Pizza	170	7	2.5	310	21	2	2	7
Philly Cheese Steak Pizza	210	6	3	530	28	1	2	12
Sweet Chili Chicken Pizza	170	4	1.5	420	27	2	8	8

Medium, 1 slice

Gluten Free Pizza, Crust Only	80	1.5	0.2	190	16	0	1	1
Bacon Double Cheeseburger Pizza	220	7	3.5	650	29	1	2	11
Big Bacon Bonanza Pizza	220	7	3.5	650	29	1	2	10
Cheese Pizza	200	5	3	480	29	1	1	9
Canadian Eh! Pizza	230	7	3	690	30	2	2	11
Classic Super Pizza	210	6	2.5	580	30	2	2	10
Garden Veggie Pizza	190	4.5	2	440	30	2	2	8
New York Pepperoni Pizza	230	8	3.5	600	29	2	1	10
Pepperoni Pizza	210	6	2.5	580	29	1	1	10
Pepperoni & Mushroom Pizza	210	6	2.5	580	30	2	2	10
Spicy BBQ Chicken Pizza	200	4.5	2	510	30	2	2	10
Tropical Hawaiian Pizza	220	7	3	630	30	1	3	10
Bacon Chicken Mushroom Melt Pizza	270	12	3	590	29	1	1	12

Description & Serving	Cal	Fat	Sfat	Sod	Carb	Fiber	Sugar	Prot
Chicken Bruschetta Parm Pizza	180	6	2.5	560	22	1	2	10
Meat Supreme Pizza	290	13	5	880	30	1	2	14
Mediterranean Vegetarian Pizza	210	6	2.5	590	31	2	2	9
Pesto Amore Pizza	170	7	2.5	310	19	2	2	8
Philly Cheese Steak Pizza	230	6	3	570	31	2	2	12
Sweet Chili Chicken Pizza	170	4.5	2	440	26	2	8	9
Large, 1 slice								
Bacon Double Cheeseburger Pizza	250	9	4	750	32	2	2	12
Big Bacon Bonanza Pizza	250	9	4	720	32	1	2	12
Cheese Pizza	230	7	3.5	530	32	1	1	11
Canadian Eh! Pizza	260	9	4	780	33	2	2	13
Classic Super Pizza	240	8	3.5	650	33	2	2	12
Garden Veggie Pizza	220	6	3	500	33	2	2	10
New York Pepperoni Pizza	260	9	4	660	32	2	1	12
Pepperoni Pizza	240	8	3.5	650	32	1	1	11
Pepperoni & Mushroom Pizza	250	8	3.5	660	32	2	2	12
Spicy BBQ Chicken Pizza	230	6	3	570	33	2	2	12
Tropical Hawaiian Pizza	260	9	4	760	34	2	3	13
Bacon Chicken Mushroom Melt Pizza	310	14	4	670	32	1	2	13
Chicken Bruschetta Parm Pizza	220	8	3.5	630	25	1	2	12
Meat Supreme Pizza	320	14	6	970	33	2	2	16
Mediterranean Vegetarian Pizza	240	8	3	670	34	2	2	9
Pesto Amore Pizza	200	8	3.5	370	23	3	3	9
Philly Cheese Steak Pizza	270	8	4	650	34	2	3	15
Sweet Chili Chicken Pizza	200	6	2.5	470	28	3	7	10
X-Large, 1 slice								
Bacon Double Cheeseburger Pizza	270	9	4.5	800	35	2	2	13
Big Bacon Bonanza Pizza	280	10	4.5	790	35	2	2	13
Cheese Pizza	240	6	3	560	35	2	2	11
Canadian Eh! Pizza	280	9	4	820	36	2	2	14
Classic Super Pizza	260	8	3.5	690	36	2	2	12
Garden Veggie Pizza	240	6	2.5	540	36	2	2	10
New York Pepperoni Pizza	270	10	4.5	720	35	2	2	12
Pepperoni Pizza	260	8	3.5	690	35	2	2	12
Pepperoni & Mushroom Pizza	260	8	3.5	690	35	2	2	12
Spicy BBQ Chicken Pizza	250	6	3	610	36	2	2	12
Tropical Hawaiian Pizza	280	9	4	750	37	2	3	13
Bacon Chicken Mushroom Melt Pizza	320	14	3.5	690	35	2	2	14
Chicken Bruschetta Parm Pizza	240	8	4	670	28	1	2	13
Meat Supreme Pizza	350	15	6	1030	36	2	2	17
Mediterranean Vegetarian Pizza	250	8	3	690	38	2	2	10
Pesto Amore Pizza	210	8	3	370	26	3	3	9
Philly Cheese Steak Pizza	280	8	4	670	37	2	3	15
Sweet Chili Chicken Pizza	220	6	2.5	490	32	3	9	10
Square, 1 slice								
Cheese Pizza	430	11	5	1000	64	3	3	19
Classic Super Pizza	460	13	6	1160	66	3	3	21

Description & Serving	Cal	Fat	Sfat	Sod	Carb	Fiber	Sugar	Prot
Garden Veggie Pizza	430	10	5	970	67	4	4	19
Mediterranean Vegetarian Pizza	500	16	7	1340	69	4	3	21
Pepperoni Pizza	450	13	6	1160	65	3	3	20
Tropical Hawaiian Pizza	470	13	6	1240	68	3	6	21

Pie, 1 slice

Bacon Double Cheeseburger Pizza	670	22	10	1920	87	4	4	32
Big Bacon Bonanza Pizza	710	26	11	2090	88	4	5	34
Cheese Pizza	570	14	7	1340	86	4	4	25
Canadian Eh! Pizza	680	22	10	2000	88	4	5	33
Classic Super Pizza	640	19	9	1710	89	5	5	30
Garden Veggie-Classic Dough	620	16	7	1120	93	6	8	27
Garden Veggie-WWMDough	620	18	7	1070	90	14	8	27
New York Pepperoni Pizza	680	24	11	1770	87	5	4	30
Pepperoni Pizza	630	19	9	1710	87	4	4	29
Spicy BBQ Chicken Pizza	620	15	7	1540	91	5	6	31
Tropical Hawaiian Pizza	660	20	9	1860	90	4	7	31
Bacon Chicken Mushroom Melt Pizza	830	39	10	1770	88	4	4	34
Chicken Bruschetta Parm Pizza	730	24	10	1990	91	4	5	38
Meat Supreme Pizza	810	33	13	2400	89	4	4	39
Mediterranean Vegetarian Pizza	650	21	8	1820	94	6	5	25
Pesto Amore Pizza	680	28	11	1260	81	8	9	32
Philly Cheese Steak Pizza	700	20	10	1730	93	5	8	37
Quatro Formaggio Pizza	640	19	9	1190	90	5	6	27
Sweet Chili Chicken Pizza	650	17	7	1420	99	9	25	30

Chicken

9 Cut Chicken Drumstick, 1 pc	160	9	1.5	520	6	0	0	14
9 Cut Chicken Thigh, 1 pc	440	34	7	950	9	0	0	23
9 Cut Chicken Breast, 1 pc	350	21	3	950	13	0	0	27
9 Cut Chicken Keel, 1 pc	270	13	2	750	7	3	0	33
9 Cut Chicken Wing, 1 pc	190	12	2	570	10	1	0	12
Classic Chicken Wings, 6	422	30	8	1180	0	0	0	40
Crispy Breaded Wings, 6	720	46	10	1320	22	0	1	46
Boneless Chicken Bites, 3	230	11	2	450	14	1	0	19
Chicken Strips, 3	320	14	1.5	900	23	2	0	23

Sandwich

Bacon Cheeseburger Stuffed Sandwich	350	12	6	990	44	2	2	17
Basic Cheese & Sauce Stuffed Sandwich	300	8	4	750	44	2	2	14
Classic Super Stuffed Sandwich	340	11	5	940	45	3	3	16
Garden Veggie Stuffed Sandwich	310	8	4	750	45	3	3	14
Mediterranean Vegetarian Stuffed Sandwich	390	15	6	1130	49	3	3	16
Pepperoni Stuffed Sandwich	330	10	5	940	44	2	2	16
Tropical Hawaiian Stuffed Sandwich	360	12	5	1050	47	2	5	17

Salad

Caesar Salad	110	4	0.2	230	4	2	4	4
Garden Salad	50	0	0.1	25	3	3	6	3
Mediterranean Greek Salad	170	11	4.5	740	8	3	6	8

Description & Serving	Cal	Fat	Sfat	Sod	Carb	Fiber	Sugar	Prot
Dressing/Condiment								
Renee's Spring Herb Italian Light, 30 ml	70	7	0.5	310	0	0	0	0
Renee's Caesar, 30 ml	190	20	2	210	1	0	0	1
Renee's Light Caesar, 30 ml	100	10	1	190	1	0	0	1
Hot Wing Sauce, 2 oz	60	0.5	0.1	1030	13	1	9	1
Mild Wing Sauce, 2 oz	70	0.5	0.1	830	15	1	11	1
Texas BBQ Sauce, 2 oz	100	0.1	0	480	23	1	18	1
Honey Mustard Sauce, 2 oz	79	0.3	0.1	138	18	0	16	1
Honey Garlic Sauce, 2 oz	91	0	0.1	259	22	0	17	0
Plum Sauce, 2 oz	94	0.3	0	222	23	0	19	0
Sweet Chili Thai Sauce, 2 oz	96	0.2	0.1	463	23	0	22	0
Blue Cheese Sauce, 2 oz	204	22	2.4	414	2	0	0	2
Homestyle Pizzaletto Sauce, 2 oz	40	1.5	0	180	5	1	3	1
Cheddar Jalapeno Dipping Sauce, 2 oz	180	18	1.8	325	4	0	2	2
Garlic Parmesan Dipping Sauce, 2 oz	311	34	2.2	250	2	0	1	0
Italian Marinara Dipping Sauce, 2 oz	30	1	0.1	125	4	1	2	1
Classic Tomato Sauce	20	0.1	0	284	4	1	2	1
Homestyle Pizzaletto Tomato Sauce	40	1.5	0	190	5	0	4	1
Pesto Tomato Sauce	160	15	3.5	310	2	1	0	5
Bruschetta Tomato Sauce	50	4.2	0	317	3	0	1	0
Side/Dessert								
Garlic Stix, 2	358	12.7	2	600	7.3	1.8	5.6	7.3
Garlic Bread/Toast, 2	242	8.5	1.8	432	6.5	1.3	3.3	6.5
Fries, reg	412	20	1.6	928	55	6	1	4
Fries, jumbo	1318	64	5.1	2970	176	19	3	13
Onion Rings	236	13	2	547	27	2	2	4
Shrimp, 5	230	13	1.5	270	15	1	0	10
Two-Bite Brownies	86	5	1.2	59	10	1	6	1
Apple Pie/Turnover	180	5	2	320	31	1	8	3

Pizza Pro

Large Pizza, 1 slice								
Cheese	46	5	3	313	24	1	2	7
Pepperoni	99	11	5	540	24	1	2	10
Sausage	70	8	4	337	25	2	3	10
Italian Sausage	68	7	4	423	24	1	3	9
Beef	64	7	4	508	24	2	3	17
Ham	53	7	4	692	24	1	3	12
Pro Special	119	13	7	800	26	2	3	17
Pro Deluxe	109	12	6	540	26	2	3	12
Meat To Please	119	13	7	828	25	1	3	17
Veggie	64	7	5	416	25	2	3	9
Large School Pizza, 1 slice								
Cheese	257	7	5	471	35	2	4	11
Pepperoni	352	16	8	810	35	2	4	14
Sausage	314	12	6	506	37	3	4	15
Italian Sausage	303	11	6	634	36	2	4	13

Description & Serving	Cal	Fat	Sfat	Sod	Carb	Fiber	Sugar	Prot
Beef	304	10	6	762	37	2	4	25
Ham	333	10	6	1037	36	2	4	19
Pro Special	644	20	10	1200	38	3	5	25
Pro Deluxe	391	18	10	806	38	3	5	18
Meat To Please	425	20	10	1241	37	2	4	26
Veggie	303	11	7	642	38	4	4	13

Medium Pizza, 1 slice

Cheese	176	5	23	304	26	2	3	7
Pepperoni	239	10	5	528	26	2	3	9
Sausage	211	7	4	326	27	3	3	10
Italian Sausage	204	7	4	403	26	2	3	9
Beef	204	6	4	479	26	2	3	16
Ham	227	7	4	682	26	2	3	12
Pro Special	288	12	6	769	28	2	4	16
Pro Deluxe	141	12	6	511	28	2	3	12
Meat To Please	276	12	6	773	26	2	3	16
Veggie	208	7	4	412	27	2	3	9

Personal Pizza, 1 slice

Cheese	117	3	2	199	17	1	2	5
Pepperoni	152	7	3	324	17	1	2	6
Sausage	132	5	2	209	17	1	2	6
Italian Sausage	129	6	2	243	17	1	2	7
Beef	129	4	2	277	17	1	2	9
Ham	145	5	2	405	17	1	2	8
Pro Special	183	8	4	464	17	2	2	11
Pro Deluxe	157	7	3	273	17	2	2	7
Meat To Please	178	8	4	466	16	2	2	11
Veggie	135	5	2	228	17	2	2	6

Side

Cheesestick, 1	84	2	1	118	12	1	1	3

Sandwich, 1/2 of sub

Ham & Cheese Hot Sub Sandwich	345	8	2	3947	35	2	4	10
Italian Club Hot Sub Sandwich	364	11	3	3831	36	2	5	8
Chicken Fajita Hot Sub Sandwich	369	9	3	3860	39	3	4	131

Popeyes

Chicken

Chicken Pieces

Mild Chicken Wing	150	10	3.5	690	5	0	0	9
Mild Chicken Leg	110	7	2.5	280	3	0	0	11
Mild Chicken Thigh	280	20	7	710	7	0	0	16
Mild Chicken Breast	350	20	7	1130	8	0	0	33
Mild Chicken Wing, Skinless	40	1.5	0.5	400	0	<1	0	7
Mild Chicken Leg, Skinless	50	2	0.5	190	0	0	0	9
Mild Chicken Thigh, Skinless	80	4	1	230	0	0	0	11
Mild Chicken Breast, Skinless	120	2	1	540	0	0	0	24

Description & Serving	Cal	Fat	Sfat	Sod	Carb	Fiber	Sugar	Prot
Spicy Chicken Wing	140	9	3.5	290	5	0	0	8
Spicy Chicken Leg	100	5	2	230	3	0	0	9
Spicy Chicken Thigh	300	24	8	490	7	0	0	15
Spicy Chicken Breast	360	22	8	760	8	1	0	31
Spicy Chicken Wing, Skinless	40	2	0.5	125	0	<1	0	6
Spicy Chicken Leg, Skinless	50	1.5	0.5	135	0	0	0	9
Spicy Chicken Thigh, Skinless	80	3	1	170	2	0	0	12
Spicy Chicken Breast, Skinless	120	2	1	380	<1	<1	0	25
Strips/Nuggets/Tenders/Wings								
Mild Chicken Strips, 2	130	2.5	1	620	3	0	0	25
Louisiana Nuggets, 6	220	12	5	500	13	<1	0	15
Louisiana Mild Tenders, 3	375	17	7	1620	24	0	0	33
Louisiana Spicy Tenders, 3	405	17	7	2160	30	0	0	33
Cajun Wings Segments, 6	595	43	15	1274	19	0	0	34
Sandwich/Wrap								
Loaded Chicken Wrap	400	17	6	1100	44	4	0	19
Delta Mini	300	13	4	780	30	1	4	15
Chicken Biscuit	350	20	9	930	30	<1	0	13
Crispy Chicken Sandwich	560	23	8	1690	56	3	12	33
Grilled Chicken Sandwich	359	9.5	2	978	46	2	6	21
Po Boy Sandwich	330	17	3	560	36	0	10	8
Other Entrée								
Crawfish Etouffee	180	5	1	640	25	2	0	7
Popcorn Shrimp	280	16	6	1110	22	<1	0	12
Butterfly Shrimp	310	19	8	800	22	2	0	13
Chicken Sausage Jambalaya	220	11	3	760	20	1	3	10
Smothered Chicken	210	8	2	743	24	1	0	10
Chicken Etouffee	160	10	3	870	6	2	1	12
Chicken Bowl	570	29	10	1600	44	8	2	35
Side/Dessert								
Biscuit	240	13	7	490	26	1	2	4
French Fries	310	17	7	660	35	3	1	4
Corn on the Cob	190	2	0.5	0	37	4	7	6
Mashed Potatoes w/o Gravy	100	3	1	380	17	<1	3	1
Mashed Potatoes & Gravy	120	4	2	570	18	2	0	3
Red Beans & Rice	320	19	6	710	31	17	2	10
Cajun Rice	170	6	2	530	22	2	1	8
Coleslaw	260	23	3.5	260	14	9	15	<1
Green Beans	70	1	0	400	14	2	1	2
Cinnamon Apple Turnover	250	12	4	320	34	2	11	3

Port of Subs

Sandwich

	Cal	Fat	Sfat	Sod	Carb	Fiber	Sugar	Prot
5" Roast Beef Sandwich w/ horseradish sauce & w/o mustard or mayo	739	24	12	186	85	3	1	43
5" Ham Turkey Sub w/o mustard or mayo	328	5	2	1327	46	3	4	22

Description & Serving	Cal	Fat	Sfat	Sod	Carb	Fiber	Sugar	Prot
5" Smoked Ham Turkey Sub w/o mustard or mayo	320	5	1	1343	46	3	6	21
5" Vegetarian Sub w/o cheese, mustard, or mayo	238	2	1	865	44	4	3	7
5" Roast Beef Sub w/o mustard or mayo	315	4	1	884	43	3	3	23
5" Turkey Sub w/o mustard or mayo	315	4	1	1233	47	3	3	21
5" Peppered Pastrami Sub w/o mustard or mayo	293	4	2	708	44	3	4	16
5" Roasted Chicken Breast Sub w/o mustard or mayo	304	3	1	1130	44	3	5	24
5" Smoked Ham Sub w/o mustard or mayo	301	4	2	1184	44	3	3	18
5" Roast Beef Turkey Sub w/o mustard or mayo	315	4	1	1059	45	3	4	22
5" Ham Salami Capicolla Pepperoni Provolone Sub w/o mustard or mayo	532	26	10	1676	45	3	3	28
5" Ham Turkey Provolone Sub w/o mustard or mayo	434	15	5	1467	46	3	4	26
5" Salami Turkey Provolone Sub w/o mustard or mayo	465	20	7	1371	46	3	3	23
5" Ham Salami Provolone Sub w/o mustard or mayo	469	21	8	1465	45	3	3	24
5" Smoked Ham Turkey Smokey Cheddar Sub w/o mustard or mayo	431	15	5	1599	47	3	6	25
5" Vegetarian Sub w/o mustard or mayo	599	33	14	1555	49	4	5	24
5" Roast Beef Provolone Sub w/o mustard or mayo	421	14	4	1024	43	3	3	27
5" Turkey Provolone Sub w/o mustard or mayo	421	14	4	1373	47	3	3	25
5" Peppered Chicken Breast Provolone Sub w/o mustard or mayo	439	17	7	766	44	3	4	21
5" Roasted Chicken Provolone Sub w/o mustard or mayo	410	13	4	1270	45	3	5	28
5" Ham American Sub w/o mustard or mayo	382	20	8	1814	45	3	5	29
5" Salami Provolone Sub w/o mustard or mayo	479	25	9	1228	45	3	3	22
5" Peppered Pastrami Turkey Swiss Sub w/o mustard or mayo	511	26	13	834	44	3	3	23
5" Smoked Ham Swiss Sub w/o mustard or mayo	447	17	7	1242	45	3	3	23
5" Salami Pepperoni Provolone Sub w/o mustard or mayo	511	27	11	1265	45	3	3	26
5" Bacon Lettuce & Tomato Sub w/o mustard or mayo	519	30	7	1205	43	3	3	20
5" Tuna Sub w/o cheese, mustard, or mayo	422	18	4	760	45	3	5	19
5" Roast Beef Turkey Provolone Sub w/o mustard or mayo	421	14	4	1199	45	3	3	26

Specialty Sandwich/Wrap

5" Grilled Chicken Griller	518	13	5	1848	58	3	1	40
5" Hot Pastrami Griller	538	15	7	1824	58	3	1	39
5" BBQ Pork Griller	782	18	8	2746	104	9	28	53
5" N.Y. Steak & Cheese Griller	615	18	8	887	57	3	1	51
5" Italian Griller	553	21	9	2107	58	3	2	30
Turkey & Bacon Ranch Wrap	589	38	8	1771	34	17	1	43
Chicken Caesar Wrap	632	34	5	1711	35	18	4	56
Hot Grilled Chicken & Smokey Cheddar Wrap	484	18	4	1782	35	18	1	59

Description & Serving	Cal	Fat	Sfat	Sod	Carb	Fiber	Sugar	Prot
Salad								
Macaroni Salad	440	30	5	1027	36	3	11	7
Potato Salad	360	26	4	980	54	6	14	4
Caesar Salad w/ Caesar dressing	333	30	7	853	7	2	4	3
Grilled Chicken Caesar Salad w/ Caesar dressing	541	34	8	1830	15	5	6	37
Grilled Chicken Salad w/ vinegar & olive oil	300	10	1	1023	16	3	6	36
Garden Salad w/ vinegar & olive oil	93	5	1	45	10	2	5	2
Tuna Salad w/ vinegar & olive oil	311	23	3	495	12	2	6	16
Chef Salad w/ vinegar & olive oil	388	25	12	1409	13	2	5	26
Kids								
4" Turkey Sandwich	190	3	0.5	710	4	1	2	8
4" Ham Sandwich	200	3	0.5	521	4	1	2	10
4" Salami Sandwich	254	9	1.9	599	4	1	2	9
Dessert								
Brownie	300	10	3	320	48	<1	32	4

Pretzelmaker/Pretzel Time

	Cal	Fat	Sfat	Sod	Carb	Fiber	Sugar	Prot
Pretzel								
Plain Pretzel	290	2	0	15	61	2	11	7
Original Pretzel	340	7	1	220	61	2	11	7
Garlic Pretzel	350	7	1	790	64	2	12	7
Caramel Nut Pretzel	390	7	1	55	74	2	17	7
Ranch Pretzel	240	7	1	930	63	2	11	7
Cinnamon Sugar Pretzel	370	8	1	15	68	2	17	7
Parmesan Pretzel	360	9	2	290	61	2	11	9
Pretzel Bites, sml	450	11	1.5	360	8	3	15	9
Pretzel Bites, med	640	16	2	500	112	4	21	13
Pretzel Bites, lrg (2 servings)	510	13	1.5	400	88	3	17	10
Cinnamon Sugar Pretzel Bites	520	12	1.5	20	95	3	28	9
PT Pretzel Dog	440	27	10	1120	34	1	8	15
Condiment								
Cheddar Cheese, 1.5 oz	70	5	1	420	6	0	2	1
Ketchup, 2 packets	20	0	0	200	4	0	4	0
Mustard, 2 packets	5	0	0	125	1	0	0	0
Nacho Cheese, 1.5 oz	80	5	1	530	7	0	2	1
Pizza Sauce, 1.5 oz	30	0.5	0	250	6	2	3	1
Caramel, 1.5 oz	140	0	0	160	35	0	27	1
Cream Cheese, 1.5 oz	200	20	14	200	4	0	2	2
Cream Cheese Icing, 1.5 oz	180	9	6	85	22	0	21	1
Beverage								
Strawberry Banana Breezer, 20 oz	650	20	13	100	115	0	108	6
Raspberry Breezer, 20 oz	650	20	13	100	117	0	112	6
Peach Breezer, 20 oz	650	20	13	110	117	0	115	6
Coffee Breezer, 20 oz	640	21	14	100	107	0	106	6

Description & Serving	Cal	Fat	Sfat	Sod	Carb	Fiber	Sugar	Prot
Mocha Breezer, 20 oz	620	20	13	100	106	0	104	6
MFC Lemonade, 20 oz	160	0	0	15	92	0	87	0

Qdoba

Breakfast

10" Breakfast Burrito w/ Spicy Mexican Chorizo w/o toppings or condiments	290	11	3	610	36	1	1	16
13" Breakfast Burrito w/ Spicy Mexican Chorizo w/o toppings or condiments	530	21	8	1380	57	3	4	27
10" Breakfast Burrito w/ Grilled Chicken w/o toppings or condiments	400	16	5	800	36	1	1	31
13" Breakfast Burrito w/ Grilled Chicken w/o toppings or condiments	520	18	6	520	55	2	2	34
Naked Burrito w/ Spicy Mexican Chorizo w/o toppings or condiments, sml	80	4.5	1	150	1	0	0	10
Naked Burrito w/ Spicy Mexican Chorizo w/o toppings or condiments, lrg	190	10	3	340	1	0	0	25
Naked Burrito w/ Grilled Chicken w/o toppings or condiments, sml	200	13	4.5	670	3	1	2	18
Naked Burrito w/ Grilled Chicken w/o toppings or condiments, lrg	190	10	3	450	1	0	0	25
10" Breakfast Quesadilla w/ Spicy Mexican Chorizo w/o toppings or condiments	730	47	26	1270	37	1	2	44
13" Breakfast Quesadilla w/ Spicy Mexican Chorizo w/o toppings or condiments	970	57	31	2040	58	3	5	55
10" Breakfast Quesadilla w/ Grilled Chicken w/o toppings or condiments	840	52	28	1460	37	1	2	59
13" Breakfast Quesadilla w/ Grilled Chicken w/o toppings or condiments	960	54	29	1710	56	2	3	62
10" Breakfast Quesadilla w/ Cheese w/o toppings or condiments	650	42	25	1120	36	1	2	34
13" Breakfast Quesadilla w/ Cheese w/o toppings or condiments	770	44	26	1370	55	2	3	37

Entrée

Beef

Ground Beef Queso Burrito w/o toppings or condiments	890	38	16	2070	98	5	3	35
Naked Ground Beef Queso Burrito w/o toppings or condiments	560	30	13	1360	44	3	1	26
Shredded Beef Queso Burrito w/o toppings or condiments	840	29	13	2100	102	4	3	39
Naked Shredded Beef Queso Burrito w/o toppings or condiments	510	21	10	1390	48	2	1	30
Ground Beef Fajita Ranchera Burrito w/o toppings or condiments	810	30	11	2000	97	5	4	32
Naked Ground Beef Fajita Ranchera Burrito w/o toppings or condiments	480	22	8	1290	43	3	2	23

Description & Serving	Cal	Fat	Sfat	Sod	Carb	Fiber	Sugar	Prot
Shredded Beef Fajita Ranchera Burrito w/o toppings or condiments	760	21	8	2030	101	4	4	36
Naked Shredded Beef Fajita Ranchera Burrito w/o toppings or condiments	430	13	4.5	1320	47	2	2	27
Ground Beef Poblano Pesto Burrito w/o toppings or condiments	850	35	12	2130	98	5	3	33
Naked Ground Beef Poblano Pesto Burrito w/o toppings or condiments	520	27	9	1420	44	3	1	24
Shredded Beef Poblano Pesto Burrito w/o toppings or condiments	800	26	9	2160	102	4	3	37
Naked Shredded Beef Poblano Pesto Burrito w/o toppings or condiments	470	18	6	1450	48	2	1	28
Ground Beef Ancho Chile BBQ Burrito w/o toppings or condiments	890	33	12	2320	112	5	21	33
Naked Ground Beef Ancho Chile BBQ Burrito w/o toppings or condiments	560	25	9	1610	58	3	19	24
Shredded Beef Ancho Chile BBQ Burrito w/o toppings or condiments	840	24	9	2350	116	4	21	37
Naked Shredded Beef Ancho Chile BBQ Burrito w/o toppings or condiments	510	16	6	1640	62	2	19	28
Ground Beef Grilled Veggie Burrito w/o toppings or condiments	790	30	11	1780	95	4	2	32
Naked Ground Beef Grilled Veggie Burrito w/o toppings or condiments	460	22	8	1070	41	2	0	23
Shredded Beef Grilled Veggie Burrito w/o toppings or condiments	740	21	8	1810	99	3	2	36
Naked Shredded Beef Grilled Veggie Burrito w/o toppings or condiments	410	13	4.5	1100	45	1	0	27
Ground Beef Burrito w/o toppings or condiments	790	30	11	1780	95	4	2	32
Naked Ground Beef Burrito w/o toppings or condiments	460	22	8	1070	41	2	0	23
Shredded Beef Burrito w/o toppings or condiments	740	21	8	1810	99	3	2	36
Naked Shredded Beef Burrito w/o toppings or condiments	410	13	4.5	1100	45	1	0	27
Ground Beef Crispy Taco w/o toppings or condiments, 1	140	9	3	210	8	1	0	7
Shredded Beef Crispy Taco w/o toppings or condiments, 1	120	6	2	220	10	1	0	8
Ground Beef Soft Taco w/o toppings or condiments, 1	170	8	3.5	380	15	0	1	9
Shredded Beef Soft Taco w/o toppings or condiments, 1	150	4.5	2.5	390	17	0	1	10
Ground Beef Grilled Quesadilla w/o toppings or condiments	1010	61	33	1900	56	3	3	57
Shredded Beef Grilled Quesadilla w/o toppings or condiments	960	52	30	1930	60	2	3	61

Chicken

Description & Serving	Cal	Fat	Sfat	Sod	Carb	Fiber	Sugar	Prot
Grilled Chicken Queso Burrito w/o toppings or condiments	840	31	12	1880	98	4	3	40
Naked Grilled Chicken Queso Burrito w/o toppings or condiments	510	23	9	1170	44	2	1	31

Description & Serving	Cal	Fat	Sfat	Sod	Carb	Fiber	Sugar	Prot
Grilled Chicken Fajita Ranchera Burrito w/o toppings or condiments	760	23	7	1810	97	4	4	37
Naked Grilled Chicken Fajita Ranchera Burrito w/o toppings or condiments	430	15	4	1100	43	2	2	28
Grilled Chicken Poblano Pesto Burrito w/o toppings or condiments	800	28	8	1940	98	4	3	38
Naked Grilled Chicken Poblano Pesto Burrito w/o toppings or condiments	470	20	5	1230	44	2	1	29
Grilled Chicken Ancho Chile BBQ Burrito w/o toppings or condiments	840	26	8	2130	112	4	21	38
Naked Grilled Chicken Ancho Chile BBQ Burrito w/o toppings or condiments	510	18	5	1420	58	2	19	29
Grilled Chicken Grilled Veggie Burrito w/o toppings or condiments	800	27	8	1690	100	6	4	38
Naked Grilled Chicken Grilled Veggie Burrito w/o toppings or condiments	470	19	5	980	46	4	2	29
Grilled Chicken Burrito w/o toppings or condiments	740	23	7	1590	95	3	2	37
Naked Grilled Chicken Burrito w/o toppings or condiments	410	15	4	880	41	1	0	28
Grilled Chicken Crispy Taco w/o toppings or condiments, 1	120	7	1.5	140	8	1	0	8
Grilled Chicken Soft Taco w/o toppings or condiments, 1	150	6	2	320	15	0	1	10
Grilled Chicken Grilled Quesadilla w/o toppings or condiments	960	54	29	1710	56	2	3	62
Pork								
Pulled Pork Queso Burrito w/o toppings or condiments	810	26	11	1930	107	4	4	34
Naked Pulled Pork Queso Burrito w/o toppings or condiments	480	18	8	1220	53	2	2	25
Pulled Pork Fajita Ranchera Burrito w/o toppings or condiments	730	18	6	1860	106	4	5	31
Naked Pulled Pork Fajita Ranchera Burrito w/o toppings or condiments	400	10	3	1150	52	2	3	22
Pulled Pork Poblano Pesto Burrito w/o toppings or condiments	770	23	7	1990	107	4	4	32
Naked Pulled Pork Poblano Pesto Burrito w/o toppings or condiments	440	15	4	1280	53	2	2	23
Pulled Pork Ancho Chile BBQ Burrito w/o toppings or condiments	810	20	7	2180	121	4	22	32
Naked Pulled Pork Ancho Chile BBQ Burrito w/o toppings or condiments	480	12	4	1470	67	2	20	23
Pulled Pork Grilled Veggie Burrito w/o toppings or condiments	770	21	7	1740	109	6	5	32
Naked Pulled Pork Grilled Veggie Burrito w/o toppings or condiments	440	13	4	1030	55	4	3	23
Pulled Pork Burrito w/o toppings or condiments	710	18	6	1640	104	3	3	31
Naked Pulled Pork Burrito w/o toppings or condiments	380	10	3	930	50	1	1	22
Pulled Pork Crispy Taco w/o toppings or condiments, 1	110	4.5	1	160	11	1	0	6

Description & Serving	Cal	Fat	Sfat	Sod	Carb	Fiber	Sugar	Prot
Pulled Pork Soft Taco w/o toppings or condiments, 1	140	3.5	1.5	330	18	0	1	8
Pulled Pork Grilled Quesadilla w/o toppings or condiments	930	49	28	1760	65	2	4	56
Steak								
Grilled Steak Queso Burrito w/o toppings or condiments	840	31	13	1820	97	4	3	38
Naked Grilled Steak Queso Burrito w/o toppings or condiments	510	23	10	1110	43	2	1	29
Grilled Steak Fajita Ranchera Burrito w/o toppings or condiments	760	23	8	1750	96	4	4	35
Naked Grilled Steak Fajita Ranchera Burrito w/o toppings or condiments	430	15	5	1040	42	2	2	26
Grilled Steak Poblano Pesto Burrito w/o toppings or condiments	800	28	9	1880	97	4	3	36
Naked Grilled Steak Poblano Pesto Burrito w/o toppings or condiments	470	20	6	1170	43	2	1	27
Grilled Steak Ancho Chile BBQ Burrito w/o toppings or condiments	840	26	9	2070	111	4	21	36
Naked Grilled Steak Ancho Chile BBQ Burrito w/o toppings or condiments	510	18	6	1360	57	2	19	27
Grilled Steak Grilled Veggie Burrito w/o toppings or condiments	800	27	9	1630	99	6	4	36
Naked Grilled Steak Grilled Veggie Burrito w/o toppings or condiments	470	19	6	920	45	4	2	27
Grilled Steak Burrito w/o toppings or condiments	740	23	8	1530	94	3	2	35
Naked Grilled Steak Burrito w/o toppings or condiments	410	15	5	820	40	1	0	26
Grilled Steak Crispy Taco w/o toppings or condiments, 1	120	7	2	120	8	1	0	8
Grilled Steak Soft Taco w/o toppings or condiments, 1	150	6	2.5	300	15	0	1	10
Grilled Steak Grilled Quesadilla w/o toppings or condiments	960	54	30	1650	55	2	3	60
Vegetarian								
Grilled Vegetable Queso Burrito w/o toppings or condiments	710	25	10	1640	102	7	5	16
Naked Grilled Vegetable Queso Burrito w/o toppings or condiments	380	17	7	930	48	5	3	7
Grilled Vegetables Fajita Ranchera Burrito w/o toppings or condiments	570	13	4	1470	96	4	4	12
Naked Grilled Vegetables Fajita Ranchera Burrito w/o toppings or condiments	240	5	1	760	42	2	2	3
Grilled Vegetables Poblano Pesto Burrito w/o toppings or condiments	610	18	5	1600	97	4	3	13
Naked Grilled Vegetables Poblano Pesto Burrito w/o toppings or condiments	280	10	2	890	43	2	1	4
Grilled Vegetables Ancho Chile BBQ Burrito w/o toppings or condiments	650	16	5	1790	111	4	21	13

Description & Serving	Cal	Fat	Sfat	Sod	Carb	Fiber	Sugar	Prot
Naked Grilled Vegetables Ancho Chile BBQ Burrito w/o toppings or condiments	320	8	2	1080	57	2	19	4
Grilled Vegetables Grilled Veggie Burrito w/o toppings or condiments	610	17	5	1350	99	6	4	13
Naked Grilled Vegetables Grilled Veggie Burrito w/o toppings or condiments	280	9	2	640	45	4	2	4
Grilled Vegetables Burrito w/o toppings or condiments	610	17	5	1350	99	6	4	13
Naked Grilled Vegetables Burrito w/o toppings or condiments	280	9	2	640	45	4	2	4
Grilled Vegetables Crispy Taco w/o toppings or condiments, 1	80	4.5	0.5	60	10	2	1	0
Grilled Vegetables Soft Taco w/o toppings or condiments, 1	110	3.5	1	240	17	1	2	2
Cheese Grilled Quesadilla w/o toppings or condiments	770	44	26	1370	55	2	3	37
Grilled Vegetables Grilled Quesadilla w/o toppings or condiments	830	48	27	1470	60	5	5	38

Salad

Description & Serving	Cal	Fat	Sfat	Sod	Carb	Fiber	Sugar	Prot
Grilled Chicken Taco Salad w/o toppings or dressing	600	32	8	500	44	5	3	32
Naked Grilled Chicken Taco Salad w/o toppings or dressing	210	10	3	350	4	2	2	26
Ground Beef Taco Salad w/o toppings or dressing	650	39	12	690	44	6	3	27
Naked Ground Beef Taco Salad w/o toppings or dressing	260	17	7	540	4	3	2	21
Pulled Pork Taco Salad w/o toppings or dressing	570	27	7	550	53	5	4	26
Naked Pulled Pork Taco Salad w/o toppings or dressing	180	4.5	2	400	13	2	3	20
Shredded Beef Taco Salad w/o toppings or dressing	600	30	8	720	48	5	3	31
Naked Shredded Beef Taco Salad w/o toppings or dressing	210	8	3.5	570	8	2	2	25
Grilled Vegetables Taco Salad w/o toppings or dressing	470	26	6	260	48	8	5	8
Naked Grilled Vegetables Taco Salad w/o toppings or dressing	80	3.5	1	110	8	5	4	2
Grilled Steak Taco Salad w/o toppings or dressing	600	32	9	440	43	5	3	30
Naked Grilled Steak Taco Salad w/o toppings or dressing	210	10	4	290	3	2	2	24

Soup

Description & Serving	Cal	Fat	Sfat	Sod	Carb	Fiber	Sugar	Prot
Grilled Chicken Mexican Gumbo	280	14	4	1320	10	1	2	28
Ground Beef Mexican Gumbo	330	21	8	1510	10	2	2	23
Pulled Pork Mexican Gumbo	250	9	3	1370	19	1	3	22
Shredded Beef Mexican Gumbo	280	12	4.5	1540	14	1	2	27
Grilled Vegetables Mexican Gumbo	150	8	2	1080	14	4	4	4
Grilled Steak Mexican Gumbo	280	14	5	1260	9	1	2	26

Description & Serving	Cal	Fat	Sfat	Sod	Carb	Fiber	Sugar	Prot
Grilled Chicken Tortilla Soup	150	8	2	1100	9	1	2	11
Grilled Chicken Tortilla Soup w/ Crispy Tortilla Strips	220	11	2.5	1130	18	2	2	12

Nachos/Chips

Description & Serving	Cal	Fat	Sfat	Sod	Carb	Fiber	Sugar	Prot
Grilled Chicken 3-Cheese Nachos w/o toppings or condiments	940	52	19	1160	82	10	4	37
Ground Beef 3-Cheese Nachos w/o toppings or condiments	990	59	23	1350	82	11	4	32
Pulled Pork 3-Cheese Nachos w/o toppings or condiments	910	47	18	1210	91	10	5	31
Shredded Beef 3-Cheese Nachos w/o toppings or condiments	940	50	19	1380	86	10	4	36
Grilled Vegetables 3-Cheese Nachos w/o toppings or condiments	810	46	17	920	86	13	6	13
Grilled Steak 3-Cheese Nachos w/o toppings or condiments	940	52	20	1100	81	10	4	35
Homemade Tortilla Chips, sml	280	13	2.5	115	37	4	1	3
Homemade Tortilla Chips, lrg	560	26	4.5	230	75	9	2	6

Kids

Description & Serving	Cal	Fat	Sfat	Sod	Carb	Fiber	Sugar	Prot
Homemade Tortilla Chips	280	13	2.5	115	37	4	1	3
Pinto Beans & Cheese	90	2.5	1.5	170	11	4	0	5
Black Beans & Cheese	100	2.5	1.5	150	12	6	0	6
Lil' Naked Chicken Burrito w/o toppings or condiments	190	7	1	410	21	0	0	10
Grilled Chicken Crispy Taco w/o toppings or condiments	140	8	1.5	180	9	1	0	10
Grilled Chicken Soft Taco w/o toppings or condiments	170	7	2	350	16	0	1	12
Ground Beef Crispy Taco w/o toppings or condiments	140	9	3	210	8	1	0	7
Ground Beef Soft Taco w/o toppings or condiments	170	8	3.5	380	15	0	1	9
Pulled Pork Crispy Taco w/o toppings or condiments	110	4.5	1	160	11	1	0	6
Pulled Pork Soft Taco w/o toppings or condiments	140	3.5	1.5	330	18	0	1	8
Shredded Beef Crispy Taco w/o toppings or condiments	120	6	2	220	10	1	0	8
Shredded Beef Soft Taco w/o toppings or condiments	150	4.5	2.5	390	17	0	1	10
Grilled Steak Crispy Taco w/o toppings or condiments	120	7	2	120	8	1	0	8
Grilled Steak Soft Taco w/o toppings or condiments	150	6	2.5	300	15	0	1	10
Grilled Vegetables Crispy Taco w/o toppings or condiments	80	4.5	0.5	60	10	2	1	0
Grilled Vegetables Soft Taco w/o toppings or condiments	110	3.5	1	240	17	1	2	2

Description & Serving	Cal	Fat	Sfat	Sod	Carb	Fiber	Sugar	Prot
Cheese Quesadilla w/o toppings or condiments	350	19	11	650	31	1	1	15
Grilled Chicken Quesadilla w/o toppings or condiments	430	23	12	800	32	1	1	25

Quiznos

Breakfast

	Cal	Fat	Sfat	Sod	Carb	Fiber	Sugar	Prot
Black Angus Steak, Cheddar Breakfast Sandwich	390	17.5	9	1040	36	3	2	30
Egg & Cheddar Breakfast Sandwich	350	20	11	720	36	3	2	19
Bacon, Egg, Cheddar Breakfast Sandwich	440	25.5	12	1120	36	4	2	25
Ham, Egg, Cheddar Breakfast Sandwich	350	16.5	8	1100	37	4	3	23
Garden Vegetable w/ Cheddar Breakfast Sandwich	310	15.5	8	630	38	4	3	17
Fruit Parfait w/ Yogurt	200	2.5	1.5	115	37	3	30	9

Sandwich

	Cal	Fat	Sfat	Sod	Carb	Fiber	Sugar	Prot
Prime Rib & Peppercorn Premium Sub w/ cheese & dressing, sml	590	35	10.5	1100	46	3	6	25
Prime Rib Cheesesteak Premium Sub w/ cheese & dressing, sml	670	41	10	1085	46	3	5	29
Black Angus Steak Premium Sub w/ cheese & dressing, sml	490	16.5	8	1460	52	2	13	34
Mesquite Chicken w/ Bacon Premium Sub w/ cheese & dressing, sml	510	23.5	7.5	1180	42	3	2	30
Baja Chicken w/ Bacon Premium Sub w/ cheese & dressing, sml	500	21.5	7	1270	45	2	7	30
Honey Mustard Chicken Premium Sub w/ cheese & dressing, sml	530	26	5.5	1085	45	3	7	30
Chicken Carbonara Premium Sub w/ cheese & dressing, sml	520	25	7	1230	42	2	5	30
Classic Italian Sub w/ cheese & dressing, sml	570	28	10.5	1590	44	3	5	22
The Traditional Sub w/ cheese & dressing, sml	440	19.5	6	1360	45	3	7	20
The Classic Club Sub w/ cheese & dressing, sml	570	33.5	9	1420	43	3	6	24
Turkey Ranch & Swiss Sub w/ cheese & dressing, sml	410	17	2.5	1230	45	3	5	20
Tuscan Turkey Sub w/ cheese & dressing, sml	410	17	3.5	1160	46	2	6	21
Turkey Bacon Guacamole Sub w/ cheese & dressing, sml	530	27	7	1630	45	5	7	25
Honey Bourbon Chicken Sub w/ cheese & dressing, sml	320	4.5	0.5	920	50	3	11	22
Steakhouse Beef Dip Sub w/ cheese & dressing, sml	440	18	3.5	1900	47	2	5	23
Honey Bacon Club Sub w/ cheese & dressing, sml	510	24	5	1420	53	3	13	24
Veggie Sub w/ cheese & dressing, sml	550	27	8	1270	44	5	6	17
Turkey & Cheddar Sub w/ cheese & dressing, sml	480	25.5	6	1260	43	3	4	20
Honey-Cured Ham & Swiss Sub w/ cheese & dressing, sml	500	27	5	1120	44	3	6	20
Roast Beef & Cheddar Sub w/ cheese & dressing, sml	490	25	6	1270	43	3	5	21
Tuna Melt Sub w/ cheese & dressing, sml	750	55.5	10.5	930	41	3	4	22
The 5 Meat Stack Sub w/ cheese & dressing, sml	550	32.5	12	1660	42	2	5	25

Description & Serving	Cal	Fat	Sfat	Sod	Carb	Fiber	Sugar	Prot
Primo Meatball Sub w/ cheese & dressing, sml	480	22	8	1500	48	6	6	27
Pesto Turkey Torpedo w/ cheese & dressing	650	18	4.5	1870	82	4	5	29
Italian Torpedo w/ cheese & dressing	810	31	9	2050	82	4	6	30
Turkey Club Torpedo w/ cheese & dressing	780	31	8	2050	82	3	5	33
Beef Bacon & Cheddar Torpedo w/ cheese & dressing	760	28.5	9.5	1855	80	4	4	38
Big Kahuna Tuna Torpedo w/ cheese & dressing	980	50.5	10	1670	80	3	5	35

Specialty Sandwich

Sonoma Turkey Sammie w/ cheese & dressing	280	14	4	740	26	1	1	12
Italiano Sammie w/ cheese & dressing	305	18	6.5	805	24	1	1	14
Alpine Chicken Sammie w/ cheese & dressing	295	14.5	3	560	25	1	1	17
Bistro Steak Melt Sammie w/ cheese & dressing	280	13	4	645	26	1	1	14
Cantina Chicken Sammie w/ cheese & dressing	205	4	0.5	455	29	2	4	12
Roadhouse Steak Sammie w/ cheese & dressing	195	4	1	575	29	1	4	11
Veggie Sammie w/ cheese & dressing	285	14.5	4.5	635	28	2	3	9

Salad

Raspberry Chipotle Chicken Flatbread Salad w/o dressing	620	27	8.5	1370	56	6	5	40
Chicken Caesar Flatbread Salad w/o dressing	540	19	5	1160	56	6	4	37
Classic Cob Flatbread Salad w/o dressing	560	23	6.5	1300	56	6	4	33
Chicken w/ Honey Mustard Flatbread Salad w/o dressing	570	23	6.5	1230	56	6	4	36
Black & Bleu Flatbread Salad w/o dressing	550	22	6.5	1520	57	6	5	32
Side Chopped Salad w/o dressing	15	0	0	5	3	1	1	1

Soup

Chili Bread Bowl	760	22	7	1800	107	8	7	36
Country Fresh Bread Bowl	760	26	12	1760	103	5	6	32
Broccoli Cheese Soup	140	10	6	580	8	1	3	5
Chili	140	7	2	620	12	4	4	9
Chicken Noodle Soup	130	3	0.5	1290	18	0	1	6

Kids

Tasty Turkey Sammie	190	6	2	620	24	1	1	10
Ham Melt Sammie	200	7	2.5	620	25	1	2	10
Just Cheese Sammie	180	6	3	350	23	1	1	11
Cheesy Pepperoni Pizza Sub	230	10	4	640	24	1	2	11
Cheese Pizza Sub	170	4.5	2	390	24	1	2	8
Toasty Turkey & Cheese Sub	180	4.5	1.5	635	25	1	2	11
Toasty Ham & Cheese Sub	190	6	2.5	605	25	1	3	11
Cheesy Toasted Cheese Sub	170	7	2.5	360	24	1	1	8
Cheesy Toasted Cheese Sub on Flatbread	370	15	6	740	48	2	2	18

Dessert

Chocolate Chunk Cookie	380	15	8	300	58	1	32	5
Double Chocolate Chunk Cookie	370	15	7	230	58	3	34	5
Cinnamon Sugar Cookie	400	16	8	280	59	0	36	3
Oatmeal Raisin Cookie	340	11	5	290	59	2	36	5

Description & Serving	Cal	Fat	Sfat	Sod	Carb	Fiber	Sugar	Prot
Dressing								
Buttermilk Ranch Dressing	350	35	5	590	5	0	3	1
Honey Mustard Dressing	500	50	7	540	13	0	11	1
Peppercorn Caesar Dressing	480	50	9	960	5	1	4	3
Fat Free Balsamic Vinaigrette Dressing	120	0	0	1310	29	1	18	0
Raspberry Chipotle Dressing	210	6	1	510	40	3	33	0

Red Lobster

Appetizer

	Cal	Fat	Sfat	Sod	Carb	Fiber	Sugar	Prot
Buffalo Chicken Wings	680	39	9	1750	0	NP	NP	NP
Chicken Breast Strips	414	24	2	1320	28	NP	NP	NP
Chilled Jumbo Shrimp Cocktail	120	1	0	590	9	NP	NP	NP
Crispy Calamari & Vegetables	1520	98	12	3060	116	NP	NP	NP
Fried Crawfish	1180	75	8	2050	88	NP	NP	NP
Fried Oysters	590	32	3.5	1100	58	NP	NP	NP
Hand-Shucked Oysters, 12	100	2	0	340	8	NP	NP	NP
Lobster Pizza	720	30	13	1390	69	NP	NP	NP
Lobster, Artichoke & Seafood Dip	1200	74	20	1950	101	NP	NP	NP
Lobster, Crab & Seafood Stuffed Mushrooms	380	21	11	1050	20	NP	NP	NP
Mozzarella Cheesesticks	680	39	14	1910	49	NP	NP	NP
New England Seafood Sampler	760	42	11	2270	46	NP	NP	NP
Pan-Seared Crab Cakes	360	22	3.5	1200	15	NP	NP	NP
Parrot Bay Jumbo Coconut Shrimp	588	33	7	1170	54	NP	NP	NP
Peach-Bourbon BBQ Scallops	580	35	5	1880	40	NP	NP	NP
Southwestern Lobster Rolls	870	51	13	1430	74	NP	NP	NP
Steamed Clams	430	15	3.5	1120	10	NP	NP	NP
Ultimate Fondue	1490	80	40	3580	124	NP	NP	NP

Lunch

	Cal	Fat	Sfat	Sod	Carb	Fiber	Sugar	Prot
Farm-Raised Catfish-Blackened	190	9	1.5	150	0	NP	NP	NP
Farm-Raised Catfish-Fried	220	12	1.5	280	2	NP	NP	NP
Flounder-Broiled	140	1.5	0.37	660	0	NP	NP	NP
Flounder-Fried	220	8	0.5	260	2	NP	NP	NP
Frozen Walleye-Beer Battered	350	21	2	600	12	NP	NP	NP
Frozen Walleye-Blackened	150	4	0.5	210	5	NP	NP	NP
Frozen Walleye-Broiled	130	2	0.39	280	0	NP	NP	NP
Frozen Walleye-Fried	300	15	1.5	500	18	NP	NP	NP
Seafood-Stuffed Flounder	160	6	1.5	780	6	NP	NP	NP
Bay Scallops-Broiled	70	1	0.27	490	2	NP	NP	NP
Bay Scallops-Fried	140	7	0.5	780	9	NP	NP	NP
Crunch-Fried Fish	410	24	2	1200	27	NP	NP	NP
Fried Crawfish	425	29	3.5	655	24	NP	NP	NP
Garlic Shrimp Scampi	130	9	1.5	690	1	NP	NP	NP
Hand-Breaded Shrimp	228	12	1	690	15	NP	NP	NP
Lightly Breaded Clam Strips	370	22	2	820	31	NP	NP	NP
Sailor's Platter	263	5.5	0.72	1006	5	NP	NP	NP
Crunch-Fried Fish Sandwich	730	37	9	1540	68	NP	NP	NP

Description & Serving	Cal	Fat	Sfat	Sod	Carb	Fiber	Sugar	Prot
Crunchy Popcorn Shrimp	280	14.5	1.5	1072	26	NP	NP	NP
Maple-Glazed Chicken	410	6.5	1.5	1300	62	NP	NP	NP

Entrée

Chicken

Honey BBQ Grilled Chicken & Shrimp	710	30	12	2630	26	NP	NP	NP
Maple-Glazed Chicken	570	10	2.5	1950	62	NP	NP	NP
Shrimp & Wood-Grilled Chicken w/ Garlic Shrimp Scampi	390	7.5	1.75	1690	36	NP	NP	NP
Shrimp & Wood-Grilled Chicken w/ Hand-Breaded Shrimp	530	17.5	2.5	2310	43	NP	NP	NP
Shrimp & Wood-Grilled Chicken w/ Wood-Grilled Shrimp Skewer	390	8	1.5	1460	34	NP	NP	NP
Wood-Grilled Chicken BLT w/ Freshly Cooked Chips	1030	58	11	2480	68	NP	NP	NP
Chicken Breast Strips	690	40	3.5	2200	46	NP	NP	NP

Crab

North Pacific King Crab Legs, 1 lb	390	3	0	3570	3	NP	NP	NP
North Pacific King Crab Legs, 1/2 lb	130	1	0	1190	1	NP	NP	NP
Snow Crab Legs, 1 lb	160	1	0	1900	0	NP	NP	NP
Snow Crab Legs, 1/2 lb	80	0.5	0	950	0	NP	NP	NP
Steamed Snow Crab Legs	80	0.5	0	950	0	NP	NP	NP
Crab Crackin' Monday, 1 lb	160	1	0	1900	0	NP	NP	NP

Fish

Arctic Char, half portion	335	19.5	4	255	10	NP	NP	NP
Arctic Char, full portion	625	38.5	8	310	14	NP	NP	NP
Barramundi, half portion	235	5.5	1.5	275	9	NP	NP	NP
Barramundi, full portion	425	1.5	3	350	12	NP	NP	NP
Cobia, half portion	405	27.5	9	255	6	NP	NP	NP
Cobia, full portion	765	54.5	18	310	6	NP	NP	NP
Cod, half portion	175	2	0.26	270	8	NP	NP	NP
Cod, full portion	305	3.5	0.52	340	10	NP	NP	NP
Corvina, half portion	185	1.5	0.33	305	8	NP	NP	NP
Corvina, full portion	325	2.5	0.66	410	10	NP	NP	NP
Flounder, half portion	195	1.5	0.16	350	9	NP	NP	NP
Flounder, full portion	345	2.5	0.32	500	12	NP	NP	NP
Grouper, half portion	205	1.5	0.29	285	6	NP	NP	NP
Grouper, full portion	365	2.5	0.58	370	6	NP	NP	NP
Haddock, half portion	175	1.5	0.21	270	6	NP	NP	NP
Haddock, full portion	305	2.5	0.44	340	6	NP	NP	NP
Mahi-Mahi, half portion	205	1	0.16	305	6	NP	NP	NP
Mahi-Mahi, full portion	365	1.5	0.32	410	6	NP	NP	NP
Monchong, half portion	195	1.5	21	290	8	NP	NP	NP
Monchong, full portion	345	2.5	42	380	10	NP	NP	NP
Opah, half portion	275	12.5	3	290	6	NP	NP	NP
Opah, full portion	505	24.5	6	380	6	NP	NP	NP
Perch, half portion	175	2	0.32	290	6	NP	NP	NP
Perch, full portion	305	3.5	0.66	380	6	NP	NP	NP
Pompano, half portion	235	6.5	2.5	295	7	NP	NP	NP
Pompano, full portion	425	12.5	5	390	8	NP	NP	NP

Description & Serving	Cal	Fat	Sfat	Sod	Carb	Fiber	Sugar	Prot
Red Rockfish, half portion	175	2.5	0.43	290	8	NP	NP	NP
Red Rockfish, full portion	305	4.5	0.86	380	10	NP	NP	NP
Salmon, half portion	265	8.5	2	320	8	NP	NP	NP
Salmon, full portion	485	16.5	4	440	10	NP	NP	NP
Seabass, half portion	225	6.5	1.5	280	6	NP	NP	NP
Seabass, full portion	405	12.5	3	360	6	NP	NP	NP
Snapper, half portion	205	1.5	0.28	335	8	NP	NP	NP
Snapper, full portion	365	2.5	0.56	470	10	NP	NP	NP
Sole, half portion	145	2	0.37	260	6	NP	NP	NP
Sole, full portion	245	3.5	0.74	320	6	NP	NP	NP
Tilapia, half portion	205	3	1	235	9	NP	NP	NP
Tilapia, full portion	365	5.5	2	270	12	NP	NP	NP
Trout, Rainbow, half portion	225	9.5	2.5	390	6	NP	NP	NP
Trout, Rainbow, full portion	405	18.5	5	580	6	NP	NP	NP
Tuna, half portion	205	1	0.14	420	7	NP	NP	NP
Tuna, full portion	365	1.5	0.28	640	8	NP	NP	NP
Wahoo, half portion	225	2	0.5	390	8	NP	NP	NP
Wahoo, full portion	405	3.5	1	580	10	NP	NP	NP
Walleye, half portion	175	2	0.35	410	8	NP	NP	NP
Walleye, full portion	305	3.5	0.7	620	10	NP	NP	NP
Farm-Raised Catfish-Blackened	380	18	3	300	0	NP	NP	NP
Farm-Raised Catfish-Fried	440	24	3	560	5	NP	NP	NP
Flounder-Broiled	280	3	0.64	560	0	NP	NP	NP
Flounder-Fried	440	16	1	520	4	NP	NP	NP
Frozen Walleye-Beer Battered	700	42	4	1200	24	NP	NP	NP
Frozen Walleye-Blackened	300	8	1	420	10	NP	NP	NP
Frozen Walleye-Broiled	260	4	1	560	0	NP	NP	NP
Frozen Walleye-Fried	600	39	3	1000	36	NP	NP	NP
Seafood-Stuffed Flounder	320	11	3.5	1550	13	NP	NP	NP
Fried Oysters	590	32	3.5	1100	58	NP	NP	NP
Fried Crawfish	755	46	5	1395	64	NP	NP	NP
Seafood-Stuffed Flounder	160	6	1.5	780	6	NP	NP	NP
Wood-Grilled Fresh Salmon	210	9	2	235	<1	NP	NP	NP
Wood-Grilled Salmon BLT w/ Freshly Cooked Chips	1110	63	11	1890	73	NP	NP	NP
Lobster								
NY Strip & Rock Lobster Tail	570	27	11	1330	0	NP	NP	NP
Steak Lobster-&-Shrimp Oscar	990	60	26	2410	20	NP	NP	NP
Live Maine Lobster	45	0.48	0.12	350	0	NP	NP	NP
Rock Lobster Tail	90	1	0.2	300	2	NP	NP	NP
Rockzilla	125	1	0	475	2.5	NP	NP	NP
Maine Lobster Tail	60	0.5	0	610	0	NP	NP	NP
Pasta								
Chef's Signature Lobster & Shrimp Pasta, half portion	510	25	11	1090	43	NP	NP	NP
Chef's Signature Lobster & Shrimp Pasta, full portion	1020	50	22	2180	86	NP	NP	NP
Crab Linguini Alfredo, half portion	560	25	12	1310	47	NP	NP	NP
Crab Linguini Alfredo, full portion	1120	50	24	2620	94	NP	NP	NP

Description & Serving	Cal	Fat	Sfat	Sod	Carb	Fiber	Sugar	Prot
Shrimp Linguini Alfredo, half portion	550	29	10	1580	41	NP	NP	NP
Shrimp Linguini Alfredo, full portion	1100	58	20	3160	82	NP	NP	NP
Cajun Chicken Linguini Afredo, half portion	630	27	10	1550	45	NP	NP	NP
Cajun Chicken Linguini Afredo, full portion	1260	54	20	3100	90	NP	NP	NP
Shrimp								
Garlic-Grilled Jumbo Shrimp	365	6	1.5	1850	42	NP	NP	NP
Jumbo Shrimp w/ Lobster Butter	590	23	12	2260	61	NP	NP	NP
Maui Luau Shrimp & Salmon	790	16	3.5	2150	161	NP	NP	NP
Peach-Bourbon BBQ Shrimp & Scallops	490	12	3.5	1880	55	NP	NP	NP
Wood-Grilled Lobster, Shrimp & Scallops	720	33	17	2630	59	NP	NP	NP
Wood-Grilled Scallops, Shrimp & Chicken	580	10	2.5	2580	58	NP	NP	NP
Maple-Glazed Shrimp Skewer	60	0.5	0	370	0	NP	NP	NP
Crunchy Popcorn Shrimp	560	29	3	2144	52	NP	NP	NP
Parrot Bay Jumbo Coconut Shrimp	980	36	8	1038	50	NP	NP	NP
Coconut Shrimp Bites	290	18	3	830	19	NP	NP	NP
Fried Shrimp	190	11	1	1010	9	NP	NP	NP
Popcorn Shrimp	180	9	1	670	16	NP	NP	NP
Shrimp Scampi	130	9	1.5	690	1	NP	NP	NP
Walt's Favorite Shrimp	700	40	3	2440	52	NP	NP	NP
Shrimp Lover's Tuesday Coconut Shrimp Bites	290	18	3	830	19	NP	NP	NP
Shrimp Lover's Tuesday Fried Shrimp	190	11	1	560	9	NP	NP	NP
Shrimp Lover's Tuesday Popcorn Shrimp	180	9	1	670	16	NP	NP	NP
Shrimp Lover's Tuesday Shrimp Scampi	130	9	1.5	690	1	NP	NP	NP
Beer-Battered Shrimp & Chips	540	34	3.5	1170	40	NP	NP	NP
Wood-Grilled Shrimp Skewers	365	5.5	0.5	1850	42	NP	NP	NP
Steak								
Center-Cut NY Strip Steak	480	26	11	820	0	NP	NP	NP
Wood-Grilled Sirloin & Shrimp	500	12	4	1750	35	NP	NP	NP
Wood-Grilled Sirloin	250	7	3	640	0	NP	NP	NP
Miscellaneous Seafood								
Broiled Seafood Platter	280	8	2.02	1660	10	NP	NP	NP
Classic Fried Seafood Platter	1090	62	6.5	2830	90	NP	NP	NP
Admiral's Feast	1506	93.4	8.63	4662	101	NP	NP	NP
Seaside Shrimp Trio	1030	58	13	3490	68	NP	NP	NP
Ultimate Feast	638	40.18	16.4	2524	20	NP	NP	NP
Kids								
Broiled Fish	150	1	0.16	150	3	NP	NP	NP
Chicken Fingers	414	24	2.1	1320	28	NP	NP	NP
Grilled Chicken	215	4	1.25	705	14	NP	NP	NP
Macaroni & Cheese	280	7	2	590	42	NP	NP	NP
Popcorn Shrimp	140	7	1	620	12	NP	NP	NP
Snow Crab Legs	80	0.5	0	950	0	NP	NP	NP
Baked Potato	190	1	0	900	40	NP	NP	NP
Butter, Baked Potato Topping	90	10	6	80	1	NP	NP	NP
Sour Cream, Baked Potato Topping	30	2.5	1.5	10	1	NP	NP	NP
Caesar Salad	270	21	4.5	560	13	NP	NP	NP
Cheddar Bay Biscuit	150	8	2.5	350	16	NP	NP	NP

Description & Serving	Cal	Fat	Sfat	Sod	Carb	Fiber	Sugar	Prot
Fresh Broccoli	45	0.5	0	200	6	NP	NP	NP
Fries	330	17	1.5	740	40	NP	NP	NP
Garden Salad	90	3	0.46	105	13	NP	NP	NP
Home-Style Mashed Potatoes	180	9	4	610	22	NP	NP	NP
Wild Rice Pilaf	180	3	0.5	650	34	NP	NP	NP
Surf's Up Sundae	170	9	6	45	20			

Side

Baked Potato	190	1	0	900	40	NP	NP	NP
Butter, Baked Potato Topping	90	10	6	80	1	NP	NP	NP
Sour Cream, Baked Potato Topping	30	2.5	1.5	10	1	NP	NP	NP
Caesar Salad	270	21	4.5	560	13	NP	NP	NP
Petite Shrimp Salad Topping	15	0	0	130	0	NP	NP	NP
Cheddar Bay Biscuit	150	8	2.5	350	16	NP	NP	NP
Coleslaw	200	15	2.5	250	13	NP	NP	NP
Creamy Lobster-Topped Baked Potato	370	12	7	1110	48	NP	NP	NP
Creamy Lobster-Topped Mashed Potatoes	360	22	12	1110	23	NP	NP	NP
Fresh Asparagus	60	3	1.5	270	5	NP	NP	NP
Fresh Broccoli	45	0.5	0	200	6	NP	NP	NP
Fries	330	17	1.5	740	40	NP	NP	NP
Garden Salad	90	3	0.46	105	13	NP	NP	NP
Home-Style Mashed Potatoes	180	9	4	610	22	NP	NP	NP
Saltines	25	0.5	0	80	4	NP	NP	NP
Wild Rice Pilaf	180	3	0.5	650	34	NP	NP	NP

Salad

Hand-Tossed Caesar Salad	520	48	9	1060	14	NP	NP	NP
Hand-Tossed Caesar Salad w/ Wood-Grilled Chicken	670	51	10	1710	14	NP	NP	NP
Hand-Tossed Caesar Salad w/ Grilled Shrimp	620	51	10	1370	14	NP	NP	NP

Soup

Bayou Seafood Gumbo, cup	190	6	2	1130	15	NP	NP	NP
Bayou Seafood Gumbo, bowl	380	12	3.5	2260	31	NP	NP	NP
Creamy Potato Bacon Soup, cup	220	15	9	790	19	NP	NP	NP
Creamy Potato Bacon Soup, bowl	440	30	18	1580	38	NP	NP	NP
Manhattan Clam Chowder, cup	80	1	0	690	12	NP	NP	NP
Manhattan Clam Chowder, bowl	160	2	1	1380	24	NP	NP	NP
New England Clam Chowder, cup	240	16	10	680	13	NP	NP	NP
New England Clam Chowder, bowl	480	33	19	1360	26	NP	NP	NP
Seafood Gumbo, cup	230	8	2.5	1180	26	NP	NP	NP
Seafood Gumbo, bowl	470	17	5	2360	51	NP	NP	NP
Spicy Shrimp Soup, cup	160	6	2.5	1010	15	NP	NP	NP
Spicy Shrimp Soup, bowl	320	12	5	2020	30	NP	NP	NP

Dessert

Chocolate Wave	1490	81	25	950	172	NP	NP	NP
Key Lime Pie	580	22	12	450	88	NP	NP	NP
New York-Style Cheesecake w/ Strawberries	520	36	21	270	39	NP	NP	NP
Warm Apple Crumble a la Mode	770	31	13	200	117	NP	NP	NP
Warm Chocolate Chip Lava Cookie	1070	51	23	470	142	NP	NP	NP

Description & Serving	Cal	Fat	Sfat	Sod	Carb	Fiber	Sugar	Prot
Dressing/Condiment/Topping								
Balsamic Vinaigrette	60	5	0.5	190	4	NP	NP	NP
Blue Cheese Dressing	170	18	3.5	190	1	NP	NP	NP
Caesar Dressing	200	21	3.5	370	<1	NP	NP	NP
French Dressing	120	11	1.5	300	7	NP	NP	NP
Honey Mustard Dressing	100	11	2	160	5	NP	NP	NP
Ranch Dressing	110	11	2	210	1	NP	NP	NP
Fat-Free Ranch Dressing	40	0	0	340	10	NP	NP	NP
Thousand Island Dressing	130	13	2	180	5	NP	NP	NP
Cocktail Sauce	25	0	0	320	6	NP	NP	NP
Honey Mustard Sauce	240	22	4	320	10	NP	NP	NP
Ketchup	30	0	0	310	8	NP	NP	NP
Marinara Sauce	30	1	0	220	6	NP	NP	NP
Pico de Gallo	10	0	0	170	2	NP	NP	NP
Pina Colada Sauce, 2 oz	120	5	4	20	16	NP	NP	NP
Remoulade	150	15	2.5	150	4	NP	NP	NP
Sweet & Spicy Glaze	90	0	0	220	21	NP	NP	NP
Tartar Sauce	130	13	2	110	4	NP	NP	NP
Melted Butter	230	25	15	20	1	NP	NP	NP
Blackened w/ Cajun Spices	40	0.5	0	140	1	NP	NP	NP
New Orleans	250	19	8	770	0	NP	NP	NP
Topped w/ Honey BBQ Shrimp	180	11	4.5	890	11	NP	NP	NP
Topped w/ Lobster Butter Sauce	260	12.5	7	660	21.5	NP	NP	NP
Topped w/ Maple-Glaze & Shrimp	200	10	2	685	17	NP	NP	NP
Beverage								
Kids								
Berry Strawberry Banana Smoothie	340	9	6	85	63	NP	NP	NP
Cherry Wave Slushy	290	0	0	10	74	NP	NP	NP
Sunset Strawberry Smoothie	250	6	4	45	47	NP	NP	NP
Juice	115-135	0	0	0-25	25-30	NP	NP	NP
Milk	146	7.9	4.6	98	11	NP	NP	NP
Nonalcoholic								
Raspberry Lemonade	178	0	0	20	30	NP	NP	NP
Red Rockin' Shirley T	170	0	0	0	43	NP	NP	NP
Boston Iced Tea	50	0	0	10	13	NP	NP	NP
Harbor Café Coffee	3	0	0	5	0	NP	NP	NP
Bahama Mama	230	0	0	25	57	NP	NP	NP
Berry Mango Daiquiri	210	0	0	20	52	NP	NP	NP
Classic Margarita, Frozen	278	0	0	560	75	NP	NP	NP
Classic Margarita, On the Rocks	150	0	0	750	22	NP	NP	NP
Pina Colada	280	8	7	20	53	NP	NP	NP
Raspberry Margarita	330	0	0	0	81	NP	NP	NP
Smoothie - Banana Bay Chocolate	460	14	9	10	78	NP	NP	NP
Smoothie - Berry Strawberry Banana	340	9	6	85	63	NP	NP	NP
Smoothie - Sunset Strawberry	250	6	4	45	47	NP	NP	NP
Strawberry Daiquiri	230	0	0	5	56	NP	NP	NP

Description & Serving	Cal	Fat	Sfat	Sod	Carb	Fiber	Sugar	Prot
Strawberry Margarita	330	0	0	20	70	NP	NP	NP
Sunset Passion Colada	330	8	7	25	62	NP	NP	NP
Tropcial Freeze - Orange	250	6	5	20	49	NP	NP	NP
Tropical Freeze - Pineapple	250	5	4.5	180	50	NP	NP	NP
Alcoholic								
Amaretto Sour	170	0	0	0	30	NP	NP	NP
Biscayne Bay Breeze	240	0	0	10	47	NP	NP	NP
Bloody Mary	140	0	0	1170	16	NP	NP	NP
Malibu Hurricane	200	0	0	15	36	NP	NP	NP
Screwdriver	100	0	0	0	8	NP	NP	NP
Tequila Sunrise	170	0	0	10	24	NP	NP	NP
Top-Shelf Long Island Iced Tea	190	0	0	0	22	NP	NP	NP
Caramel Appletini	160	0	0	10	18	NP	NP	NP
Classic Martini w/ Gin	140	1.5	0.33	330	<1	NP	NP	NP
Classic Martini w/ Vodka	130	2	0	400	1	NP	NP	NP
Cosmopolitan	220	0	0	0	15	NP	NP	NP
Manhattan w/ Bourbon	150	0	0	0	5	NP	NP	NP
Manhattan w/ Whiskey	150	0	0	0	5	NP	NP	NP
Rob Roy	160	0	0	10	3	NP	NP	NP
Cognac	73	0	0	0	0	NP	NP	NP
Liqueurs	86	0	0	6	6-15	NP	NP	NP
Single Malt Scotches	69	0	0	0	0	NP	NP	NP
80 Proof Distilled Spirits	96	0	0	0	0	NP	NP	NP
Alotta colada	700	16	14	55	95	NP	NP	NP
Bahama Mama	350	0	0	20	51	NP	NP	NP
Big Berry Daiquiri	350	0.45	0.36	30	62	NP	NP	NP
Mudslide	520	21	13	160	52	NP	NP	NP
Pina Colada	320	6	5	35	55	NP	NP	NP
Red Passion Colada	310	4.5	4	35	56	NP	NP	NP
Strawberry Daiquiri	250	0	0	15	47	NP	NP	NP
Sunset Passion Colada	360	8	7	15	62	NP	NP	NP
Classic Margarita - Frozen	470	0	0	590	96	NP	NP	NP
Classic Margarita - On the Rocks	246	0	0	770	22	NP	NP	NP
Frozen Raspberry Margarita	320	0	0	0	61	NP	NP	NP
Frozen Strawberry Margarita	350	0	0	20	68	NP	NP	NP
Lobsterita - Strawberry	700	0	0	55	135	NP	NP	NP
Lobsterita - Traditional	890	0	0	890	183	NP	NP	NP
Lobsterita - Raspberry	690	0.47	0.31	50	131	NP	NP	NP
Top-Shelf Margarita - Frozen	520	0	0	640	97	NP	NP	NP
Top-Shelf Margarita - On the Rocks	296	0	0	810	25	NP	NP	NP
Baileys & Coffee	180	8	5	50	15	NP	NP	NP
Baileys & Irish Cream	270	4.5	0	0	5.7	NP	NP	NP
Coffee Nudge	130	2	1.5	15	14	NP	NP	NP
Disaronno Amaretto	80	0	0	0	12	NP	NP	NP
Frangelico	70	0	0	0	12.3	NP	NP	NP
Grand Mariner	76	0	0	0	6.5	NP	NP	NP
Irish Coffee	90	2	1	25	4	NP	NP	NP
Kahula	90	0	0	3	14.7	NP	NP	NP

Description & Serving	Cal	Fat	Sfat	Sod	Carb	Fiber	Sugar	Prot
				Red Robin				
Appetizer								
Bueno Con Queso	1433	89	NP	5740	106	7	NP	49
Creamy Artichoke & Spinach Dip	1207	73	NP	2080	101	17	NP	39
Fresh-Fried Cheese Sticks	1171	67	NP	2895	90	6	NP	52
Guacamole, Salsa & Chips	812	47	NP	1628	88	13	NP	9
Just-In-Quesadilla	1071	55	NP	3034	69	9	NP	59
Vegetarian Just-In-Quesadilla	872	48	NP	2275	68	9	NP	30
Nacho Ordinary Chili Nachos w/ Chicken	2084	134	NP	4045	132	33	NP	87
Nacho Ordinary Chili Nachos	1954	132	NP	3526	130	22	NP	62
RR's Buzzard Wings	1076	84	NP	2345	4	3	NP	79
Towering Onion Rings	1819	122	NP	3789	160	10	NP	18
Salad								
Fajita Fiesta Pollo Salad	1000	62	NP	1408	59	10	NP	51
Asian Chicken Salad	600	15	NP	1945	73	8	NP	41
Cobb Salad	736	38	NP	1841	42	8	NP	54
Crispy Chicken Tender Salad	1400	91	NP	2250	91	6	NP	58
Apple Harvest Chicken Salad	587	34	NP	1544	40	7	NP	36
Mighty Caesar - Grilled Chicken	945	61	NP	1504	47	8	NP	43
Mighty Caesar - Blackened	945	61	NP	2044	47	8	NP	43
Mighty Caesar - Salmon	1010	64	NP	1319	47	8	NP	50
Mighty Caesar	793	57	NP	1229	47	8	NP	14
Side Salad	57	2	NP	30	9	2	NP	1
Side Caesar Salad	350	22	NP	582	27	4	NP	7
Dinner Salad	212	13	NP	227	15	3	NP	9
Soup								
Chicken Tortilla Soup, cup	173	9	NP	562	11	2	NP	10
Clamdigger's Clam Chowder, cup	346	20	NP	965	26	1	NP	13
French Onion Soup, cup	276	11	NP	1413	26	2	NP	11
Red's Homemade Chili Chili, cup	289	18	NP	827	13	5	NP	20
Burger								
Beef								
Whiskey River BBQ Burger	1114	69	NP	1805	68	4	NP	49
The Banzai Burger	1033	63	NP	1912	65	3	NP	48
Monster Burger	1151	69	NP	2141	57	3	NP	74
Bleu Ribbon Burger	1052	63	NP	1925	69	3	NP	46
Royal Red Robin Burger	1191	83	NP	2090	48	3	NP	60
Red Robin Gourmet Cheeseburger	850	49	NP	1893	58	3	NP	46
Red Robin Bacon Cheeseburger	1030	70	NP	1920	48	3	NP	52
Sauted 'Shroom Burger	961	57	NP	1342	55	6	NP	60
Guacamole Bacon Burger	1160	77	NP	1460	52	4	NP	62
Santa Fe Burger	1095	68	NP	1508	66	5	NP	47
A.1. Peppercorn Burger	1433	97	NP	5618	92	3	NP	54
Burnin' Love Burger	989	66	NP	2041	54	3	NP	44

Description & Serving	Cal	Fat	Sfat	Sod	Carb	Fiber	Sugar	Prot
Natural Burger	570	25	NP	979	48	2	NP	38
Blackened Bayou Burger	919	61	NP	1949	50	4	NP	45
Chili Chili Cheeseburger	963	55	NP	1678	54	7	NP	60
Lettuce-Wrap Your Burger	422	27	NP	398	8	2	NP	34
Prime Rib Dip	998	55	NP	2756	72	5	NP	53
Chicken/Turkey								
Bruschetta Chicken Burger	832	48	NP	1466	53	4	NP	48
Whiskey River BBQ Chicken	965	53	NP	1832	68	4	NP	50
Teriyaki Chicken Burger	905	49	NP	1606	61	3	NP	57
Crispy Chicken Burger	929	56	NP	1966	71	4	NP	37
California Chicken Burger	946	57	NP	2002	49	4	NP	55
Blackened Chicken Burger	748	41	NP	1841	49	2	NP	47
Jamaican Jerk'd Chicken Burger	704	36	NP	1790	53	2	NP	44
Grilled Turkey Burger	694	43	NP	849	49	3	NP	29
Fish								
Crispy Fish Burger	605	30	NP	1892	58	3	NP	28
Grilled Salmon Burger	856	50	NP	1244	53	4	NP	47
Steak								
Steak Sliders	1208	73	NP	2040	88	9	NP	98
Vegetarian								
The Garden Burger	538	23	NP	1600	62	10	NP	23
Boca Burger	606	29	NP	1985	60	11	NP	37
Sandwich/Wrap								
BLTA Croissant	719	41	NP	1656	56	5	NP	32
Caesar's Chicken Wrap	852	43	NP	1862	69	4	NP	40
Whiskey River BBQ Chicken Wrap	1112	62	NP	2532	84	5	NP	51
Entrée								
Chicken								
Chicken Fajitas	970	38	NP	2135	77	5	NP	70
Clucks & Fries, 4 Tenders	1389	85	NP	2200	105	6	NP	50
Clucks & Fries Buffalo Style, 4 tenders	1633	113	NP	4406	105	6	NP	52
Ensenada Chicken Platter, 2 Chicken Breasts	781	45	NP	1669	22	3	NP	70
Ensenada Chicken Platter, 1 Chicken Breast	629	41	NP	1394	22	3	NP	40
Fish								
Arctic Cod Fish & Chips	1118	67	NP	2764	83	6	NP	44
Salmon & Chips	1081	69	NP	1751	80	5	NP	33
Shrimp & Cod Duo	1418	83	NP	3206	131	12	NP	41
Jumbo Shrimp & Slaw Platter, 13 shrimp	1239	56	NP	3266	146	13	NP	43
Pasta/Rice								
Chicken Parmigiano Pasta	1480	56	NP	3661	166	10	NP	77
Southwest Chicken Pasta	1483	83	NP	1861	118	4	NP	65
Southwest Pasta	1331	79	NP	1586	118	4	NP	35
Red's Rice Bowl - Chicken	808	8	NP	1619	140	6	NP	39
Red's Rice Bowl - Vegetarian	656	6	NP	890	135	6	NP	13

Description & Serving	Cal	Fat	Sfat	Sod	Carb	Fiber	Sugar	Prot
Side
Apple Slices	40	0	NP	0	16	4	NP	0
Celery	11	0	NP	54	2	1	NP	1
Chipotle Beans	111	1	NP	448	21	6	NP	5
Coleslaw	252	18	NP	676	23	4	NP	3
Garlic Parmesan Steak Fries	587	35	NP	679	64	4	NP	7
Melon Wedges	61	0	NP	29	15	2	NP	2
Onion Rings	724	54	NP	1504	62	4	NP	7
Red Robin Steak Fries	434	18	NP	444	60	4	NP	6
Slice Focaccia Bread	300	6	NP	570	48	2	NP	10
Steamed Veggies	55	0	NP	49	12	4	NP	2
Texas Toast	65	0	NP	235	14	0	NP	2
Kids
Carnival Corn Dog	295	12	NP	623	36	1	NP	11
Cheesy Mac 'n Cheesy	420	22	NP	980	42	2	NP	13
Chick-Chick-Chicken Fingers	338	18	NP	670	22	1	NP	22
Chick-n-Cheese Quesadilla	568	26	NP	1364	33	2	NP	43
Grilled Cheesewich	440	29	NP	1600	30	1	NP	15
Chick On A Stick	152	4	NP	275	0	0	NP	30
Parmesan Noodles	427	24	NP	241	43	0	NP	9
Rad Boca Burger	340	12	NP	1295	35	9	NP	31
Rad Chicken Burger	292	6	NP	525	25	1	NP	34
Rad Garden Burger	272	6	NP	580	37	8	NP	17
Rad Robin Burger	276	12	NP	370	25	1	NP	17
Rad Turkey Burger	393	22	NP	595	26	1	NP	24
Red Robinetti Spaghetti	297	2	NP	671	56	3	NP	11
Red's Cheese Pizza	605	27	NP	1465	58	6	NP	29
Red's Pizzeria Pizza	690	35	NP	1773	58	6	NP	32
Kid's Apple Slices	20	0	NP	0	8	2	NP	0
Kid's Baby Carrots & Ranch	280	0	NP	44	5	2	NP	0
Kid's Mandarin Oranges	28	0	NP	4	7	0	NP	0
Kid's Melon Wedges	61	0	NP	29	15	2	NP	2
Kid's Side Broccoli	20	0	NP	23	4	2	NP	1
Kid's Side Salad	57	2	NP	21	8	2	NP	2
Kid's Steak Fries	217	9	NP	222	30	2	NP	3
Kid's Sundae	378	19	NP	149	48	1	NP	5
Kid's Chocolate Milkshake	431	16	NP	173	70	2	NP	6
Kid's Raspberry Milkshake	499	15	NP	155	88	0	NP	5
Kid's Strawberry Smoothie	122	0	NP	12	30	2	NP	0
Kid's Freckled Lemonade Light	34	0	NP	3	8	0	NP	1
Kid's Rookie Magic	586	27	NP	439	83	0	NP	23
Kid's Hawaiian Heart Throb Smoothie	287	1	NP	7	69	9	NP	0
Kid's Groovy Smoothie	225	2	NP	20	52	1	NP	1
Kid's Raspberry Limeade	112	0	NP	10	29	1	NP	0
Dessert
Hot Fudge Sundae	803	38	NP	327	110	1	NP	10
Hot Apple Crisp	784	13	NP	480	165	12	NP	8

Description & Serving	Cal	Fat	Sfat	Sod	Carb	Fiber	Sugar	Prot
Mountain High Mudd Pie	1373	63	NP	640	184	6	NP	19
Birthday Sundae	378	19	NP	149	48	1	NP	5

Beverage

Alcoholic

Description & Serving	Cal	Fat	Sfat	Sod	Carb	Fiber	Sugar	Prot
Absolut Lemonade	198	0	NP	26	30	0	NP	0
Bailey's Irish Cream Shake	375	17	NP	117	39	0	NP	12
Banana Daiquiri	310	0	NP	0	55	2	NP	0
Gold Margarita - Frozen	172	0	NP	1111	18	2	NP	0
Gold Margarita - Peach	348	0	NP	0	61	2	NP	1
Gold Margarita - Raspberry	368	0	NP	24	65	0	NP	0
Gold Margarita - Rocks	192	0	NP	1115	22	2	NP	0
Gold Margarita - Strawberry	228	0	NP	0	32	1	NP	1
Mango Margarita	331	0	NP	1	59	2	NP	0
Nuclear Ice Tea	280	0	NP	20	24	2	NP	0
One Great Margarita - Frozen	210	0	NP	1115	25	2	NP	0
One Great Margarita - Peach	365	0	NP	0	64	2	NP	1
One Great Margarita - Raspberry	602	0	NP	30	90	0	NP	0
One Great Margarita - Rocks	230	0	NP	1119	30	2	NP	0
One Great Margarita - Strawberry	277	0	NP	0	43	2	NP	1
Peach Daiquiri	310	0	NP	0	55	2	NP	1
Raspberry Daiquiri	556	0	NP	32	84	1	NP	0
Sand In Your Shorts	357	0	NP	11	51	2	NP	1
Strawberry Daiquiri	231	0	NP	2	36	2	NP	1
Tropical Mai Tai	289	0	NP	19	41	1	NP	0
Ultimate Margarita - Frozen	208	0	NP	1117	24	2	NP	0
Ultimate Margarita - Peach	325	0	NP	0	59	2	NP	1
Ultimate Margarita - Raspberry	562	0	NP	30	85	0	NP	0
Ultimate Margarita - Rocks	228	0	NP	1121	28	2	NP	0
Ultimate Margarita - Strawberry	237	0	NP	0	38	2	NP	1

Nonalcoholic

Description & Serving	Cal	Fat	Sfat	Sod	Carb	Fiber	Sugar	Prot
Banana Milkshake	372	15	NP	131	58	1	NP	5
Dreamy Orange Smoothie	411	12	NP	80	74	1	NP	5
Freckled Lemonade	80	0	NP	20	21	0	NP	0
Freckled Lemonade Light	68	0	NP	3	17	1	NP	0
Groovy Smoothie	342	2	NP	23	81	3	NP	1
Hawaiian Heart Throb Smoothie	414	1	NP	10	100	14	NP	1
Iced Tea	3	0	NP	0	1	0	NP	0
Monster Malt - Banana	809	30	NP	411	128	2	NP	15
Monster Malt - Chocolate	898	31	NP	474	147	3	NP	17
Monster Malt - Peach	809	30	NP	411	128	2	NP	16
Monster Malt - Raspberry	1099	30	NP	441	167	1	NP	15
Monster Malt - Strawberry	743	30	NP	411	112	2	NP	16
Monster Malt - Vanilla	751	32	NP	425	112	1	NP	16
Monster Shake - Banana	640	27	NP	244	98	1	NP	10
Monster Shake - Chocolate	729	28	NP	307	117	2	NP	12
Monster Shake- Peach	640	27	NP	244	98	1	NP	11
Monster Shake - Raspberry	930	27	NP	274	137	0	NP	10
Monster Shake - Strawberry	573	27	NP	244	82	1	NP	10

Description & Serving	Cal	Fat	Sfat	Sod	Carb	Fiber	Sugar	Prot
Monster Shake - Vanilla	582	29	NP	258	82	0	NP	10
Peach Iced Tea	103	0	NP	0	26	0	NP	0
Peach Milkshake	372	15	NP	131	58	1	NP	6
Peachy Keen Splash	217	0	NP	27	56	1	NP	0
Pomegranate Iced Tea	96	0	NP	0	23	0	NP	0
Raspberry Iced Tea	103	0	NP	0	26	0	NP	0
Rookie Magic	884	41	NP	623	127	1	NP	32
Root Beer Float	456	9	NP	146	101	0	NP	3
Strawberry Milkshake	328	15	NP	131	47	1	NP	6
Vanilla Milkshake	315	15	NP	131	44	0	NP	5
Very Berry Raspberry Limeade	204	0	NP	18	52	0	NP	0

Rita's

Italian Ice

Description & Serving	Cal	Fat	Sfat	Sod	Carb	Fiber	Sugar	Prot
Italian Ice, reg cup (avg all flavors)	320	0	0	35	80	0	77	0
Sugar Free Ice, reg cup (avg all flavors)	80	0	0	25	20	0	0	0

Ice Cream/Custard

Description & Serving	Cal	Fat	Sfat	Sod	Carb	Fiber	Sugar	Prot
Cream Ice, reg cup (avg all flavors)	380	5	4	105	85	1	79	1
Custard, reg cup (avg all flavors)	330	17	11	100	40	0	31	6
Slenderita Fat Free Soft Serve, reg cup	230	0	0	260	49	1	33	8

Gelati

Description & Serving	Cal	Fat	Sfat	Sod	Carb	Fiber	Sugar	Prot
Cherry Light Gelati, reg	170	0	0	190	37	1	23	6
Chocolate Light Gelati, reg	260	0.5	0	210	57	2	23	7
Mango-Peach Light Gelati, reg	230	0	0	190	51	1	23	6
Pineapple Light Gelati, reg	230	0	0	200	51	1	23	6
Pink Lemonade Light Gelati, reg	170	0	0	190	37	1	23	6
Root Beer Light Gelati, reg	170	0	0	190	37	1	23	6
Tangerine Light Gelati, reg	170	0	0	190	37	1	23	6
Gelati w/ Italian Ice, reg (avg all flavors)	390	12	8	170	68	0	60	5
Vanilla Gelati w/ Italian Ice, reg	390	12	8	180	66	0	59	5
Chocolate Gelati w/ Italian Ice, reg	400	11	7	150	71	0	62	5
Strawberry Gelati w/ Italian Ice, reg	390	12	7	170	69	0	62	4
Coffee Gelati w/ Italian Ice, reg	380	12	8	170	67	0	59	4
Orange Cream Gelati w/ Italian Ice, reg	380	12	8	170	66	0	59	4
Gelati w/ Cream Ice, reg (avg all flavors)	420	14	10	200	71	0	61	6
Vanilla Gelati w/ Cream Ice, reg	420	15	10	210	69	0	60	5
Chocolate Gelati w/ Cream Ice, reg	430	14	9	180	73	0	63	5
Strawberry Gelati w/ Cream Ice, reg	420	14	9	200	71	0	63	10
Coffee Gelati w/ Cream Ice, reg	420	15	10	210	70	0	60	5
Orange Cream Gelati w/ Cream Ice, reg	420	15	10	210	69	0	60	5

Frozen Treat

Description & Serving	Cal	Fat	Sfat	Sod	Carb	Fiber	Sugar	Prot
Cherry Light Nilla Blendini	370	3	1.5	430	76	1	44	10
Chocolate Light Nilla Blendini	430	3.5	1.5	450	89	2	44	11
Mango-Peach Light Nilla Blendini	410	3	1.5	430	85	1	45	10
Pineapple Light Nilla Blendini	410	3	1.5	430	85	1	45	10

Description & Serving	Cal	Fat	Sfat	Sod	Carb	Fiber	Sugar	Prot
Pink Lemonade Light Nilla Blendini	370	3	1.5	430	76	1	44	10
Root Beer Light Nilla Blendini	370	3	1.5	430	76	1	44	10
Tangerine Light Nilla Blendini	370	3	1.5	430	76	1	44	10
Cherry Light Oreo Blendini	380	5	1.5	440	73	2	46	10
Chocolate Light Oreo Blendini	440	6	2	450	86	3	46	10
Mango-Peach Light Oreo Blendini	420	5	1.5	440	82	2	46	10
Pineapple Light Oreo Blendini	420	5	1.5	440	82	2	46	10
Pink Lemonade Light Oreo Blendini	380	5	1.5	440	73	2	46	10
Root Beer Light Oreo Blendini	380	5	1.5	440	73	2	46	10
Tangerine Light Oreo Blendini	380	5	1.5	440	73	2	46	10
Cherry Light Pretzel Blendini	360	1	0	650	77	2	35	11
Chocolate Light Pretzel Blendini	420	1.5	0	660	90	3	35	12
Mango-Peach Light Pretzel Blendini	400	1	0	650	86	2	35	11
Pineapple Light Pretzel Blendini	400	1	0	650	86	2	35	11
Pink Lemonade Light Pretzel Blendini	360	1	0	650	77	2	35	11
Root Beer Light Pretzel Blendini	360	1	0	650	77	2	35	11
Tangerine Light Pretzel Blendini	360	1	0	650	77	2	35	11
Cherry Light M&Ms Blendini	390	7	4	300	73	2	52	10
Chocolate Light M&Ms Blendini	440	7	4	310	86	3	52	11
Mango-Peach Light M&Ms Blendini	420	7	4	300	82	2	52	10
Pineapple Light M&Ms Blendini	420	7	4	300	82	2	52	10
Pink Lemonade Light M&Ms Blendini	390	7	4	300	73	2	52	10
Root Beer Light M&Ms Blendini	390	7	4	300	73	2	52	10
Tangerine Light M&Ms Blendini	390	7	4	300	73	2	52	10
Feature Blendini Flavor (avg all varieties)	590	23	13	410	90	1	68	8

Frozen Beverage

Vanilla Misto w/ Italian Ice, reg	480	8	5	140	103	0	96	3
Chocolate Misto w/ Italian Ice, reg	510	7	4.5	120	106	0	98	6
Vanilla Misto w/ Cream Ice, reg	560	13	10	210	109	1	98	4
Chocolate Misto w/ Cream Ice, reg	560	12	9	190	112	1	100	4
Feature Misto Flavor, reg (avg all varieties)	510	9	6	150	106	0	98	3
Ritaccino	780	20	14	340	147	0	131	7

Kids

Italian Ice, kids cup (avg all flavors)	200	0	0	20	50	0	48	0
Sugar Free Ice, kids cup (avg all flavors)	50	0	0	15	12	0	0	0
Cream Ice, kids cup (avg all flavors)	240	3	2.5	65	53	0	49	0
Custard, kids cup (avg all flavors)	230	12	8	150	28	0	22	4
Slenderita Fat Free Soft Serve, kids cup	160	0	0	180	34	1	23	6

Cone/Topping

Cake Cone	10	0	0	15	2	0	0	0
Waffle Cone	40	0.5	0	0	8	0	3	1
Hot Fudge, 1 oz	90	3	3	50	15	0	14	1
Hot Caramel, 1 oz	90	1	0.5	50	20	0	13	1
Rainbow Sprinkles, 1 oz	140	6	2.5	0	21	0	10	0
Chocolate Sprinkles, 1 oz	140	6	2.5	0	21	0	10	0
Oreos, 1 oz	140	5	1.5	160	20	1	12	1

Description & Serving	Cal	Fat	Sfat	Sod	Carb	Fiber	Sugar	Prot
Nilla Wafers, 1 oz	120	3	1.5	150	22	0	10	1
M&Ms Minis, 1 oz	140	7	4	20	19	1	18	1
Snyder's Pretzel Snaps, 1 oz	110	1	0	370	24	1	1	3

Romano's Macaroni Grill

Appetizer

	Cal	Fat	Sfat	Sod	Carb	Fiber	Sugar	Prot
Tomato Bruschetta w/ sauce & garnish	630	15	5	1750	96	NP	NP	28
Tapenade Trio w/ sauce & garnish	940	34	7	2910	130	NP	NP	29
Roasted Vegetables w/ sauce & garnish	330	21	3	440	32	NP	NP	6
Mozzarella Alla Caprese w/ sauce & garnish	330	16	9	550	33	NP	NP	13
Calamari Fritti w/ sauce & garnish	960	81	14	1700	30	NP	NP	27
Shrimp & Artichoke Dip w/ sauce & garnish	810	46	19	2130	64	NP	NP	35
Crab-Stuffed Mushrooms w/ sauce & garnish	580	42	12	960	26	NP	NP	25
Mozzarella Fritta w/ sauce & garnish	640	38	14	1440	49	NP	NP	24
Romano's Sampler w/ sauce & garnish	1200	71	19	2620	96	NP	NP	42

Pizza

	Cal	Fat	Sfat	Sod	Carb	Fiber	Sugar	Prot
Margherita Pizza, whole	970	25	13	2850	134	NP	NP	52
Pesto Chicken Pizza, whole	1550	72	24	3710	148	NP	NP	78
BBQ Chicken Pizza, whole	1090	24	12	3400	150	NP	NP	68
Sicilian Pizza, whole	1390	60	28	4070	133	NP	NP	79
Roma Sicilian Mio Pizza, half (Romano's Duo & Trio)	700	30	14	2040	67	NP	NP	40
Roma Margherita Mio Pizza, half (Romano's Duo & Trio)	490	13	7	1430	67	NP	NP	26

Salad & Soup

	Cal	Fat	Sfat	Sod	Carb	Fiber	Sugar	Prot
Warm Spinach Salad w/ dressing	380	20	8	1010	22	NP	NP	18
Side Garden Salad w/ dressing	240	16	4	740	20	NP	NP	5
Garden Salad (Romano's Duo & Trio)	240	16	4	740	20	NP	NP	5
Side Caesar Salad w/ dressing	240	18	4	510	13	NP	NP	5
Caesar Salad (Romano's Duo & Trio)	240	18	4	510	13	NP	NP	5
Parmesan-Crusted Chicken Salad w/ dressing	960	63	16	1990	49	NP	NP	51
Chicken Caesar Salad w/ dressing	700	53	12	1880	19	NP	NP	38
Chicken Florentine Salad w/ dressing	1020	76	17	2830	47	NP	NP	36
Insalata Blu w/ dressing	620	56	16	1430	8	NP	NP	19
Insalata Blu w/ Chicken w/ dressing	750	59	17	1990	12	NP	NP	42
Insalata Blu (Romano's Duo & Trio)	310	28	8	715	4	NP	NP	10
Scallops & Spinach Salad w/ dressing	420	19	4	1510	26	NP	NP	36
Chicken Toscana Soup, cup	220	11	5	1350	19	NP	NP	14
Chicken Toscana Soup, bowl	500	24	10	2500	43	NP	NP	28
Tomato & Cheese Tortellini Soup, cup	240	13	6	1090	21	NP	NP	9
Tomato & Cheese Tortellini Soup, bowl	440	18	9	2180	51	NP	NP	18

Lunch Portion

Pasta & Chicken

	Cal	Fat	Sfat	Sod	Carb	Fiber	Sugar	Prot
Carmela's Chicken Rigatoni	1130	68	29	1390	85	NP	NP	33
Pasta Milano	1210	77	32	3220	95	NP	NP	50

Description & Serving	Cal	Fat	Sfat	Sod	Carb	Fiber	Sugar	Prot
Penne Rustica	1350	81	32	3480	71	NP	NP	83
Shrimp Portofino	560	34	14	1050	37	NP	NP	26
Spaghetti Bolognese	840	50	24	1760	63	NP	NP	33
Eggplant Parmigiana	1110	61	31	2220	101	NP	NP	39
Chicken Cannelloni	590	29	17	1710	41	NP	NP	39
Spaghetti & Meatballs w/ Tomato Sauce	1150	71	33	3530	89	NP	NP	43
Spaghetti & Meatballs w/ Bolognese Sauce	1290	83	37	3500	80	NP	NP	57
Chicken Parmigiana	1020	55	16	1550	85	NP	NP	43
Layers of Lasagna	720	39	17	1940	45	NP	NP	47
Chicken Marsala	1050	61	21	2030	97	NP	NP	26
Chicken Scaloppine	1280	103	40	2700	64	NP	NP	34
Parmesan-Crusted Sole	1190	71	30	2180	101	NP	NP	37
Honey Balsamic Chicken	540	13	3	2040	54	NP	NP	51
Sandwich & Chips								
Formaggio Melts, 2 (Romano's Duo & Trio)	820	50	11	550	87	NP	NP	12
Formaggio Melts	1220	70	16	820	130	NP	NP	18
1/2 Brick Oven Meatball (Romano's Duo & Trio)	540	30	12	1780	43	NP	NP	24
Brick Oven Meatball	1040	57	24	3310	83	NP	NP	46
1/2 Grilled Chicken & Artichoke (Romano's Duo & Trio)	490	28	7	1120	38	NP	NP	23
Grilled Chicken & Artichoke	980	55	13	2240	76	NP	NP	45
Romano's Parmesan Chips	320	21	7	610	22	NP	NP	10

Entrée (Dinner Portion)

Prepared Pasta								
Carmela's Chicken Rigatoni	1430	89	36	1650	104	NP	NP	37
Pasta Milano	1530	98	44	4350	125	NP	NP	58
Penne Rustica	1590	92	38	4000	93	NP	NP	96
Shrimp Portofino	560	35	14	1190	37	NP	NP	30
Spaghetti Bolognese	1120	69	33	2290	83	NP	NP	42
Eggplant Parmigiana	1270	69	33	2610	117	NP	NP	44
Chicken Cannelloni	880	44	25	2540	61	NP	NP	59
Spaghetti & Meatballs w/ Tomato Sauce	1500	91	41	4710	118	NP	NP	59
Spaghetti & Meatballs w/ Bolognese Sauce	1810	118	54	4900	109	NP	NP	78
Chicken Parmigiana	1650	98	30	2500	116	NP	NP	74
Layers of Lasagna	1030	57	26	2640	69	NP	NP	60
Chicken Marsala	1180	70	23	2320	101	NP	NP	34
Chicken Scaloppine	1410	112	42	3000	68	NP	NP	42
Parmesan-Crusted Sole	1710	105	39	2830	131	NP	NP	62
Cappellini Pomodoro	390	14	2	980	55	NP	NP	10
Sausage Salentino	900	50	14	1970	67	NP	NP	47
Pollo Caprese	550	20	5	1660	45	NP	NP	46
Pollo Limone Rustica	1230	71	38	1770	100	NP	NP	42
Seafood Linguine	615	20	3	1280	60	NP	NP	48
Lobster Spaghetti	650	27	5	1480	65	NP	NP	37
Mushroom Ravioli	790	44	19	990	70	NP	NP	26

Description & Serving	Cal	Fat	Sfat	Sod	Carb	Fiber	Sugar	Prot
Lobster Ravioli	650	39	17	1400	46	NP	NP	27
Fettuccine Alfredo	1220	93	53	2060	71	NP	NP	28
Fettuccine Alfredo w/ Chicken	1370	98	55	2580	72	NP	NP	53
Fettuccine Alfredo w/ Shrimp	1265	93	53	2620	71	NP	NP	38
Mama's Trio	1750	96	46	4660	118	NP	NP	109
Create Your Own Handcrafted Pasta								
Pasta	390	4	0	260	79	NP	NP	12
Pomodoro Sauce (tomato basil sauce)	160	11	2	580	11	NP	NP	3
Arrabbiatta Sauce (spicy red sauce)	180	13	2	650	14	NP	NP	3
Bolognese Sauce (meat sauce)	1000	89	34	2070	20	NP	NP	31
Roasted Garlic Cream Sauce	360	29	13	1160	18	NP	NP	7
Alfredo Sauce	610	59	31	960	9	NP	NP	10
Grilled Sliced Chicken	150	5	2	520	1	NP	NP	25
Sauteed Shrimp	45	0	0	560	0	NP	NP	10
Italian Sausage	330	22	8	1270	3	NP	NP	30
Meatballs	450	33	14	1740	18	NP	NP	24
Grape Tomatoes	5	0	0	0	1	NP	NP	0
Sun-Dried Tomatoes	60	0	0	420	11	NP	NP	3
Fresh Broccoli	10	0	0	10	1	NP	NP	1
Fresh Mushrooms	10	0	0	5	1	NP	NP	1
Roasted Garlic	60	1	0	35	11	NP	NP	3
Chicken & Seafood								
Honey Balsamic Chicken	640	15	3	2380	54	NP	NP	74
Grilled Chicken Spiedini	360	10	2	1150	17	NP	NP	51
Simple Salmon	420	22	5	770	6	NP	NP	50
Grilled Halibut	770	34	11	1100	58	NP	NP	59
Grilled Salmon	750	35	8	1550	55	NP	NP	54
Jumbo Shrimp Spiedini	230	5	1	670	15	NP	NP	31
Pork & Steak								
Grilled Pork Chops	1380	77	39	4040	98	NP	NP	74
Bistecca Filet	450	17	6	880	26	NP	NP	50
Calabrese Strip	720	35	11	960	35	NP	NP	67
Kids								
Chicken Fingerias w/o Fries	360	41	4	1460	31	NP	NP	37
Fettuccine Alfredo	890	67	38	1480	53	NP	NP	20
Grilled Chicken & Broccoli	390	8	2	1020	54	NP	NP	25
Macaroni & Cheese	670	32	21	1980	63	NP	NP	30
Mona Lisa's Cheese Masterpizza	480	14	8	1300	62	NP	NP	26
Mona Lisa's Pepperoni Masterpizza	560	18	11	1560	62	NP	NP	28
Spaghetti & Meatballs w/ Meat Sauce	610	29	10	1550	63	NP	NP	27
Spaghetti & Meatballs w/ Tomato Sauce	570	25	8	1550	65	NP	NP	22
Vanilla Ice Cream w/ Chocolate Sauce	420	23	15	110	45	NP	NP	4
Side Fries	270	9	4	640	28	NP	NP	3
Side Macaroni & Cheese	330	16	10	990	30	NP	NP	15
Side Steamed Broccoli	25	0	0	220	4	NP	NP	3

Description & Serving	Cal	Fat	Sfat	Sod	Carb	Fiber	Sugar	Prot
Kid's Caesar della Casa w/ Caesar Dressing	130	10	2	240	6	NP	NP	3
Kid's Garden della Casa w/ Creamy Italian Dressing	120	8	2	150	9	NP	NP	3

Dressing/Condiment

	Cal	Fat	Sfat	Sod	Carb	Fiber	Sugar	Prot
Balsamic Vinaigrette Dressing, 1 oz	90	9	2	320	2	NP	NP	0
Caesar Dressing, 1 oz	150	16	3	260	2	NP	NP	0
Creamy Italian Dressing, 1 oz	110	10	2	35	5	NP	NP	0
Fat-Free Creamy Italian Dressing, 1 oz	20	0	0	440	5	NP	NP	0
Honey Mustard Dressing, 1 oz	120	11	2	150	6	NP	NP	0
Italian Dressing, 1 oz	80	8	2	480	2	NP	NP	0
Low-Fat Caesar Dressing, 1 oz	30	2	0	330	3	NP	NP	1
Parmesan Peppercorn Dressing, 1 oz	120	12	3	270	2	NP	NP	2
Roasted Garlic Lemon Vinaigrette Dressing, 1 oz	120	11	2	170	4	NP	NP	0
Toscana Dressing, 1 oz	160	17	3	380	1	NP	NP	0
Basil Aioli Sauce, 1 oz	160	17	3	160	1	NP	NP	0
Pizzaiola Sauce, 1 oz	40	4	0	115	3	NP	NP	1

Dessert

	Cal	Fat	Sfat	Sod	Carb	Fiber	Sugar	Prot
Amaretto Apple Crispetti	1210	41	24	480	200	NP	NP	10
Fresh Berry Tiramisu	470	26	15	130	55	NP	NP	5
Italian Sorbetto w/ Biscotti	220	2	1	20	48	NP	NP	2
Lemon Passion	1100	63	34	710	122	NP	NP	12
New York Cheesecake	1090	73	44	650	93	NP	NP	16
New York Cheesecake w/ Caramel Fudge Sauce	1630	95	54	980	174	NP	NP	21
Simple Lemon Pound Cake	250	11	6	170	35	NP	NP	3
Smothered Chocolate Cake	1580	102	47	1030	147	NP	NP	18
Tiramisu	1120	80	48	135	88	NP	NP	12

Round Table Pizza

Appetizer

	Cal	Fat	Sfat	Sod	Carb	Fiber	Sugar	Prot
Garlic Parmesan Twist, 1	170	NP	2	460	26	NP	NP	NP
Buffalo Wings, 1	70	NP	1.5	290	1	NP	NP	NP
Honey BBQ Wings, 1	80	NP	1.5	180	2	NP	NP	NP
Garlic Bread, 1	360	NP	9	600	72	NP	NP	NP
Garlic Bread w/ Cheese, 1	540	NP	13	960	72	NP	NP	NP
Side of Grilled Chicken	100	NP	1	580	0	NP	NP	NP
Creamy Garlic/Ranch Dipping Sauce, 2 oz	200	NP	5	420	2	NP	NP	NP
Pizza Sauce Dipping Sauce, 2 oz	30	NP	0	130	6	NP	NP	NP

Pizza, 1 slice

	Cal	Fat	Sfat	Sod	Carb	Fiber	Sugar	Prot
Skinny Crust Cheese Pizza, personal	130	NP	3.5	290	11	NP	NP	NP
Skinny Crust Cheese Pizza, sml	170	NP	4.5	380	16	NP	NP	NP
Skinny Crust Cheese Pizza, med	210	NP	5	460	19	NP	NP	NP
Skinny Crust Cheese Pizza, lrg	190	NP	5	420	18	NP	NP	NP
Original Crust Cheese Pizza, personal	150	NP	3.5	340	16	NP	NP	NP
Original Crust Cheese Pizza, sml	200	NP	4.5	450	22	NP	NP	NP
Original Crust Cheese Pizza, med	250	NP	5	540	27	NP	NP	NP

Description & Serving	Cal	Fat	Sfat	Sod	Carb	Fiber	Sugar	Prot
Original Crust Cheese Pizza, lrg	230	NP	5	500	25	NP	NP	NP
Original Crust Cheese Pizza, xlrg	220	NP	5	490	24	NP	NP	NP
Pan Crust Cheese Pizza, personal	210	NP	3.5	460	27	NP	NP	NP
Pan Crust Cheese Pizza, sml	290	NP	5	640	36	NP	NP	NP
Pan Crust Cheese Pizza, med	330	NP	6	730	41	NP	NP	NP
Pan Crust Cheese Pizza, lrg	300	NP	6	670	38	NP	NP	NP
Pan Crust Cheese Pizza, xlrg	310	NP	6	680	38	NP	NP	NP
Skinny Crust Italian Garlic Supreme Pizza, personal	170	NP	4	410	12	NP	NP	NP
Skinny Crust Italian Garlic Supreme Pizza, sml	230	NP	6	560	16	NP	NP	NP
Skinny Crust Italian Garlic Supreme Pizza, med	260	NP	6	610	20	NP	NP	NP
Skinny Crust Italian Garlic Supreme Pizza, lrg	240	NP	6	570	18	NP	NP	NP
Original Crust Italian Garlic Supreme Pizza, personal	190	NP	4.5	460	16	NP	NP	NP
Original Crust Italian Garlic Supreme Pizza, sml	260	NP	6	630	23	NP	NP	NP
Original Crust Italian Garlic Supreme Pizza, med	300	NP	6	700	27	NP	NP	NP
Original Crust Italian Garlic Supreme Pizza, lrg	270	NP	6	640	25	NP	NP	NP
Original Crust Italian Garlic Supreme Pizza, xlrg	260	NP	6	620	24	NP	NP	NP
Pan Crust Italian Garlic Supreme Pizza, personal	250	NP	4.5	590	28	NP	NP	NP
Pan Crust Italian Garlic Supreme Pizza, sml	350	NP	7	830	37	NP	NP	NP
Pan Crust Italian Garlic Supreme Pizza, med	390	NP	7	900	42	NP	NP	NP
Pan Crust Italian Garlic Supreme Pizza, lrg	360	NP	7	840	39	NP	NP	NP
Pan Crust Italian Garlic Supreme Pizza, xlrg	360	NP	7	830	39	NP	NP	NP
Skinny Crust Guinevere's Garden Delight Pizza, personal	120	NP	2.5	270	12	NP	NP	NP
Skinny Crust Guinevere's Garden Delight Pizza, sml	170	NP	3.5	380	17	NP	NP	NP
Skinny Crust Guinevere's Garden Delight Pizza, med	200	NP	4	450	21	NP	NP	NP
Skinny Crust Guinevere's Garden Delight Pizza, lrg	180	NP	4	420	19	NP	NP	NP
Original Crust Guinevere's Garden Delight Pizza, personal	140	NP	2.5	320	17	NP	NP	NP
Original Crust Guinevere's Garden Delight Pizza, sml	200	NP	3.5	450	24	NP	NP	NP
Original Crust Guinevere's Garden Delight Pizza, med	240	NP	4	540	28	NP	NP	NP
Original Crust Guinevere's Garden Delight Pizza, lrg	220	NP	4	500	26	NP	NP	NP
Original Crust Guinevere's Garden Delight Pizza, xlrg	210	NP	4	490	25	NP	NP	NP
Pan Crust Guinevere's Garden Delight Pizza, personal	200	NP	2.5	450	28	NP	NP	NP
Pan Crust Guinevere's Garden Delight Pizza, sml	280	NP	4.5	640	37	NP	NP	NP
Pan Crust Guinevere's Garden Delight Pizza, med	320	NP	5	720	42	NP	NP	NP
Pan Crust Guinevere's Garden Delight Pizza, lrg	300	NP	5	670	39	NP	NP	NP
Pan Crust Guinevere's Garden Delight Pizza, xlrg	300	NP	5	680	39	NP	NP	NP
Skinny Crust Maui Zaui (Zesty Red Sauce) Pizza, personal	140	NP	3.5	380	13	NP	NP	NP
Skinny Crust Maui Zaui (Zesty Red Sauce) Pizza, sml	200	NP	4.5	520	18	NP	NP	NP
Skinny Crust Maui Zaui (Zesty Red Sauce) Pizza, med	230	NP	5	640	22	NP	NP	NP
Skinny Crust Maui Zaui (Zesty Red Sauce) Pizza, lrg	220	NP	5	590	20	NP	NP	NP
Original Crust Maui Zaui (Zesty Red Sauce) Pizza, personal	170	NP	3.5	430	17	NP	NP	NP
Original Crust Maui Zaui (Zesty Red Sauce) Pizza, sml	230	NP	4.5	600	25	NP	NP	NP
Original Crust Maui Zaui (Zesty Red Sauce) Pizza, med	270	NP	5	720	29	NP	NP	NP
Original Crust Maui Zaui (Zesty Red Sauce) Pizza, lrg	250	NP	5	660	27	NP	NP	NP

Description & Serving	Cal	Fat	Sfat	Sod	Carb	Fiber	Sugar	Prot
Original Crust Maui Zaui (Zesty Red Sauce) Pizza, xlrg	240	NP	5	650	26	NP	NP	NP
Pan Crust Maui Zaui (Zesty Red Sauce) Pizza, personal	220	NP	3.5	560	29	NP	NP	NP
Pan Crust Maui Zaui (Zesty Red Sauce) Pizza, sml	320	NP	6	790	38	NP	NP	NP
Pan Crust Maui Zaui (Zesty Red Sauce) Pizza, med	360	NP	6	920	44	NP	NP	NP
Pan Crust Maui Zaui (Zesty Red Sauce) Pizza, lrg	330	NP	6	850	41	NP	NP	NP
Pan Crust Maui Zaui (Zesty Red Sauce) Pizza, xlrg	340	NP	6	850	41	NP	NP	NP
Skinny Crust Maui Zaui (Polynesian Sauce) Pizza, personal	150	NP	3.5	420	15	NP	NP	NP
Skinny Crust Maui Zaui (Polynesian Sauce) Pizza, sml	200	NP	4.5	570	20	NP	NP	NP
Skinny Crust Maui Zaui (Polynesian Sauce) Pizza, med	240	NP	5	680	24	NP	NP	NP
Skinny Crust Maui Zaui (Polynesian Sauce) Pizza, lrg	220	NP	5	630	22	NP	NP	NP
Original Crust Maui Zaui (Polynesian Sauce) Pizza, personal	170	NP	3.5	470	19	NP	NP	NP
Original Crust Maui Zaui (Polynesian Sauce) Pizza, sml	230	NP	4.5	640	26	NP	NP	NP
Original Crust Maui Zaui (Polynesian Sauce) Pizza, med	280	NP	5	770	32	NP	NP	NP
Original Crust Maui Zaui (Polynesian Sauce) Pizza, lrg	260	NP	5	710	29	NP	NP	NP
Original Crust Maui Zaui (Polynesian Sauce) Pizza, xlrg	250	NP	5	690	28	NP	NP	NP
Pan Crust Maui Zaui (Polynesian Sauce) Pizza, personal	230	NP	3.5	600	31	NP	NP	NP
Pan Crust Maui Zaui (Polynesian Sauce) Pizza, sml	320	NP	6	840	40	NP	NP	NP
Pan Crust Maui Zaui (Polynesian Sauce) Pizza, med	370	NP	6	970	46	NP	NP	NP
Pan Crust Maui Zaui (Polynesian Sauce) Pizza, lrg	340	NP	6	900	43	NP	NP	NP
Pan Crust Maui Zaui (Polynesian Sauce) Pizza, xlrg	340	NP	6	900	43	NP	NP	NP
Skinny Crust Montague's All Meat Marvel Pizza, personal	170	NP	4.5	430	12	NP	NP	NP
Skinny Crust Montague's All Meat Marvel Pizza, sml	230	NP	6	580	16	NP	NP	NP
Skinny Crust Montague's All Meat Marvel Pizza, med	290	NP	7	730	20	NP	NP	NP
Skinny Crust Montague's All Meat Marvel Pizza, lrg	260	NP	7	650	18	NP	NP	NP
Original Crust Montague's All Meat Marvel Pizza, personal	190	NP	4.5	480	16	NP	NP	NP
Original Crust Montague's All Meat Marvel Pizza, sml	260	NP	6	660	23	NP	NP	NP
Original Crust Montague's All Meat Marvel Pizza, med	330	NP	7	820	27	NP	NP	NP
Original Crust Montague's All Meat Marvel Pizza, lrg	290	NP	7	730	25	NP	NP	NP
Original Crust Montague's All Meat Marvel Pizza, xlrg	290	NP	7	720	24	NP	NP	NP
Pan Crust Montague's All Meat Marvel Pizza, personal	250	NP	4.5	610	27	NP	NP	NP
Pan Crust Montague's All Meat Marvel Pizza, sml	330	NP	6	790	36	NP	NP	NP
Pan Crust Montague's All Meat Marvel Pizza, med	380	NP	7	920	41	NP	NP	NP
Pan Crust Montague's All Meat Marvel Pizza, lrg	360	NP	7	850	38	NP	NP	NP
Pan Crust Montague's All Meat Marvel Pizza, xlrg	360	NP	7	850	38	NP	NP	NP
Skinny Crust King Arthur Supreme Pizza, personal	160	NP	4	380	12	NP	NP	NP
Skinny Crust King Arthur Supreme Pizza, sml	220	NP	5	510	17	NP	NP	NP
Skinny Crust King Arthur Supreme Pizza, med	260	NP	6	640	21	NP	NP	NP
Skinny Crust King Arthur Supreme Pizza, lrg	240	NP	6	570	19	NP	NP	NP
Original Crust King Arthur Supreme Pizza, personal	180	NP	4	430	17	NP	NP	NP
Original Crust King Arthur Supreme Pizza, sml	250	NP	5	590	24	NP	NP	NP

Description & Serving	Cal	Fat	Sfat	Sod	Carb	Fiber	Sugar	Prot
Original Crust King Arthur Supreme Pizza, med	300	NP	6	720	28	NP	NP	NP
Original Crust King Arthur Supreme Pizza, lrg	270	NP	6	650	26	NP	NP	NP
Original Crust King Arthur Supreme Pizza, xlrg	260	NP	6	640	25	NP	NP	NP
Pan Crust King Arthur Supreme Pizza, personal	220	NP	3.5	530	28	NP	NP	NP
Pan Crust King Arthur Supreme Pizza, sml	310	NP	6	740	37	NP	NP	NP
Pan Crust King Arthur Supreme Pizza, med	360	NP	7	850	42	NP	NP	NP
Pan Crust King Arthur Supreme Pizza, lrg	340	NP	6	790	39	NP	NP	NP
Pan Crust King Arthur Supreme Pizza, xlrg	340	NP	6	800	39	NP	NP	NP
Skinny Crust Smokehouse Combo: Pepperoni Pizza, personal	160	NP	4	430	13	NP	NP	NP
Skinny Crust Smokehouse Combo: Pepperoni Pizza, sml	220	NP	5	550	18	NP	NP	NP
Skinny Crust Smokehouse Combo: Pepperoni Pizza, med	270	NP	7	690	21	NP	NP	NP
Skinny Crust Smokehouse Combo: Pepperoni Pizza, lrg	250	NP	6	640	20	NP	NP	NP
Original Crust Smokehouse Combo: Pepperoni Pizza, personal	180	NP	4	480	17	NP	NP	NP
Original Crust Smokehouse Combo: Pepperoni Pizza, sml	250	NP	5	630	24	NP	NP	NP
Original Crust Smokehouse Combo: Pepperoni Pizza, med	310	NP	7	770	29	NP	NP	NP
Original Crust Smokehouse Combo: Pepperoni Pizza, lrg	290	NP	6	720	26	NP	NP	NP
Original Crust Smokehouse Combo: Pepperoni Pizza, xlrg	280	NP	6	700	26	NP	NP	NP
Pan Crust Smokehouse Combo: Pepperoni Pizza, personal	240	NP	4	600	29	NP	NP	NP
Pan Crust Smokehouse Combo: Pepperoni Pizza, sml	340	NP	6	820	38	NP	NP	NP
Pan Crust Smokehouse Combo: Pepperoni Pizza, med	390	NP	7	960	43	NP	NP	NP
Pan Crust Smokehouse Combo: Pepperoni Pizza, lrg	370	NP	7	900	40	NP	NP	NP
Pan Crust Smokehouse Combo: Pepperoni Pizza, xlrg	370	NP	7	900	40	NP	NP	NP
Skinny Crust Smokehouse Combo: Chicken Pizza, personal	160	NP	3.5	420	13	NP	NP	NP
Skinny Crust Smokehouse Combo: Chicken Pizza, sml	220	NP	5	550	18	NP	NP	NP
Skinny Crust Smokehouse Combo: Chicken Pizza, med	260	NP	6	650	21	NP	NP	NP
Skinny Crust Smokehouse Combo: Chicken Pizza, lrg	240	NP	5	590	19	NP	NP	NP
Original Crust Smokehouse Combo: Chicken Pizza, personal	180	NP	3.5	480	17	NP	NP	NP
Original Crust Smokehouse Combo: Chicken Pizza, sml	250	NP	5	630	24	NP	NP	NP
Original Crust Smokehouse Combo: Chicken Pizza, med	300	NP	6	740	29	NP	NP	NP
Original Crust Smokehouse Combo: Chicken Pizza, lrg	270	NP	5	670	26	NP	NP	NP
Original Crust Smokehouse Combo: Chicken Pizza, xlrg	260	NP	5	640	25	NP	NP	NP

Description & Serving	Cal	Fat	Sfat	Sod	Carb	Fiber	Sugar	Prot
Pan Crust Smokehouse Combo: Chicken Pizza, personal	240	NP	3.5	600	29	NP	NP	NP
Pan Crust Smokehouse Combo: Chicken Pizza, sml	340	NP	6	830	38	NP	NP	NP
Pan Crust Smokehouse Combo: Chicken Pizza, med	380	NP	7	920	43	NP	NP	NP
Pan Crust Smokehouse Combo: Chicken Pizza, lrg	360	NP	6	850	40	NP	NP	NP
Pan Crust Smokehouse Combo: Chicken Pizza, xlrg	360	NP	6	830	40	NP	NP	NP
Skinny Crust Gourmet Veggie Pizza, personal	130	NP	3	350	13	NP	NP	NP
Skinny Crust Gourmet Veggie Pizza, sml	180	NP	4	460	17	NP	NP	NP
Skinny Crust Gourmet Veggie Pizza, med	220	NP	5	560	21	NP	NP	NP
Skinny Crust Gourmet Veggie Pizza, lrg	200	NP	4.5	540	20	NP	NP	NP
Original Crust Gourmet Veggie Pizza, personal	160	NP	3	400	18	NP	NP	NP
Original Crust Gourmet Veggie Pizza, sml	220	NP	4	530	24	NP	NP	NP
Original Crust Gourmet Veggie Pizza, med	260	NP	5	650	29	NP	NP	NP
Original Crust Gourmet Veggie Pizza, lrg	240	NP	4.5	620	27	NP	NP	NP
Original Crust Gourmet Veggie Pizza, xlrg	230	NP	4.5	600	26	NP	NP	NP
Pan Crust Gourmet Veggie Pizza, personal	210	NP	3	540	29	NP	NP	NP
Pan Crust Gourmet Veggie Pizza, sml	310	NP	5	730	38	NP	NP	NP
Pan Crust Gourmet Veggie Pizza, med	350	NP	6	850	43	NP	NP	NP
Pan Crust Gourmet Veggie Pizza, lrg	320	NP	5	810	41	NP	NP	NP
Pan Crust Gourmet Veggie Pizza, xlrg	320	NP	6	810	40	NP	NP	NP
Skinny Crust Chicken & Garlic Gourmet Pizza, personal	140	NP	3	350	12	NP	NP	NP
Skinny Crust Chicken & Garlic Gourmet Pizza, sml	200	NP	4.5	480	17	NP	NP	NP
Skinny Crust Chicken & Garlic Gourmet Pizza, med	230	NP	6	580	20	NP	NP	NP
Skinny Crust Chicken & Garlic Gourmet Pizza, lrg	220	NP	5	540	18	NP	NP	NP
Original Crust Chicken & Garlic Gourmet Pizza, personal	160	NP	3	400	17	NP	NP	NP
Original Crust Chicken & Garlic Gourmet Pizza, sml	230	NP	4.5	560	23	NP	NP	NP
Original Crust Chicken & Garlic Gourmet Pizza, med	270	NP	5	670	27	NP	NP	NP
Original Crust Chicken & Garlic Gourmet Pizza, lrg	250	NP	5	620	25	NP	NP	NP
Original Crust Chicken & Garlic Gourmet Pizza, xlrg	240	NP	5	600	24	NP	NP	NP
Pan Crust Chicken & Garlic Gourmet Pizza, personal	220	NP	3.5	530	28	NP	NP	NP
Pan Crust Chicken & Garlic Gourmet Pizza, sml	320	NP	5	650	37	NP	NP	NP
Pan Crust Chicken & Garlic Gourmet Pizza, med	360	NP	6	870	42	NP	NP	NP
Pan Crust Chicken & Garlic Gourmet Pizza, lrg	340	NP	6	810	39	NP	NP	NP
Pan Crust Chicken & Garlic Gourmet Pizza, xlrg	340	NP	6	810	39	NP	NP	NP
Skinny Crust Ulti-Meat Pizza, personal	180	NP	4.5	480	12	NP	NP	NP
Skinny Crust Ulti-Meat Pizza, sml	240	NP	6	660	16	NP	NP	NP
Skinny Crust Ulti-Meat Pizza, med	290	NP	7	750	20	NP	NP	NP
Skinny Crust Ulti-Meat Pizza, lrg	270	NP	7	690	18	NP	NP	NP
Original Crust Ulti-Meat Pizza, personal	200	NP	5	530	16	NP	NP	NP
Original Crust Ulti-Meat Pizza, sml	280	NP	6	730	23	NP	NP	NP
Original Crust Ulti-Meat Pizza, med	330	NP	7	830	27	NP	NP	NP
Original Crust Ulti-Meat Pizza, lrg	300	NP	7	770	25	NP	NP	NP
Original Crust Ulti-Meat Pizza, xlrg	300	NP	7	750	24	NP	NP	NP
Pan Crust Ulti-Meat Pizza, personal	260	NP	5	660	27	NP	NP	NP
Pan Crust Ulti-Meat Pizza, sml	370	NP	7	930	37	NP	NP	NP

Description & Serving	Cal	Fat	Sfat	Sod	Carb	Fiber	Sugar	Prot
Pan Crust Ulti-Meat Pizza, med	410	NP	8	1020	41	NP	NP	NP
Pan Crust Ulti-Meat Pizza, lrg	390	NP	8	950	38	NP	NP	NP
Pan Crust Ulti-Meat Pizza, xlrg	390	NP	8	950	39	NP	NP	NP
Skinny Crust Wombo Combo Pizza, personal	160	NP	4	430	12	NP	NP	NP
Skinny Crust Wombo Combo Pizza, sml	220	NP	5	590	17	NP	NP	NP
Skinny Crust Wombo Combo Pizza, lrg	270	NP	6	750	21	NP	NP	NP
Skinny Crust Wombo Combo Pizza, xlrg	250	NP	6	710	20	NP	NP	NP
Original Crust Wombo Combo Pizza, personal	180	NP	4	480	17	NP	NP	NP
Original Crust Wombo Combo Pizza, sml	250	NP	5	660	24	NP	NP	NP
Original Crust Wombo Combo Pizza, med	300	NP	7	840	29	NP	NP	NP
Original Crust Wombo Combo Pizza, lrg	280	NP	6	790	26	NP	NP	NP
Original Crust Wombo Combo Pizza, xlrg	270	NP	6	770	26	NP	NP	NP
Pan Crust Wombo Combo Pizza, personal	240	NP	4	610	28	NP	NP	NP
Pan Crust Wombo Combo Pizza, sml	340	NP	6	860	38	NP	NP	NP
Pan Crust Wombo Combo Pizza, med	390	NP	7	1030	43	NP	NP	NP
Pan Crust Wombo Combo Pizza, lrg	360	NP	7	970	40	NP	NP	NP
Pan Crust Wombo Combo Pizza, xlrg	370	NP	7	980	40	NP	NP	NP
Skinny Crust Hawaiian Pizza, personal	120	NP	2.5	330	13	NP	NP	NP
Skinny Crust Hawaiian Pizza, sml	170	NP	3.5	480	18	NP	NP	NP
Skinny Crust Hawaiian Pizza, med	210	NP	4.5	550	22	NP	NP	NP
Skinny Crust Hawaiian Pizza, lrg	190	NP	4	510	20	NP	NP	NP
Original Crust Hawaiian Pizza, personal	150	NP	3	380	17	NP	NP	NP
Original Crust Hawaiian Pizza, sml	210	NP	3.5	550	25	NP	NP	NP
Original Crust Hawaiian Pizza, med	240	NP	4.5	640	29	NP	NP	NP
Original Crust Hawaiian Pizza, lrg	220	NP	4	590	27	NP	NP	NP
Original Crust Hawaiian Pizza, xlrg	220	NP	4	580	26	NP	NP	NP
Pan Crust Hawaiian Pizza, personal	200	NP	3	500	28	NP	NP	NP
Pan Crust Hawaiian Pizza, sml	290	NP	5	720	38	NP	NP	NP
Pan Crust Hawaiian Pizza, med	330	NP	5	810	43	NP	NP	NP
Pan Crust Hawaiian Pizza, lrg	300	NP	5	760	40	NP	NP	NP
Pan Crust Hawaiian Pizza, xlrg	310	NP	5	760	40	NP	NP	NP
Skinny Crust Pepperoni Pizza, lrg	210	11	5	590	18	1	0	10
Original Crust Pepperoni Pizza, lrg	240	11	8	670	24	1	1	11
Pan Crust Pepperoni Pizza, lrg	320	12	8	810	38	2	1	14

Salad, w/o dressing

	Cal	Fat	Sfat	Sod	Carb	Fiber	Sugar	Prot
Garden Salad, sml	45	NP	0	95	7	NP	NP	NP
Garden Salad, lrg	90	NP	0	190	14	NP	NP	NP
Garden Salad, party size	270	NP	0	570	42	NP	NP	NP
Caesar Salad, sml	60	NP	1	170	5	NP	NP	NP
Caesar Salad, lrg	120	NP	2.5	350	9	NP	NP	NP
Caesar Salad, party size	360	NP	7.5	1050	27	NP	NP	NP

Sandwich

	Cal	Fat	Sfat	Sod	Carb	Fiber	Sugar	Prot
Chicken Club Sandwich	700	NP	14	2190	77	NP	NP	NP
Ham Club Sandwich	640	NP	14	2330	78	NP	NP	NP
Turkey Club Sandwich	620	NP	14	1980	77	NP	NP	NP
Turkey Pesto Sandwich	610	NP	14	1490	74	NP	NP	NP

Description & Serving	Cal	Fat	Sfat	Sod	Carb	Fiber	Sugar	Prot
Turkey Santa Fe Sandwich	630	NP	14	1550	75	NP	NP	NP
RT Veggie Sandwich	530	NP	11	1630	83	NP	NP	NP

Dessert

Dessert Pizza, 1 slice	210	NP	1.5	250	32	NP	NP	NP
Cinnamon Twist, 1	180	NP	0	290	34	NP	NP	NP

Rubio's Mexican Grill

Entrée

Chicken

	Cal	Fat	Sfat	Sod	Carb	Fiber	Sugar	Prot
Big Burrito Especial Chicken	830	32	7	2030	99	7	9	38
Baja Grill Burrito Chicken	620	26	9	1890	53	4	7	46
HealthMex Chicken Burrito	500	10	2.5	1700	70	6	7	34
Grilled Chicken Taco	280	15	4	450	22	3	2	15
Grilled Chicken Taco w/ Flour Tortilla	300	17	5	720	23	1	3	16
HealthMex Chicken Taco	150	1.5	0	400	21	3	2	12
HealthMex Chicken Taco w/ Flour Tortilla	170	3.5	1	670	22	1	3	13
Chicken Street Tacos	100	4	0.5	240	9	2	1	10
Grilled Chicken Taco	360	21	7	670	23	3	2	22
Grilled Chicken Taco w/ Flour Tortilla	380	23	8	940	24	1	3	23
Chicken Grilled Grande Bowl w/o dressing	550	18	7	1540	61	8	8	40
Chicken Enchilada	390	21	12	800	23	3	2	27
Chicken Quesadilla	1190	69	29	2370	87	8	6	61

Pork

Carnitas Rajas Burrito	740	39	13	1970	75	4	10	34
Carnitas Rajas Taco	210	11	2	420	23	3	3	9
Carnitas Rajas Taco w/ Flour Tortilla	230	13	3	690	24	1	4	10
Carnitas Street Tacos	100	5	1.5	250	9	2	2	7
Carnitas Enchilada	380	23	13	810	24	3	3	23

Seafood

Grilled Mesquite Shrimp Burrito	710	34	11	2100	72	5	5	30
Mahi Mahi Burrito	700	42	12	1150	49	4	5	34
Fish Burrito	710	40	8	1520	71	6	10	25
HealthMex Mahi Mahi Burrito	510	15	3	1190	68	6	6	29
World Famous Fish Taco	270	14	2	420	29	3	3	10
World Famous Fish Taco w/ Flour Tortilla	290	16	3	690	30	1	4	11
Fish Taco Especial	330	20	4.5	510	30	4	4	13
Fish Taco Especial w/ Flour Tortilla	350	22	5.5	780	31	2	5	14
Grilled Mahi Mahi Taco	300	17	4	250	22	4	2	15
Grilled Mahi Mahi Taco w/ Flour Tortilla	320	19	5	520	23	2	3	16
Grilled Mesquite Shrimp Taco	230	12	2	540	22	3	1	9
Grilled Mesquite Shrimp Taco w/ Flour Tortilla	250	14	3	810	23	1	2	10
HealthMex Mahi Mahi Taco	160	4	0.5	200	21	3	2	12
HealthMex Mahi Mahi Taco w/ Flour Tortilla	180	6	1.5	470	22	1	3	13
Garlic Herb Shrimp Taco	360	22	7	580	23	3	1	19
Garlic Herb Shrimp Taco w/ Flour Tortilla	380	24	8	850	24	1	2	20

Description & Serving	Cal	Fat	Sfat	Sod	Carb	Fiber	Sugar	Prot
Steak								
Big Burrito Especial Steak	870	38	11	2360	99	7	8	32
Baja Grill Burrito Steak	670	34	14	2320	53	4	6	38
Steak Quesadilla	1230	75	32	2710	87	8	5	55
Grilled Steak Taco	220	10	4	520	22	3	1	13
Grilled Steak Taco w/ Flour Tortilla	240	12	5	790	23	1	2	14
Steak Street Taco	120	6	2	380	9	2	0	8
Grilled Steak Taco	370	23	8	800	23	3	1	20
Grilled Steak Taco w/ Flour Tortilla	390	25	9	1070	24	1	2	21
Vegetarian								
Bean & Cheese Burrito	700	33	17	1750	75	12	5	29
Grilled Veggie Burrito	630	29	9	1290	73	4	7	19
Cheese Enchilada	340	21	12	570	23	3	2	17
Cheese Quesadilla	1070	67	28	1820	85	8	5	38
Grilled Portobello & Poblano Taco	310	19	6	340	25	4	3	12
Grilled Portobello & Poblano Taco w/ Flour Tortilla	330	21	7	710	26	2	4	13
Kids								
Cheese Quesadilla	500	27	14	1030	44	1	3	23
Chicken Taquitos, 2	230	10	4.5	270	21	2	0	15
Bean & Cheese Burrito	530	23	11	1200	63	8	3	20
Mini Churro	80	4	1	70	11	0	5	1
Side								
Rice, reg	120	1	0	220	25	1	1	2
Rice, lrg	310	3	0	580	67	2	2	5
Pinto Beans, reg	110	2	0.5	340	22	8	0	2
Pinto Beans, lrg	300	2.5	1	940	65	24	1	5
Black Beans, reg	100	1	0	340	17	2	2	6
Black Beans, lrg	280	0.5	0	950	50	7	7	17
Chips, reg	260	13	1	290	33	4	0	3
Chips, lrg	570	29	2.5	650	74	9	0	7
Guacamole & Chips	790	49	6	920	85	16	2	10
Salad								
Chicken Chopped Salad w/ dressing	570	33	9	1480	34	7	10	36
Chicken Chopped Salad w/o dressing	410	17	6	1100	31	7	8	35
Chicken Tropical Salad w/ dressing	410	23	3.5	720	25	5	18	27
Chicken Tropical Salad w/o dressing	210	5	0.5	580	17	4	12	26
Chicken Chipotle Ranch Salad w/ dressing	520	35	6	1460	24	6	9	30
Chicken Chipotle Ranch Salad w/o dressing	460	20	3	1080	40	8	8	30
Chicken Fiesta Salad w/ dressing	590	46	11	1130	13	4	7	32
Chicken Fiesta Salad w/o dressing	300	15	5	910	11	4	6	32
Chicken Grilled Grande Bowl	700	33	9	1650	61	8	8	40
Wrap								
Chicken Chopped Wrapsalada w/ dressing	800	40	10	2070	72	9	9	41
Chicken Chopped Wrapsalada w/o dressing	640	25	10	1540	68	7	6	39

Description & Serving	Cal	Fat	Sfat	Sod	Carb	Fiber	Sugar	Prot
Chicken Tropical Wrapsalada w/ dressing	650	30	5	1320	64	8	18	32
Chicken Tropical Wrapsalada w/o dressing	450	13	5	1020	55	5	11	31
Chicken Chipotle Ranch Wrapsalada w/ dressing	770	42	8	2070	65	9	10	36
Chicken Chipotle Ranch Wrapsalada w/o dressing	560	21	3.5	1610	61	7	6	33
Chicken Fiesta Wrapsalada w/ dressing	830	53	12	1740	53	8	7	38
Chicken Fiesta Wrapsalada w/o dressing	540	23	10	1360	51	6	7	36

Nachos/Snack

Description & Serving	Cal	Fat	Sfat	Sod	Carb	Fiber	Sugar	Prot
Nachos Grande	1270	78	27	1850	112	20	2	37
Chicken Nachos Grande	1390	80	28	2400	114	20	3	60
Steak Nachos Grande	1430	87	31	2730	114	20	2	54
Chicken Taquitos, 3	270	8	2	360	33	4	1	16

Dressing/Condiment

Description & Serving	Cal	Fat	Sfat	Sod	Carb	Fiber	Sugar	Prot
Chipotle Dressing, 2 oz	160	15	2.5	380	3	1	2	1
Creamy Mandarin, 2 oz	180	18	2.5	135	6	0	5	0
Chipotle Ranch, 2 oz	210	21	4	390	2	0	2	1
Salsa Picante	20	1	0	200	2	1	0	1
Salsa Roasted Chipotle	5	0	0	120	1	0	1	0
Salsa Verde	5	0	0	150	1	0	0	0
Salsa Regular	5	0	0	180	1	0	1	0

Dessert

Description & Serving	Cal	Fat	Sfat	Sod	Carb	Fiber	Sugar	Prot
Brownie	430	22	6	270	57	2	37	6
Churro	170	8	2	140	22	0	9	2

Ruby Tuesday

Appetizer

	Cal	Fat	Sfat	Sod	Carb	Fiber	Sugar	Prot
Asian Dumplings, 1 serving (4 per item)	110	5	NP	NP	11	1	NP	NP
Buffalo Shrimp, 1 serving (4 per item)	126	6	NP	NP	11	1	NP	NP
Cheddar Fries, 1 serving (4 per item)	314	18	NP	NP	24	2	NP	NP
Chicken Quesadilla, 1 serving (4 per item)	139	7	NP	NP	10	0	NP	NP
Barbecue Chicken Strips, 1 serving (4 per item)	203	9	NP	NP	17	1	NP	NP
Buffalo Chicken Strips, 1 serving (4 per item)	236	14	NP	NP	13	2	NP	NP
Thai Phoon Chicken Strips, 1 serving (4 per item)	262	18	NP	NP	12	1	NP	NP
Traditional Chicken Strips, 1 serving (4 per item)	177	9	NP	NP	11	1	NP	NP
Fire Wings, 1 serving (4 per item)	159	9	NP	NP	1	1	NP	NP
Four Way Sampler, 1 serving (4 per item)	354	20	NP	NP	20	2	NP	NP
Fresh Avocado Quesadilla, 1 serving (4 per item)	215	14	NP	NP	11	2	NP	NP
Fresh Guacamole Dip, 1 serving (4 per item)	347	23	NP	NP	22	9	NP	NP
Fried Mozzarella, 1 serving (4 per item)	182	11	NP	NP	11	2	NP	NP
Jumbo Lump Crab Cake, 1 serving (4 per item)	68	4	NP	NP	3	1	NP	NP
Queso Dip, 1 serving (4 per item)	306	19	NP	NP	25	3	NP	NP
Southwestern Spring Rolls, 1 serving (4 per item)	173	10	NP	NP	14	1	NP	NP
Spinach Artichoke Dip, 1 serving (4 per item)	300	19	NP	NP	23	2	NP	NP
Thai Phoon Shrimp, 1 serving (4 per item)	191	13	NP	NP	11	1	NP	NP

Description & Serving	Cal	Fat	Sfat	Sod	Carb	Fiber	Sugar	Prot
Salad								
Grilled Chicken Salad	489	28	NP	NP	4	3	NP	NP
Carolina Chicken Salad	1129	71	NP	NP	28	8	NP	NP
Club House Salad	840	53	NP	NP	2	7	NP	NP
Signature House Salad	391	30	NP	NP	19	3	NP	NP
Soup/Chili								
White Bean Chicken Chili	318	11	NP	NP	29	11	NP	NP
Broccoli & Cheese Soup	403	29	NP	NP	21	1	NP	NP
Burger								
Beef								
Alpine Swiss Burger	1207	83	NP	NP	64	3	NP	NP
Bacon Cheeseburger	1227	86	NP	NP	62	3	NP	NP
Boston Blue Burger	1424	96	NP	NP	84	6	NP	NP
Brewmaster Burger	1221	82	NP	NP	74	3	NP	NP
Classic Cheeseburger	1160	81	NP	NP	62	3	NP	NP
Ruby's Classic Burger	1090	75	NP	NP	61	3	NP	NP
Smokehouse Burger	1434	97	NP	NP	84	5	NP	NP
Three Cheese Burger	1320	94	NP	NP	62	3	NP	NP
Triple Prime Bacon Cheddar Burger	1226	88	NP	NP	48	2	NP	NP
Triple Prime Burger	998	69	NP	NP	48	2	NP	NP
Triple Prime Cheddar Burger	1158	83	NP	NP	48	2	NP	NP
Triple Prime Havarti Burger	1306	94	NP	NP	48	2	NP	NP
Bison								
Bison Bacon Cheeseburger	1107	71	NP	NP	62	3	NP	NP
Chicken								
Buffalo Chicken Burger	1127	68	NP	NP	75	5	NP	NP
Chicken BLT	1145	67	NP	NP	75	5	NP	NP
The Ultimate Chicken	1161	66	NP	NP	59	3	NP	NP
Fish								
Jumbo Lump Crab Burger	820	54	NP	NP	54	5	NP	NP
Blackened Fish	861	53	NP	NP	44	2	NP	NP
Minis								
Buffalo Chicken Minis Combo	573	23	NP	NP	54	5	NP	NP
Ruby Minis Combo, 2 pack	589	36	NP	NP	37	2	NP	NP
Turkey Minis Combo, 2 pack	529	29	NP	NP	40	3	NP	NP
Bacon Cheese Minis, 4 pack	1268	79	NP	NP	75	4	NP	NP
Buffalo Chicken Minis, 4 pack	1146	46	NP	NP	107	10	NP	NP
Double Bacon Cheese Minis	987	69	NP	NP	38	2	NP	NP
Double Ruby Minis	897	62	NP	NP	38	2	NP	NP
Double Smokehouse Minis	1045	70	NP	NP	49	2	NP	NP
Double Turkey Minis	853	54	NP	NP	40	4	NP	NP
Mini Trio	856	47	NP	NP	64	5	NP	NP
Ruby Minis, 4 pack	1178	72	NP	NP	75	4	NP	NP
Turkey Minis, 4 pack	1058	58	NP	NP	79	6	NP	NP

Description & Serving	Cal	Fat	Sfat	Sod	Carb	Fiber	Sugar	Prot
Turkey								
Avocado Turkey Burger	1130	68	NP	NP	62	5	NP	NP
Bella Turkey Burger	1008	56	NP	NP	65	3	NP	NP
Turkey Burger	890	48	NP	NP	62	3	NP	NP
Veggie								
Veggie Burger	952	53	NP	NP	95	3	NP	NP
Wrap								
Grilled Chicken Wrap	436	17	NP	NP	40	2	NP	NP
Turkey Burger Wrap	551	19	NP	NP	44	2	NP	NP
Entrée								
Chicken								
Chicken Bella	387	17	NP	NP	6	0	NP	NP
Grilled Chicken	257	7	NP	NP	0	0	NP	NP
Chicken & Broccoli Quiche	721	48	NP	NP	33	2	NP	NP
Chicken & Broccoli Pasta	1167	55	NP	NP	90	11	NP	NP
Chicken Fresco	426	22	NP	NP	8	1	NP	NP
Chicken Piccata	1405	76	NP	NP	104	14	NP	NP
Chicken Tender Dinner	650	25	NP	NP	35	5	NP	NP
Parmesan Chicken Pasta	1450	76	NP	NP	105	12	NP	NP
Fish								
Creole Catch	320	16	NP	NP	1	1	NP	NP
New Orleans Seafood	443	25	NP	NP	2	0	NP	NP
Grilled Salmon	365	23	NP	NP	0	0	NP	NP
Louisiana Fried Shrimp	423	17	NP	NP	38	2	NP	NP
Asian Glazed Salmon	433	27	NP	NP	8	1	NP	NP
Chesapeake Catch	536	32	NP	NP	7	1	NP	NP
Crab Cake Dinner	271	17	NP	NP	10	3	NP	NP
Herb Crusted Tilapia	402	24	NP	NP	9	2	NP	NP
Parmesan Shrimp Pasta	1030	48	NP	NP	85	9	NP	NP
Asian Salmon & Shrimp	466	28	NP	NP	7	0	NP	NP
Clam Chowder	437	28	NP	NP	23	2	NP	NP
Lobster Entrée	225	7	NP	NP	0	0	NP	NP
Lobster Ravioli	853	53	NP	NP	56	5	NP	NP
Lobster Tail Add-On	113	3	NP	NP	0	0	NP	NP
Shrimp Scampi & Steak	1049	54	NP	NP	73	6	NP	NP
Steak & Lobster Tail	411	19	NP	NP	2	0	NP	NP
Ribs								
Classic Barbecue Full-Rack	986	65	NP	NP	29	0	NP	NP
Classic Barbecue Half-Rack	493	32	NP	NP	14	0	NP	NP
Memphis Dry Rub Full-Rack	1076	80	NP	NP	7	0	NP	NP
Memphis Dry Rub Half-Rack	538	40	NP	NP	3	0	NP	NP
Ribs & Louisiana Fried Shrimp	916	49	NP	NP	53	2	NP	NP
Triple Play	1094	56	NP	NP	55	4	NP	NP

Description & Serving	Cal	Fat	Sfat	Sod	Carb	Fiber	Sugar	Prot
Steak								
Plain Grilled Petite Sirloin	206	5	NP	NP	2	0	NP	NP
Plain Grilled Top Sirloin	256	6	NP	NP	2	0	NP	NP
House Sirloin	298	15	NP	NP	2	0	NP	NP
Bayou Sirloin	387	16	NP	NP	5	0	NP	NP
Cowboy Rib Eye	932	56	NP	NP	28	4	NP	NP
Peppercorn Mushroom Sirloin	414	18	NP	NP	10	0	NP	NP
Petite Sirloin	298	15	NP	NP	2	0	NP	NP
Rib Eye	683	45	NP	NP	5	1	NP	NP
Top Sirloin	349	16	NP	NP	2	0	NP	NP
Vegetarian								
Spinach & Mushroom Quiche	673	44	NP	NP	39	15	NP	NP
Tomato Basil Quiche	734	44	NP	NP	52	11	NP	NP
Side								
Fresh Steamed Broccoli	89	6	NP	NP	5	3	NP	NP
White Cheddar Mashed Potatoes	130	7	NP	NP	15	2	NP	NP
Creamy Mashed Cauliflower	136	8	NP	NP	9	5	NP	NP
Premium Baby Green Beans	85	5	NP	NP	5	3	NP	NP
Brown-Rice Pilaf	226	7	NP	NP	33	2	NP	NP
Sauteed Baby Portabella Mushrooms	75	4	NP	NP	6	0	NP	NP
Entrée Bread	140	7	NP	NP	14	1	NP	NP
Fresh Steamed Broccoli	89	6	NP	NP	5	3	NP	NP
Piping-Hot Fries	359	13	NP	NP	52	5	NP	NP
Plain Baked Potato	329	2	NP	NP	54	12	NP	NP
Baked Potato w/ Butter & Sour Cream	488	17	NP	NP	56	12	NP	NP
Loaded Baked Potato	668	31	NP	NP	56	12	NP	NP
Cole Slaw	159	13	NP	NP	8	1	NP	NP
Onion Straws	298	21	NP	NP	20	4	NP	NP
Kids								
Kids Butter Pasta	622	25	NP	NP	74	8	NP	NP
Kids Cheese Sticks	704	34	NP	NP	73	9	NP	NP
Kids Chicken Breast	217	9	NP	NP	5	3	NP	NP
Kids Chicken Tenders	714	31	NP	NP	74	7	NP	NP
Kids Chop Steak	403	30	NP	NP	15	2	NP	NP
Kids Fried Shrimp	571	21	NP	NP	71	6	NP	NP
Kids Grilled Cheese	749	32	NP	NP	90	7	NP	NP
Kids Minis	917	46	NP	NP	88	7	NP	NP
Kids Turkey Minis	873	41	NP	NP	88	8	NP	NP
Kids Mac & Cheese	680	37	NP	NP	58	3	NP	NP
Kids Pasta Marinara	490	6	NP	NP	79	10	NP	NP
Kids Sundae	574	29	NP	NP	70	1	NP	NP
Dressing/Condiment								
Lite Ranch Dressing, 1 oz	47	5	NP	NP	1	0	NP	NP
Asian BBQ Sauce, 1 oz	60	3	NP	NP	7	0	NP	NP
Balsamic Vinaigrette Dressing, 1 oz	35	3	NP	NP	4	0	NP	NP

Description & Serving	Cal	Fat	Sfat	Sod	Carb	Fiber	Sugar	Prot
BBQ Sauce, 1 oz	47	0	NP	NP	12	0	NP	NP
Blue Cheese Dressing, 1 oz	170	18	NP	NP	1	0	NP	NP
French Dressing, 1 oz	113	10	NP	NP	6	0	NP	NP
Honey Mustard Dressing, 1 oz	85	8	NP	NP	5	0	NP	NP
Italian Dressing, 1 oz	60	6	NP	NP	2	0	NP	NP
Lemon Butter Sauce, 1 oz	88	9	NP	NP	1	0	NP	NP
Marinara Sauce, 1 oz	17	1	NP	NP	1	1	NP	NP
Orange Peanut Sauce, 1 oz	62	3	NP	NP	8	0	NP	NP
Parmesan Cream Sauce, 1 oz	60	5	NP	NP	1	0	NP	NP
Ranch Dressing, 1 oz	94	10	NP	NP	1	0	NP	NP
Salsa, 1 oz	9	0	NP	NP	1	0	NP	NP
Steak Sauce (made w/ Sam Adams), 1 oz	51	0	NP	NP	12	0	NP	NP
Signature Parmesan Dressing, 1 oz	150	16	NP	NP	1	0	NP	NP
Sour Cream, 1 oz	22	1	NP	NP	2	0	NP	NP
Sweet Chile Sauce, 1 oz	170	17	NP	NP	2	0	NP	NP
Thousand Island Dressing, 1 oz	70	7	NP	NP	3	0	NP	NP

Beverage

Description & Serving	Cal	Fat	Sfat	Sod	Carb	Fiber	Sugar	Prot
Freshly Made Lemonade - Blackberry	190	0	NP	NP	46	2	NP	NP
Freshly Made Lemonade - Mixed Berry	190	0	NP	NP	46	1	NP	NP
Freshly Made Lemonade - Pomegranate	235	0	NP	NP	59	0	NP	NP
Freshly Made Lemonade - Raspberry	185	0	NP	NP	46	0	NP	NP
Freshly Made Lemonade - Strawberry	192	0	NP	NP	48	1	NP	NP
Handcrafted Fruit Tea - Blackberry	162	0	NP	NP	39	2	NP	NP
Handcrafted Fruit Tea - Mango	104	0	NP	NP	26	1	NP	NP
Handcrafted Fruit Tea - Mixed Berry	162	0	NP	NP	39	1	NP	NP
Handcrafted Fruit Tea - Peach	162	0	NP	NP	41	0	NP	NP
Handcrafted Fruit Tea - Raspberry	162	0	NP	NP	39	2	NP	NP
RT Palmer	125	0	NP	NP	31	1	NP	NP
Ruby T	114	0	NP	NP	29	0	NP	NP
Classic Coke Float	384	14	NP	NP	64	0	NP	NP
Dream Cream Soda - Orange Creamsicle	202	7	NP	NP	33	0	NP	NP
Dream Cream Soda - Peaches 'n Cream	244	7	NP	NP	44	0	NP	NP
Dream Cream Soda - Strawberry	245	7	NP	NP	44	1	NP	NP
Ruby's Root Beer Float	399	14	NP	NP	68	0	NP	NP

Dessert

Description & Serving	Cal	Fat	Sfat	Sod	Carb	Fiber	Sugar	Prot
Blondie for One	626	27	NP	NP	86	2	NP	NP
Blondie for Two	1054	44	NP	NP	149	3	NP	NP
Mini Chocolate Chip Cookie	80	4	NP	NP	10	1	NP	NP
Chocolate Chip Cookie	320	15	NP	NP	40	2	NP	NP
Chocolate Tallcake	1276	60	NP	NP	173	2	NP	NP
Double Chocolate Cake	988	50	NP	NP	118	6	NP	NP
New York Cheesecake	736	60	NP	NP	82	2	NP	NP
Strawberries & Ice Cream	900	50	NP	NP	98	4	NP	NP
Mini White Chocolate Macadamia Nut Cookie	85	5	NP	NP	10	0	NP	NP
White Chocolate Macadamia Nut Cookie	340	20	NP	NP	38	1	NP	NP

Description & Serving	Cal	Fat	Sfat	Sod	Carb	Fiber	Sugar	Prot
Ryan's								
Salad								
Black-Eyed Pea Salad, 1 spoon	40	0	0	140	7	2	2	2
Bowtie Pasta Salad w/ Vegetables, 1 spoon	110	7	1.5	330	10	<1	2	3
Broccoli & Cauliflower Salad w/ Raisins, 1 spoon	120	8	1	290	11	2	8	3
Caesar Salad, 1 spoon	130	12	2	340	3	1	2	3
Cole Slaw, 1 spoon	180	6	2	540	11	1	10	<1
Corn Salad, 1 spoon	100	5	1	300	11	1	4	4
Greek Pasta Salad, 1 spoon	110	7	1.5	230	11	1	2	3
Greek Salad, 1 spoon	90	8	2	430	3	1	1	2
Homemade Tuna Salad, 1 spoon	50	7	1	320	8	0	0	13
Italian Salad, 1 spoon	50	4.5	0.5	260	4	1	2	<1
Lettuce-Iceberg, 1 oz	5	0	0	0	0	0	0	0
Lettuce-Romaine, 1 oz	5	0	0	0	0	0	0	0
Macaroni Salad, 1 spoon	140	6	1	350	2	1	7	3
Marinated Seven Bean Salad, 1 spoon	120	0	0	290	29	4	18	4
Marinated Vegetable Salad, 1 spoon	50	3.5	0.5	190	5	1	3	1
Potato Salad, 1 spoon	110	4.5	1	420	16	1	3	2
Rotini Pasta Salad w/ Vegetables, 1 spoon	90	4	0.5	260	12	1	2	2
Shell Pasta Salad w/ Vegetables, 1 spoon	90	4.5	0.5	260	11	1	2	2
Spinach & Strawberry Salad, 1 spoon	70	4	0.5	180	7	1	5	1
Tomato & Onion Salad, 1 spoon	40	2.5	0.5	135	5	1	3	<1
Soup								
Chicken Gumbo Soup, 4 oz	50	1.5	0.5	540	7	<1	1	2
Chicken Noodle Soup, 4 oz	50	1	0	550	8	0	1	3
Clam Chowder, 4 oz	90	3	1	620	11	<1	2	4
Cream of Broccoli w/ Cheese Soup, 4 oz	70	3	1.5	500	9	<1	5	3
Cream of Potato Soup, 4 oz	70	3	1	440	11	<1	2	1
Vegetable Beef Soup, 4 oz	45	0.5	0	500	8	1	2	2
Entrée								
Beef								
Corn Dog, 1	240	11	3.5	420	28	1	8	6
Grilled Hot Dog Weiner, 1	140	13	5	470	1	0	0	5
Homestyle Chuck Roast w/ Vegetables, 1 spoon	150	7	2.5	270	4	<1	2	16
Meatloaf, 1 slice	100	6	2.5	300	6	0	3	6
Mexican Casserole, 1 spoon	190	9	4	550	21	2	4	8
Taco Meat, 1.25 oz	70	4	1.5	180	3	1	0	5
Chicken/Turkey								
BBQ Chicken, 1 spoon	150	6	2	270	9	0	0	15
Bourbon Chicken, 1 spoon	70	3	0.5	230	3	0	1	9
Chicken & Dumplings, 1 spoon	60	2	0	560	3	0	0	8
Chicken Fajitas, 1 spoon	90	2.5	0.5	650	4	1	3	13
Chicken Pot Pie, 1 spoon	290	18	5	440	24	1	1	8
Fried Chicken Breast, 1	270	12	3	200	1	1	0	39
Fried Chicken Leg, 1	160	10	2.5	110	1	1	0	17

Description & Serving	Cal	Fat	Sfat	Sod	Carb	Fiber	Sugar	Prot
Fried Chicken Thigh, 1	220	13	3.5	150	2	2	0	23
Fried Chicken Wing, 1	70	3	1	50	0	0	0	10
Grilled Chicken Breast, plain, 1	180	4	1	85	0	0	0	35
Grilled Teriyaki Chicken Thighs, 1 pc	60	2.5	0.5	180	4	0	1	6
Rotisserie Chicken Breast, 1	280	13	3.5	230	<1	0	0	40
Rotisserie Chicken Leg, 1	120	9	2.5	160	<1	0	0	13
Rotisserie Chicken Thigh, 1	250	16	4.5	260	1	0	0	25
Carved Turkey Breast, 1 slice	90	3.5	1	135	0	0	0	14
White Turkey w/ Gravy, 1 spoon	90	2	1	400	4	0	<1	15
Pasta/Pizza								
Macaroni & Beef w/ Tomatoes, 1 spoon	120	4.5	2	580	15	2	6	6
Macaroni & Cheese, 1 spoon	120	2.5	1	530	19	<1	1	4
Meat Lasagna, 1 pc	250	11	5	670	22	2	5	18
Spaghetti, 1 spoon	130	2.5	0.5	90	23	1	1	4
Cheese Pizza, 1 slice	200	8	3	310	21	<1	1	10
Pepperoni Pizza, 1 slice	250	13	5	480	21	<1	1	12
Pork/Ribs								
BBQ Pork, 1 spoon	230	16	6	370	5	1	3	17
Grilled Pork Chop-BBQ, 1	190	9	3	150	4	0	0	22
Grilled Pork Chop-Plain, 1	170	9	3	45	0	0	0	22
Grilled Pork Chop-Teriyaki, 1	190	10	3	260	3	0	3	22
Grilled Sliced Sausage in BBQ Sauce, 1 spoon	210	17	8	620	8	0	2	7
Grilled Sausage in Peppers & Onions, 1 spoon	200	17	8	460	4	<1	3	7
BBQ Ribs, 1	180	12	5	560	7	0	6	10
Seafood								
Baked Whole Salmon, 1 pc	140	10	2	120	0	0	0	14
Crab Cakes, 1	120	5	1.5	270	15	1	2	3
Fried Breaded Catfish Fillet, 1	340	16	2	450	12	1	0	36
Fried Fish, 1 pc	90	5	1	160	4	0	0	9
Fried Shrimp, 11	150	8	1.5	470	16	1	<1	6
Fried Tilapia, 1 pc	70	2.5	0.5	115	4	0	0	7
Steak								
Chicken Fried Steak w/o Gravy, 1 pc	210	13	4	630	15	<1	0	9
Chicken Fried Steak w/ Gravy, 1 pc	220	13	4	700	16	<1	0	9
Sirloin Steak, 3 oz	180	9	3.5	170	0	0	0	25
Side								
Biscuit, 1	190	9	2.5	620	22	<1	2	4
Blueberry Bagel, half	120	0.5	0	225	25	1	2	4
Cinnamon Roll, 1	210	7	1.5	270	34	1	15	3
English Muffin, half	70	1	0	150	13	<1	<1	2
Wheat Roll, 1	190	3	0.5	170	35	2	1	6
White Roll, 1	190	2.5	0.5	150	37	1	9	5
4" Hamburger Bun w/ Sesame Seeds, 1 roll	180	3.5	1	310	31	<1	4	6
Hot Dog Bun, 1	130	2	0	250	24	<1	3	4
Yellow Corn Taco Shells, 2	110	4	1	100	17	2	2	2
Yellow Corn Tortilla Chips, 11	150	7	1	115	20	2	0	2

Description & Serving	Cal	Fat	Sfat	Sod	Carb	Fiber	Sugar	Prot
Low Fat Cottage Cheese, 1 oz	25	0.5	0	115	1	0	0	4
Lowfat Blueberry Yogurt, 1 oz	25	0	0	10	5	0	4	1
Cantaloupe, 1 spoon	25	0	0	10	6	<1	7	<1
Pineapple, 1 spoon	35	0	0	0	10	1	7	0
Red Grapes, 1 spoon	60	0	0	0	15	<1	12	<1
Strawberries, 1 spoon	25	0	0	0	6	1	4	<1
Watermelon, 1 spoon	25	0	0	0	6	0	5	<1
Baby Lima Beans w/ Sauce, 1 spoon	50	1	0	200	10	2	1	2
Baked Beans, 1 spoon	90	1	0	420	20	5	3	6
Baked Potato-Plain, 1 ea	180	0	0	10	31	4	1	4
Breaded Fried Okra, 1 spoon	220	12	1	590	28	3	2	3
Brussel Sprouts, 1 spoon	40	2	0.5	30	6	2	1	2
Candied Sweet Potatoes w/ Marshmallows, 1 spoon	130	1.5	0	270	31	2	17	1
Chopped Collard Greens in Sauce, 1 spoon	20	1	0	240	3	2	1	1
Corn Cobbet, 1	90	3	0.5	420	4	2	2	2
Cornbread Stuffing, 1 spoon	100	5	1	440	13	1	1	2
Cream Corn, 1 spoon	40	0	0	80	10	1	3	1
Cut Corn, 1 spoon	50	2	0	330	9	1	1	1
Fried Onion Rings, 6	230	14	2.5	290	25	2	3	3
Fried Potatoes, 1 spoon	110	3.5	0.5	240	5	2	0	3
Garlic Mashed Potatoes, 1 spoon	90	4	1	230	11	1	<1	3
Glazed Baby Carrots w/ Sauce, 1 spoon	60	3	0.5	120	7	1	5	<1
Green Beans-Plain, 1 spoon	10	0	0	5	2	1	1	<1
Grilled Vegetables w/ Broccoli, 1 spoon	40	3	1	210	2	<1	1	1
Grilled Vegetables w/ Cauliflower, 1 spoon	40	3.5	1	230	2	<1	1	1
Pinto Beans, 1 spoon	70	1	0	270	14	4	0	5
Rice Pilaf, 1 spoon	60	1	0	180	12	0	0	1
Seasoned Green Beans, 1 spoon	25	2	0	140	3	1	1	0
Steamed Broccoli Spears, 1 spoon	40	2.5	0.5	350	<1	1	3	2
Steamed Cabbage w/ Bacon, 1 spoon	60	5	2	220	2	1	1	1
Stewed Tomatoes w/ Okra & Corn, 1 spoon	25	0	0	270	6	1	4	<1
Yellow Squash w/ Onions, 1 spoon	40	3.5	1	15	2	1	1	0

Dressing/Condiment

Description & Serving	Cal	Fat	Sfat	Sod	Carb	Fiber	Sugar	Prot
Blue Cheese Dressing, 1 oz	150	16	3	320	2	0	2	1
Fat Free French Dressing, 1 oz	45	0	0	290	11	0	5	0
Fat Free Catalina Dressing, 1 oz	50	0	0	350	11	0	7	0
Fat Free Creamy Italian Dressing, 1 oz	15	0	0	330	3	<1	1	0
Fat Free Ranch Dressing, 1 oz	50	0	0	330	11	0	3	0
Fat Free Thousand Island Dressing, 1 oz	45	0	0	260	10	0	5	0
French Dressing, 1 oz	120	12	1.5	220	4	0	4	0
Golden Italian Dressing, 1 oz	90	8	1	430	4	0	3	0
Light Raspberry Vinaigrette, 1 oz	60	4	0	270	5	0	5	0
Ranch Dressing-House Blend, 1 oz	140	15	2.5	240	2	0	<1	0
Thousand Island Dressing, 1 oz	80	8	1.5	115	3	0	3	0
Brown Gravy, 2 oz	25	1	0.5	360	4	0	2	0
Brown Gravy w/ Mushrooms, 2 oz	25	1	0.5	320	4	0	2	0
Cheddar Cheese Sauce, 2 oz	50	2	1	390	7	0	1	1

Description & Serving	Cal	Fat	Sfat	Sod	Carb	Fiber	Sugar	Prot
Cocktail Sauce, 1 oz	40	1	0.5	350	9	0	8	<1
Cranberry Sauce, 1 oz	55	0	0	10	14	0	13	0
Giblet Gravy, 2 oz	40	2.5	1	270	4	0	0	<1
Half & Half Creamer, 1	15	1	0	10	0	0	0	0
Honey Spread, 1 container	60	6	1	65	2	0	1	3
Horseradish Cream Sauce, 1 oz	140	13	2	250	6	0	5	0
Salsa, 1 oz	10	0	0	150	2	0	0	0
Sour Cream, 1 tbsp	25	2.5	1.5	5	<1	0	0	0
Sour Cream, light, 1 tbsp	15	1.5	1	10	1	0	0	<1
Spaghetti Sauce w/ Meat, 2 oz	140	8	3.5	660	10	<1	6	8
Tartar Sauce, 1 oz	170	17	15	150	4	0	2	0
Whipped Margarine, 1 tbsp	100	11	2	110	0	0	0	0
White Pepper Gravy, 2 oz	45	2	0.5	320	7	0	0	0

Topping

Description & Serving	Cal	Fat	Sfat	Sod	Carb	Fiber	Sugar	Prot
Cheddar Cheese, cubed, 1 spoon	60	5	3	95	0	0	0	4
White Cheese w/ Pepper, cubed, 1 spoon	60	5	3	100	0	0	0	4
White Cheese, shredded, 1 spoon	40	3.5	2	60	0	0	0	3
Yellow/Orange Cheese, shredded, 1 spoon	40	3.5	2	60	0	0	0	3
Cauliflower, 1 spoon	5	0	0	5	1	0	0	0
Cherry Tomatoes, 1	5	0	0	0	1	0	0	0
Cucumbers, 1 oz	5	0	0	0	1	0	0	0
Green Peppers, 1 spoon	5	0	0	0	1	0	0	0
Hard Cooked Diced Eggs, 1 oz	45	3	1	70	<1	0	0	3
Julienne Turkey Ham, 1 oz	40	1	0.5	300	<1	0	0	6
Julienne White Turkey, 1 oz	45	2.5	0.5	250	1	0	0	4
Kosher Deli Pickle Spear, 1	5	0	0	370	1	0	1	0
Onion, diced, 1 spoon	5	0	0	0	2	0	0	0
Sliced Green Olives, 1 spoon	15	1.5	0	130	1	<1	0	0
Sliced Pepperoni, 1 oz	140	13	3	480	<1	0	0	5
Sliced Ripe Olives, 1 spoon	15	1.5	0	130	1	<1	0	0

Dessert

Description & Serving	Cal	Fat	Sfat	Sod	Carb	Fiber	Sugar	Prot
Apple Cinnamon Cookie	140	7	2.5	70	17	0	10	1
Banana Pudding, 1 spoon	170	7	1	60	28	1	17	1
Butter Pecan Frozen Yogurt, no sugar added, 4 oz	60	0	0	85	16	0	3	2
Cheesecake, plain, 1 pc	370	19	10	450	45	<1	35	5
Chocolate Chip Cookie	130	7	2	110	16	1	9	1
Chocolate Soft Serve Ice Cream, reduced fat, 4 oz	120	3	2.5	70	21	<1	15	2
Coconut Meringue Pie, 1 pc	190	6	4	150	32	1	23	2
Gelatin, sugar free, 3 oz	5	0	0	45	0	0	0	1
Ice Cream Cone, flat bottom, 1	15	0	0	15	3	0	<1	0
Ice Cream Cone, sugar, 1	50	0.5	0	55	10	0	4	1
Key Lime Pie, 1 pc	280	12	7	140	39	<1	31	3
Lemon Crème Cake, sugar free, 1 pc	170	15	3	230	9	0	0	3
Oatmeal Raisin Cookie	120	5	1.5	100	16	1	8	1
Orange Lowfat Frozen Yogurt, 4 oz	90	1	0.5	55	17	0	15	3
Pudding, sugar free, 1 spoon	40	1	0.5	210	7	0	4	<1

Description & Serving	Cal	Fat	Sfat	Sod	Carb	Fiber	Sugar	Prot
Ranger Cookie	120	5	2.5	65	16	0	9	1
Red Velvet Cream Cake, 1 pc	170	8	2	220	23	2	13	3
Strawberry No Fat Frozen Yogurt, 4 oz	90	0	0	55	22	0	9	3
Sugar Cookie	120	5	1	150	17	0	10	1
Vanilla Soft Serve Ice Cream, 4 oz	130	5	3.5	65	19	0	12	2
White Chocolate Macadamia Nut Cookie	90	4.5	1.5	110	13	0	7	1

Dessert Topping

Description & Serving	Cal	Fat	Sfat	Sod	Carb	Fiber	Sugar	Prot
Candy Corn, 12 pc	80	0	0	55	19	0	17	0
Chocolate Candy Buttons, 2 tbsp	130	6	3.5	15	19	<1	17	1
Chocolate Covered Raisins, 2 tbsp	90	3.5	2	5	14	0	12	1
Cocoa Drop, 2 tbsp	120	7	4	<5	14	1	12	1
Gummy Bears, 8 pc	70	0	0	20	17	0	12	0
Orange Candy Slices, 2	80	0	0	0	20	0	15	0
Spiced Jelly Drops, 7 pc	80	0	0	<5	19	0	13	0
Tiny Jelly Beans, 16 pc	80	0	0	0	19	0	15	0
Caramel Sundae Topping, 2 tbsp	130	3	1	50	24	0	21	<1
Crushed Chocolate Cookie Topping, 2 tbsp	90	3	1	115	14	<1	6	1
Granulated Peanuts, 2 tbsp	90	8	1.5	65	3	2	1	4
Maraschino Cherry Halves, 2	10	0	0	0	2	0	2	0
Old Fashioned Fudge Topping, 2 tbsp	120	3	1	55	23	<1	19	1
Pineapple Sundae Topping, 2 tbsp	50	0	0	10	12	0	11	0
Rainbow Sprinkles, 1 tbsp	70	2	1.5	0	13	0	11	0
Strawberry Sundae Topping, 2 tbsp	60	0	0	0	14	0	9	0
Whipped Topping, 1 tbsp	35	3	2.5	10	2	0	2	0
Whipped Topping, sugar free, 1 tbsp	5	0	0	0	<1	0	0	0

Schlotzsky's

Sandwich, small

Description & Serving	Cal	Fat	Sfat	Sod	Carb	Fiber	Sugar	Prot
The Original Sandwich	559	26	12	1834	52	3	4	28
Ham & Cheese Original-Style Sandwich	508	19	9	2033	54	3	5	31
Turkey Original-Style Sandwich	602	27	11	1832	54	3	5	34
Smoked Turkey Breast Sandwich	353	6	1	1070	52	2	4	20
Angus Roast Beef & Cheese Sandwich	534	22	11	1424	50	2	3	33
Turkey Bacon Club Sandwich	561	25	10	1660	51	3	4	32
Chicken Breast Sandwich	342	4	0	1341	52	3	4	26
Fresh Veggie Sandwich	342	10	5	751	50	4	4	14
Albuquerque Turkey Sandwich	694	37	12	1819	57	4	6	34
Chipotle Chicken Sandwich	379	10	2	1094	47	3	3	27
Homestyle Tuna Sandwich	375	11	2	998	48	3	3	22
Turkey & Guacamole Sandwich	368	7	1	1073	54	4	4	21
Chicken & Pesto Sandwich	384	9	1	1122	49	3	3	27
Dijon Chicken Sandwich	378	7	1	1514	52	5	5	29
Angus Corned Beef Sandwich	390	9	2	1557	53	4	5	27
Angus Pastrami & Swiss Sandwich	606	24	12	1646	56	4	5	43
Angus Pastrami Reuben Sandwich	618	26	13	1510	54	4	4	41
Angus Beef & Provolone Sandwich	501	19	6	1350	55	3	7	27
Angus Corned Beef Reuben Sandwich	618	27	13	1530	54	4	4	40
Smoked Turkey Reuben Sandwich	608	26	11	1505	57	4	6	34

Description & Serving	Cal	Fat	Sfat	Sod	Carb	Fiber	Sugar	Prot
Santa Fe Chicken Sandwich	427	10	4	1456	53	3	4	31
Cheese Original-Style Sandwich	562	27	15	1183	51	3	3	28
BLT Sandwich	369	14	4	877	49	2	2	14
Deluxe Original-Style Sandwich	738	38	16	3124	55	3	6	43
Texas Schlotzsky's Sandwich	540	23	12	1976	51	2	5	32

Sandwich, medium

Description & Serving	Cal	Fat	Sfat	Sod	Carb	Fiber	Sugar	Prot
The Original Sandwich	771	34	15	2634	78	4	6	40
Ham & Cheese Original-Style Sandwich	733	27	12	2980	80	4	7	44
Turkey Original-Style Sandwich	831	35	14	2529	80	4	7	47
Smoked Turkey Breast Sandwich	519	9	1	1568	77	4	6	29
Angus Roast Beef & Cheese Sandwich	784	32	15	2188	75	4	5	47
Turkey Bacon Club Sandwich	787	32	13	2383	77	5	6	47
Chicken Breast Sandwich	513	6	0	2046	78	5	6	39
Fresh Veggie Sandwich	484	12	5	1159	77	6	6	19
Albuquerque Turkey Sandwich	974	51	16	2609	81	6	8	48
Chipotle Chicken Sandwich	551	14	3	1595	68	4	4	39
Homestyle Tuna Sandwich	563	16	3	1468	73	5	4	33
Turkey & Guacamole Sandwich	563	13	1	1604	82	7	6	31
Chicken & Pesto Sandwich	568	14	2	1653	73	4	4	40
Dijon Chicken Sandwich	576	11	1	2329	79	8	8	44
Angus Corned Beef Sandwich	581	13	3	2346	78	6	7	40
Angus Pastrami & Swiss Sandwich	904	36	18	2480	83	6	8	64
Angus Pastrami Reuben Sandwich	909	39	19	2170	80	5	6	60
Angus Beef & Provolone Sandwich	762	29	10	2015	81	4	9	41
Angus Corned Beef Reuben Sandwich	909	40	19	2200	80	5	6	59
Smoked Turkey Reuben Sandwich	895	38	17	2163	84	5	8	51
Santa Fe Chicken Sandwich	622	15	7	2104	76	5	5	46
Cheese Original-Style Sandwich	791	38	20	1698	76	4	5	39
BLT Sandwich	559	21	6	1353	74	4	4	21
Deluxe Original-Style Sandwich	956	46	18	4084	80	5	10	55
Texas Schlotzsky's Sandwich	756	31	15	2853	73	4	8	45

Panini/Wrap

Description & Serving	Cal	Fat	Sfat	Sod	Carb	Fiber	Sugar	Prot
Grilled Chicken Romano Panini	570	16	8	1567	62	1	2	70
Panini Italiano	736	32	15	2406	67	2	4	43
Smoked Ham Crostini Panini	644	23	12	1978	67	2	4	39
Classic Swiss & Tomato Panini	624	26	15	1081	63	1	3	33
Mozzarella & Portobello Panini	485	15	8	1158	63	2	4	24
Smoked Turkey & Guacamole Panini	602	21	6	1735	69	5	4	32
Asian Chicken Wrap	537	12	3	2143	80	5	26	56
Parmesan Chicken Caesar Wrap	556	21	6	1728	61	5	5	61
Homestyle Tuna Wrap	457	17	4	1320	55	4	5	23
Feta & Portobello Wrap	618	39	10	1295	55	4	6	14
Grilled Chicken & Guacamole Wrap	689	36	10	1404	60	8	4	63

Pizza, 8"

Description & Serving	Cal	Fat	Sfat	Sod	Carb	Fiber	Sugar	Prot
Pepperoni & Double Cheese Pizza	685	30	13	1741	74	3	4	31
BBQ Chicken & Jalapeno Pizza	715	16	8	2447	99	3	19	69
Combination Special Pizza	639	25	10	1691	76	4	5	27
Vegetarian Special Pizza	540	17	7	1370	74	4	4	22

Description & Serving	Cal	Fat	Sfat	Sod	Carb	Fiber	Sugar	Prot
Mediterranean Pizza	560	20	9	1581	74	4	5	21
Grilled Chicken & Pesto Pizza	683	22	9	1891	75	4	4	72
Smoked Turkey & Jalapeno Pizza	653	21	8	2038	78	4	6	36
Thai Chicken Pizza	724	23	9	2008	85	4	12	71
Bacon Tomato & Portobello Pizza	619	23	9	1624	75	4	4	28
Double Cheese Pizza	597	21	10	1374	74	3	4	27
Baby Spinach Salad Pizza	454	7	3	1552	80	4	9	18
Fresh Tomato & Pesto Pizza	556	19	8	1335	73	3	4	25

Kids

Description & Serving	Cal	Fat	Sfat	Sod	Carb	Fiber	Sugar	Prot
Cheese Sandwich	394	15	8	772	48	2	2	17
Cheese Pizza	479	13	5	1060	73	3	3	18
Pepperoni Pizza	523	17	6	1246	73	3	3	20
Ham & Cheese Sandwich	424	16	8	1147	49	2	3	21
Turkey Sandwich	300	5	1	750	49	2	2	13

Soup

Description & Serving	Cal	Fat	Sfat	Sod	Carb	Fiber	Sugar	Prot
Boston Clam Chowder, sml	175	11	2	1014	20	0	0	4
Boston Clam Chowder, med	261	17	3	1503	29	1	0	7
Broccoli Cheese, sml	172	14	5	997	12	1	2	4
Broccoli Cheese, med	278	22	8	1661	19	2	3	7
Chicken Tortilla, sml	143	6	3	1690	15	1	5	8
Chicken Tortilla, med	214	8	4	2535	22	2	7	12
Hearty Vegetable Beef, sml	60	3	1	568	7	1	2	3
Hearty Vegetable Beef, med	91	4	2	863	10	2	3	5
Old Fashioned Chicken Noodle, sml	83	2	1	1022	12	1	1	6
Old Fashioned Chicken Noodle, med	125	2	1	1534	18	2	1	8
Potato w/ Bacon, sml	177	10	1	1054	22	1	2	4
Potato w/ Bacon, med	265	15	2	1571	34	2	3	5
Timberline Chili, sml	275	9	4	890	31	7	9	18
Timberline Chili, med	417	14	5	1027	47	11	14	27
Tomato Basil, sml	200	5	2	1220	30	2	6	6
Tomato Basil, med	304	8	3	1853	46	3	9	9
Vegetarian Vegetable, sml	98	1	0	1042	22	5	5	2
Vegetarian Vegetable, med	141	1	0	1500	32	7	7	4
Wisconsin Cheese, sml	263	20	4	1154	20	0	8	4
Wisconsin Cheese, med	394	30	6	1731	30	1	12	7

Salad

Description & Serving	Cal	Fat	Sfat	Sod	Carb	Fiber	Sugar	Prot
Grilled Chicken Caesar Salad	221	8	2	759	12	3	3	53
Caesar Salad	103	5	2	289	10	3	3	6
Garden Salad	51	1	0	291	12	4	4	3
Turkey Chef Salad	309	18	7	1412	14	4	6	26
Baby Spinach & Feta Salad	113	7	5	448	6	3	2	8
Chicken Salad	292	15	4	898	12	3	4	61
Greek Salad	137	8	5	655	13	4	6	7
Ham & Turkey Chef Salad	254	13	6	1340	14	4	7	22
Side Salad	26	1	0	236	7	2	2	1
Potato Salad	242	13	3	515	29	3	8	3
Pasta Salad	68	3	0	293	12	1	10	0

Description & Serving	Cal	Fat	Sfat	Sod	Carb	Fiber	Sugar	Prot
Beverage								
Schlotzsky's Lemonade, kids	146	0	0	62	39	0	23	0
Schlotzsky's Lemonade, sml	243	0	0	103	45	0	45	0
Schlotzsky's Lemonade, med	388	0	0	164	104	0	91	0
Schlotzsky's Raspberry Lemonade, kids	146	0	0	62	39	0	23	0
Schlotzsky's Raspberry Lemonade, sml	243	0	0	103	45	0	45	0
Schlotzsky's Raspberry Lemonade, med	388	0	0	164	104	0	91	0
Dessert								
Brownie	417	22	9	208	54	3	39	5
New York-Style Cheesecake	350	23	13	200	30	1	19	6
Carrot Cake	717	42	6	767	80	3	56	7
Chocolate Chip Cookie	160	8	5	160	22	1	13	2
Fudge Chocolate Chip Cookie	160	8	5	190	22	1	14	2
Oatmeal Raisin Cookie	150	6	3	115	22	1	14	2
Sugar Cookie	160	7	4	200	22	0	11	2
White Chocolate Macadamia Cookie	170	9	5	170	21	1	13	2

Sheetz

Description & Serving	Cal	Fat	Sfat	Sod	Carb	Fiber	Sugar	Prot
Breakfast								
Egg & Cheese Shmuffin w/o condiments & toppings	325	16	7	846	28	2	3	16
Bacon, Egg & Cheese Shmuffin w/o condiments & toppings	526	33	14	1537	31	2	3	28
Sausage, Egg & Cheese Shmuffin w/o condiments & toppings	500	33	13	1239	28	2	3	21
Ham, Egg & Cheese Shmuffin w/o condiments & toppings	424	19	8	1541	32	2	6	29
Steak, Egg & Cheese Shmuffin w/o condiments & toppings	509	24	9	1195	29	2	4	33
Egg & Cheese Shmiscuit w/o condiments & toppings	455	26	9	1505	38	1	5	17
Bacon, Egg & Cheese Shmiscuit w/o condiments & toppings	656	43	16	2196	41	1	5	29
Sausage, Egg & Cheese Shmiscuit w/o condiments & toppings	630	43	15	1898	38	1	5	22
Ham, Egg & Cheese Shmiscuit w/o condiments & toppings	554	29	10	2200	42	1	8	30
Steak, Egg & Cheese Shmiscuit w/o condiments & toppings	639	34	11	1854	39	1	6	34
Egg & Cheese Shmagel w/o condiments & toppings	446	18	7	1097	52	2	1	21
Bacon, Egg & Cheese Shmagel w/o condiments & toppings	647	35	14	1788	55	2	1	33
Sausage, Egg & Cheese Shmagel w/o condiments & toppings	621	35	13	1490	52	2	1	26
Ham, Egg & Cheese Shmagel w/o condiments & toppings	538	21	8	1742	56	2	4	33

Description & Serving	Cal	Fat	Sfat	Sod	Carb	Fiber	Sugar	Prot
Steak, Egg & Cheese Shmagel w/o condiments & toppings	630	26	9	1446	53	2	2	38
Egg & Cheese Meltz w/o condiments & toppings	426	19	8	847	48	1	7	17
Bacon, Egg & Cheese Meltz w/o condiments & toppings	627	36	15	1538	51	1	7	29
Sausage, Egg & Cheese Meltz w/o condiments & toppings	601	36	14	1240	48	1	7	22
Ham, Egg & Cheese Meltz w/o condiments & toppings	525	22	9	1542	52	1	10	30
Steak, Egg & Cheese Meltz w/o condiments & toppings	610	27	10	1196	49	1	8	34
Egg & Cheese Croissant w/o condiments & toppings	329	24	9	765	29	1	3	13
Bacon, Egg & Cheese Croissant w/o condiments & toppings	405	31	12	1027	30	1	3	17
Sausage, Egg & Cheese Croissant w/o condiments & toppings	504	41	15	1158	29	1	3	18
Ham, Egg & Cheese Croissant w/o condiments & toppings	428	27	10	1460	33	1	6	26
Steak, Egg & Cheese Croissant w/o condiments & toppings	421	28	10	940	30	1	4	22
Spicy Sausage Breakfast Burrito	270	13	5	540	10	1	1	11
Sausage Breakfast Burrito	300	16	6	760	29	1	0	11
Hashbrowns	130	8	4	250	14	3	0	1
Sausage Biscuit w/o cheese	434	28	8	1291	35	1	4	11
Sausage Dipper	354	22	7	334	27	1	8	12
Chicken Biscuit w/o cheese & condiments	378	15	2	1415	46	3	4	15
Plain Biscuit	259	11	2	898	35	<1	4	6
Plain Bagel	250	3	0	490	49	2	0	10
Plain English Muffin	129	<1	0	239	25	2	2	5
Blueberry Muffin	440	24	4	400	50	2	28	6
Carrot Cake Muffin	440	20	4	420	60	2	40	6
Chocolate Chip Muffin	520	28	14	460	64	4	44	6

Sandwich

	Cal	Fat	Sfat	Sod	Carb	Fiber	Sugar	Prot
Lil' Pork BBQ w/o cheese, pickles, or onions	246	9	2	682	30	1	9	13
Big Ol' Pork BBQ on Wheat Burger Bun w/o cheese, pickles, or onions	463	16	6	1305	54	4	19	27
Big Ol' Pork BBQ on Corn Dusted Bun w/o cheese, pickles, or onions	483	17	6	1265	56	2	19	25
6" Meatball Sub on Wheat w/o cheese, condiments, or toppings	415	13	4	846	60	3	4	17
6" Meatball Sub on White w/o cheese, condiments, or toppings	396	12	4	832	55	2	4	16
6" Steak Sub on Wheat w/o cheese, condiments, or toppings	460	10	2	858	57	3	4	28
6" Steak Sub on White w/o cheese, condiments, or toppings	441	9	2	844	52	2	4	27
6" Chicken Sub on Wheat w/o cheese, condiments, or toppings	393	6	1	1145	56	3	3	33

Description & Serving	Cal	Fat	Sfat	Sod	Carb	Fiber	Sugar	Prot
6" Chicken Sub on White w/o cheese, condiments, or toppings	374	5	1	1131	51	2	3	32
6" Pepperoni Sub on Wheat w/o cheese, condiments, or toppings	473	20	6	1162	56	3	3	20
6" Pepperoni Sub on White w/o cheese, condiments, or toppings	454	19	6	1148	51	2	3	19
6" Turkey Sub on Wheat w/o cheese, condiments, or toppings	327	4	0	985	58	3	4	20
6" Turkey Sub on White w/o cheese, condiments, or toppings	308	3	0	971	53	2	4	19
6" Ham Sub on Wheat w/o cheese, condiments, or toppings	347	4	1	1005	59	3	5	20
6" Ham Sub on White w/o cheese, condiments, or toppings	328	3	1	991	54	2	5	19
6" Italian Sub on Wheat w/o cheese, condiments, or toppings	397	10	3	1127	58	3	4	21
6" Italian Sub on White w/o cheese, condiments, or toppings	378	9	3	1113	53	2	4	20
6" Roast Beef Sub on Wheat w/o cheese, condiments, or toppings	316	4	1	722	57	3	3	17
6" Roast Beef Sub on White w/o cheese, condiments, or toppings	297	3	1	708	52	2	3	16
6" Chicken Salad Sub on Wheat w/o cheese, condiments, or toppings	526	23	4	955	65	3	7	18
6" Chicken Salad Sub on White w/o cheese, condiments, or toppings	507	22	4	941	60	2	7	17
6" BLT Sub on Wheat w/o cheese, condiments, or toppings	487	19	7	1205	61	3	4	23
6" BLT Sub on White w/o cheese, condiments, or toppings	468	18	7	1191	56	2	4	22
6" Deli Sub on Wheat w/o cheese, condiments, or toppings	418	13	4	965	58	3	4	18
6" Deli Sub on White w/o cheese, condiments, or toppings	399	12	4	951	53	2	4	17
6" Cheese Sub on Wheat w/ Cheddar Cheese & w/o condiments	387	11	5	681	57	3	3	18
6" Cheese Sub on White w/ Cheddar Cheese & w/o condiments	368	10	5	667	52	2	3	17
6" Club Sub on Wheat w/o cheese, condiments, or toppings	327	4	0	985	58	3	4	20
6" Club Sub on White w/o cheese, condiments, or toppings	308	3	0	971	53	2	4	19
6" Tuna Salad Sub on Wheat w/o cheese, condiments, or toppings	490	18	3	884	65	3	7	22
6" Tuna Salad Sub on White w/o cheese, condiments, or toppings	471	17	3	870	60	2	7	21
Ham & Cheese Sandwich on Wheat w/o condiments or toppings	323	14	6	1333	26	1	5	22
Deli Sandwich on Wheat w/o cheese, condiments, or toppings	302	17	5	892	24	1	3	13

Description & Serving	Cal	Fat	Sfat	Sod	Carb	Fiber	Sugar	Prot
Turkey Sandwich on Wheat	164	4	0	762	23	1	3	13
Roast Beef Sandwich on Wheat	167	4	1	569	22	1	2	12
Tuna Salad on Wheat	327	18	3	661	30	1	6	15
Italian Sandwich on Wheat	275	13	4	1107	24	1	3	17
Chicken Salad Sandwich on Wheat	363	23	4	732	30	1	6	11
Chicken Breast Sandwich on Wheat Bun w/o cheese, condiments, or toppings	340	6	2	980	41	5	5	32

Specialty Sandwich/Wrap

Description & Serving	Cal	Fat	Sfat	Sod	Carb	Fiber	Sugar	Prot
Ham Melt w/o cheese, condiments, or toppings	422	7	3	857	70	2	11	18
Bacon Melt	552	22	9	1052	70	2	9	21
Roast Beef Melt	351	5	2	361	67	2	9	9
Club Melt	402	7	2	837	69	2	10	18
Turkey Melt	402	7	2	837	69	2	10	18
Chicken Salad Ciabatta Sandwich w/o cheese, condiments, or toppings	481	25	5	1097	51	3	6	15
Tuna Salad Ciabatta Sandwich	445	20	4	1026	51	3	6	19
Turkey Ciabatta Sandwich	282	6	1	1127	44	3	3	17
Deli Ciabatta Sandwich	373	15	5	1107	44	3	3	15
Roast Beef Ciabatta Sandwich	231	4	1	651	42	3	2	8
Ham Ciabatta Sandwich	302	6	2	1147	45	3	4	17
Italian Ciabatta Sandwich	231	4	1	651	42	3	2	8
Steak Wrap w/o cheese, condiments, or toppings	326	11	2	831	24	9	2	29
Grilled Chicken Wrap w/o cheese, condiments, or toppings	259	7	1	1118	23	9	1	34
Turkey Wrap w/o cheese, condiments, or toppings	213	6	0	1118	27	9	3	24
Grilled Chicken Caesar Wrap	527	32	6	1870	31	9	2	36

Burger/Hot Dog

Description & Serving	Cal	Fat	Sfat	Sod	Carb	Fiber	Sugar	Prot
Gourmet Burger w/o cheese, condiments, or toppings	551	31	12	475	40	4	5	28
Jr. Burger w/o cheese, condiments, or toppings	230	11	3	359	22	1	2	10
Double Burger w/o cheese, condiments, or toppings	230	11	3	359	22	1	2	10
Hot Dog w/o cheese, condiments, or toppings	260	15	5	670	24	1	3	9
Deli Dog w/o cheese, condiments, or toppings	627	35	11	1635	56	2	4	22

Salad

Description & Serving	Cal	Fat	Sfat	Sod	Carb	Fiber	Sugar	Prot
Garden Salad w/o dressing or toppings	27	0	0	27	7	2	4	2
Grilled Chicken Salad w/o dressing or toppings	144	4	1	663	7	2	4	24
Steak Salad w/o dressing or toppings	211	8	2	376	8	2	5	19
Crispy Chicken Salad w/o dressing or toppings	269	8	1	1060	30	2	4	22
Taco Salad w/o dressing or toppings	254	10	2	173	38	5	4	5
Chef Salad w/o dressing or toppings	149	4	1	999	12	2	7	20
Grilled Chicken Caesar Salad w/o croutons	478	42	7	1418	2	0	0	24

Entrée

Description & Serving	Cal	Fat	Sfat	Sod	Carb	Fiber	Sugar	Prot
Steak Fajita	522	14	4	986	61	4	5	27
Chicken Fajita	396	8	3	953	60	4	4	21
Regular Chicken Strips (3 pc)	242	8	1	1033	23	0	0	20

Description & Serving	Cal	Fat	Sfat	Sod	Carb	Fiber	Sugar	Prot
Nachos/Side								
Nachos Bueno	504	23	4	738	65	6	0	7
Nachos Grande w/ all toppings	724	39	12	1630	83	6	3	11
Small Cheese Nachoz	274	13	3	564	34	3	0	4
Cinnamon Sugar Pretzel	595	110	2	752	107	3	13	16
Salted Pretzel	564	13	2	2350	97	3	3	16
Jalapeno Filled Pretzels	484	12	6	1392	76	3	3	18
Plain Pretzel w/o salt	470	2	0	752	97	3	3	16
Bag of Fryz	162	6	2	356	23	2	0	2
Cup of Fryz	258	10	3	568	36	3	0	3
Bucket of Fryz	526	21	5	1158	74	7	0	7
Grande Fryz w/ all toppings	727	35	12	2194	91	6	0	9
Cheese Fryz	652	30	8	2274	81	7	0	9
Shmokehouse Fryz	973	52	16	2862	103	7	8	17
Small Cheese Fryz	452	19	5	1309	60	5	0	6
Garlic Fryz	554	49	33	1186	102	35	24	35
Mac & Cheese	129	6	3	934	14	0	2	5
Chili Mac & Cheese	129	6	3	934	14	0	2	5
Three Cheese Mac & Cheese	185	11	6	1025	15	0	2	9
Cole Slaw	198	9	1	184	28	1	26	1
Dessert								
Chocolate Chunk Cookie	210	10	4	170	28	1	17	2
Chocolate No Bakes	180	8	2	60	24	1	17	4
Oatmeal Raisin Cookie	200	9	2	160	27	1	14	2
Peanut Butter Cookie	230	14	4	130	23	1	14	4
Peanut Butter No Bakes	180	8	2	60	24	1	18	3
Pink Iced Cookie	270	12	4	210	37	0	24	2
Raisin Filled Cookie	220	8	2	125	35	0	21	2
Cinnamon Roll w/ Cream Cheese Icing	460	18	8	440	66	2	34	6
Cinnamon Roll, Glazed	380	14	7	400	58	2	26	6
Cinnamon Roll w/ Peanut Butter Icing	440	16	7	420	68	2	36	6
Cinnamon Roll w/ Vanilla Icing	440	16	7	400	68	2	38	6
Apple Fritter	450	25	6	280	49	1	20	5
Chocolate Iced Custard Filled	380	17	4	340	51	1	25	5
Chocolate Iced Glazed Ring	350	16	4	300	47	1	22	4
Chocolate Iced Glazed Ring w/ Sprinkles	370	17	4	300	49	1	24	4
Cream Filled Chocolate Iced	420	20	5	340	57	1	31	5
Cream Filled Glazed	360	17	4	310	47	1	23	4
Glazed Ring	290	14	3	280	35	0	12	4
Old Fashion Chocolate Cake	530	33	7	360	54	2	33	4
Old Fashion Vanilla Cake	480	26	6	370	57	1	34	3
Raspberry Filled Glazed	330	14	3	310	46	1	18	4
Vanilla Iced Glazed Ring w/ Sprinkles	360	16	4	290	49	0	24	4
Beverage								
Hot								
Breakfast Blend Coffee, 12 oz	8	0	0	0	2	0	0	0
Colombian Coffee, 12 oz	8	0	0	0	2	0	0	0
Decaf House Blend Coffee, 12 oz	8	0	0	0	2	0	0	0

Description & Serving	Cal	Fat	Sfat	Sod	Carb	Fiber	Sugar	Prot
House Blend Coffee, 12 oz	8	0	0	0	2	0	0	0
Serious Dark Roast Coffee, 12 oz	8	0	0	0	2	0	0	0
Vanilla Nut Cream Coffee, 12 oz	8	0	0	0	2	0	0	0
Almond-Honey, 12 oz	195	5	2	180	38	0	35	2
Butterscotch Krimpet, 12 oz	225	8	2	113	38	0	29	0
Chocolate Covered Pretzel, 12 oz	195	5	2	330	38	2	33	2
Cotton Candy, 12 oz	210	5	2	173	39	0	33	2
Creme Brulee Cupo'ccino, 12 oz	210	6	2	114	38	0	30	2
Fat Free French Vanilla Cupo'ccino, 12 oz	105	0	0	110	26	0	18	2
French Vanilla Cupo'ccino, 12 oz	213	8	2	116	38	0	32	2
Hot Chocolate, 12 oz	186	3	0	0	39	2	35	3
Sugar Free Caramel Pecan, 12 oz	168	5	<1	162	34	0	1	1
Plain Latte w/ 2% milk & w/o whipped cream, Regular (12 oz)	101	4	2	92	11	0	9	7
Caramel Vanilla Latte w/ 2% milk & w/o whipped cream, Regular (12 oz)	175	4	2	92	29	0	27	7
Raspberry Vanilla Latte w/ 2% milk & w/o whipped cream, Regular (12 oz)	177	4	2	92	29	0	27	7
Sugar Free Caramel Vanilla Latte w/ 2% milk & w/o whipped cream, Regular (12 oz)	101	4	2	92	11	0	9	7
Caramel Hazelnut Latte w/ 2% milk & w/o whipped cream, Regular (12 oz)	172	4	2	92	29	0	27	7
Very Vanilla Latte w/ 2% milk & w/o whipped cream, Regular (12 oz)	252	4	2	92	48	0	46	7
Hot Chai Latte w/ 2% milk & w/o whipped cream, Regular (12 oz)	280	6	4	154	45	0	44	10
Plain Dark Chocolate Mocha w/ 2% milk & w/o whipped cream, Regular (12 oz)	141	4	2	100	20	1	18	8
Plain White Chocolate Mocha w/ 2% milk & w/o whipped cream, Regular (12 oz)	141	4	2	122	21	0	18	7
Plain Sugar Free Mocha w/ 2% milk & w/o whipped cream, Regular (12 oz)	141	4	2	110	23	0	9	7
Black & White Mocha w/ 2% milk & w/o whipped cream, Regular (12 oz)	181	4	2	130	30	1	27	8
Caramel Mocha w/ 2% milk & w/o whipped cream, Regular (12 oz)	143	4	2	101	20	1	18	8
Chocolate Chip Cookie Americano, Regular (12 oz)	5	0	0	0	19	0	18	1
Peanut Butter Americano, Regular (12 oz)	80	0	0	9	20	0	18	1
Sugar Free Amaretto Americano, Regular (12 oz)	5	0	0	0	1	0	0	1
Banana Americano, Regular (12 oz)	82	0	0	0	20	0	18	1
Caramel Americano, Regular (12 oz)	77	0	0	0	19	0	18	1
Sugar Free Caramel Americano, Regular (12 oz)	5	0	0	0	1	0	0	1
Sugar Free Vanilla Americano, Regular (12 oz)	5	0	0	0	1	0	0	1
Hazelnut Americano, Regular (12 oz)	74	0	0	0	18	0	17	1
Raspberry Americano, Regular (12 oz)	81	0	0	0	20	0	19	1
Vanilla Americano, Regular (12 oz)	80	0	0	0	20	0	19	1
Chai Americano, Regular (12 oz)	65	0	0	0	15	0	14	1
Toasted Marshmallow Americano, Regular (12 oz)	80	0	0	0	19	0	18	1
Americano, Regular (12 oz)	5	0	0	0	1	0	0	1

Description & Serving	Cal	Fat	Sfat	Sod	Carb	Fiber	Sugar	Prot
Chocolate Chip Cappuccino w/ 2% milk, Regular (12 oz)	69	2	1	62	19	0	18	5
Sugar Free Amaretto Cappuccino w/ 2% milk, Regular (12 oz)	69	2	1	62	7	0	6	5
Banana Cappuccino w/ 2% milk, Regular (12 oz)	120	2	1	62	19	0	18	5
Caramel Cappuccino w/ 2% milk, Regular (12 oz)	117	2	1	62	19	0	18	5
Sugar Free Caramel Cappuccino w/ 2% milk, Regular (12 oz)	69	2	1	62	7	0	6	5
Sugar Free Hazelnut Cappuccino w/ 2% milk, Regular (12 oz)	69	2	1	62	7	0	6	5
Sugar Free Vanilla Cappuccino w/ 2% milk, Regular (12 oz)	69	2	1	62	7	0	6	5
Hazelnut Cappuccino w/ 2% milk, Regular (12 oz)	115	2	1	62	19	0	18	5
Raspberry Cappuccino w/ 2% milk, Regular (12 oz)	120	2	1	62	20	0	19	5
Vanilla Cappuccino w/ 2% milk, Regular (12 oz)	119	2	1	62	19	0	18	5
Cappuccino w/ 2% milk, Regular (12 oz)	69	2	1	62	7	0	6	5
Chocolate Chip Red Alert, Regular (12 oz)	11	0	0	0	20	0	18	1
Peanut Butter Red Alert, Regular (12 oz)	86	0	0	9	21	0	18	1
Sugar Free Amaretto Red Alert, Regular (12 oz)	11	0	0	0	2	0	0	1
Banana Red Alert, Regular (12 oz)	88	0	0	0	21	0	18	1
Caramel Red Alert, Regular (12 oz)	83	0	0	0	20	0	18	1
Sugar Free Caramel Red Alert, Regular (12 oz)	11	0	0	0	2	0	0	1
Sugar Free Vanilla Red Alert, Regular (12 oz)	11	0	0	0	2	0	0	1
Hazelnut Red Alert, Regular (12 oz)	80	0	0	0	19	0	17	1
Raspberry Red Alert, Regular (12 oz)	87	0	0	0	21	0	19	1
Vanilla Red Alert, Regular (12 oz)	86	0	0	0	21	0	19	1
Toasted Red Alert, Regular (12 oz)	86	0	0	0	20	0	18	1
Red Alert, Regular (12 oz)	11	0	0	0	2	0	0	1
Dark Hot Chocolate w/ 2% milk & w/o whipped cream, Regular (12 oz)	224	6	3	154	32	1	31	10
White Hot Chocolate w/ 2% milk & w/o whipped cream, Regular (12 oz)	224	6	3	199	34	0	30	9
Sugar Free Hot Chocolate w/ 2% milk & w/o whipped cream, Regular (12 oz)	224	6	3	174	38	1	13	10
Chocolate Chip Steamer w/ 2% milk & w/o whipped cream, Regular (12 oz)	160	6	4	154	52	0	51	10
Peanut Butter Steamer w/ 2% milk & w/o whipped cream, Regular (12 oz)	310	6	4	172	54	0	51	10
Sugar Free Amaretto Steamer w/ 2% milk & w/o whipped cream, Regular (12 oz)	160	6	4	154	16	0	15	10
Banana Steamer w/ 2% milk & w/o whipped cream, Regular (12 oz)	313	6	4	154	53	0	52	10
Caramel Steamer w/ 2% milk & w/o whipped cream, Regular (12 oz)	304	6	4	154	52	0	51	10
Sugar Free Caramel Steamer w/ 2% milk & w/o whipped cream, Regular (12 oz)	160	6	4	154	16	0	15	10
Sugar Free Vanilla Steamer w/ 2% milk & w/o whipped cream, Regular (12 oz)	160	6	4	154	16	0	15	10
Hazelnut Steamer w/ 2% milk & w/o whipped cream, Regular (12 oz)	299	6	4	154	51	0	50	10

Description & Serving	Cal	Fat	Sfat	Sod	Carb	Fiber	Sugar	Prot
Raspberry Steamer w/ 2% milk & w/o whipped cream, Regular (12 oz)	313	6	4	154	54	0	53	10
Vanilla Steamer w/ 2% milk & w/o whipped cream, Regular (12 oz)	311	6	4	154	53	0	52	10
Toasted Steamer w/ 2% milk & w/o whipped cream, Regular (12 oz)	310	6	4	154	52	0	51	10
Single Espresso Shot	5	0	0	0	1	0	0	1
Double Espresso Shot	10	0	0	0	2	0	0	2
Cold								
Iced Latte w/ 2% milk, Regular (16 oz)	212	4	3	108	35	0	25	8
Iced Caramel Vanilla Latte w/ 2% milk, Regular (16 oz)	286	4	3	108	53	0	43	8
Iced Chai Latte w/ 2% milk, Regular (16 oz)	252	4	3	108	44	0	43	7
Iced Sugar Free Caramel Vanilla Latte w/ 2% milk, Regular (16 oz)	212	4	3	108	35	0	25	8
Iced Caramel Hazelnut Latte w/ 2% milk, Regular (16 oz)	283	4	3	108	53	0	43	8
Iced Dark Chocolate Mocha w/ 2% milk, Regular (16 oz)	292	4	3	123	53	1	43	9
Iced White Chocolate Mocha w/ 2% milk, Regular (16 oz)	292	4	3	168	55	0	42	8
Iced Sugar Free Dark Chocolate Mocha w/ 2% milk, Regular (16 oz)	292	4	3	143	59	1	25	9
Frozen Latte w/ 2% milk & w/o whipped cream, Regular (16 oz)	268	10	7	87	44	0	33	7
Frozen Caramel & Vanilla Latte, Regular (16 oz)	317	10	7	87	56	0	45	7
Frozen Soy Milk Latte, Regular (16 oz)	175	3	0	59	34	1	23	5
Frozen Sugar Free Caramel Vanilla Latte, Regular (16 oz)	268	10	7	87	44	0	33	7
Frozen Caramel & Hazelnut Latte, Regular (16 oz)	315	10	7	87	56	0	45	7
Frozen Dark Chocolate Mocha, Regular (16 oz)	348	10	7	102	62	1	51	8
Frozen White Chocolate Mocha, Regular (16 oz)	348	10	7	147	64	0	50	7
Frozen Sugar Free Dark Chocolate Mocha, Regular (16 oz)	348	10	7	122	68	1	33	8
Frozen Vanilla Cream, Regular (16 oz)	244	14	10	124	28	0	27	8
Frozen Dark Chocolate Cream, Regular (16 oz)	324	14	10	139	46	1	45	9
Frozen White Chocolate Cream, Regular (16 oz)	324	14	10	184	48	0	44	8
Frozen Sugar Free Dark Chocolate Cream, Regular (16 oz)	324	14	10	159	52	1	27	9
Frozen Cookies N Cream Cream, Regular (16 oz)	764	35	17	738	108	5	74	13
Chocolate Covered Strawberry Smoothie, Regular (16 oz)	329	0	0	21	80	6	64	1
PB & J Smoothie, Regular (16 oz)	378	0	0	62	92	2	88	4
PB & B Smoothie, Regular (16 oz)	389	0	0	25	96	5	48	0
Wildberry Banana Smoothie, Regular (16 oz)	349	0	0	4	83	4	59	0
Orange Smoothie, Regular (16 oz)	318	8	6	120	61	2	56	7
Strawberry Lemonade Smoothie, Regular (16 oz)	288	0	0	13	71	4	51	0
Wildberry Lemonade Smoothie, Regular (16 oz)	349	0	0	4	83	3	64	0
Strawberry Banana Smoothie, Regular (16 oz)	288	0	0	13	71	5	46	0

Description & Serving	Cal	Fat	Sfat	Sod	Carb	Fiber	Sugar	Prot
Add-On								
Whipped Cream	15	2	1	0	1	0	1	0
Power Shake Smoothie Addition	118	1	1	76	11	1	2	16
Yogurt Smoothie Addition	97	<1	0	67	17	0	7	3
Protein Smoothie Addition	12	0	0	0	0	0	0	3
Fat-Burner Smoothie Addition	0	0	0	0	0	0	0	0
Multivitamin Smoothie Addition	0	0	0	0	0	0	0	0
Cream Base Smoothie Addition	180	12	9	62	22	0	21	4
Dressing/Condiment								
Italian Romano Dressing (for salad)	140	14	2	740	4	0	3	1
Ranch Dressing (for salad)	260	28	4	240	2	0	2	1
Fat Free Italian Dressing (for salad)	20	0	0	700	5	0	3	0
Blue Cheese Dressing (for salad)	300	31	5	650	3	0	3	1
Honey Mustard Dressing (for salad)	186	16	2	301	10	0	9	0
BBQ Sauce (for 6" sub, burger, wrap, or sandwich)	35	0	0	156	9	0	9	0
Buffalo Sauce (for 6" sub, burger, wrap, or sandwich)	5	0	0	414	0	0	0	0
Butter	202	22	16	172	0	0	0	0
Chili Sauce	46	4	2	132	2	<1	0	2
Grape Jelly	106	0	0	0	27	0	24	0
Honey Mustard Dressing (for 6" sub, burger, wrap, or sandwich)	11	0	0	57	5	2	2	0
Italian Romano Dressing (for 6" sub, burger, wrap, or sandwich)	57	6	<1	295	2	0	1	<1
Ketchup (for 6" sub, burger, wrap, or sandwich)	15	0	0	190	4	0	4	0
Marinara Sauce (for 6" sub, burger, wrap, or sandwich)	11	<1	0	96	1	<1	<1	<1
Mayonnaise (for 6" sub, burger, wrap, or sandwich)	142	16	3	128	0	0	0	0
Ranch Dressing (for 6" sub, burger, wrap, or sandwich)	151	16	2	142	2	0	<1	<1
Relish	27	0	0	107	5	0	5	0
Salsa	9	0	0	151	2	0	0	0
Sauerkraut	9	0	0	323	2	2	2	0
Sour Cream (for salad)	111	11	6	46	4	0	2	2
Strawberry Jelly	106	0	0	0	27	0	24	27
Syrup	120	0	0	35	31	0	17	0
Taco Sauce	9	0	0	111	2	0	<1	0
Yellow Mustard (for 6" sub, burger, wrap, or sandwich)	12	0	0	119	0	0	0	0
Topping								
Hot Pepper Cheese (for 6" sub, burger, wrap, or sandwich)	101	8	5	172	1	0	0	7
Cheddar Cheese (for 6" sub, burger, wrap, or sandwich)	111	9	5	172	1	0	0	7
Provolone Cheese (for 6" sub, burger, wrap, or sandwich)	101	8	4	243	1	0	0	7

Description & Serving	Cal	Fat	Sfat	Sod	Carb	Fiber	Sugar	Prot
Swiss Cheese (for 6" sub, burger, wrap, or sandwich)	101	8	5	61	1	0	0	8
Yellow American Cheese (for 6" sub, burger, wrap, or sandwich)	116	9	5	387	1	0	0	6
Nacho Cheese (for 6" sub, burger, wrap, or sandwich)	50	4	1	446	3	0	0	<1
Parmesan Cheese (for 6" sub, burger, wrap, or sandwich)	3	<1	<1	13	<1	0	<1	<1
Pickles (for 6" sub, burger, wrap, or sandwich)	0	0	0	222	<1	0	<1	0
Bacon (for 6" sub, burger, wrap, or sandwich)	150	12	4	723	2	0	0	12
Cooked Peppers (for 6" sub, burger, wrap, or sandwich)	24	1	0	151	2	<1	<1	0
Cooked Onions (for 6" sub, burger, wrap, or sandwich)	19	<1	0	57	2	0	<1	0
Jalapeño Peppers (for 6" sub, burger, wrap, or sandwich)	6	0	0	272	<1	0	0	0
Mild Pepper Rings (for 6" sub, burger, wrap, or sandwich)	3	0	0	267	<1	0	0	0
Shredded Lettuce (for 6" sub, burger, wrap, or sandwich)	4	0	0	3	<1	<1	<1	<1
Black Olives (for 6" sub, burger, wrap, or sandwich)	12	1	<1	64	<1	<1	0	<1
Green Peppers (for 6" sub, burger, wrap, or sandwich)	4	<1	0	<1	<1	<1	0	<1
Sliced Tomatoes (for 6" sub, burger, wrap, or sandwich)	6	<1	0	2	1	0	0	<1
Diced Onions (for 6" sub, burger, wrap, or sandwich)	6	<1	0	<1	1	0	0	<1
Shredded Jack Cheese (for salad)	111	9	6	182	1	0	0	7
Crackers (for salad)	24	<1	<1	92	4	8	0	0
Pickles (for salad)	0	0	0	222	<1	0	<1	0
Jalapeño Peppers (for salad)	6	0	0	272	<1	0	0	0
Mild Pepper Rings (for salad)	3	0	0	267	<1	0	0	0
Green Peppers (for salad)	4	<1	0	<1	<1	<1	0	<1
Bacon Bits (for salad)	38	3	1	170	0	0	0	2
Black Olives (for salad)	12	1	<1	64	<1	<1	0	<1
Diced Tomatoes (for salad)	4	<1	0	2	<1	0	0	<1
Diced Onions (for salad)	6	<1	0	<1	1	0	0	<1

Sizzler

Prepared Salad

	Cal	Fat	Sfat	Sod	Carb	Fiber	Sugar	Prot
Ambrosia Salad, 4 oz	123	4	4	30	22	2	16	1
Caesar Salad, 2 oz	25	2	0	35	1	0	0	1
Carrot Raisin Salad, 2 oz	55	3	1	37	6	1	5	0
Creamy Cole Slaw, 2 oz	34	2	0	104	3	0	3	0
Cucumber Tomato Salad, 2 oz	12	0	0	148	2	0	1	0
Greek Salad, 2 oz	22	2	0	104	1	0	0	1
Hearts of Palm Pasta Salad, 2 oz	26	0	0	42	5	1	1	1
Macaroni Salad, 4 oz	224	12	2	564	27	1	9	3

Description & Serving	Cal	Fat	Sfat	Sod	Carb	Fiber	Sugar	Prot
Potato Salad, 4 oz	325	27	5	638	18	1	8	2
Seafood Salad, 4 oz	159	11	2	536	11	0	3	6
Sicilian Pasta Salad, 2 oz	64	4	1	117	6	0	1	1
Spinach Cranberry Salad, 2 oz	18	1	0	6	2	0	2	0
Strawberry Banana Salad, 4 oz	82	0	0	9	19	2	11	1
Three Bean Salad, 1 oz	25	1	0	70	5	1	2	1
Tuna Pasta Salad, 4 oz	207	19	3	374	1	0	1	8
Waldorf Salad, 4 oz	124	8	1	41	13	1	11	1

Salad Bar

Description & Serving	Cal	Fat	Sfat	Sod	Carb	Fiber	Sugar	Prot
Artichoke Hearts, 2 oz	52	3	0	188	4	0	0	2
Baby Corn, 2 oz	13	0	0	140	2	1	1	1
Bacon Bits, 1 oz	54	3	1	313	3	1	1	4
Bean Sprouts, 2 oz	6	0	0	19	1	0	0	0
Beets, Pickled, 2 oz	8	0	0	53	2	1	1	0
Bell Peppers, Green, 2 oz	5	0	0	1	1	0	1	0
Black Olives, Sliced, 1 oz	30	3	0	140	1	0	0	0
Blue Cheese Crumbles, 1 oz	51	4	3	192	0	0	0	3
Broccoli Florets, 2 oz	6	0	0	5	1	0	0	1
Cantaloupe, 1 wedge	27	0	0	11	6	1	6	1
Carrots, 2 oz	12	0	0	19	3	1	1	0
Cauliflower, 2 oz	8	0	0	8	1	1	1	0
Cheddar Cheese, 2 oz	111	9	6	182	0	0	0	7
Cherry Tomatoes, 2 oz	8	0	0	2	1	0	1	0
Cottage Cheese, Low Fat, 1 oz	25	1	0	95	1	0	1	4
Croutons, 1 oz	30	1	0	90	5	0	0	1
Cucumbers, Sliced, 2 oz	5	0	0	1	1	0	0	0
Eggs, Chopped, 2 oz	51	4	1	42	0	0	0	4
Garbanzo Beans, 1 oz	25	0	0	125	4	2	0	2
Grapes, 4 oz	15	0	0	0	4	0	3	0
Green Beans, 1 oz	5	0	0	1	1	0	0	0
Green Onions, 1 oz	5	0	0	2	1	0	0	0
Honeydew Melon, 1 wedge	23	0	0	10	5	0	5	0
Jicama, 2 oz	6	0	0	1	1	1	0	0
Kidney Beans, 1 oz	25	0	0	130	4	2	1	1
Mushrooms, 2 oz	5	0	0	1	1	0	0	1
Parmesan Cheese, 1 oz	51	4	2	218	1	0	1	5
Peas, 1 oz	15	0	0	1	3	1	1	1
Pineapple, 1 slice	30	0	0	1	7	1	5	0
Radishes, 2 oz	5	0	0	11	1	0	1	0
Raisins, 1 oz	65	0	0	5	16	1	15	1
Red Cabbage, 2 oz	6	0	0	5	1	0	1	0
Red Onions, 2 oz	13	0	0	1	3·	0	1	0
Roasted Corn & Peppers, 1 oz	27	1	0	27	5	1	1	1
Romaine & Iceberg Lettuce Mix, 2 oz	2	0	0	1	0	0	0	0
Spinach, 2 oz	2	0	0	6	0	0	0	0
Spring Lettuce Mix, 2 oz	3	0	0	9	1	0	0	0
Strawberries, 1 berry	4	0	0	0	1	0	1	0
Sunflower Seeds, 1 oz	118	11	1	115	3	2	0	4
Turkey Ham, 1 oz	38	3	1	169	1	0	1	2

Description & Serving	Cal	Fat	Sfat	Sod	Carb	Fiber	Sugar	Prot
Watermelon, 1 wedge	19	0	0	1	4	0	4	0
Zucchini, 2 oz	6	0	0	3	1	0	1	0

Soup

Description & Serving	Cal	Fat	Sfat	Sod	Carb	Fiber	Sugar	Prot
Broccoli Cheese Soup, 1 bowl	305	19	15	563	28	0	3	5
Chicken Noodle Soup, 1 bowl	98	2	0	623	14	0	0	5
Chicken Tortilla Soup, 1 bowl	102	3	0	1071	15	3	3	3
Clam Chowder, 1 bowl	327	18	14	830	35	0	2	5
French Onion Soup, 1 bowl	53	2	0	527	6	0	5	2
Menudo, 1 bowl	68	2	1	426	7	2	0	6
Minestrone Soup, 1 bowl	68	1	0	683	14	2	3	3
Split Pea Soup, 1 bowl	113	1	0	782	19	2	3	7
Vegetable Steak Soup, 1 bowl	109	6	2	651	9	1	2	5
Vegetable Soup, 1 bowl	53	0	0	653	10	2	6	2

Burger/Sandwich

Description & Serving	Cal	Fat	Sfat	Sod	Carb	Fiber	Sugar	Prot
Mega Bacon Cheeseburger, 1/2 lb	1008	61	25	2486	48	3	8	64
Sizzler Burger, 1/3 lb	618	30	9	1355	47	3	8	36
Sizzler Burger, 1/2 lb	760	40	13	1394	47	3	8	49
Crispy Chicken Sandwich	592	27	4	1052	61	4	7	26
Grilled Chicken Club	666	31	10	1350	48	3	8	45
Malibu Chicken Sandwich	643	32	10	1296	57	3	8	30

Entrée

Chicken

Description & Serving	Cal	Fat	Sfat	Sod	Carb	Fiber	Sugar	Prot
Grilled Chicken Fettuccine Alfredo	1018	59	36	2219	62	2	9	50
Chicken Breast Strips	510	24	4	2173	45	0	15	27
Hibachi Chicken, single	201	7	1	704	7	0	5	26
Lemon Herb Chicken, single	215	11	3	596	1	0	0	26
Malibu Chicken, single	303	20	8	607	10	0	1	20

Pork

Description & Serving	Cal	Fat	Sfat	Sod	Carb	Fiber	Sugar	Prot
Ribs, half rack	623	39	15	1105	37	0	24	28
Ribs, full rack	1157	79	30	1609	51	0	34	57

Seafood

Description & Serving	Cal	Fat	Sfat	Sod	Carb	Fiber	Sugar	Prot
Grilled Salmon w/ Rice Pilaf	532	20	4	921	40	1	1	47
Fish 'n Chips	1037	49	10	2839	111	4	8	40
Fisherman's Platter	819	34	6	2413	82	5	8	45
Grilled Shrimp Fettuccini Alfredo	986	55	35	2082	64	2	9	53
Grilled Shrimp Skewers	543	26	5	1332	42	2	1	33
Half Dozen Fried Shrimp	216	6	1	1131	24	1	1	15
Shrimp Fry Dozen	433	12	1	2263	48	2	2	29
Shrimp, Shrimp, Shrimp	970	41	11	3210	92	5	4	51
Unlimited Shrimp, 12 pc	267	7	1	1392	30	1	1	18

Steak

Description & Serving	Cal	Fat	Sfat	Sod	Carb	Fiber	Sugar	Prot
Chopped Steak, 8 oz	519	30	11	1402	17	1	2	42
Classic Steak, 6 oz	256	12	2	1475	2	0	0	32
Classic Steak, 8 oz	318	14	3	1578	2	0	1	41
Filet Mignon, 6 oz	466	35	13	1183	1	0	0	34
Flat Iron Steak, 10 oz	798	65	25	1288	1	0	0	48

Description & Serving	Cal	Fat	Sfat	Sod	Carb	Fiber	Sugar	Prot
Porterhouse, 18 oz	1363	107	41	1363	1	0	0	92
Prime Rib w/ Au Jus & Horseradish, 10 oz	782	63	25	326	1	0	0	50
Rib Eye, 12 oz	949	62	23	1278	1	0	0	91
Bacon Wrapped Sirloin Filets	553	35	11	2324	5	1	1	49
Burgundy Mushroom Sirloin Tips w/ Rice Pilaf	869	36	10	3197	85	3	4	47
Steak Combination								
Big Appetite Trio	1058	46	12	4511	68	2	7	82
Classic Trio	698	32	10	3025	32	1	1	64
Steak & Colossal Shrimp	625	19	4	2513	43	2	1	66
Steak & Grilled Shrimp Skewers	639	27	5	2513	43	2	1	51
Steak & Half Dozen Fried Shrimp	472	17	3	2607	26	1	1	47
Steak & Hibachi Chicken	457	19	4	2179	9	0	5	58
Steak & Lemon Herb Chicken	471	23	5	2071	4	0	0	58
Steak & Lobster Tail	369	13	2	1939	4	1	0	56
Steak & Malibu Chicken	559	32	10	2082	12	0	1	52
Steak & Shrimp Fry Dozen	689	23	4	3738	50	2	2	61
Steak & Shrimp Scampi w/ Rice Pilaf	920	60	11	2808	44	1	2	44
Steak & Unlimited Shrimp, 12 pc	523	19	3	2867	32	1	1	50
Ultimate Sizzlin' Trio	1410	86	21	4281	74	9	10	83
Side								
Baked Potato	265	4	1	15	51	4	2	6
Broccoli, 5 oz	51	0	0	38	7	3	2	4
Cheese Toast, 1 slice	237	19	4	416	13	1	0	5
French Fries, 5 oz	286	13	3	783	42	3	0	3
Rice Pilaf, 5 oz	224	4	1	743	39	1	1	5
Smashed Potatoes, 6 oz	158	6	2	486	24	2	1	2
Kids								
Cheese Pizza, 4 slices	390	16	8	720	47	2	4	15
Classic Steak, 6 oz	256	12	2	1475	2	0	0	32
Dino Chicken Nuggets	283	16	3	640	17	1	1	15
Fried Shrimp	334	18	4	704	31	1	0	12
Grilled Cheese	399	26	10	1142	28	0	2	12
Macaroni & Cheese	490	16	5	1190	68	3	16	17
Sizzler Burger, 1/3 lb	607	30	9	1192	45	2	7	35
Dressing/Condiment								
Balsamic Vinaigrette, 1 oz	90	8	1	300	4	0	3	0
Signature Blue Cheese Dressing, 1 oz	106	11	4	156	1	0	1	1
Caesar Dressing, 1 oz	160	17	3	240	1	0	0	1
French Dressing, 1 oz	130	12	2	270	6	0	6	0
Italian Dressing, 1 oz	80	8	1	330	2	0	2	0
Low Fat Italian Dressing, 1 oz	40	3	1	270	3	0	2	0
Honey Mustard Dressing, 1 oz	110	8	1	270	9	0	8	0
Ranch Dressing, 1 oz	113	12	3	197	1	0	1	0
Thousand Island Dressing, 1 oz	97	9	2	355	5	0	5	1
BBQ Sauce, 1.5 oz	90	0	0	600	23	0	15	0
Burger Sauce, 1 oz	156	16	3	195	3	0	2	0
Burgundy Mushroom Sauce, 2 oz	41	3	1	357	3	0	1	1

Description & Serving	Cal	Fat	Sfat	Sod	Carb	Fiber	Sugar	Prot
Cocktail Sauce, 1.5 oz	42	0	0	452	10	1	9	1
Dill Tartar Sauce, 1.5 oz	210	23	4	256	1	0	0	0
Garlic Margarine, 1.5 oz	263	29	5	325	1	0	0	0
Hibachi Sauce, 1 oz	46	0	0	727	10	0	7	1
Lemon Herb Sauce, 1 oz	45	4	2	256	1	0	0	0
Malibu Sauce, 1.5 oz	270	30	5	241	0	0	0	0
Savory Butter, 1.5 oz	383	43	5	0	0	0	0	0

Skyline Chili

Chili Bowl

	Cal	Fat	Sfat	Sod	Carb	Fiber	Sugar	Prot
Chili Bowl	270	16	NP	1110	6	1	3	25
Chili Cheese Bowl	440	30	NP	1380	6	1	3	35
Chili Bean Bowl	270	12	NP	840	17	6	3	23
Loaded Chili Bowl	580	40	NP	1450	18	4	5	38
Coney Bowl	870	69	NP	2170	9	2	4	54
Vegetarian Black Beans & Rice Bowl	320	9	NP	1090	46	8	3	12

Chili & Spaghetti/Rice

	Cal	Fat	Sfat	Sod	Carb	Fiber	Sugar	Prot
Chili Spaghetti 3-Way, sml	380	22	NP	1420	22	2	2	23
Chili Spaghetti 3-Way, reg	760	44	NP	2850	43	3	4	46
Chili Spaghetti 3-Way, lrg	1070	64	NP	3880	58	5	5	65
Chili Spaghetti 4-Way Onion, sml	390	22	NP	1420	23	2	2	23
Chili Spaghetti 4-Way Onion, reg	770	44	NP	2850	46	4	5	47
Chili Spaghetti 4-Way Onion, lrg	1090	64	NP	3890	62	5	7	66
Chili Spaghetti 4-Way Bean, sml	420	23	NP	1440	29	4	2	26
Chili Spaghetti 4-Way Bean, reg	850	45	NP	2880	59	9	5	52
Chili Spaghetti 4-Way Bean, lrg	1230	67	NP	4070	61	12	7	76
Chili Spaghetti 5-Way, sml	420	22	NP	1420	29	4	3	25
Chili Spaghetti 5-Way, reg	840	45	NP	2850	58	9	6	51
Chili Spaghetti 5-Way, lrg	1230	65	NP	4130	87	13	9	73
Chili Spaghetti, sml	230	9	NP	1230	22	2	2	14
Chili Spaghetti, reg	450	18	NP	2460	43	4	4	28
Chili Spaghetti, lrg	620	26	NP	3370	58	5	5	40
Chili Spaghetti Onion, sml	230	9	NP	1230	23	2	2	14
Chili Spaghetti Onion, reg	470	17	NP	2570	51	4	5	26
Chili Spaghetti Onion, lrg	640	26	NP	3370	62	5	7	40
Chili Spaghetti Bean, sml	260	9	NP	1230	28	4	2	16
Chili Spaghetti Bean, reg	520	17	NP	2570	61	9	4	30
Chili Spaghetti Bean, lrg	730	23	NP	3590	87	13	6	42
Chili Spaghetti Bean & Onion, sml	270	9	NP	1280	32	5	3	15
Chili Spaghetti Bean & Onion, reg	530	17	NP	2570	64	9	6	31
Chili Spaghetti Bean & Onion, lrg	750	24	NP	3590	92	14	8	42
Black Bean & Rice Spaghetti, sml	250	6	NP	1280	40	5	2	8
Black Bean & Rice Spaghetti, reg	490	12	NP	2550	79	9	3	16
Black Bean & Rice Spaghetti, lrg	680	16	NP	3570	110	13	4	23
Black Bean & Rice 3-Way, sml	420	20	NP	1540	40	5	2	19
Black Bean & Rice 3-Way, reg	800	40	NP	2830	74	9	4	36
Black Bean & Rice 3-Way, lrg	1160	58	NP	4110	105	12	5	53
Black Bean & Rice 4-Way, sml	430	20	NP	1540	44	5	4	19

Description & Serving	Cal	Fat	Sfat	Sod	Carb	Fiber	Sugar	Prot
Black Bean & Rice 4-Way, reg	810	40	NP	2830	77	9	5	37
Black Bean & Rice 4-Way, lrg	1170	58	NP	4110	109	13	7	54
Black Bean & Rice 5-Way, sml	470	20	NP	1540	50	8	4	21
Black Bean & Rice 5-Way, reg	880	40	NP	2830	89	14	6	41
Black Bean & Rice 5-Way, lrg	1240	58	NP	3860	121	20	8	59

Hot Dog

Description & Serving	Cal	Fat	Sfat	Sod	Carb	Fiber	Sugar	Prot
Regular Coney w/o cheese	220	12	NP	560	17	1	3	11
Cheese Coney	340	22	NP	730	17	1	3	18

Burrito

Description & Serving	Cal	Fat	Sfat	Sod	Carb	Fiber	Sugar	Prot
Black Bean Burrito	600	25	NP	1090	67	9	4	25
Black Bean Burrito Deluxe	690	30	NP	1190	75	11	9	27
Chili Bean Mix Burrito	610	30	NP	960	54	8	4	30
Chili Bean Mix Burrito Deluxe	700	36	NP	1060	62	10	10	33
All Chili Burrito	560	30	NP	1100	37	3	4	34
All Chili Burrito Deluxe	650	35	NP	1200	45	6	9	37
Chili Cheese Melt	350	16	NP	390	33	2	2	17

Sandwich/Wrap

Description & Serving	Cal	Fat	Sfat	Sod	Carb	Fiber	Sugar	Prot
Regular Chili Sandwich w/o cheese	180	7	NP	580	17	1	3	12
Chili Cheese Sandwich	290	17	NP	760	17	1	3	19
Classic Chicken Wrap w/o dressing	510	21	NP	1300	55	3	3	31
Greek Chicken Wrap w/o dressing	510	21	NP	2070	54	7	7	29
Buffalo Chicken Wrap w/o dressing	520	21	NP	1460	55	3	3	31
Southwest Chicken Wrap w/o dressing	670	30	NP	2040	65	6	8	34

Salad

Description & Serving	Cal	Fat	Sfat	Sod	Carb	Fiber	Sugar	Prot
Greek Salad w/o dressing	60	3.5	NP	210	5	2	3	3
Garden Salad w/o dressing	80	5	NP	105	6	2	3	5
Classic Chicken Salad w/o dressing	150	7	NP	480	8	2	4	17
Greek Chicken Salad w/o dressing	170	8	NP	2830	9	8	5	18
Buffalo Chicken Salad w/o dressing	150	7	NP	640	7	2	4	17
Southwest Chicken Salad w/o dressing & tortilla chips	460	16	NP	1260	18	5	6	25
Southwest Chicken Salad w/ tortilla chips & w/o dressing	760	44	NP	1570	66	8	5	30

Side

Description & Serving	Cal	Fat	Sfat	Sod	Carb	Fiber	Sugar	Prot
Plain Potato	310	0	NP	25	72	6	5	7
Chili Potato	440	8	NP	580	74	7	6	19
Sour Cream Potato	570	27	NP	290	72	6	5	7
Cheddar Potato	740	41	NP	590	72	6	5	21
3-Way Potato	870	49	NP	1140	75	7	6	33
4-Way Potato	890	49	NP	1150	78	7	7	33
5-Way Potato	950	50	NP	1150	90	12	9	37
French Fries	630	33	NP	430	79	6	1	8
Side of Cheese	230	19	NP	350	1	0	0	14
Side of Chili	130	8	NP	560	3	1	1	12
Bowl of Crackers	100	3	NP	300	20	<1	0	3
Garlic Bread Half	200	15	NP	240	16	0	0	3
Cheddar Bread Half	260	20	NP	320	16	0	0	6

Description & Serving	Cal	Fat	Sfat	Sod	Carb	Fiber	Sugar	Prot
Kids								
Kids P'sghetti Special	280	16	NP	1010	19	1	1	14
Kids 3-Way Special	380	22	NP	1420	22	2	2	23
Kids Single Wiener Hot Doggy Special w/o cheese	160	9	NP	260	14	0	2	5
Kids Single Wiener Hot Doggy Special w/ cheese	270	18	NP	430	15	0	2	12
Kids Double Wiener Hot Doggy Special w/o cheese	250	17	NP	430	15	0	3	8
Kids Double Wiener Hot Doggy Special w/ cheese	360	26	NP	600	16	0	3	15
Kids Coney Special w/o cheese	210	12	NP	480	15	1	3	10
Kids Coney Special w/ cheese	330	22	NP	650	16	1	3	17
Dressing/Condiment								
Honey French Dressing	210	18	NP	310	14	0	13	0
Light Italian Dressing	20	1	NP	770	2	0	2	0
Dijon Honey Mustard Dressing	180	17	NP	240	8	0	7	1
Chili Ranch Dressing	275	29	NP	606	0	0	2	0
Greek Salad Dressing	250	28	NP	470	1	0	0	0
Light Ranch Dressing	70	4	NP	310	8	0	3	1
Buttermilk Ranch Dressing	230	24	NP	390	2	0	2	1

Smoothie King

Description & Serving	Cal	Fat	Sfat	Sod	Carb	Fiber	Sugar	Prot
Stay Healthy Smoothies								
Blueberry Heaven, 20 oz	325	1	0	259	73	2	64	7
Cranberry Cooler, 20 oz	496	0	0	38	120	3	89	1
Cranberry Supreme, 20 oz	554	1	0	87	130	3	96	4
Hearty Apple, 20 oz	405	1	0	271	86	2	75	9
Immune Builder, 20 oz	380	1	0	57	89	6	77	5
Kiwi Island Treat, 20 oz	498	1	0	147	116	0	96	6
Mangosteen Madness, 20 oz	383	0	0	29	94	2	92	1
Orange Ka-BAM, 20 oz	465	0	0	190	117	3	108	1
Pomegranate Punch, 20 oz	464	0	0	9	110	1	108	1
Yerba Maté - Mango, 20 oz	372	0	0	13	91	2	75	1
Yerba Maté - Mixed Berry, 20 oz	348	0	0	22	84	3	81	2
Yerba Maté - Pomegranate, 20 oz	372	0	0	9	91	2	73	1
Trim Down Smoothies								
Angel Food, 20 oz	354	0	0	50	84	6	75	4
Blackberry Dream, 20 oz	365	1	0	8	88	2	68	2
Celestial Cherry High, 20 oz	341	0	0	7	82	3	53	2
Island Impact, 20 oz	312	0	0	142	73	2	67	4
Island Treat, 20 oz	333	0	0	11	81	6	69	3
Low-Carb Banana, 20 oz	268	9	4	176	7	1	3	39
Low-Carb Chocolate, 20 oz	268	9	4	176	7	1	3	39
Low-Carb Strawberry, 20 oz	268	9	4	176	7	1	3	39
Low-Carb Vanilla, 20 oz	268	9	4	176	7	1	3	39
MangoFest, 20 oz	285	0	0	10	72	1	69	0
Muscle Punch, 20 oz	364	1	0	50	84	6	75	5
Muscle Punch Plus, 20 oz	366	1	0	57	84	6	75	5
Passion Passport, 20 oz	395	0	0	10	96	2	92	2
Peach Slice, 20 oz	314	0	0	63	72	2	55	4

Description & Serving	Cal	Fat	Sfat	Sod	Carb	Fiber	Sugar	Prot
Pineapple Pleasure, 20 oz	280	0	0	21	66	3	61	2
Raspberry Collider, 20 oz	344	0	0	102	88	4	74	1
Raspberry Sunrise, 20 oz	392	0	0	22	95	2	73	2
The Shredder - Chocolate, 20 oz	311	3	0	315	36	1	19	39
The Shredder - Strawberry, 20 oz	356	1	0	329	56	3	41	30
The Shredder - Vanilla, 20 oz	283	2	0	592	30	0	12	36
Slim-N-Trim Chocolate, 20 oz	297	2	0	165	57	3	48	15
Slim-N-Trim Orange-Vanilla, 20 oz	215	1	0	259	46	0	38	7
Slim-N-Trim Strawberry, 20 oz	375	1	0	259	84	5	72	8
Slim-N-Trim Vanilla, 20 oz	253	1	0	259	53	3	42	7
Strawberry Kiwi Breeze, 20 oz	376	0	0	131	90	3	84	4
Youth Fountain, 20 oz	253	0	0	29	61	3	54	3

Get Energy Smoothies

Açaí Adventure, 20 oz	435	5	1	163	92	4	75	5
Coffee Smoothie Caramel, 20 oz	340	1	0	236	66	0	56	14
Coffee Smoothie Mocha, 20 oz	260	2	0	226	43	1	36	17
Coffee Smoothie Vanilla, 20 oz	347	1	0	236	69	0	65	14
Go Goji, 20 oz	433	0	0	38	104	0	104	1
Green Tea Tango, 20 oz	304	4	2	130	54	2	41	8
Instant Vigor, 20 oz	366	0	0	139	86	4	72	4
Pep Upper, 20 oz	411	0	0	131	97	3	85	4
Power Punch, 20 oz	428	1	0	50	101	6	76	5
Power Punch Plus, 20 oz	500	1	0	59	113	6	85	8
Super Punch, 20 oz	395	0	0	194	100	6	90	2
Super Punch Plus, 20 oz	459	0	0	194	116	6	90	2

Build Up Smoothies

The Activator - Chocolate, 20 oz	404	1	0	119	83	5	56	19
The Activator - Strawberry, 20 oz	556	1	0	209	121	8	89	19
The Activator - Vanilla, 20 oz	406	1	0	209	83	5	54	18
Gladiator, 20 oz	180	NP	NP	150	1	NP	NP	45
High Protein Almond Mocha, 20 oz	366	9	1	195	42	2	37	30
High Protein Banana, 20 oz	322	9	1	297	32	4	23	27
High Protein Chocolate, 20 oz	366	9	1	194	42	2	37	30
High Protein Lemon, 20 oz	372	9	1	297	44	1	40	26
High Protein Pineapple, 20 oz	320	9	1	336	29	2	23	28
The Hulk - Chocolate, 20 oz	905	35	16	363	123	7	88	28
The Hulk - Strawberry, 20 oz	1044	35	16	351	157	8	120	26
The Hulk - Vanilla, 20 oz	901	35	16	358	120	5	86	26

Snack Right Smoothies

Banana Berry Treat, 20 oz	370	0	0	129	88	6	75	4
Berry Punch, 20 oz	367	0	0	95	93	4	84	0
Caribbean Way, 20 oz	395	0	0	4	97	6	88	2
Cherry Picker, 20 oz	439	0	0	237	103	2	51	5
Fruit Fusion, 20 oz	360	0	0	129	84	2	73	4
Grape Expectations, 20 oz	398	0	0	9	95	3	90	2
Grape Expectations II, 20 oz	548	0	0	9	133	6	125	2
Lemon Twist Banana, 20 oz	358	0	0	9	87	3	82	2
Lemon Twist Strawberry, 20 oz	438	0	0	9	107	3	103	1

Description & Serving	Cal	Fat	Sfat	Sod	Carb	Fiber	Sugar	Prot
Light & Fluffy, 20 oz	395	0	0	0	99	6	89	1
Peach Slice Plus, 20 oz	464	0	0	63	110	5	90	4
Pineapple Surf, 20 oz	461	1	0	279	104	4	92	7
Strawberry X-Treme, 20 oz	366	0	0	7	92	6	70	1
Indulge Smoothies								
Banana Boat, 20 oz	550	14	8	309	95	6	77	12
Coconut Surprise, 20 oz	460	7	6	145	90	3	83	7
Malts, 20 oz	755	39	24	213	82	0	77	17
Mo'cuccino Vanilla, 20 oz	551	14	8	311	91	0	85	10
Mo'cuccino Caramel, 20 oz	596	14	8	311	101	0	88	10
Mo'cuccino Mocha, 20 oz	470	14	8	135	72	1	69	11
Peanut Power, 20 oz	562	25	6	64	74	3	59	11
Peanut Power Plus Chocolate, 20 oz	730	30	6	376	98	3	63	20
Peanut Power Plus Grape, 20 oz	762	25	6	64	122	3	107	11
Peanut Power Plus Strawberry, 20 oz	712	25	6	64	112	6	94	11
Pina Colada Island, 20 oz	600	10	8	438	110	3	98	13
Shakes, 20 oz	745	39	24	213	80	0	76	17
Yogurt D-Lite, 20 oz	356	4	2	309	61	0	48	14
Kids' Kups								
Berry Interesting, 12 oz	277	0	0	11	69	3	62	1
Choc-A-Laka, 12 oz	252	3	1	161	45	2	32	12
CW, Jr., 12 oz	270	0	0	3	68	5	59	1
Gimme-Grape, 12 oz	265	0	0	9	64	2	59	1
Lil' Angel, 12 oz	223	0	0	7	56	5	47	1
Smarti Tarti, 12 oz	200	0	0	9	49	0	46	1

Sonic

Breakfast

	Cal	Fat	Sfat	Sod	Carb	Fiber	Sugar	Prot
Breakfast Toaster - Sausage, Egg & Cheese	620	42	13	1380	40	2	6	20
Breakfast Toaster - Bacon, Egg & Cheese	530	32	10	1440	40	2	7	20
Breakfast Burrito - Sausage, Egg & Cheese	480	31	11	1200	38	1	2	18
Breakfast Burrito - Bacon, Egg & Cheese	450	27	10	1290	38	1	2	19
SuperSonic Breakfast Burrito	570	36	12	1650	48	3	3	19
CroisSonic Breakfast Sandwich - Bacon, Egg & Cheese	510	36	15	1060	29	0	5	18
CroisSonic Breakfast Sandwich - Sausage, Egg & Cheese	600	46	18	1000	29	0	5	19
Sausage Biscuit Dippers w/ gravy, 3 pc	690	44	18	1770	57	0	7	16
Steak & Egg Breakfast Burrito	590	34	12	1370	47	5	3	28
French Toast Sticks, 4 pc	500	31	5	490	49	2	9	7
Jr. Breakfast Burrito	320	21	7	810	25	0	1	12

Burger/Hot Dog

	Cal	Fat	Sfat	Sod	Carb	Fiber	Sugar	Prot
Sonic Burger w/ mayonnaise	650	37	10	720	55	5	11	26
Sonic Burger w/ mustard	560	26	9	750	54	5	11	26
Sonic Burger w/ ketchup	560	26	9	820	57	5	14	26
Sonic Cheeseburger w/ mayonnaise	720	42	14	1040	56	5	12	29
Sonic Cheeseburger w/ mustard	620	31	12	1070	55	5	12	29

Description & Serving	Cal	Fat	Sfat	Sod	Carb	Fiber	Sugar	Prot
Sonic Cheeseburger w/ ketchup	630	31	12	1140	59	5	15	29
Sonic Bacon Cheeseburger w/ mayo	780	48	16	1300	57	5	12	33
SuperSonic Cheeseburger w/ mayo	980	64	24	1430	58	5	13	46
SuperSonic Cheeseburger w/ mustard	890	53	22	1460	57	5	13	46
SuperSonic Cheeseburger w/ ketchup	900	53	22	1540	60	5	16	46
Jr. Burger	310	15	5	610	30	3	7	15
Jr. Deluxe Burger	350	20	6	440	28	3	4	15
Jr. Bacon Cheeseburger	410	23	10	1060	31	3	8	20
Hickory Burger	580	26	9	850	60	5	16	25
California Cheeseburger	690	39	13	1060	57	5	13	29
SuperSonic Jalapeño Cheeseburger	890	53	22	1600	56	5	12	46
Thousand Island Burger	610	32	10	810	56	5	13	26
Jalapeño Cheeseburger	620	31	12	1200	54	5	11	28
Jalapeño Burger	550	26	9	880	53	5	10	25
Green Chili Cheeseburger	630	31	12	1070	56	5	12	29
Chili Cheeseburger	660	35	14	990	56	5	11	31
Hickory Cheeseburger	640	31	12	1170	61	5	17	28
Jr. Double Cheeseburger	570	35	16	1290	33	3	9	30
Bacon Cheeseburger Toaster Sandwich	670	39	14	1390	52	3	13	29
Ex-Long Chili Cheese Coney	660	39	15	1860	55	4	7	28
Corn Dog	210	11	3.5	530	23	2	4	6
Ex-Long Slaw Dog	670	38	12	1770	60	4	8	24
Regular Coney	390	23	9	1090	32	2	4	17

Sandwich/Wrap

Chicken Club Toaster Sandwich	740	46	11	1740	55	4	7	29
BLT Toaster Sandwich	500	29	7	950	45	2	7	17
Country Fried Steak Toaster Sandwich	670	37	10	1370	71	4	6	14
Grilled Chicken Bacon Ranch Sandwich	470	22	7	1620	35	3	10	35
Crispy Chicken Bacon Ranch Sandwich	610	34	9	1730	48	4	10	30
Grilled Chicken Sandwich	400	19	2.5	960	32	3	8	28
Crispy Chicken Sandwich	550	32	4.5	1070	46	4	8	22
Grilled Chicken Wrap	400	14	3.5	1420	39	2	5	28
Crispy Chicken Wrap	480	21	4.5	1360	54	3	5	20
Fritos Chili Cheese Wrap	670	39	13	1420	66	4	3	21
Jr. Fritos Chili Cheese Wrap	330	17	6	690	34	3	2	12

Salad

Grilled Chicken Salad	250	10	6	1070	12	3	6	29
Jumbo Popcorn Chicken Salad	420	25	8	1410	32	5	7	21
Santa Fe Grilled Chicken Salad	310	12	6	1160	22	6	6	31

Entrée

Chicken Strip Dinner, 4 pc	930	43	8	1610	100	7	7	36
Jumbo Popcorn Chicken, sml	380	22	5	1250	27	3	1	18
Jumbo Popcorn Chicken, lrg	560	32	6	1890	41	5	2	27

Snack/Side

Onion Rings, med	440	21	3.5	430	55	3	14	6
Onion Rings, lrg	640	31	5	630	80	4	20	9
Tater Tots, sml	200	13	2.5	440	20	2	0	2

Description & Serving	Cal	Fat	Sfat	Sod	Carb	Fiber	Sugar	Prot
Tater Tots, med	320	21	4	700	32	3	0	2
Tater Tots, lrg	530	34	6	1140	52	6	0	4
Tater Tots w/ cheese, sml	270	18	6	750	22	2	1	5
Tater Tots w/ cheese, med	420	28	9	1170	35	3	1	7
Tater Tots w/ cheese, lrg	660	44	13	1770	55	6	2	10
Tater Tots w/ chili & cheese, sml	290	21	7	710	23	3	1	7
Tater Tots w/ chili & cheese, med	490	34	11	1180	38	5	2	13
Tater Tots w/ chili & cheese, lrg	760	53	16	1830	61	7	2	18
French Fries, sml	200	8	1.5	270	30	2	0	2
French Fries, med	330	13	2.5	440	48	4	0	4
French Fries, lrg	450	18	3.5	600	67	5	0	5
French Fries w/ cheese, sml	270	13	5	590	32	2	1	5
French Fries w/ cheese, med	420	21	7	910	51	4	1	8
French Fries w/ cheese, lrg	580	28	10	1230	70	5	2	11
French Fries w/ chili & cheese, sml	300	16	6	540	33	3	1	8
French Fries w/ chili & cheese, med	490	27	10	920	54	5	1	14
French Fries w/ chili & cheese, lrg	690	37	13	1290	75	7	2	19
Pickle-O's	310	16	3	1020	36	2	2	5
Mozzarella Sticks	440	22	9	1050	40	2	1	19
Ched 'R' Peppers, 4 pc	330	17	6	1110	36	2	2	8
Fritos Chili Cheese Pie, med	470	32	9	770	36	3	1	13
Fritos Chili Cheese Pie, lrg	940	64	18	1540	72	6	3	25
Burrito	370	18	6	480	40	6	0	10
Burrito Deluxe	420	22	7	640	43	6	1	13
2 Tacos	340	20	6	360	35	4	1	8
Apple Slices	35	0	0	0	9	2	7	0
Apple Slices w/ Fat-Free Caramel Dipping Sauce	120	0	0	60	27	2	23	0

Kids

Description & Serving	Cal	Fat	Sfat	Sod	Carb	Fiber	Sugar	Prot
Jr. Burger	117	15	5	610	30	3	7	15
Corn Dog	74	11	3.5	530	23	2	4	6
Grilled Cheese Sandwich	110	20	8	1010	39	2	6	12
Chicken Strips, 2 pc	70	11	2	470	10	1	0	14
Apple Slices w/ Fat-Free Caramel Dipping Sauce	96	0	0	60	27	2	23	0
Lemon Real Fruit Slush, Wacky Pack size (12 oz)	170	0	0	25	46	0	44	0
Lemon-Berry Real Fruit Slush, Wacky Pack size (12 oz)	180	0	0	30	48	0	45	0
Lime Real Fruit Slush, Wacky Pack size (12 oz)	170	0	0	25	46	0	44	0
Strawberry Real Fruit Slush, Wacky Pack size (12 oz)	180	0	0	30	48	0	45	0
Cherry Slush, Wacky Pack size (12 oz)	170	0	0	25	46	0	46	0
Grape Slush, Wacky Pack size (12 oz)	170	0	0	30	45	0	45	0
Orange Slush, Wacky Pack size (12 oz)	170	0	0	30	45	0	45	0
Blue Coconut Slush, Wacky Pack size (12 oz)	170	0	0	25	45	0	44	0
Watermelon Slush, Wacky Pack size (12 oz)	170	0	0	30	46	0	45	0
Green Apple Slush, Wacky Pack size (12 oz)	180	0	0	30	48	0	46	0
Bubble Gum Slush, Wacky Pack size (12 oz)	170	0	0	30	45	0	45	0
Raspberry Iced Tea, Wacky Pack size (12 oz)	5	0	0	15	1	0	0	0
Peach Iced Tea, Wacky Pack size (12 oz)	5	0	0	15	1	0	0	0

Description & Serving	Cal	Fat	Sfat	Sod	Carb	Fiber	Sugar	Prot
Cranberry Iced Tea, Wacky Pack size (12 oz)	20	0	0	10	6	0	5	0
Limeade, Wacky Pack size (12 oz)	110	0	0	25	30	0	29	0
Low-Cal Diet Lime Limeade, Wacky Pack size (12 oz)	5	0	0	5	1	0	0	0
Cherry Limeade, Wacky Pack size (12 oz)	140	0	0	30	37	0	36	0
Low-Cal Diet Cherry Limeade, Wacky Pack size (12 oz)	10	0	0	10	2	0	1	0
Strawberry Limeade, Wacky Pack size (12 oz)	140	0	0	30	36	0	33	0
Minute Maid Apple Juice Limeade, Wacky Pack size (12 oz)	120	0	0	25	33	0	33	0
Minute Maid Cranberry Limeade, Wacky Pack size (12 oz)	120	0	0	25	33	0	32	0
Powerade Add-In Flavor, Wacky Pack amt	25	0	0	20	6	0	6	0
Vanilla Add-In Flavor, Wacky Pack amt	20	0	0	0	5	0	5	0
Cherry Add-In Flavor, Wacky Pack amt	30	0	0	0	8	0	7	0
Low-Cal Diet Cherry Add-In Flavor, Wacky Pack amt	5	0	0	0	2	0	1	0
Grape Add-In Flavor, Wacky Pack amt	20	0	0	5	5	0	5	0
Green Apple Add-In Flavor, Wacky Pack amt	30	0	0	0	7	0	6	0
Orange Add-In Flavor, Wacky Pack amt	20	0	0	0	5	0	4	0
Blue Coconut Add-In Flavor, Wacky Pack amt	20	0	0	0	1	0	4	0
Watermelon Add-In Flavor, Wacky Pack amt	25	0	0	0	6	0	4	0
Fresh Lemon Add-In Flavor, Wacky Pack amt	0	0	0	0	1	0	0	0
Fresh Lime Add-In Flavor, Wacky Pack amt	0	0	0	0	1	0	0	0
Minute Maid Apple Juice Add-In Flavor, Wacky Pack amt	15	0	0	0	4	0	4	0
Minute Maid Cranberry Add-In Flavor, Wacky Pack amt	20	0	0	0	5	0	5	0
Chocolate Topping, Wacky Pack amt	50	0	0	40	12	0	8	0
Strawberry Topping, Wacky Pack amt	35	0	0	0	8	0	5	0
Pineapple Topping, Wacky Pack amt	30	0	0	5	7	0	4	0

Dressing/Condiment

Description & Serving	Cal	Fat	Sfat	Sod	Carb	Fiber	Sugar	Prot
Original Ranch Dressing, 42.5 g	190	20	3.5	380	2	0	1	1
Original Light Ranch Dressing, 42.5 g	110	5	1	590	14	0	3	3
Honey Mustard, 42.5 g	180	16	2.5	240	10	0	8	1
Fat-Free Italian, 42.5 g	40	0	0	450	10	0	3	0
Thousand Island , 42.5 g	190	19	3	440	7	0	5	1
Ranch Sauce, 28 g	150	16	2.5	210	1	0	1	0
Honey Mustard Sauce, 29 g	90	7	1	190	7	0	5	0
BBQ Sauce, 30 g	45	0	0	390	11	0	7	0
Syrup	80	0	0	0	21	21	19	0
Mustard, 6 g	5	0	0	55	0	0	0	0
Mayonnaise, 12 g	80	9	1.5	60	0	0	0	0
Ketchup, 9 g	10	0	0	110	2	0	2	0
Marinara Sauce, 28 g	15	0	0	270	3	1	2	0
Picante Sauce, 14 g	5	0	0	140	1	0	0	0
Hickory Sauce, 26 g	40	0	0	410	9	0	8	0

Description & Serving	Cal	Fat	Sfat	Sod	Carb	Fiber	Sugar	Prot
Topping/Flavoring								
Cheese	60	5	3	310	2	0	1	3
Bacon	70	5	2	260	0	0	0	4
Chili	50	3.5	1.5	160	2	1	1	3
Jalapeño	5	0	0	280	1	1	0	0
Green Chilies	5	0	0	5	1	0	0	0
Slaw	45	3	0.5	45	4	1	1	0
Grilled Onions	25	2	0	200	2	1	1	0
Bubble Gum Add-In Flavor, sml	20	0	0	10	5	0	4	0
Powerade Add-In Flavor, sml	25	0	0	20	6	0	6	0
Vanilla Add-In Flavor, sml	20	0	0	0	5	0	5	0
Cherry Add-In Flavor, sml	30	0	0	0	8	0	7	0
Low-Cal Diet Cherry Add-In Flavor, sml	5	0	0	0	2	0	1	0
Grape Add-In Flavor, sml	20	0	0	5	5	0	5	0
Green Apple Add-In Flavor, sml	30	0	0	0	7	0	6	0
Orange Add-In Flavor, sml	20	0	0	0	5	0	4	0
Blue Coconut Add-In Flavor, sml	20	0	0	0	1	0	4	0
Watermelon Add-In Flavor, sml	25	0	0	0	6	0	4	0
Fresh Lemon Add-In Flavor, sml	0	0	0	0	1	0	0	0
Fresh Lime Add-In Flavor, sml	0	0	0	0	1	0	0	0
Minute Maid Apple Juice Add-In Flavor, sml	15	0	0	0	4	0	4	0
Minute Maid Cranberry Add-In Flavor, sml	20	0	0	0	5	0	5	0
Chocolate Topping, sml amt	50	0	0	40	12	0	8	0
Strawberry Topping, sml amt	35	0	0	0	8	0	5	0
Pineapple Topping, sml amt	30	0	0	5	7	0	4	0
Fruit Drink								
Tropical Fruit Smoothie, 14 oz	500	0	0	170	124	4	98	1
Strawberry Fruit Smoothie, 14 oz	540	0	0	120	134	3	99	4
Strawberry-Banana Fruit Smoothie, 14 oz	440	0	0	100	110	3	83	3
Lemon Real Fruit Slush, 14 oz	200	0	0	30	53	0	50	0
Lemon-Berry Real Fruit Slush, 14 oz	210	0	0	30	55	0	52	0
Lime Real Fruit Slush, 14 oz	200	0	0	30	52	0	50	0
Strawberry Real Fruit Slush, 14 oz	210	0	0	30	55	0	52	0
Cherry Slush, 14 oz	200	0	0	30	53	0	53	0
Grape Slush, 14 oz	190	0	0	35	52	0	52	0
Orange Slush, 14 oz	200	0	0	30	52	0	51	0
Blue Coconut Slush, 14 oz	190	0	0	30	52	0	51	0
Watermelon Slush, 14 oz	200	0	0	30	53	0	51	0
Green Apple Slush, 14 oz	200	0	0	30	54	0	53	0
Bubble Gum Slush, 14 oz	190	0	0	35	52	0	51	0
Raspberry Iced Tea, 14 oz	5	0	0	15	1	0	0	0
Peach Iced Tea, 14 oz	5	0	0	15	1	0	0	0
Cranberry Iced Tea, 14 oz	20	0	0	10	6	0	5	0
Limeade, 14 oz	140	0	0	30	38	0	37	0
Low-Cal Diet Lime Limeade, 14 oz	5	0	0	10	1	0	0	0
Cherry Limeade, 14 oz	170	0	0	35	45	0	44	0
Low-Cal Diet Cherry Limeade, 14 oz	10	0	0	10	2	0	1	0
Strawberry Limeade, 14 oz	170	0	0	35	45	0	41	0

Description & Serving	Cal	Fat	SFat	Sod	Carb	Fiber	Sugar	Prot
Minute Maid Apple Juice Limeade, 14 oz	160	0	0	35	42	0	41	0
Minute Maid Cranberry Limeade, 14 oz	150	0	0	35	41	0	41	0

Coffee Drink

Description & Serving	Cal	Fat	SFat	Sod	Carb	Fiber	Sugar	Prot
Coffee, 14 oz	10	0	0	35	2	1	0	1
Caramel Iced Latte, 14 oz	260	8	6	190	44	0	38	3
Hazelnut Iced Latte, 14 oz	260	7	5	90	44	0	40	3
Mocha Iced Latte, 14 oz	260	7	5	150	45	0	36	3
Mocha/Caramel Iced Latte, 14 oz	260	8	5	170	45	0	0	3
Caramel/Hazelnut Iced Latte, 14 oz	260	8	5	140	44	0	39	3
Mocha Hazelnut Iced Latte, 14 oz	250	7	5	120	45	0	38	3
Caramel Java Chiller, 14 oz	540	18	12	300	86	0	74	7
Hazelnut Java Chiller, 14 oz	530	18	11	250	86	0	75	7
Mocha Java Chiller, 14 oz	540	18	11	260	87	0	73	7
Mocha/Caramel Java Chiller, 14 oz	540	18	11	280	85	0	73	7
Caramel/Hazelnut Java Chiller, 14 oz	530	18	11	230	85	0	74	7
Mocha/Hazelnut Java Chiller, 14 oz	540	18	11	250	86	0	75	7
Sonic Boom Espresso Shot	5	0	0	5	1	0	0	0

Frozen Dessert

Description & Serving	Cal	Fat	SFat	Sod	Carb	Fiber	Sugar	Prot
Oreo Sonic Blast, 14 oz	540	21	12	280	80	1	67	7
M&M's Sonic Blast, 14 oz	600	24	15	210	88	1	78	8
Reese's Peanut Butter Cups Sonic Blast, 14 oz	560	19	12	250	89	1	74	9
Butterfinger Sonic Blast, 14 oz	580	22	13	240	88	0	72	8
Vanilla Shake, 14 oz	470	17	11	200	71	0	62	7
Chocolate Shake, 14 oz	540	16	10	270	89	0	74	6
Strawberry Shake, 14 oz	510	16	10	200	83	1	69	7
Banana Shake, 14 oz	470	16	10	190	76	1	63	7
Pineapple Shake, 14 oz	500	16	10	200	80	0	66	6
Caramel Shake, 14 oz	530	17	11	320	88	0	76	6
Peanut Butter Shake, 14 oz	640	34	13	300	75	0	63	10
Peanut Butter Fudge Shake, 14 oz	610	28	14	280	81	1	68	8
Hot Fudge Shake, 14 oz	570	21	14	240	85	1	71	6
Strawberry Creamslush Treat, 14 oz	450	12	7	150	84	1	72	5
Orange Creamslush Treat, 14 oz	430	13	8	160	77	0	70	5
Cherry Creamslush Treat, 14 oz	440	13	8	160	77	0	71	5
Grape Creamslush Treat, 14 oz	430	13	8	160	76	0	70	5
Watermelon Creamslush Treat, 14 oz	440	13	8	160	77	0	70	5
Blue Coconut Creamslush Treat, 14 oz	430	13	8	160	76	0	69	5
Lemon Creamslush Treat, 14 oz	430	13	8	160	77	0	69	5
Lemon-Berry Creamslush Treat, 14 oz	460	12	7	150	85	1	73	5
Lime Creamslush Treat, 14 oz	430	13	8	160	77	0	69	5
Coca-Cola Float/Blended Float, 14 oz	290	8	5	95	54	0	50	3
Diet Coke Float/Blended Float, 14 oz	220	8	5	100	33	0	29	3
Dr. Pepper Float/Blended Float, 14 oz	310	8	5	120	58	0	54	3
Diet Dr. Pepper Float/Blended Float, 14 oz	220	8	5	130	33	0	29	3
Barq's Root Beer Float/Blended Float, 14 oz	300	8	5	110	56	0	52	3
Sprite Float/Blended Float, 14 oz	290	8	5	110	53	0	49	3
Sprite Zero Float/Blended Float, 14 oz	220	8	5	100	33	0	29	3
Banana Split	420	9	6	140	80	2	57	4

Description & Serving	Cal	Fat	Sfat	Sod	Carb	Fiber	Sugar	Prot
Hot Fudge Cake Sundae	500	20	12	310	73	2	55	5
Banana Fudge Sundae	440	16	11	170	70	2	54	4
Hot Fudge Sundae	440	18	13	170	63	1	52	4
Peanut Butter Sundae	510	31	12	230	53	0	44	8
Peanut Butter Fudge Sundae	470	25	13	200	58	1	48	6
Strawberry Sundae	380	13	9	120	61	1	49	4
Chocolate Sundae	410	13	9	190	67	0	55	4
Pineapple Sundae	370	13	9	125	58	0	47	4
Caramel Sundae	390	13	9	240	64	0	55	4
Jr. Butterfinger Sundae	170	6	3.5	65	26	0	20	2
Jr. M&M's Sundae	180	7	4.5	55	26	0	23	2
Jr. Oreo Sundae	150	5	3	90	22	0	17	2
Jr. Reese's Sundae	160	4.5	3	75	27	0	21	3
Nuts Add-On	20	1.5	0	0	1	0	0	1
Vanilla Cone	180	6	4	80	30	0	22	2
Vanilla Dish	240	9	5	100	36	0	32	3

Sonny's Real Pit Bar-B-Q

Appetizer

Chicken Tenders	697	40	7	2240	48	5	<1	38

Salad

Backyard Garden Salad	30	<1	<1	10	6	2	4	2
Caesar Salad w/ Chicken Tenders	1014	68	13	2916	67	9	5	44
Caesar Salad w/ Chargrilled Chicken	586	39	7	1577	30	5	5	42
Big Salad w/ Chicken Tenders	734	36	6	2044	71	9	8	38
Big Salad w/ Chargrilled Chicken	306	7	1	704	34	6	9	36
Big Salad w/ Sliced Beef	412	16	6	343	33	6	8	40
Big Salad w/ Sliced Pork	472	23	8	358	33	6	8	38
Big Salad w/ Sliced Smoked Turkey	253	5	1	1062	34	6	8	23
Big Salad w/ Pulled Pork	590	33	11	564	34	6	8	46
Big Salad w/ Pulled Beef Brisket	692	42	15	767	45	6	8	38
Big Salad w/ Pulled Chicken	461	18	11	603	33	6	8	31

Sandwich/Burger

Sliced Beef Sandwich on Bun	436	14	7	481	39	1	6	38
Sliced Beef Sandwich on Garlic Bread	596	26	9	681	54	2	1	40
Sliced Pork Sandwich on Bun	496	22	9	496	38	1	6	36
Sliced Pork Sandwich on Garlic Bread	656	33	11	696	53	2	1	38
Smoked Turkey Sandwich on Bun	277	4	4	1200	39	1	6	22
Smoked Turkey Sandwich on Garlic Bread	437	15	3	1400	54	2	1	29
Pulled Pork Sandwich on Bun	614	31	11	702	39	1	10	44
Pulled Pork Sandwich on Garlic Bread	774	43	13	902	54	2	1	46
Pulled Beef Brisket Sandwich on Bun	716	41	15	905	50	1	6	37
Pulled Beef Brisket Sandwich on Garlic Bread	876	52	17	1105	65	2	1	39
Pulled Chicken Sandwich on Bun	486	17	9	741	39	1	6	29
Pulled Chicken Sandwich on Garlic Bread	646	28	11	1051	56	2	<1	66
Charbroiled Chicken Sandwich on Bun	384	6	1	1031	40	1	7	46

Description & Serving	Cal	Fat	Sfat	Sod	Carb	Fiber	Sugar	Prot
Charbroiled Chicken Sandwich on Garlic Bread	490	18	3	1042	54	2	2	36
Catfish Sandwich on Bun	361	8	3	1052	52	2	8	19
Catfish Sandwich on Garlic Bread	521	19	5	1252	67	3	3	21
Hamburger on Bun	815	43	16	560	38	1	6	64
Cheeseburger on Bun w/ American Cheese	865	47	18	815	38	1	6	67

Lunch Portion

Beef

	Cal	Fat	Sfat	Sod	Carb	Fiber	Sugar	Prot
Sliced Beef	236	12	6	91	1	0	0	32
Pulled Beef Brisket	516	38	15	515	12	0	0	31

Chicken/Turkey

	Cal	Fat	Sfat	Sod	Carb	Fiber	Sugar	Prot
Chicken Tenders	558	32	6	1792	38	4	<1	30
Charbroiled Chicken	130	3	<1	452	1	0	1	23
Pulled Chicken	286	14	9	351	1	0	0	23
Smoked Turkey	77	1	1	810	1	0	0	16

Fish

	Cal	Fat	Sfat	Sod	Carb	Fiber	Sugar	Prot
Breaded Catfish	266	16	3	657	16	<1	2	14

Pork

	Cal	Fat	Sfat	Sod	Carb	Fiber	Sugar	Prot
Sliced Pork	296	19	8	106	<1	0	0	30
Pulled Pork	414	29	11	312	1	0	0	38

Ribs

	Cal	Fat	Sfat	Sod	Carb	Fiber	Sugar	Prot
Sweet & Smokey Ribs	739	61	24	509	3	0	2	43
Baby Back Ribs	635	39	17	993	19	0	13	50

Entrée (Dinner Portion)

Beef

	Cal	Fat	Sfat	Sod	Carb	Fiber	Sugar	Prot
Sliced Beef	354	18	9	137	1	0	0	49
Pulled Beef Brisket	929	69	27	927	22	0	0	55

Chicken/Turkey

	Cal	Fat	Sfat	Sod	Carb	Fiber	Sugar	Prot
Chicken Tenders	837	47	9	2687	58	6	<1	45
Chicken Wings w/ Bar-B-Q Sauce, 10 pc	1125	70	19	1694	3	<1	<1	121
Bar-B-Q Chicken, 1/4 chicken	270	13	9	281	0	0	0	78
Bar-B-Q Chicken, 1/2 chicken	540	27	18	561	0	0	0	156
Bar-B-Q Chicken, whole chicken	1080	55	35	1121	0	0	0	312
Charbroiled Chicken	260	5	1	904	2	0	1	56
Pulled Chicken	515	26	17	561	2	0	0	58
Smoked Turkey	116	2	1	1214	2	0	0	23

Combination

	Cal	Fat	Sfat	Sod	Carb	Fiber	Sugar	Prot
Super Combo (Sliced Pork, Sliced Beef, Bar-B-Q Chicken, Sweet & Smokey Ribs)	1181	68	35	761	3	0	2	153
Bar-B-Q Chicken & Ribs	1038	64	33	789	3	0	2	121
Bar-B-Q Chicken & Sliced Pork	595	32	17	386	<1	0	<1	108
Bar-B-Q Chicken & Pulled Pork	713	42	20	592	1	0	1	116

Fish

	Cal	Fat	Sfat	Sod	Carb	Fiber	Sugar	Prot
Breaded Catfish	533	33	6	1313	33	1	3	28
Breaded Shrimp	533	26	9	1618	46	0	0	29

Description & Serving	Cal	Fat	Sfat	Sod	Carb	Fiber	Sugar	Prot
Pork								
Sliced Pork	444	29	12	159	<1	0	0	45
Pulled Pork	745	51	20	561	2	0	0	69
Pork 3 Ways	1449	109	43	926	4	0	3	112
Ribs								
Sweet & Smokey Ribs	1364	113	45	939	6	0	4	79
Baby Back Ribs	1270	79	33	1987	39	0	25	101
Rib Sampler	1544	115	46	1616	23	0	15	103
Side								
Bar-B-Q Beans	147.61	1.86	0.5	639.72	25.32	4.69	8.43	8.06
Potato Salad	216	16	1	962	14	5	4	3
Mustard Potato Salad	69	8	1	479	21	4	6	3
Macaroni & Cheese	213	10	5	755	23	1	3	10
Onion Rings, half order	724	41	8	1568	80	5	10	9
Onion Rings, full order	1345	76	14	2913	148	10	18	17
French Fries	363	17	4	148	47	5	0	5
Fried Okra	417	29	5	871	34	6	6	5
Corn Nuggets	608	29	5	1213	79	6	2	7
Corn on the Cob	140	2	<1	20	34	2	NP	5
Southern Green Beans	95	5	1	469	11	4	5	3
Coleslaw	216	16	2	307	19	3	14	2
Baked Potato	264	<1	<1	14	61	4	5	6
Baked Sweet Potato	293	<1	<1	117	68	11	21	7
Garlic Bread, 1 slice	180	7	1	295	27	1	<1	4
Cornbread, 1 loaf	259	9	2	561	43	<1	16	4
Dressing/Condiment								
Lo-Cal French Dressing, 2 tbsp	35	1	0	300	7	0	6	0
Lo-Cal Red French Dressing, 2 tbsp	40	2	0	240	5	0	5	0
Lo-Cal Italian Dressing, 2 tbsp	40	3	0	360	4	0	3	0
Fat Free Ranch Dressing, 2 tbsp	45	0	0	340	9	0	5	1
Fat Free Honey Mustard, 2 tbsp	60	0	0	280	13	<1	12	0
Creamy Italian Dressing, 2 tbsp	100	10	2	250	4	0	3	0
Thousand Island Dressing, 2 tbsp	110	10	1	320	6	0	6	0
Caesar Dressing, 2 tbsp	140	15	3	420	2	0	1	2
Ranch Dressing, 2 tbsp	110	11	2	180	2	0	<1	<1
Blue Cheese Dressing, 2 tbsp	180	19	3	320	0	0	0	<1
Golden Italian Dressing, 2 tbsp	120	11	2	380	5	0	4	0
French Dressing, 2 tbsp	120	11	2	240	6	0	5	0
Sweet Bar-B-Q Sauce, 2 tbsp	60	0	0	460	14	0	13	0
Sizzlin' Sweet Bar-B-Q Sauce, 2 tbsp	50	0.5	0	480	10	0	11	0
Smokin' Bar-B-Q Sauce, 2 tbsp	45	0	0	460	10	0	8	0
Mild Bar-B-Q Sauce, 2 tbsp	40	1	0	410	6	0	4	<1
Mustard Bar-B-Q Sauce, 2 tbsp	25	0.5	0	350	4	0	4	0
Dessert								
Banana Pudding	367	12	5	228	63	1	25	1
Peach Cobbler	333	20	7	380	60	<1	45	2
Blueberry Cobbler	348	22	8	431	62	2	45	3

Description & Serving	Cal	Fat	Sfat	Sod	Carb	Fiber	Sugar	Prot
Apple Cobbler	339	22	8	446	61	1	44	3
Double Chocolate Brownie Bliss	1470	61	38	302	226	5	170	13

Starbucks

Cold Beverage

	Cal	Fat	Sfat	Sod	Carb	Fiber	Sugar	Prot
Blended Strawberry Lemonade, Tall (12 oz)	200	0	0	0	49	1	47	1
Caffè Vanilla Frappuccino Blended Coffee w/o whip, Tall (12 oz)	230	2.5	1.5	180	49	0	43	4
Caffè Vanilla Frappuccino Blended Coffee w/ whip, Tall (12 oz)	320	10	6	190	52	0	45	4
Caffè Vanilla Frappuccino Light Blended Coffee, Tall (12 oz)	140	0.5	0	180	30	2	23	4
Caramel Frappuccino Blended Coffee w/o whip, Tall (12 oz)	220	3	2	180	44	0	38	4
Caramel Frappuccino Blended Coffee w/ whip, Tall (12 oz)	300	11	7	190	46	0	39	4
Caramel Frappuccino Light Blended Coffee, Tall (12 oz)	130	1	0	180	25	2	18	4
Cinnamon Dolce Frappuccino Blended Coffee w/o whip, Tall (12 oz)	210	2.5	1.5	180	43	0	37	4
Cinnamon Dolce Frappuccino Blended Coffee w/ whip, Tall (12 oz)	290	10	6	190	45	0	39	4
Cinnamon Dolce Frappuccino Light Blended Coffee, Tall (12 oz)	120	0.5	0	180	24	2	17	4
Coffee Frappuccino Blended Coffee, Tall (12 oz)	180	2.5	1.5	170	37	0	31	4
Coffee Frappuccino Light Blended Coffee, Tall (12 oz)	90	0.5	0	160	18	2	12	4
Double Chocolaty Chip Frappuccino Blended Crème w/o whip, Tall (12 oz)	300	6	2.5	230	57	2	43	10
Double Chocolaty Chip Frappuccino Blended Crème w/ whip, Tall (12 oz)	380	14	8	240	59	2	45	11
Espresso Frappuccino Blended Coffee, Tall (12 oz)	140	1.5	1	125	27	0	22	3
Espresso Frappuccino Light Blended Coffee, Tall (12 oz)	80	0	0	140	16	2	10	4
Iced Apple Chai Infusion, Tall (12 oz)	170	0	0	10	44	0	40	1
Iced Berry Chai Infusion, Tall (12 oz)	150	0	0	0	37	0	33	1
Iced Brewed Coffee, Tall (12 oz)	60	0	0	0	15	0	15	0
Iced Caffè Americano, Tall (12 oz)	10	0	0	5	2	0	0	1
Iced Caffè Latte w/ 2% milk, Tall (12 oz)	100	3.5	2.5	80	10	0	9	6
Iced Caffè Mocha w/ 2% milk & w/o whip, Tall (12 oz)	150	4.5	2	60	26	1	20	7
Iced Caffè Mocha w/ 2% milk & whip, Tall (12 oz)	230	12	7	70	29	1	21	7
Iced Caramel Macchiato w/ 2% milk, Tall (12 oz)	170	5	3	95	24	0	22	7
Iced Coffee w/ 2% Milk, Tall (12 oz)	90	1	0.5	25	18	0	18	2
Iced Espresso Truffle w/o whip, Tall (12 oz)	190	5	3.5	70	27	3	18	7
Iced Espresso Truffle w/ whip, Tall (12 oz)	270	13	8	75	29	3	20	8
Iced Gingersnap Latte w/ 2% milk & w/o whip, Tall (12 oz)	160	3	2	70	27	0	22	6

Description & Serving	Cal	Fat	Sfat	Sod	Carb	Fiber	Sugar	Prot
Iced Gingersnap Latte w/ 2% milk & whip, Tall (12 oz)	240	11	7	80	29	0	24	6
Iced Peppermint Mocha Twist w/ 2% milk & w/o whip, Tall (12 oz)	200	4.5	2	55	39	2	32	6
Iced Peppermint Mocha Twist w/ 2% milk & whip, Tall (12 oz)	280	13	7	65	41	2	34	6
Iced Peppermint White Chocolate Mocha w/ 2% milk & w/o whip, Tall (12 oz)	310	7	5	140	54	0	52	7
Iced Peppermint White Chocolate Mocha w/ 2% milk & whip, Tall (12 oz)	390	15	10	150	56	0	53	8
Iced Pumpkin Spice Latte w/ 2% milk & w/o whip, Tall (12 oz)	190	3	2	130	33	0	32	8
Iced Pumpkin Spice Latte w/ 2% milk & whip, Tall (12 oz)	270	11	7	135	35	0	34	8
Iced Sugar-Free Syrup Flavored Latte w/ 2% milk, Tall (12 oz)	90	3	2	85	9	0	7	6
Iced Syrup Flavored Latte w/ 2% milk, Tall (12 oz)	140	3	2	70	23	0	21	6
Iced Tazo Green Tea Latte w/ 2% milk, Tall (12 oz)	190	4	2.5	85	31	1	30	7
Iced Vanilla Latte w/ 2% milk, Tall (12 oz)	140	3	2	70	23	0	21	6
Iced White Chocolate Mocha w/ 2% milk & w/o whip, Tall (12 oz)	260	7	5	150	41	0	39	8
Iced White Chocolate Mocha w/ 2% milk & whip, Tall (12 oz)	340	15	10	150	43	0	41	8
Java Chip Frappuccino Blended Coffee w/o whip, Tall (12 oz)	260	6	4	180	50	1	40	5
Java Chip Frappuccino Blended Coffee w/ whip, Tall (12 oz)	340	14	9	180	52	1	42	6
Java Chip Frappuccino Light Blended Coffee, Tall (12 oz)	160	3.5	2	180	30	3	20	5
Lemonade Blended Beverage, Tall (12 oz)	190	0	0	5	49	1	47	0
Lemonade Blended Beverage w/ Tazo Zen Green Tea, Tall (12 oz)	160	0	0	0	39	1	37	0
Mint Chocolaty Chip Frappuccino Blended Crème w/o whip, Tall (12 oz)	310	5	2	240	61	2	50	9
Mint Chocolaty Chip Frappuccino Blended Crème w/ Chocolate Whipped Cream, Tall (12 oz)	400	14	8	250	64	2	52	10
Mint Mocha Chip Frappuccino Blended Coffee w/o whip, Tall (12 oz)	270	5	3.5	200	54	1	45	5
Mint Mocha Chip Frappuccino Blended Coffee w/ Chocolate Whipped Cream, Tall (12 oz)	360	14	9	210	57	1	47	6
Mint Mocha Chip Frappuccino Light Blended Coffee w/o whip, Tall (12 oz)	170	3	1.5	180	32	3	23	5
Mocha Frappuccino Blended Coffee w/o whip, Tall (12 oz)	200	3	1.5	170	41	0	34	4
Mocha Frappuccino Blended Coffee w/ whip, Tall (12 oz)	280	11	6	180	43	0	36	5
Mocha Frappuccino Light Blended Coffee, Tall (12 oz)	110	1	0	170	23	2	15	4

Description & Serving	Cal	Fat	Sfat	Sod	Carb	Fiber	Sugar	Prot
Peppermint Mocha Twist Frappuccino Blended Coffee w/o whip, Tall (12 oz)	290	4.5	2.5	250	60	1	54	5
Peppermint Mocha Twist Frappuccino Blended Coffee w/ whip, Tall (12 oz)	380	1	7	260	63	1	55	5
Pumpkin Spice Frappuccino Blended Coffee w/o whip, Tall (12 oz)	230	2.5	1.5	210	47	0	41	5
Pumpkin Spice Frappuccino Blended Coffee w/ whip, Tall (12 oz)	310	11	7	210	49	0	43	5
Pumpkin Spice Frappuccino Light Blended Coffee, Tall (12 oz)	120	0.5	0	190	25	2	19	5
Pumpkin Spice Frappuccino Blended Crème w/o whip, Tall (12 oz)	280	2	0	270	55	0	47	10
Pumpkin Spice Frappuccino Blended Crème w/ whip, Tall (12 oz)	360	10	5	280	58	0	49	10
Starbucks Doubleshot on Ice + Energy Beverage w/ 2% milk, Tall (12 oz)	70	0.5	0	15	14	0	12	3
Starbucks Doubleshot on Ice Beverage w/ 2% milk, Tall (12 oz)	70	0.5	0	15	14	0	12	2
Strawberries & Crème Frappuccino Blended Crème w/o whip, Tall (12 oz)	280	2	1	300	56	1	44	9
Strawberries & Crème Frappuccino Blended Crème w/ whip, Tall (12 oz)	360	10	6	310	58	1	46	9
Tazo Black Shaken Iced Tea, Tall (12 oz)	60	0	0	10	16	0	15	0
Tazo Black Shaken Iced Tea Lemonade, Tall (12 oz)	100	0	0	10	25	0	25	0
Tazo Chai Frappuccino Blended Crème w/o whip, Tall (12 oz)	260	1.5	0	220	52	0	44	8
Tazo Chai Frappuccino Blended Crème w/ whip, Tall (12 oz)	340	10	5	230	55	0	45	9
Tazo Chai Iced Tea Latte w/ 2% milk, Tall (12 oz)	180	3	2	70	33	0	31	5
Tazo Green Shaken Iced Tea, Tall (12 oz)	60	0	0	10	16	0	15	0
Tazo Green Shaken Iced Tea Lemonade, Tall (12 oz)	100	0	0	10	25	0	25	0
Tazo Green Tea Frappuccino Blended Crème w/o whip, Tall (12 oz)	290	2	0	230	60	1	51	9
Tazo Green Tea Frappuccino Blended Crème w/ whip, Tall (12 oz)	370	10	5	240	62	1	53	9
Tazo Passion Shaken Iced Tea, Tall (12 oz)	60	0	0	10	16	0	15	0
Tazo Passion Shaken Iced Tea Lemonade, Tall (12 oz)	100	0	0	10	25	0	25	0
Vanilla Bean Frappuccino Blended Crème w/o whip, Tall (12 oz)	260	2	0	230	53	0	44	9
Vanilla Bean Frappuccino Blended Crème w/ whip, Tall (12 oz)	340	10	5	240	55	0	45	9
White Chocolate Mocha Frappuccino Blended Coffee w/o whip, Tall (12 oz)	240	3.5	2.5	200	47	0	41	5
White Chocolate Mocha Frappuccino Blended Coffee w/ whip, Tall (12 oz)	320	12	7	210	49	0	43	5
White Chocolate Mocha Frappuccino Light Blended Coffee, Tall (12 oz)	140	1.5	1	190	27	2	21	5

Description & Serving	Cal	Fat	Sfat	Sod	Carb	Fiber	Sugar	Prot
Hot Beverage								
Apple Chai Infusion, Tall (12 oz)	240	0	0	15	61	0	55	1
Berry Chai Infusion, Tall (12 oz)	190	0	0	5	47	0	43	1
Caffè Americano w/ 2% milk, Tall (12 oz)	10	0	0	5	2	0	0	1
Caffè Latte w/ 2% milk, Tall (12 oz)	150	6	3.5	115	14	0	13	10
Caffè Misto/Café Au Lait w/ 2% milk, Tall (12 oz)	80	3	2	70	7	0	7	5
Caffè Mocha w/ 2% milk & w/o whip, Tall (12 oz)	200	6	3.5	100	31	1	24	10
Caffè Mocha w/ 2% milk & whip, Tall (12 oz)	270	12	7	105	33	1	26	10
Cappuccino w/ 2% milk, Tall (12 oz)	90	3.5	2	70	9	0	8	6
Caramel Apple Spice w/o whip, Tall (12 oz)	240	0	0	20	57	0	51	0
Caramel Apple Spice w/ whip, Tall (12 oz)	300	7	4	25	59	0	52	0
Caramel Macchiato w/ 2% milk, Tall (12 oz)	180	5	3.5	100	25	0	23	8
Cinnamon Dolce Crème w/ 2% milk & w/o whip, Tall (12 oz)	210	6	3.5	120	31	0	31	9
Cinnamon Dolce Crème w/ 2% milk & whip, Tall (12 oz)	270	12	7	125	32	0	32	10
Cinnamon Dolce Latte w/ 2% milk & w/o whip, Tall (12 oz)	200	5	3	110	30	0	29	9
Cinnamon Dolce Latte w/ 2% milk & whip, Tall (12 oz)	270	11	7	115	32	0	31	9
Cinnamon Dolce Latte w/ Sugar-Free Syrup, 2% milk, & whip, Tall (12 oz)	140	5	3.5	125	14	0	12	9
Coffee of the Week, Tall (12 oz)	5	0	0	10	0	0	0	0
Decaf Coffee of the Week, Tall (12 oz)	5	0	0	10	0	0	0	0
Espresso Truffle w/o whip, Tall (12 oz)	300	9	5	110	43	5	3	11
Espresso Truffle w/ whip, Tall (12 oz)	360	15	9	115	45	5	31	15
Gingersnap Latte w/ 2% milk & w/o whip, Tall (12 oz)	210	5	3	110	31	0	27	9
Gingersnap Latte w/ 2% milk & whip, Tall (12 oz)	270	11	7	115	33	0	28	9
Hot Chocolate w/ 2% milk & w/o whip, Tall (12 oz)	230	7	3.5	110	37	1	31	10
Hot Chocolate w/ 2% milk & whip, Tall (12 oz)	290	13	7	115	39	1	32	11
Peppermint Mocha Twist w/ 2% milk & w/o whip, Tall (12 oz)	260	7	3.5	95	44	2	37	9
Peppermint Mocha Twist w/ 2% milk & whip, Tall (12 oz)	320	13	7	100	46	2	38	10
Peppermint White Chocolate Mocha w/ 2% milk & w/o whip, Tall (12 oz)	360	9	6	180	59	0	57	11
Peppermint White Chocolate Mocha w/ 2% milk & whip, Tall (12 oz)	420	15	10	190	61	0	58	11
Pumpkin Spice Crème w/ 2% milk & w/o whip, Tall (12 oz)	250	6	3.5	180	38	0	38	11
Pumpkin Spice Crème w/ 2% milk & whip, Tall (12 oz)	310	12	7	180	40	0	39	12
Pumpkin Spice Latte w/ 2% milk & w/o whip, Tall (12 oz)	240	5	3	170	38	0	36	11
Pumpkin Spice Latte w/ 2% milk & whip, Tall (12 oz)	300	11	7	170	39	0	38	11

Description & Serving	Cal	Fat	Sfat	Sod	Carb	Fiber	Sugar	Prot
Salted Caramel Signature Hot Chocolate w/ 2% milk & w/o whip, Tall (12 oz)	420	18	11	230	60	5	51	11
Salted Caramel Signature Hot Chocolate w/ 2% milk & whip, Tall (12 oz)	480	24	15	230	62	5	52	11
Steamed Apple Juice, Tall (12 oz)	170	0	0	15	43	0	39	0
Syrup Flavored Latte w/ 2% milk, Tall (12 oz)	190	5	3.5	110	27	0	26	9
Tazo Awake Tea Latte w/ 2% milk, Tall (12 oz)	150	4	2	70	24	0	24	6
Tazo Chai Tea Latte w/ 2% milk, Tall (12 oz)	180	3	2	75	33	0	31	6
Tazo Earl Grey Tea Latte w/ 2% milk, Tall (12 oz)	150	4	2	70	24	0	24	6
Tazo Green Tea Latte w/ 2% milk, Tall (12 oz)	260	6	4	120	41	1	40	10
Tazo Tea w/ 2% milk, Tall (12 oz)	0	0	0	0	0	0	0	0
Vanilla Crème w/ 2% milk & w/o whip, Tall (12 oz)	200	6	3.5	115	28	0	27	9
Vanilla Crème w/ 2% milk & whip, Tall (12 oz)	260	12	7	125	29	0	28	10
Vanilla Latte w/ 2% milk, Tall (12 oz)	190	5	3.5	110	27	0	26	9
Vanilla Latte + Protein w/ 2% milk, Tall (12 oz)	200	4.5	3	130	27	1	24	13
Vanilla Rooibos Tea Latte w/ 2% milk, Tall (12 oz)	150	4	2	70	24	0	24	6
White Chocolate Mocha w/ 2% milk & w/o whip, Tall (12 oz)	310	9	6	180	46	0	44	11
White Chocolate Mocha w/ 2% milk & whip, Tall (12 oz)	370	15	10	190	48	0	45	12
White Hot Chocolate w/ 2% milk & w/o whip, Tall (12 oz)	310	9	7	190	46	0	45	12
White Hot Chocolate w/ 2% milk & whip, Tall (12 oz)	380	15	10	200	48	0	47	12
Espresso, Doppio, 2 oz	10	0	0	0	2	0	0	1
Espresso con Panna, Doppio, 2 oz	35	2.5	1.5	0	3	0	1	1
Espresso Macchiato, Doppio, 2 oz	15	0	0	0	2	0	0	1
Espresso, Solo, 1 oz	5	0	0	0	1	0	0	0
Espresso con Panna, Solo, 1 oz	30	2.5	1.5	0	2	0	1	0
Espresso Macchiato, Solo, 1 oz	10	0	0	0	1	0	0	1

Breakfast

Description & Serving	Cal	Fat	Sfat	Sod	Carb	Fiber	Sugar	Prot
Blueberry Oat Bar w/ Organic Blueberries	250	10	6	90	35	4	15	3
Greek Yogurt Honey Parfait	290	12	6	100	43	1	32	8
Strawberry Blueberry Yogurt Parfait	350	4.5	0.5	100	66	4	35	10
Butter Croissant	310	18	11	290	32	<1	4	5
Multigrain Bagel	320	4	0	220	62	4	8	12
Plain Bagel	300	1	0	460	64	2	8	10
Apple Fritter	420	20	9	360	59	1	27	5
Cheese Danish	420	25	16	370	39	<1	16	7
Classic Glazed Old-Fashioned Doughnut	420	21	10	260	57	<1	34	4
Double Iced Cinnamon Roll	490	20	12	480	70	3	34	7
Morning Bun	350	16	9	330	45	2	19	6
Apple Bran Muffin w/ Omega 3's & 7g Fiber	350	9	2.5	520	64	7	34	6
Blueberry Struesel Muffin	360	11	6	390	59	2	33	7
Lowfat Raspberry Sunshine Muffin	340	6	1.5	500	65	2	37	7
Perfect Oatmeal	140	2.5	0.5	105	25	4	0	5
Perfect Oatmeal Topping - Brown Sugar	50	0	0	0	13	0	13	0
Perfect Oatmeal Topping - Dried Fruit	100	0	0	10	24	2	20	1

Description & Serving	Cal	Fat	Sfat	Sod	Carb	Fiber	Sugar	Prot
Perfect Oatmeal Topping - Nut Medley	100	9	1	0	2	1	1	2
Bacon, Gouda Cheese, Egg Frittata on Artisan Roll	380	20	8	1050	31	0	1	19
Classic Sausage, Egg & Aged Cheddar Breakfast Sandwich	500	29	9	980	42	2	3	20
Egg White, Spinach & Feta Wrap	280	9	3.5	1140	35	8	4	19
Ham, Egg Frittata, Cheddar Cheese on Artisan Roll	370	16	6	730	32	0	1	23
Portobello Mushroom Piadini	370	18	9	650	39	2	4	14
Reduced-Fat Egg White Turkey Bacon Breakfast Sandwich	340	10	3	750	47	3	6	22
Sausage Piadini	500	32	15	740	36	1	3	19

Salad/Fruit

Chop Chop Pasta Salad	480	26	8	1340	32	2	2	30
Farmers Market Salad w/ Dressing	300	20	5	350	24	4	16	8
Fruit & Cheese Plate	380	21	11	530	37	3	24	15

Sandwich/Mixed Plate

Cobb Salad Sandwich	460	18	4.5	1340	42	3	5	34
Egg Salad Sandwich	450	26	5	740	36	2	5	19
Hickory Ham & Cheddar	450	14	5	1500	55	3	16	21
Protein Plate w/ Peanut Butter	370	17	5	600	39	5	17	17
Rosemary Ham & Swiss	410	22	9	1070	30	1	2	23
Tarragon Chicken Salad Sandwich	490	12	2	1330	62	4	15	35
Turkey & Swiss Sandwich w/ Mayonnaise	390	13	4.5	1180	36	2	5	34
Turkey Cranberry Pesto	400	19	2	980	35	2	6	24

Dessert

Black & White Cookies, 2	240	12	1	160	32	1	22	2
Chocolate Chunk Cookie	360	17	10	170	50	2	31	4
Double Chocolate Brownie	410	24	7	75	46	3	30	6
Marshmallow Dream Bar	210	4	2.5	250	43	0	15	1
Outrageous Oatmeal Cookie	370	14	8	170	56	3	36	5
Rich Toffee Pecan Bar	380	22	8	120	48	<1	17	4
Starbucks Indulgent Cookie	320	19	11	85	40	3	31	4
Strawberry Rhubarb Cookie	290	14	6	190	38	1	18	4
Tropical Paradise Bar w/ Coconut & Passionfruit	300	16	11	135	37	1	26	3
Cheery Cherry Pie	370	19	11	410	46	2	21	4
Gluten-Free Valencia Orange Cake w/ Almonds	290	16	2	40	32	4	23	9
Luscious Lemon Tart	410	25	14	25	42	<1	23	5
Banana Nut Bread	480	19	2.5	210	73	4	44	7
Marble Loaf	330	12	5	480	50	1	32	6
Pumpkin Loaf	320	12	2	400	50	1	32	5
Reduced-Fat Banana Chocolate Chip Coffee Cake	380	7	4	490	77	3	50	5
Reduced-Fat Cinnamon Swirl Coffee Cake	290	7	3.5	390	55	2	34	4
Reduced-Fat Very Berry Coffee Cake	320	9	3.5	470	54	4	28	6
Starbucks Classic Coffee Cake	420	19	10	530	59	1	34	6
Blueberry Scone	500	23	13	640	68	2	21	7
Cinnamon Chip Scone	470	18	10	390	63	2	26	8
Maple Oat Pecan Scone	470	21	11	270	64	5	16	7
Petite Vanilla Bean Scone	140	5	2.5	90	21	0	10	0

Description & Serving	Cal	Fat	Sfat	Sod	Carb	Fiber	Sugar	Prot

Subway

Breakfast

Black Forest Ham & Cheese Breakfast Sandwich	450	19	7	1450	47	5	5	27
Cheese Breakfast Sandwich	420	18	7	1060	46	5	4	22
Double Bacon & Cheese Breakfast Sandwich	520	25	11	1440	47	5	4	29
Mega Breakfast Sandwich	720	45	18	1580	47	5	4	33
Sausage & Cheese Breakfast Sandwich	670	41	16	1390	46	5	4	30
Steak & Cheese Breakfast Sandwich	490	20	8	1400	48	5	5	31
Western w/ Cheese Breakfast Sandwich	450	19	7	1460	48	5	5	27
Black Forest Ham & Cheese on Flatbread	480	22	8	1530	46	3	2	27
Cheese Breakfast on Flatbread	460	21	7	1170	45	3	1	23
Double Bacon & Cheese on Flatbread	560	28	11	1540	46	3	2	30
Mega Breakfast Sandwich on Flatbread	750	48	18	1650	46	3	2	34
Sausage & Cheese on Flatbread	700	44	17	1460	46	3	1	30
Steak & Cheese on Flatbread	521	23	8	1470	48	3	2	32
Western w/ Cheese on Flatbread	490	22	8	1560	47	3	2	28
Hash Browns, 4 pc	150	9	1	440	17	2	0	1

Sandwich

6" Black Forest Ham Sandwich on wheat w/ std toppings & no cheese	290	4.5	1	1200	47	5	7	18
6" Oven Roasted Chicken Breast Sandwich on wheat w/ std toppings & no cheese	320	4.5	1	750	49	5	7	23
6" Roast Beef Sandwich on wheat w/ std toppings & no cheese	310	4.5	1.5	840	46	5	6	26
6" Subway Club Sandwich on wheat w/ std toppings & no cheese	320	5	1.5	1160	47	5	6	26
6" Sweet Onion Chicken Teriyaki on wheat w/ std toppings & no cheese	380	4.5	1	1010	60	5	17	26
6" Turkey Breast on wheat w/ std toppings & no cheese	280	3.5	1	920	47	5	6	18
6" Turkey Breast & Black Forest Ham on wheat w/ std toppings & no cheese	300	4	1	1140	47	5	6	19
6" Veggie Delite on wheat w/ std toppings & no cheese	230	2.5	0.5	410	45	5	5	8
6" Big Philly Cheesesteak Sandwich on wheat w/ cheese & std toppings	520	18	9	1570	53	6	7	39
6" BLT Sandwich on wheat w/ cheese & std toppings	360	13	6	990	45	5	5	17
6" Chicken & Bacon Ranch Sandwich on wheat w/ cheese & std toppings	570	28	10	1190	49	6	6	35
6" Cold Cut Combo Sandwich on wheat w/ cheese & std toppings	410	16	6	1450	48	5	6	21
6" Italian B.M.T. Sandwich on wheat w/ cheese & std toppings	450	20	8	1730	48	5	7	22
6" Meatball Marinara Sandwich on wheat w/ cheese & std toppings	580	23	9	1530	70	9	16	24
6" Spicy Italian Sandwich on wheat w/ cheese & std toppings	520	28	11	1830	47	5	7	22

Description & Serving	Cal	Fat	Sfat	Sod	Carb	Fiber	Sugar	Prot
6" Subway Melt Sandwich on wheat w/ cheese & std toppings	380	11	5	1530	49	5	7	25
6" The Feast Sandwich on wheat w/ cheese & std toppings	540	22	9	2470	50	5	8	39
6" Tuna Sandwich on wheat w/ cheese & std toppings	530	30	6	930	46	5	5	21

Specialty Sandwich

Description & Serving	Cal	Fat	Sfat	Sod	Carb	Fiber	Sugar	Prot
Black Forest Ham on Flatbread w/ std toppings & no cheese	320	7	1.5	1270	47	3	4	18
Oven Roasted Chicken Breast on Flatbread w/ std toppings & no cheese	250	7	1.5	820	48	3	4	24
Roast Beef on Flatbread w/ std toppings & no cheese	240	8	2	920	45	3	3	27
Subway Club on Flatbread w/ std toppings & no cheese	250	8	1.5	1230	47	3	4	26
Sweet Onion Chicken Teriyaki on Flatbread w/ std toppings & no cheese	410	7	1.5	1080	59	3	14	26
Turkey Breast on Flatbread w/ std toppings & no cheese	310	6	1	990	47	3	3	18
Turkey Breast & Black Forest Ham on Flatbread w/ std toppings & no cheese	330	7	1.5	1220	47	3	4	20
Veggie Delite on Flatbread w/ std toppings & no cheese	260	5	1	490	44	3	2	9

Salad

Description & Serving	Cal	Fat	Sfat	Sod	Carb	Fiber	Sugar	Prot
Ham Salad w/o dressing or croutons	110	3	1	850	12	4	6	12
Oven Roasted Chicken Breast Salad w/o dressing or croutons	130	2.5	0.5	280	10	4	4	20
Roast Beef Salad w/o dressing or croutons	140	3.5	1	500	10	4	5	21
Subway Club Salad w/o dressing or croutons	140	3.5	1	810	12	4	6	20
Sweet Onion Chicken Teriyaki Salad w/o dressing or croutons	200	3	1	660	25	4	16	20
Turkey Breast Salad w/o dressing or croutons	110	2	0.5	570	12	4	5	12
Turkey Breast & Ham Salad w/o dressing or croutons	120	3	0.5	790	12	4	6	14
Veggie Delite Salad w/o dressing or croutons	50	1	0	65	10	4	4	3

Soup

Description & Serving	Cal	Fat	Sfat	Sod	Carb	Fiber	Sugar	Prot
Chicken Tortilla Soup	110	1.5	0.5	440	11	3	4	6
Chipotle Chicken Corn Chowder	140	3	1.5	900	22	2	4	6
Chicken & Dumpling Soup	170	5	2	810	23	2	2	8
Chili Con Carne	340	11	5	950	35	10	7	20
Cream of Potato w/ Bacon Soup	240	13	5	870	26	3	3	5
Fire-Roasted Tomato Orzo Soup	130	1	0.5	410	24	2	4	6
Golden Broccoli & Cheese Soup	180	11	5	990	16	4	3	5
Minestrone Soup	90	1	0	910	17	3	4	4
New England Style Clam Chowder	150	5	1	990	20	4	2	6
Roasted Chicken Noodle Soup	80	2	0.5	950	12	1	2	6
Rosemary Chicken & Dumpling Soup	90	1.5	0.5	810	14	1	3	6
Spanish Style Chicken & Rice w/ Pork Soup	110	2.5	1	980	16	1	1	6

Description & Serving	Cal	Fat	Sfat	Sod	Carb	Fiber	Sugar	Prot
Tomato Garden Vegetable w/ Rotini Soup	90	0.5	0	820	20	3	8	3
Vegetable Beef Soup	100	2	0.5	960	17	3	5	5
Wild Rice w/ Chicken Soup	230	11	3.5	900	26	1	3	6

Pizza

8" Cheese Pizza	680	22	9	1070	96	4	7	32
8" Cheese & Veggies Pizza	740	25	11	NP	100	5	9	36
8" Pepperoni Pizza	790	32	13	1350	96	4	8	38
8" Sausage Pizza	820	34	14	1420	97	4	8	39

Kids

Veggie Delite Kids Pak Sandwich on mini wheat w/ std toppings & no cheese	150	1.5	0	280	30	3	3	6
Black Forest Ham Kids Pak Sandwich on mini wheat w/ std toppings & no cheese	180	2.5	0.5	670	31	3	4	10
Roast Beef Kids Pak Sandwich on mini wheat w/ std toppings & no cheese	200	3	1	500	30	4	4	15
Turkey Breast Kids Pak Sandwich on mini wheat w/ std toppings & no cheese	190	2.5	0.5	610	31	3	4	12

Dessert

Chocolate Chip Cookie	210	10	6	150	30	1	18	2
Chocolate Chunk Cookie	220	10	5	100	30	<1	17	2
Double Chocolate Chip Cookie	209.6	10	6	170	30	1	20	2
M&M Cookie	210	10	5	100	32	<1	18	2
Oatmeal Raisin Cookie	200	8	4	170	30	1	17	3
Peanut Butter Cookie	220	12	5	190	26	1	16	4
Sugar Cookie	220	12	6	140	28	<1	14	2
White Chip Macadamia Nut Cookie	220	11	5	160	29	<1	18	2
Apple Pie	250	10	2	290	37	1	25	0

Bread

6" Italian (White) Bread	200	2	0.5	390	38	1	5	7
6" 9-Grain Wheat Bread	210	2	0.5	410	41	4	3	8
6" Parmesan Oregano Bread	220	2.5	1	620	41	2	5	8
6" Honey Oat Bread	260	3	0.5	430	49	5	8	9
6" Hearty Italian Bread	220	2	1	390	41	2	5	8
6" Monterey Cheddar Bread	240	5	3	460	39	1	5	10
6" Italian Herbs & Cheese Bread	250	5	2	590	41	2	5	10
6" Roasted Garlic Bread	230	2.5	0.5	1360	45	2	7	8
Flatbread	240	5	1	480	41	2	<1	8
Mini Italian Bread	130	1.5	0	260	26	1	3	5
Mini Wheat Bread	140	1.5	0	270	28	3	2	5
Wrap	310	8	2.5	610	51	1	0	8

Topping

Bacon, 2 strips	45	3.5	1.5	190	0	0	0	3
Banana Peppers, 3 rings	0	0	0	20	0	0	0	0
Cucumbers, 3 slices	<5	0	0	0	<1	0	0	0
Green Peppers, 3 strips	0	0	0	0	0	0	0	0
Jalapeno Peppers, 3 rings	<5	0	0	70	0	0	0	0
Lettuce	<5	0	0	0	0	0	0	0

Description & Serving	Cal	Fat	Sfat	Sod	Carb	Fiber	Sugar	Prot
Onions	5	0	0	0	1	0	0	0
Pickles, 3 chips	0	0	0	115	0	0	0	0
Olives, 3 rings	<5	0	0	25	0	0	0	0
Tomatoes, 3 wheels	5	0	0	0	2	0	0	0
American, Processed Cheese, amt on 6" sandwich or salad	40	3.5	2	200	1	0	0	2
Monterey Cheddar Cheese, Shredded, amt on 6" sandwich or salad	50	4.5	3	90	1	0	0	3
Natural Cheddar, amt on 6" sandwich or salad	60	5	3	100	0	0	0	4
Pepperjack, amt on 6" sandwich or salad	50	4	2.5	140	0	0	0	3
Provolone, amt on 6" sandwich or salad	50	4	2	125	0	0	0	4
Swiss, amt on 6" sandwich or salad	50	4.5	2.5	30	0	0	0	4
Chicken Patty, Roasted, amt on 6" sandwich or salad	90	2.5	0.5	330	4	0	2	15
Chicken Strips, amt on 6" sandwich or salad	80	1.5	0.5	210	0	0	0	16
Cold Cut Combo Meats, amt on 6" sandwich or salad	140	11	3.5	830	2	0	1	10
Egg Patty, amt on 6" sandwich or salad	110	8	2	360	3	1	0	9
Ham Salad, amt on 6" sandwich or salad	60	2	0.5	790	2	0	2	9
Italian BMT Meats, amt on 6" sandwich or salad	180	14	5	1120	2	0	2	11
Meatballs, amt on 6" sandwich or salad	310	17	6	910	25	4	11	13
Roast Beef, amt on 6" sandwich or salad	80	2.5	1	430	1	0	1	18
Seafood Sensation, amt on 6" sandwich or salad	190	16	2.5	430	7	0	1	5
Steak, amt on 6" sandwich or salad	112	4	2	560	4	0	1	15
Subway Club Meats, amt on 6" sandwich or salad	90	2.5	1	750	2	0	1	17
Tuna, amt on 6" sandwich or salad	260	24	4	310	0	0	0	10
Turkey Breast, amt on 6" sandwich or salad	50	1	0	500	2	0	1	9
Veggie Patty, amt on 6" sandwich or salad	160	5	0.5	520	12	0	2	15

Dressing/Condiment

Description & Serving	Cal	Fat	Sfat	Sod	Carb	Fiber	Sugar	Prot
Fat Free Italian Salad Dressing	35	0	0	720	7	0	4	1
Ranch Salad Dressing	290	30	4.5	540	3	0	3	1
Chipotle Southwest Sauce, 21 g	100	10	1.5	220	1	0	0	0
Honey Mustard Sauce, Fat Free, 21 g	30	0	0	115	7	0	6	0
Light Mayonnaise, 1 tbsp	50	5	1	100	<1	0	0	0
Mayonnaise Packet, 1 tbsp	110	12	2	80	0	0	0	0
Mustard, yellow or deli brown, 2 tsp	5	0	0	115	<1	0	0	0
Olive Oil Blend, 1 tsp	45	5	0	0	0	0	0	0
Ranch Dressing, 21 g	110	11	1.5	200	1	0	1	0
Red Wine Vinaigrette, Fat Free, 21 g	30	0	0	340	6	0	3	0
Sweet Onion Sauce, Fat Free, 21 g	40	0	0	85	9	0	8	0
Vinegar, 1 tsp	0	0	0	0	0	0	0	0

Swiss Chalet

Appetizer

Description & Serving	Cal	Fat	Sfat	Sod	Carb	Fiber	Sugar	Prot
Hearty Chicken Minestrone Soup	160	3.5	1	680	20	6	2	17
Chalet Chicken Soup	90	3	1	190	1	0	0	15
Chicken Spring Rolls, 4	400	16	2.5	430	45	1	3	20

Description & Serving	Cal	Fat	Sfat	Sod	Carb	Fiber	Sugar	Prot
Crispy Dry Ribs	920	64	24	1880	4	0	0	76
The Garlic Cheese Loaf	860	53	19	1610	77	5	1	27
The Garlic Loaf, no cheese	650	35	9	1210	74	5	1	14
Cheese Perogies, 7	420	10	2	790	69	4	2	12
Chalet Chicken Wings, 8	550	34	7	790	23	2	9	39

Entrée

Classic Quarter Chicken Breast w/ skin	300	11	3.5	490	3	3	0	47
Classic Quarter Chicken Breast, skinless	180	3.5	1	190	0	0	0	38
Classic Quarter Chicken Leg w/ skin	310	19	6	430	2	2	0	35
Classic Quarter Chicken Leg, skinless	220	10	3	240	0	1	0	33
Classic Half Chicken w/ skin	610	31	9	920	5	5	0	82
Classic Double Leg w/ skin	630	38	12	860	4	4	0	70
Chicken Pot Pie	550	34	19	1420	63	4	7	30
Health Check Classic Quarter Chicken	360	11	3.5	745	14	8	3	50
1/3 Rack BBQ Ribs	430	28	11	300	4	2	0	40
Half Rack BBQ Ribs	650	42	16	450	6	3	1	60
Full Rack BBQ Ribs	1300	85	32	900	11	6	1	120
Crispy Tortilla Strips	150	10	1.5	180	13	1	0	2
Fresh Vegetable Stir Fry w/o rice	320	24	3.5	720	26	5	15	4
Chicken Stir Fry w/o rice	430	26	4	1180	26	5	15	29
Chicken Stir Fry w/ rice	750	30	4	2290	89	6	17	32

Side

Oven-Baked Potato	220	0	0	1	48	5	0	0
Sweet Kernel Corn	140	1	0	45	30	5	5	5
Fresh Vegetable Medley	60	2	0.2	70	11	4	5	3
Fresh, Hand Cut Fries	530	27	2	95	64	6	0	7
Real Sour Cream & Chives	70	5	3.5	35	3	0	2	2
Mashed Potatoes	150	4	1.5	410	27	3	3	3
Gravy	45	1.5	0.5	600	7	0	1	1
Creamy Coleslaw	200	14	0	460	15	3	12	2
Ramekin of Creamy Coleslaw	70	5	0	160	5	1	4	1
Seasoned Rice	240	3.5	0.3	830	48	1	1	5
Freshly Sauteed Mushrooms	220	16	2.5	350	11	2	4	6
White Roll	110	0.4	0.1	230	22	1	0	4
Multigrain Roll	110	1	0.1	200	21	1	0	4

Sandwich/Burger/Wrap

Classic Hot Chicken Sandwich, white	380	6	1.5	690	29	2	2	53
Classic Hot Chicken Sandwich, dark	450	15	4	770	29	2	2	49
Chipotle Chicken Sandwich	490	8	2.5	1160	72	3	22	32
Chicken on a Kaiser, white	440	6	1.5	730	42	2	3	56
Chicken on a Kaiser, dark	510	14	4	810	42	3	3	53
Chargrilled Hamburger, no bun	490	38	17	1150	1	0	0	35
Chargrilled Hamburger w/ bun	710	39	17	1630	43	2	3	44
Chargrilled Bacon Cheese Burger, no bun	680	52	23	1760	4	0	0	48
Chargrilled Bacon Cheese Burger w/ bun	890	54	24	2240	46	2	3	56
Chargrilled Veggie Burger, no bun	110	11	2	570	10	6	0	23
Chargrilled Veggie Burger w/ bun	330	12	2.5	1050	52	8	3	32

Description & Serving	Cal	Fat	SFat	Sod	Carb	Fiber	Sugar	Prot
Rotisserie Chicken Caesar Wrap	890	50	13	1810	62	4	6	45
Rotisserie Chicken Club Wrap	820	40	15	1730	58	3	5	59
Rotisserie Chicken Quesadilla, plain	620	23	11	1460	72	4	14	32

Salad

Garden Salad w/o dresssing	40	0	0	60	9	3	5	2
Caesar Salad w/ dressing	420	37	6	650	16	2	3	5
Greek Salad w/o dresssing	80	5	2.5	430	6	3	3	4
Side Salad w/o dressing	20	1	0	25	5	2	2	1
Side Caesar Salad w/ dressing	210	19	3	320	9	2	2	3
Side Greek Salad w/o dresssing	45	2.5	1	210	5	2	2	2
Chalet Chopped Salad	440	27	6	1250	29	7	13	23
Bacon Ranch Salad	530	37	10	1070	22	5	9	25
Chicken Caesar Salad, w/ dressing	630	41	8	1300	30	4	4	35
Chicken Caesar Salad	680	41	8	1550	42	4	12	35
Spinach Chicken Salad	170	2	0.5	530	14	5	7	28

Dressing/Condiment

World-Renowned Chalet Dipping Sauce, 100 ml	25	0.5	0.2	700	5	0	1	0.3
Fat Free Raspberry Vinaigrette, 15 ml	15	0	0	65	3	0	2	0
Ranch Dressing, 15 ml	70	7	1	120	1	0	1	0.1
Chalet Dressing, 15 ml	80	7	1	200	3	0	3	0.1
Caesar Dressing, 15 ml	90	9	1.5	105	1	0	0	0.2
Light Italian Dressing, 15 ml	15	1.5	0.1	135	1	0	0	0
Balsamic Vinaigrette, 15 ml	60	7	0.5	130	1	0	1	0
Greek Dressing, 15 ml	70	7	1	135	1	0	1	0.1
Lemon Garlic Dressing, 15 ml	40	4	0.3	110	1	0	0	0.1
Light Mayonnaise, 15 ml	45	4.5	0.5	130	1	0	0	0.1
Blue Cheese Dip, 15 ml	70	7	1	140	1	0	1	0.3
Cajun Sauce Dip, 57 g	100	9	4	290	3	0	0	2
Plum Sauce, 28 g	50	0	0	90	13	0	10	0
Sweet Chili Sauce, 57 g	100	0	0	200	24	0	19	0.4
Salsa, 40 g	20	0	0	380	4	0	3	1

Kids

Chicken Strips, 3	320	15	1.5	780	27	2	0	20
Mini Chicken Sandwiches, 3	320	8	2	500	32	2	3	30
Mini Burgers, 3	360	18	8	640	32	2	4	22
Cheesy Pizza	370	13	6	860	45	2	3	17
Chicken Thigh & Drumstick	310	19	6	430	2	2	0	35

Dessert

Colossal Caramel Fudge Cheesecake	660	41	16	340	68	2	47	7
Coconut Cream Pie	540	33	21	310	57	1	40	4
Carrot Cake	610	39	11	310	63	2	43	6
Pecan Pie	590	29	10	590	79	2	29	6
Old Fashioned Fudge Cake	720	44	12	530	81	4	49	6
Chocolate Lava Cake	430	23	7	310	53	2	31	4
Lemon Meringue Pie	400	11	5	430	73	1	44	3
Classic Apple Pie	440	19	9	430	65	3	31	4
Apple Crumble	480	10	6	330	94	4	67	10

Description & Serving	Cal	Fat	Sfat	Sod	Carb	Fiber	Sugar	Prot
Vanilla Ice Cream	120	6	2.5	50	17	0	13	1
Chocolate Ice Cream	130	5	3	35	19	1	14	1
Cranberry Raspberry Frozen Yogurt	110	2	1	50	22	0	15	3
Butterscotch Sauce	100	0	0	70	25	0	18	0.3
Chocolate Sauce	80	0	0	15	20	0	15	0.6
Strawberry Sauce	40	0	0	0	10	0	10	0

Taco Bell

Entrée

Beef

	Cal	Fat	Sfat	Sod	Carb	Fiber	Sugar	Prot
Fresco Crunchy Taco	150	7	2.5	350	13	3	1	7
Fresco Soft Taco	180	7	3	640	22	3	2	8
Crunchy Taco	170	10	3.5	330	12	3	1	8
Soft Taco	210	9	4	620	21	3	2	10
Volcano Taco	240	17	5	470	14	3	1	8
Volcano Burrito	800	42	12	2010	81	8	6	24
Crunchy Taco Supreme	200	12	5	350	15	3	2	9
Double Decker Taco	330	13	5	820	38	8	2	14
Double Decker Taco Supreme	360	15	6	840	41	8	3	15
Soft Taco Supreme	240	11	5	650	24	3	3	11
Beef Gordita Supreme	320	16	5	640	30	4	5	13
Beef Gordita Baja	360	21	5	800	30	5	5	13
Beef Gordita Nacho Cheese	320	16	3.5	780	31	4	5	12
Beef Chalupa Supreme	370	21	6	610	31	3	4	14
Beef Chalupa Baja	410	26	5	770	31	4	3	13
Beef Chalupa Nacho Cheese	370	21	3.5	750	32	3	4	12
Beef Burrito Supreme	420	15	7	1380	52	9	5	17
Beef Fiesta Burrito	380	14	5	1190	50	5	3	14
Beef Grilled Stuft Burrito	690	30	10	2130	79	12	5	27
1/2 lb Beef & Potato Burrito	510	22	6	1750	66	7	4	14
1/2 lb Beef Combo Burrito	450	18	7	1640	52	10	3	22
Crunchwrap Supreme	540	21	7	1400	71	6	7	16
Mexican Pizza	540	30	8	1020	47	8	2	21
Beef Enchirito	370	17	8	1430	35	8	2	19
MexiMelt	280	14	7	870	23	4	2	15
Cheesy Double Beef Burrito	470	20	6	1580	54	6	4	18

Chicken

	Cal	Fat	Sfat	Sod	Carb	Fiber	Sugar	Prot
Fresco Burrito Supreme – Chicken	340	8	2.5	1410	50	8	4	18
Fresco Fiesta Burrito – Chicken	340	8	2.5	1240	50	4	4	16
Fresco Ranchero Chicken Soft Taco	170	4	1.5	740	22	2	3	12
Ranchero Chicken Soft Taco	270	14	4	840	21	2	2	14
Chicken Gordita Supreme	300	13	3.5	680	29	3	5	17
Chicken Gordita Baja	340	18	3.5	840	29	3	5	17
Chicken Gordita Nacho Cheese	300	13	2	820	30	2	5	15
Chicken Chalupa Supreme	350	18	4	650	30	2	4	17
Chicken Chalupa Baja	390	23	4	800	29	2	3	17
Chicken Chalupa Nacho Cheese	350	18	2	780	30	2	4	16
Chicken Burrito Supreme	390	12	5	1420	51	7	5	21

Description & Serving	Cal	Fat	Sfat	Sod	Carb	Fiber	Sugar	Prot
Chicken Fiesta Burrito	360	10	3.5	1220	49	3	3	17
Chicken Grilled Stuft Burrito	650	23	7	2210	77	9	5	34
Chicken Enchirito	350	14	7	1470	34	7	2	22
Chicken Taquitos	320	11	4.5	1000	37	2	2	18
Chicken Quesadilla	520	27	12	1490	41	4	3	28
Grilled Chicken Burrito	440	20	5	1260	48	3	3	16
Grilled Chicken Soft Taco	200	8	3	640	19	1	1	12
Steak								
Fresco Burrito Supreme – Steak	330	8	3	1340	49	8	4	16
Fresco Grilled Steak Soft Taco	160	4.5	1.5	600	21	2	3	9
Grilled Steak Soft Taco	250	14	4	710	20	2	2	11
Steak Gordita Supreme	290	13	4	610	29	3	5	14
Steak Gordita Baja	330	18	4	760	28	3	5	14
Steak Gordita Nacho Cheese	290	13	2	740	29	2	5	13
Steak Chalupa Supreme	340	18	4	580	29	2	4	15
Steak Chalupa Baja	380	23	4	730	29	2	4	14
Steak Chalupa Nacho Cheese	340	18	2.5	710	30	2	4	13
Steak Burrito Supreme	380	12	5	1340	51	7	5	18
Steak Fiesta Burrito	350	11	4	1150	48	3	4	14
Steak Grilled Stuft Burrito	630	24	8	2060	76	9	6	28
Steak Enchirito	340	14	7	1400	33	7	2	19
Steak Taquitos	310	11	5	930	37	2	3	15
Steak Quesadilla	510	28	12	1410	41	4	3	25
Vegetarian								
Fresco Bean Burrito	340	8	2.5	1290	56	11	4	12
7-Layer Burrito	510	18	6	1410	68	12	5	18
1/2 lb Cheesy Bean & Rice Burrito	480	21	5	1440	60	7	5	13
Cheese Roll-Up	200	10	5	530	19	2	1	9
Bean Burrito	370	10	3.5	1270	55	11	3	14
Side/Nachos								
Pintos 'n Cheese	180	7	3	720	19	9	1	10
Mexican Rice	130	3.5	0	410	21	1	1	2
Cheesy Fiesta Potatoes	270	16	2.5	840	28	3	2	4
Nachos	330	21	2	520	31	2	2	4
Nachos Supreme	440	24	5	800	42	8	3	13
Nachos BellGrande	770	42	7	1300	78	15	5	20
Triple Layer Nachos	350	18	1.5	740	39	7	2	7
Salad								
Chicken Ranch Fully Loaded Taco Salad	970	57	10	1740	78	10	7	36
Chipotle Steak Fully Loaded Taco Salad	960	60	11	1780	77	9	9	30
Fiesta Taco Salad	840	43	10	1790	82	18	10	31
Fiesta Taco Salad w/o shell	470	23	9	1520	42	16	9	25
Express Taco Salad	610	31	9	1430	58	17	7	26
Condiment								
Guacamole, 21 g	35	3	0	85	2	1	0	0
Salsa, 21 g	5	0	0	80	1	0	1	0
Sour Cream, 21 g	30	2	1	20	2	0	1	1

Description & Serving	Cal	Fat	Sfat	Sod	Carb	Fiber	Sugar	Prot
Beverage								
Mango Strawberry Frutista Freeze	250	0	0	10	62	0	59	0
Strawberry Frutista Freeze	230	0	0	55	57	0	57	0
Dessert								
Cinnamon Twists	170	7	0	200	26	1	10	1
Caramel Apple Empanada	310	15	2.5	310	39	2	13	3

Taco Bueno

Breakfast

Description & Serving	Cal	Fat	Sfat	Sod	Carb	Fiber	Sugar	Prot
Bacon Egg Quesadilla	910	59	NP	2090	51	1	2	45
Bacon Egg Burrito	490	26	NP	1110	36	2	4	26
Potato Egg Burrito	460	22	NP	680	47	3	4	17
Sausage Egg Burrito	440	23	NP	720	37	2	4	21
Meat Lovers Burrito	560	32	NP	1360	37	2	4	31
Bacon Egg Taco	240	13	NP	690	18	1	2	12
Potato Egg Taco	230	10	NP	550	24	1	2	9
Sausage Egg Taco	250	15	NP	700	19	1	2	13
Meat Lovers Breakfast Taco	310	20	NP	940	19	1	2	16
Potato Stix	280	22	NP	350	18	2	0	2

Entrée

Beef

Description & Serving	Cal	Fat	Sfat	Sod	Carb	Fiber	Sugar	Prot
Beef Burrito	510	29	NP	1377	41	3	1	23
Beef Burrito w/o Cheddar Cheese	432	22	NP	1255	40	3	1	19
Beef Burrito w/o Chili	455	25	NP	1105	35	2	1	20
Beef Big Ol' Burrito	772	46	NP	1833	57	3	2	33
Beef Big Ol' Burrito w/o Cheddar Cheese	615	33	NP	1590	56	3	2	24
Beef Big Ol' Burrito w/o Chili	716	43	NP	1561	51	2	2	31
Beef Big Ol' Burrito w/o Sour Cream	715	40	NP	1814	55	3	1	32
Combination Burrito	564	29	NP	1505	54	3	1	23
Combination Burrito w/o Cheddar Cheese	486	23	NP	1384	53	3	1	18
Combination Burrito w/o Chili	509	26	NP	1234	48	2	1	20
Combination Burrito w/o Refried Beans	440	23	NP	1157	40	3	1	18
Beef Potato Burrito	358	21	NP	905	32	3	3	11
Beef Potato Burrito w/o Queso	305	17	NP	644	30	3	1	9
Beef Potato Burrito w/o Sour Cream	330	18	NP	896	31	3	2	11
Beef Muchaco	496	25	NP	877	49	2	2	17
Beef Muchaco w/o Refried Beans	392	20	NP	596	38	2	2	14
Beef Muchaco w/o Cheddar Cheese	457	22	NP	826	49	2	2	15
Beef Crispy Taco	200	14	NP	378	7	0	0	10
Beef Crispy Taco w/o Cheddar Cheese	161	11	NP	317	6	0	0	7
Beef Soft Taco	245	14	NP	620	18	1	0	11
Beef Soft Taco w/o Cheddar Cheese	206	11	NP	559	17	1	0	9
Party Taco	143	10	NP	244	5	0	0	7
Party Taco w/o Cheddar Cheese	104	7	NP	183	5	0	0	4
Beef Bueno Chilada	523	32	NP	2056	42	2	6	24
Beef Bueno Chilada w/o Chili	412	35	NP	1512	29	1	6	19

Description & Serving	Cal	Fat	Sfat	Sod	Carb	Fiber	Sugar	Prot
Beef Bueno Chilada w/o Queso	337	18	NP	1147	35	2	2	14
Beef Quesadilla	823	51	NP	1612	49	2	1	38
Chicken								
Chicken Big Ol' Burrito	607	30	NP	1640	53	5	3	31
Chicken Big Ol' Burrito w/o Cheddar Cheese	450	17	NP	1397	52	3	3	22
Chicken Big Ol' Burrito w/o Sour Cream	551	24	NP	1621	51	2	2	30
Chicken Potato Burrito	327	18	NP	928	33	3	3	11
Chicken Potato Burrito w/o Queso	274	14	NP	667	31	3	2	9
Chicken Potato Burrito w/o Sour Cream	299	15	NP	918	32	3	2	11
Chicken Ultimate Gourmet Burrito	960	26	NP	2980	135	10	5	47
Chicken Ultimate Gourmet Bowl	650	16	NP	2270	89	9	4	40
Chicken Muchaco	387	18	NP	817	40	2	2	17
Chicken Muchaco w/o Cheddar Cheese	348	14	NP	756	39	2	2	15
Chicken Crispy Taco	140	7	NP	368	8	0	1	9
Chicken Crispy Taco w/o Cheddar Cheese	100	4	NP	307	7	0	1	7
Chicken Soft Taco	184	8	NP	610	19	1	1	10
Chicken Soft Taco w/o Cheddar Cheese	145	5	NP	549	18	1	1	8
Flame-Grilled Chicken Fajita Taco	210	8	NP	600	19	1	2	15
Flame-Grilled Chicken Fajita Taco w/o Cheddar Cheese	142	4	NP	497	19	1	1	7
Chicken Bueno Chilada	477	26	NP	2090	43	2	7	24
Chicken Bueno Chilada w/o Chili	365	20	NP	1546	30	1	6	19
Chicken Bueno Chilada w/o Queso	290	12	NP	1181	36	2	2	14
Chicken Quesadilla	761	44	NP	1658	50	2	1	38
Steak								
Steak Ultimate Gourmet Burrito	1010	31	NP	2790	137	10	6	45
Steak Ultimate Gourmet Bowl	700	21	NP	2080	91	9	5	38
Flame-Grilled Steak Fajita Taco	230	11	NP	500	20	1	2	14
Flame-Grilled Steak Fajita Taco w/o Pepper Jack Cheese	156	5	NP	455	18	1	1	9
Vegetarian								
Bean Burrito	604	29	NP	1590	67	3	1	22
Bean Burrito w/o Cheddar Cheese	526	23	NP	1469	66	3	1	17
Bean Burrito w/o Chili	549	26	NP	1319	61	2	1	19
Party Burrito	374	18	NP	1002	43	1	1	13
Party Burrito w/o Cheddar Cheese	335	14	NP	941	43	1	1	11
Party Burrito w/o Chili	346	16	NP	866	40	1	1	12
Black Bean Burrito	490	15	NP	730	70	9	2	18
Cheese Quesadilla	709	42	NP	1261	48	2	1	30
Mini Cheese Quesadilla	274	15	NP	533	23	1	1	11
Side								
Black Beans, side	180	0	NP	810	36	12	0	12
Black Beans, platter	90	0	NP	405	18	6	0	6
Cilantro Lime Rice, side	280	0.5	NP	510	63	1	0	5
Cilantro Lime Rice, platter	140	0.25	NP	255	31.5	0.5	0	2.5
Refried Beans	634	34	NP	1787	60	1	1	24
Refried Beans w/o Cheddar Cheese	556	28	NP	1666	60	1	1	20

Description & Serving	Cal	Fat	Sfat	Sod	Carb	Fiber	Sugar	Prot
Refried Beans w/o Chili	578	31	NP	1516	54	0	0	22
Small Mexican Rice	235	6	NP	643	41	1	2	5
Small Refried Beans	317	17	NP	894	30	0	0	12
Small Refried Beans w/o Cheddar Cheese	278	14	NP	833	30	0	0	10
Small Refried Beans w/o Chili	289	16	NP	758	27	0	0	11

Salad

Beef Taco Salad	1043	75	NP	1705	58	12	2	36
Beef Taco Salad w/o Cheddar Cheese	886	62	NP	1462	56	12	2	27
Beef Taco Salad w/o Chili	987	72	NP	1433	51	12	2	33
Beef Taco Salad w/o Guacamole	988	70	NP	1577	56	11	2	35
Beef Taco Salad w/o Sour Cream	986	70	NP	1686	56	12	2	35
Beef Taco Salad w/o Tortilla Bowl	564	45	NP	1383	15	2	2	28
Chicken Taco Salad	838	57	NP	1325	53	12	3	30
Chicken Taco Salad w/o Cheddar Cheese	680	44	NP	1083	52	12	3	21
Chicken Taco Salad w/o Guacamole	783	52	NP	1198	51	11	3	29
Chicken Taco Salad w/o Sour Cream	781	51	NP	1307	51	12	2	29
Chicken Taco Salad w/o Tortilla Bowl	359	26	NP	1004	10	1	2	22
Beef Nacho Salad	759	48	NP	1877	58	8	6	28
Beef Nacho Salad w/o Cheddar Cheese	681	42	NP	1756	57	8	6	24
Beef Nacho Salad w/o Chili	648	41	NP	1334	45	6	5	24
Chicken Nacho Salad	713	43	NP	1911	59	8	7	28
Chicken Nacho Salad w/o Cheddar Cheese	634	37	NP	1790	58	8	7	24
Chicken Nacho Salad w/o Chili	601	36	NP	1368	46	6	6	24

Soup

Chicken Tortilla Soup, bowl	237	11	NP	1430	19	2	3	20
Chicken Tortilla Soup w/o Tortilla Strips & Cheese, bowl	148	6	NP	1382	11	2	3	17
Chicken Tortilla Soup, cup	117	6	NP	736	11	1	3	18
Chicken Tortilla Soup w/o Tortilla Strips & Cheese, cup	61	2	NP	691	7	1	3	16

Nachos/Snack

Corn Tortilla Chips, 1.5 oz	219	11	NP	25	27	4	1	3
Cheese Nachos	572	35	NP	1396	47	6	8	18
MexiDips & Chips	1086	62	NP	1862	105	12	7	29
MexiDips & Chips w/o Cheddar Cheese	1047	59	NP	1802	105	12	7	27
MexiDips & Chips w/o MexiDips Bowls	970	57	NP	1846	91	10	6	27
Beef Mucho Nachos	1567	97	NP	4105	127	11	13	57
Beef Mucho Nachos w/o Cheddar Cheese	1488	91	NP	3984	126	11	13	52
Beef Mucho Nachos w/o Chili	1399	87	NP	3290	109	9	12	50
Beef Mucho Nachos w/o Refried Beans	1233	81	NP	3176	91	11	13	45
Beef Mucho Nachos w/o Sour Cream	1510	91	NP	4086	125	11	12	56
Chicken Mucho Nachos	1505	90	NP	4150	128	11	13	57
Chicken Mucho Nachos w/o Cheddar Cheese	1426	83	NP	4029	128	11	13	53
Chicken Mucho Nachos w/o Chili	1337	80	NP	3335	110	9	12	50
Chicken Mucho Nachos w/o Refried Beans	1171	73	NP	3221	93	11	13	45
Chicken Mucho Nachos w/o Sour Cream	1448	84	NP	4131	126	11	12	56
Tostada	401	24	NP	932	32	2	1	16

Description & Serving	Cal	Fat	Sfat	Sod	Carb	Fiber	Sugar	Prot
Tostada w/o Cheddar Cheese	283	15	NP	749	31	2	1	9
Tostada w/o Chili	345	21	NP	660	26	1	0	13
Tostada w/o Refried Beans	234	16	NP	467	15	2	1	10
Kids								
Kids Cheese Quesadilla	219	11	NP	462	23	1	1	8
Topping/Condiment								
Cheddar Cheese, 0.5 oz	79	6	NP	121	1	0	0	4
Jalapenos, 0.7 oz	3	0	NP	334	1	1	0	0
Onions, 0.5 oz	7	0	NP	0	2	0	0	0
Guacamole, 0.9 oz	55	5	NP	128	2	1	0	1
Pico de Gallo, 0.5 oz	5	0	NP	10	1	0	0	0
Queso, 3.5 oz	279	21	NP	1362	10	0	7	14
Salsa, Original Red, 2 oz	14	0	NP	366	3	1	0	1
Sour Cream, 1 oz	57	6	NP	19	2	0	1	1
Dessert								
Cheesecake Chimichanga	210	11	NP	160	24	1	4	4
Cinnamon Chips	676	31	NP	254	95	4	54	8

Taco Cabana

Breakfast								
Potato & Egg Taco	220	11	2	390	23	0	1	8
Bacon & Egg Taco	200	9	2.5	530	20	0	1	11
Chorizo & Egg Taco	200	9	2.5	510	20	0	1	9
Barbacoa Taco	250	12	6	420	19	0	1	19
Potato & Egg Burrito	400	21	5	690	42	0	1	14
Bacon & Egg Burrito	370	17	5	970	35	0	1	20
Chorizo & Egg Burrito	360	17	6	930	36	0	1	18
Barbacoa Burrito	470	24	12	750	34	0	1	30
Huevos Rancheros - Scrambled Eggs	720	35	11	1880	66	7	3	33
Huevos Rancheros - Fried Eggs	850	48	14	1800	66	7	3	34
Eggs Mexicana Platter	900	51	18	2450	69	7	7	41
Steak Fajitas & Scrambled Eggs	750	33	11	1830	69	7	4	40
Steak Fajitas & Fried Eggs	880	47	13	1750	68	7	4	42
Entrée								
Beef								
Beef Soft Taco	230	9	3	710	21	<1	2	13
Carne Guisada Soft Taco	190	5	1	330	20	0	1	12
Beef Hard Taco	180	10	3.5	430	11	2	1	12
Beef Chalupa	310	16	6	640	24	5	2	16
Beef Burrito	670	30	12	2060	65	4	4	35
Beef Burrito Ultimo	760	37	16	2190	68	6	6	36
Beef Cabana Bowl	1160	62	23	2560	114	11	6	35
Beef Enchilada	225	12	5	722	13	2	1	15
Chicken								
Chicken Fajita (dark), 2 tortillas	700	21	7	2400	92	5	9	33
Chicken Fajita Platter (dark), 2 tortillas	1590	53	19	5110	200	10	19	71

Description & Serving	Cal	Fat	Sfat	Sod	Carb	Fiber	Sugar	Prot
Chicken Fajita (white), 2 tortillas	710	20	6	2470	93	5	10	36
Chicken Fajita Platter (white), 2 tortillas	1610	51	18	5240	202	10	19	76
Chicken Soft Taco	210	7	2	720	23	1	2	13
Chicken Fajita Soft Taco (dark)	180	5	1	610	20	<1	1	13
Chicken Fajita Soft Taco (white)	190	4	1	650	21	<1	1	14
Chicken Hard Taco	160	7	2.5	430	13	2	1	11
Chicken Chalupa	290	14	5	640	26	5	2	16
Chicken Burrito	620	25	10	2070	68	5	5	34
Chicken Burrito Ultimo	720	32	14	2200	71	7	6	35
Chicken Fajita Burrito (dark)	580	24	11	1850	60	2	5	31
Chicken Fajita Burrito (white)	590	23	11	1910	61	1	5	34
Chicken Fajita Quesadilla (dark), personal	670	39	18	1580	49	3	4	33
Chicken Fajita Quesadilla (dark), reg	1260	75	36	2960	84	5	7	63
Chicken Fajita Quesadilla (white), personal	670	38	18	1610	49	3	4	34
Chicken Fajita Quesadilla (white), reg	1270	74	36	3020	85	5	8	66
Chicken Fajita Taco Dinner (dark)	900	25	5	3090	125	6	8	40
Chicken Fajita Taco Dinner (white)	920	24	4.5	3180	126	6	8	43
1/4 Dark Flameante Chicken Dinner	920	41	11	3030	82	2	7	54
1/4 White Flameante Chicken Dinner	770	22	6	2690	81	2	7	60
1/2 Flameante Chicken Dinner	1220	54	15	4070	83	2	9	99
Chicken Cabana Bowl	1140	60	22	2570	116	12	6	35
Chicken Fajita Cabana Bowl (dark)	1180	61	22	2660	114	11	6	41
Chicken Fajita Cabana Bowl (white)	1190	60	22	2720	115	11	6	44
Sour Cream Chicken Enchilada	170	6	2	511	20	3	2	11
Combination								
Super Tex-Mex Dinner	1490	76	29	3180	141	19	8	59
Mexican Dinner	1130	53	21	2600	113	11	6	47
Enchilada Dinner	1270	66	29	2800	115	11	5	52
Taco Dinner	990	40	14	2390	112	11	7	41
Carne Guisada Dinner	840	28	9	1650	93	8	5	45
Steak								
Steak Fajita, 2 tortillas	730	24	8	2470	93	5	9	32
Steak Fajita Platter, 2 tortillas	1640	57	21	5240	202	10	18	70
Steak Fajita Soft Taco	200	6	1.5	650	21	0	1	12
Steak Fajita Burrito	610	26	12	1910	61	1	4	31
Steak Fajita Quesadilla, personal	680	40	19	1610	49	2	4	32
Steak Fajita Quesadilla, reg	1290	77	37	3020	85	5	7	63
Steak Fajita Taco Dinner	940	28	6	3180	126	6	7	39
Steak Fajita Cabana Bowl	1200	63	23	2720	115	11	6	40
Vegetarian								
Bean & Cheese Soft Taco	300	14	6	590	31	3	1	11
Black Bean Soft Taco	180	4	1	630	30	1	2	5
Bean & Cheese Chalupa	290	17	7	350	23	5	2	11
Guacamole Chalupa	340	21	6	610	30	9	2	9
Bean & Cheese Burrito	690	35	14	1290	71	9	2	25
Black Bean Burrito	370	7	2	1560	68	3	4	10
Cheese Quesadilla, personal	620	37	18	1340	48	2	4	26

Description & Serving	Cal	Fat	Sfat	Sod	Carb	Fiber	Sugar	Prot
Cheese Quesadilla, reg	1170	72	36	2480	82	5	7	49
Cheese Enchilada	320	23	11	630	13	2	0	17

Side

Rice	120	0.5	0	520	25	0	1	2
Refried Beans	250	13	5	420	24	6	1	8
Borracho Beans	110	3	1	520	16	0	1	5
Black Beans	40	1	0	380	6	1	1	2

Salad

Beef Taco Salad	1030	65	24	1920	69	13	6	40
Beef Taco Salad w/o shell	640	38	17	1600	37	10	5	35
Chicken Taco Salad	990	60	22	1930	72	14	6	39
Chicken Taco Salad w/o shell	600	33	14	1600	39	11	5	34
Steak Fajita Taco Salad	740	49	18	1290	45	6	4	29
Steak Fajita Taco Salad w/o shell	350	22	10	960	12	4	3	24
Chicken Fajita Taco Salad (dark)	710	47	17	1230	44	7	5	29
Chicken Fajita Taco Salad (dark) w/o shell	320	20	9	900	11	4	4	24
Chicken Fajita Taco Salad (white)	720	46	16	1290	45	7	5	32
Chicken Fajita Taco Salad (white) w/o shell	330	19	9	960	12	4	4	27

Nachos

Bean & Cheese Queso Nachos, personal	510	37	15	1300	54	8	6	19
Bean & Cheese Queso Nachos, reg	1020	75	30	2610	108	17	12	39
Beef Queso Nachos, personal	460	35	14	1470	43	5	6	24
Beef Queso Nachos, reg	930	69	28	2940	87	11	12	47
Chicken Queso Nachos, personal	440	32	13	1470	45	6	6	23
Chicken Queso Nachos, reg	880	64	26	2950	89	12	13	46
Super Beef Queso Nachos, personal	680	49	20	1810	59	10	8	29
Super Beef Queso Nachos, reg	1370	98	41	3620	117	20	16	59
Super Chicken Queso Nachos, personal	660	47	19	1810	60	10	8	29
Super Chicken Queso Nachos, reg	1320	93	38	3630	120	21	16	58
Steak Fajita Queso Nachos, personal	540	41	17	1490	46	7	7	24
Steak Fajita Queso Nachos, reg	1080	82	34	2990	93	14	14	47
Chicken Fajita Queso Nachos (dark), personal	520	40	17	1460	46	7	7	24
Chicken Fajita Queso Nachos (dark), reg	1050	80	33	2930	92	14	14	48
Chicken Fajita Queso Nachos (white), personal	530	39	16	1490	46	7	7	25
Chicken Fajita Queso Nachos (white) , reg	1060	79	33	2990	93	14	14	50
Bean & Cheese Shredded Cheese Nachos, personal	580	45	19	670	50	8	1	27
Bean & Cheese Shredded Cheese Nachos, reg	1170	90	38	1340	100	17	2	54
Beef Shredded Cheese Nachos, personal	540	42	18	840	39	5	1	31
Beef Shredded Cheese Nachos, reg	1080	84	35	1680	78	11	2	62
Chicken Shredded Cheese Nachos, personal	520	40	16	840	41	6	1	31
Chicken Shredded Cheese Nachos, reg	1030	79	33	1690	81	12	3	61
Super Beef Shredded Cheese Nachos, personal	760	57	24	1180	55	10	3	37
Super Beef Shredded Cheese Nachos, reg	1520	113	48	2360	109	20	6	74
Super Chicken Shredded Cheese Nachos, personal	730	54	23	1180	56	10	3	36

Description & Serving	Cal	Fat	Sfat	Sod	Carb	Fiber	Sugar	Prot
Super Chicken Shredded Cheese Nachos, reg	1470	108	46	2370	112	21	6	73
Steak Fajita Shredded Cheese Nachos, personal	610	49	21	860	42	7	2	31
Steak Fajita Shredded Cheese Nachos, reg	1220	97	42	1730	85	14	4	62
Chicken Fajita Shredded Cheese Nachos (dark), personal	600	47	20	830	42	7	2	31
Chicken Fajita Shredded Cheese Nachos (dark), reg	1200	95	41	1660	84	14	4	62
Chicken Fajita Shredded Cheese Nachos (white), personal	600	47	20	860	42	7	2	33
Chicken Fajita Shredded Cheese Nachos (white), reg	1200	94	40	1730	85	14	4	65
Chips & Queso, personal or w/ combo meal	380	31	12	1090	42	5	6	15
Chips & Queso, reg	900	72	31	2910	87	11	15	37

Dressing/Condiment

Southwest Ranch Dressing, 1 oz	112	11	3	155	2	0	0	1
Guacamole, 3 oz	110	9	1	340	7	4	1	1
Sour Cream, 3 oz	160	14	10	40	3	0	3	3
Queso, 3 oz	200	15	9	1080	5	0	5	10
Shredded Cheese, 1 oz	110	9	5	180	0	0	0	7
Salsa Roja, 1 oz	5	0	0	95	1	0	1	0
Salsa Verde, 1 oz	10	0	0	125	1	0	1	0
Salsa Fuego, 1 oz	5	0	0	170	1	0	1	0
Salsa Ranch, 1 oz	35	4	0.5	170	1	0	1	0

Taco Del Mar

Breakfast

Mondito Breakfast Burrito, Refried, 320 g	590	27	9	1050	60	6	3	28
Mondito Breakfast Burrito, Refried, 354 g	640	31	11	1160	62	7	3	29
Mondo Breakfast Burrito, Refried, 587 g	1080	50	16	2010	105	11	5	52
Mondo Breakfast Burrito, Refried, 658 g	1190	59	21	2240	110	13	7	54
Breakfast Flour Taco, Refried	260	15	5	640	18	1	1	13
Egg & Cheese Burrito, Refried	490	19	6	830	59	6	3	22
Egg & Cheese Flour Taco, Refried	200	10	3.5	510	17	1	1	9
Eggs, 2 oz scoop	90	7	1.5	250	1	0	0	7
Hash Browns, 1 triangle	110	6	1	140	13	2	0	1
Potatoes Diced, 1.75 oz scoop	60	1	0	20	11	1	0	2
Sausage, 1.25 oz scoop	100	8	3	220	1	0	0	6

Entrée

Beef

Beef Baja Bowl, Refried	830	35	15	2540	81	10	6	44
Beef Mondo Burrito, Refried	1070	36	12.5	2560	134	12	6	54
Beef Mondito, Refried	555	18.5	6.25	1290	70.5	6	3	28
Beef Enchilada	1030	37	16	3210	115	13	6	55
Beef Quesadilla	800	37	16	1540	66	6	5	49

Description & Serving	Cal	Fat	Sfat	Sod	Carb	Fiber	Sugar	Prot
Beef Hard Taco	270	15	6	510	17	1	1	17
Beef Soft Taco	280	11	5	590	28	4	1	18
Chicken								
Chicken Baja Bowl, Refried	790	31	12	2230	79	9	6	44
Chicken Mondo Burrito, Refried	1030	32	9	2250	131	11	6	54
Chicken Mondito, Refried	545	16.5	4.75	1130	69.5	6	3	28
Chicken Enchilada	990	33	13	2900	113	12	5	55
Chicken Quesadilla	770	33	13	1220	64	5	4	49
Chicken Hard Taco	260	13	4.5	360	16	1	1	17
Chicken Soft Taco	260	9	3.5	430	27	3	1	19
Fish								
Fish Baja Bowl, Refried	880	41	13	2330	95	9	7	31
Fish Mondo Burrito, Refried	840	30	5	1620	110	12	7	32
Fish Mondito, Refried	505	20.5	5.25	930	60.5	7	3	21
Fish Hard Taco	270	15	4	360	23	1	1	10
Fish Soft Taco	270	11	3.5	440	34	3	1	12
Pork								
Pork Baja Bowl, Refried	790	33	13	2260	81	9	5	40
Pork Mondo Burrito, Refried	920	24	5	2100	132	11	5	43
Pork Mondito, Refried	545	17.5	5.25	1140	70.5	6	3	26
Pork Enchilada	990	35	14	2930	114	12	5	51
Pork Quesadilla	770	35	14	1250	65	5	4	45
Pork Hard Taco	260	14	4.5	370	17	1	1	15
Pork Soft Taco	260	10	4	450	28	3	1	16
Vegan								
Vegan Mondo, Refried	800	19	3.5	1830	133	12	6	24
Mondito Vegan, Refried	430	11	2	940	70	6	3	13
Vegetarian								
Cheese Mondo Burrito, Refried	870	24	8	1830	130	10	5	30
Cheese Mondito, Refried	460	13	4	920	69	5	3	16
Cheese Enchilada	820	27	11	2490	112	12	5	31
Cheese Quesadilla	710	35	16	990	63	4	4	32
Veggie Soft Taco	310	8	3	640	49	5	1	11
Side								
Black Beans, 4.25 oz	140	2	0	420	24	8	2	7
Refried Beans, 4.25 oz	160	3.5	1	480	24	5	1	7
Whole Pinto Beans, 4.25 oz	90	0	0	200	20	6	1	6
Rice, 1 scoop	230	3	0	720	45	1	0	4
Rice & Black Beans, 1 tray	370	5	0.5	1190	69	9	3	12
Rice & Refried Beans, 1 tray	390	7	1.5	1260	69	6	2	12
Rice & Whole Pinto Beans, 1 tray	320	3	0	980	66	8	2	10
Salad								
Beef Taco Salad, Refried	930	49	19	2180	75	12	7	47
Chicken Taco Salad, Refried	900	45	16	1870	73	11	6	47
Fish Taco Salad, Refried	1040	61	18	2050	89	11	8	34
Pork Taco Salad, Refried	900	46	17	1900	74	11	6	43

Description & Serving	Cal	Fat	Sfat	Sod	Carb	Fiber	Sugar	Prot
Snack								
Nachos, Refried	1190	65	25	1800	110	12	6	37
Chips & Salsa	590	27	5	550	78	5	3	8
Kids								
Kids Chips & Cheese	400	22	7	350	38	2	0	10
Kids Bean & Cheese Burrito	480	17	7	800	58	7	2	20
Kids Bean & Cheese Burrito & Chips	760	31	9	970	95	9	2	24
Kids Quesadilla	320	14	6	320	34	2	1	13
Kids Quesadilla & Chips	600	27	8	490	71	4	1	17
Kids Beef Taco	270	15	6	460	16	1	1	17
Kids Chicken Taco	250	13	4.5	300	15	1	0	17
Kids Pork Taco	250	14	4.5	320	16	1	0	15
Condiment								
Enchilada Sauce, 3 oz	35	0	0	610	7	0	2	1
Guacamole, 0.75 oz	40	3.5	0.5	170	2	1	1	1
Salsa, 3 oz	15	0	0	210	4	1	2	1
Sour Cream, 0.75 oz	70	6	4	60	2	0	1	1
Green Sauce, 2 tbsp	5	0	0	45	1	0	0	0
Habanero Sauce, 2 tbsp	10	0	0	160	1	0	1	0
Red Sauce, 2 tbsp	5	0	0	45	1	0	0	0
White Sauce, 2 tbsp	120	13	2	160	1	0	1	0
Queso, 1/4 cup	80	6	2.5	450	2	0	0	3
Dessert								
Oreo Brownie	400	17	4.5	210	59	1	37	4
Butter Cookie	220	10	7	190	31	0	17	2
Chocolate Chip Cookie	240	12	8	140	34	1	23	2
Chocolate Chip Cookie w/ Nuts	240	13	7	125	30	2	20	3
Milk Chocolate Cookie	240	12	8	150	31	0	21	3
Oatmeal, Raisin, & Walnut Cookie	240	11	6	180	35	1	21	3
Peanut Butter Cookie	240	13	6	95	27	0	15	4
Triple Chocolate Cookie	230	12	8	150	31	1	18	3
White Chocolate Macadamia Cookie	270	16	8	135	30	0	12	3

Taco John's

	Cal	Fat	Sfat	Sod	Carb	Fiber	Sugar	Prot
Breakfast								
Bacon Breakfast Burrito	550	25	6	1370	56	7	5	21
Bacon Breakfast Egg Burrito	500	24	9	1120	43	5	6	26
Bacon Breakfast Taco	270	13	4	810	25	2	1	10
Bacon Potato Olés Scrambler, sml	630	41	10	1860	45	6	2	20
Bacon Scrambler Burrito	550	25	6	1370	58	7	6	21
Breakfast Egg Burrito	420	19	8	730	42	5	6	21
Sausage Breakfast Burrito	640	35	10	1300	56	7	5	23
Sausage Breakfast Egg Burrito	590	34	13	1050	42	6	6	28
Sausage Breakfast Taco	310	18	6	770	25	2	1	11
Sausage Potato Olés Scrambler, sml	720	50	14	1780	45	6	2	22
Sausage Scrambler Burrito	640	32	9	1440	58	7	7	21

Description & Serving	Cal	Fat	Sfat	Sod	Carb	Fiber	Sugar	Prot
Entrée								
Beef								
Crispy Taco	180	10	3.5	270	13	2	1	9
Softshell Taco	220	11	4.5	580	21	2	1	11
Softshell Taco w/o cheese	190	8	3	530	20	2	1	9
Taco Bravo	340	13	4.5	750	40	5	1	15
Taco Burger	270	12	4	600	28	3	4	14
Taco Burger w/o cheese	250	9	2.5	560	28	3	4	12
Super Burrito	450	18	7	920	54	9	6	19
Meat & Potato Burrito	500	23	6	1100	58	8	5	15
Beefy Burrito	440	20	7	860	45	7	5	22
Combination Burrito	400	14	5	830	50	8	5	18
Beef Grilled Burrito	600	32	13	1230	52	8	5	27
Super Potato Olés, sml	620	39	11	1270	53	7	2	14
Mexi Rolls, 2 pc w/o nacho cheese	130	5	2	190	14	2	0	6
Chicken								
Chicken Softshell Taco	190	6	3	700	19	1	0	13
Chicken & Potato Burrito	470	19	4.5	1220	56	7	5	17
Crunchy Chicken & Potato Burrito	600	28	6	1320	65	7	5	20
Chicken Grilled Burrito	590	29	11	1510	50	6	5	32
Chicken Quesadilla	500	24	13	1240	44	5	5	29
Crunchy Chicken w/o sauce	450	27	3.5	1420	24	0	0	29
Vegetarian								
Bean Burrito	380	9	3	830	58	9	5	15
Bean Burrito w/o cheese	320	4.5	0	740	58	9	5	11
Cheese Quesadilla	450	23	12	930	43	5	5	20
Side								
Chili w/ cheese	220	11	5	1240	17	4	2	14
Chili w/o cheese	160	6	2	1160	17	4	2	10
Mexican Rice	250	6	0	1080	45	0	2	5
Refried Beans w/ cheese	320	6	3.5	1020	47	11	2	18
Refried Beans w/o cheese	280	1.5	0.5	980	50	11	2	15
Potato Olés, sml	430	26	3.5	1220	45	6	1	4
Potato Olés, reg	600	36	5	1710	62	8	1	6
Potato Olés, lrg	770	46	6	2200	80	11	1	7
Salad								
Taco Salad w/o dressing	520	33	11	860	37	7	7	21
Chicken Taco Salad w/o dressing	480	27	9	1020	35	6	7	24
Crunchy Chicken Taco Salad w/o dressing	660	40	10	1180	47	6	7	29
Snack/Nachos								
Buffalo Chicken Snackarito	290	15	5	990	27	1	1	11
Ranch Chicken Snackarito	240	12	4	690	23	1	1	11
Chips & Queso	430	25	7	940	43	2	1	9
Nachos	380	23	6	750	38	1	0	6
Super Nachos, sml	450	27	9	650	38	3	1	12

Description & Serving	Cal	Fat	Sfat	Sod	Carb	Fiber	Sugar	Prot
Dressing/Condiment								
House Dressing, 1.5 oz	70	7	1	260	2	0	1	0
Ranch Dressing, 1.5 oz	140	16	2	350	3	0	1	1
Bacon Ranch Dressing, 1.5 oz	130	10	1.5	370	10	0	7	1
Creamy Italian Dressing, 1.5 oz	130	15	2	320	3	0	1	0
Mild Sauce, 1 oz	10	0	0	130	1	0	0	0
Hot Sauce, 1 oz	10	0	0	125	1	0	0	0
Super Hot Sauce, 1 oz	10	0	0	25	1	0	0	0
Pico de Gallo, 1 oz	10	0	0	90	1	0	0	0
Salsa, 2 oz	20	0	0	220	4	1	2	1
Sour Cream, 2 oz	120	12	7	30	2	0	0	2
Guacamole, 2 oz	90	6	2	115	8	2	2	0
Nacho Cheese, 3 oz	120	9	4	520	5	0	0	4
Dessert								
Cini-Sopapilla Bites	210	5	0.5	320	37	4	7	4
Churro	190	7	1.5	170	15	4	10	2
Apple Grande (seasonal)	270	12	3	420	39	2	15	5
Choco Taco (seasonal)	390	20	15	160	48	1	32	5

TacoTime

Entrée

Beef

	Cal	Fat	Sfat	Sod	Carb	Fiber	Sugar	Prot
Big Juan Burrito w/ Ground Beef	634	23	10	2708	73	13	4	30
Casita Burrito w/ Ground Beef	543	24	12	2572	46	6	5	29
Beef, Bean & Cheese Burrito	495	17	7	2308	55	11	2	26
Crisp Ground Beef Burrito	428	21	6	827	36	4	1	22
Soft Meat Burrito	426	16	7	1095	43	8	2	23
Soft Taco w/ Ground Beef	418	16	7	1016	43	9	2	23
Crisp Taco w/ Ground Beef	263	17	5	461	12	2	1	14
Crisp Taco w/ Ground Beef & Sour Cream	292	19	7	466	12	2	2	14
Super Soft Taco w/ Ground Beef	589	23	10	2383	63	12	3	29
Super Soft Taco w/ Ground Beef on Wheat Tortilla	590	23	10	2408	62	8	3	30
Ground Beef Chimichanga	646	27	13	2516	63	11	5	31
Ground Beef Enchilada	292	12	5	834	21	3	4	18
Taco Burger	456	26	8	1175	31	3	7	21
Ground Beef Tostada	375	20	6	1827	25	5	2	21
Chicken								
Big Juan Burrito w/ Chicken	575	16	8	2550	70	11	4	34
Casita Burrito w/ Chicken	485	17	10	2349	42	5	4	34
Chicken & Black Bean Burrito	487	16	6	1269	54	9	3	30
Chicken B.L.T. Burrito	694	39	10	1596	43	8	4	39
Crispy Chicken Ranchero Burrito	604	31	7	1254	51	7	3	29
Crisp Chicken Burrito	380	17	6	537	33	2	0	22
Soft Taco w/ Chicken	361	9	4	857	40	7	1	28
Super Soft Taco w/ Chicken	532	16	8	2160	60	10	2	34
Super Soft Taco w/ Chicken on Wheat Tortilla	533	16	8	2185	59	6	2	34

Description & Serving	Cal	Fat	Sfat	Sod	Carb	Fiber	Sugar	Prot
Chicken Chimichanga	606	20	11	2619	63	10	4	37
Chicken Enchilada	235	5	3	611	17	1	3	23
Chicken Tostada	317	13	4	1604	22	3	1	26
Vegetarian								
Soft Veggie Burrito	520	17	7	2531	73	12	3	19
Bean Tostada	232	13	4	1320	21	3	1	8
Kids								
Crisp Pinto Bean Burrito	363	14	3	1906	47	5	0	13
Soft Pinto Bean Burrito	369	10	5	2105	54	10	1	14
Junior Soft Taco	314	13	6	800	28	6	2	18
Cheddar Melt	250	12	7	472	25	4	0	11
Side								
Cheddar Fries, sml	349	25	8	806	26	3	1	8
Cheddar Fries, med	499	35	11	1169	39	4	1	11
Cheddar Fries, lrg	697	49	16	1578	52	5	1	16
Mexi-Fries, sml	265	18	3	669	26	3	1	3
Mexi-Fries, med	387	26	5	987	38	4	1	4
Mexi-Fries, lrg	530	36	6	1305	51	5	1	5
Stuffed Mexi-Fries, sml	321	20	6	705	29	3	3	7
Stuffed Mexi-Fries, med	463	28	8	1023	42	4	4	11
Stuffed Mexi-Fries, lrg	642	40	11	1376	57	6	6	14
Mexi-Rice	76	1	0	351	17	0	1	2
Refritos w/ Chips	227	7	3	2622	29	5	2	11
Refritos w/o Chips	208	6	3	2621	26	5	2	11
Salad								
Regular Taco Salad w/ Chicken	314	13	4	679	22	2	3	25
Regular Taco Salad w/ Ground Beef	368	20	6	815	24	4	3	20
Tostada Delight Salad w/ Chicken	446	19	7	2050	35	4	2	30
Tostada Delight Salad w/ Ground Beef	487	26	10	1969	36	6	3	24
Snack								
Nachos Grande	927	43	21	3577	96	10	9	37
Taco Chips	150	3	0	7	27	1	0	3
Dressing/Condiment								
Chipotle Ranch Dressing, 1 oz	165	18	3	157	1	0	1	1
Ranch Dressing, 1 oz	181	20	3	167	1	NP	1	1
Thousand Island Dressing, 1 oz	132	12	2	369	5	0	3	0
Sour Cream, .5 oz	28	2	2	5	0	0	0	0
Guacamole, 1 oz	50	5	1	125	2	1	1	0
Salsa Fresca, 1 oz	8	0	0	174	2	0	1	0
Salsa Nuevo, 1 oz	8	0	0	131	2	0	1	0
Salsa Verde, 1 oz	6	0	0	149	2	0	0	0
Dessert								
Plain Churro	205	16	5	160	17	0	4	2
Churro w/ Cinnamon & Sugar	245	16	5	160	27	0	14	2
Cinnamon Crustos	294	6	1	273	58	3	19	6
Apple Empanada	234	7	1	201	40	2	10	4

Description & Serving	Cal	Fat	Sfat	Sod	Carb	Fiber	Sugar	Prot
Cherry Empanada	240	7	1	190	41	2	4	4
Pumpkin Empanada	256	8	1	198	42	2	16	6

TCBY

Frozen Yogurt

98% Fat Free, small

Description & Serving	Cal	Fat	Sfat	Sod	Carb	Fiber	Sugar	Prot
Cake Batter Frozen Yogurt	220	4	3	180	46	6	32	8
Cake Batter Frozen Yogurt in Cake Cone	180	3	2	150	37	4	24	6
Cake Batter Frozen Yogurt in Premade Waffle Cone	230	4	2	225	49	4	30	7
Cake Batter Frozen Yogurt in Fresh Waffle Cone	310	6.5	3	365	58	5	37	6
Cheesecake Frozen Yogurt	240	4	2	130	46	6	30	8
Cheesecake Frozen Yogurt in Cake Cone	190	3	1.5	110	37	4	22	6
Cheesecake Frozen Yogurt in Premade Waffle Cone	250	4	1.5	185	49	4	28	7
Cheesecake Frozen Yogurt in Fresh Waffle Cone	330	6.5	2.5	325	58	5	35	6
Chocolate Frozen Yogurt	220	4	2	190	46	6	34	8
Chocolate Frozen Yogurt in Cake Cone	180	3	1.5	155	37	4	25	6
Chocolate Frozen Yogurt in Premade Waffle Cone	230	4	1.5	230	49	4	31	7
Chocolate Frozen Yogurt in Fresh Waffle Cone	310	6.5	2.5	370	58	5	38	6
Classic Tart Frozen Yogurt	180	0	0	40	42	4	30	6
Classic Tart Frozen Yogurt in Cake Cone	150	0	0	45	34	3	22	4
Classic Tart Frozen Yogurt in Premade Waffle Cone	200	1	0	120	46	3	28	5
Classic Tart Frozen Yogurt in Fresh Waffle Cone	280	3.5	1	260	55	4	35	4
Coffee Frozen Yogurt	240	3	2	160	46	6	32	8
Coffee Frozen Yogurt in Cake Cone	190	2	1.5	135	37	4	24	6
Coffee Frozen Yogurt in Premade Waffle Cone	250	3	1.5	210	49	4	30	7
Coffee Frozen Yogurt in Fresh Waffle Cone	330	5.5	2.5	350	58	5	37	6
Golden Vanilla Frozen Yogurt	240	4	2	190	50	6	34	8
Golden Vanilla Frozen Yogurt in Cake Cone	190	3	1.5	155	40	4	25	6
Golden Vanilla Frozen Yogurt in Premade Waffle Cone	250	4	1.5	230	52	4	31	7
Golden Vanilla Frozen Yogurt in Fresh Waffle Cone	330	6.5	2.5	370	61	5	38	6
Peanut Butter Frozen Yogurt	260	4	1	190	52	6	38	10
Peanut Butter Frozen Yogurt in Cake Cone	210	3	0.5	155	42	4	28	7
Peanut Butter Frozen Yogurt in Premade Waffle Cone	260	4	0.5	230	54	4	34	8
Peanut Butter Frozen Yogurt in Fresh Waffle Cone	340	6.5	1.5	370	63	5	41	7
Strawberry Frozen Yogurt	220	4	3	180	46	6	32	8
Strawberry Frozen Yogurt in Cake Cone	180	3	2	150	37	4	24	6
Strawberry Frozen Yogurt in Premade Waffle Cone	230	4	2	225	49	4	30	7
Strawberry Frozen Yogurt in Fresh Waffle Cone	310	6.5	3	365	58	5	37	6
White Chocolate Mousse Frozen Yogurt	240	4	3	130	46	6	30	8

Description & Serving	Cal	Fat	Sfat	Sod	Carb	Fiber	Sugar	Prot
White Chocolate Mousse Frozen Yogurt in Cake Cone	190	3	2	110	37	4	22	6
White Chocolate Mousse Frozen Yogurt in Premade Waffle Cone	250	4	2	185	49	4	28	7
White Chocolate Mousse Frozen Yogurt in Fresh Waffle Cone	330	6.5	3	325	58	5	35	6
Fat Free, small								
Dutch Chocolate Frozen Yogurt	220	0	0	200	48	6	36	8
Dutch Chocolate Frozen Yogurt in Cake Cone	180	0	0	165	39	4	27	6
Dutch Chocolate Frozen Yogurt in Premade Waffle Cone	230	1	0	240	51	4	33	7
Dutch Chocolate Frozen Yogurt in Fresh Waffle Cone	310	3.5	1	380	60	5	40	6
Old Fashioned Vanilla Frozen Yogurt	220	0	0	130	46	6	30	8
Old Fashioned Vanilla Frozen Yogurt in Cake Cone	180	0	0	110	37	4	22	6
Old Fashioned Vanilla Frozen Yogurt in Premade Waffle Cone	230	1	0	185	49	4	28	7
Old Fashioned Vanilla Frozen Yogurt in Fresh Waffle Cone	310	3.5	1	325	58	5	35	6
Hand-Scooped, small								
Blueberries & Cream Frozen Yogurt	200	4	2.5	95	32	1	21	4
Blueberries & Cream Frozen Yogurt in Cake Cone	220	4	2.5	110	35	1	21	4
Blueberries & Cream Frozen Yogurt in Premade Waffle Cone	270	5	2.5	185	47	1	27	5
Blueberries & Cream Frozen Yogurt in Fresh Waffle Cone	350	7.5	3.5	325	56	2	34	4
Butter Pecan Frozen Yogurt	240	12	3.5	120	28	1	19	6
Butter Pecan Frozen Yogurt in Cake Cone	260	12	3.5	135	31	1	19	6
Butter Pecan Frozen Yogurt in Premade Waffle Cone	310	13	3.5	210	43	1	25	7
Butter Pecan Frozen Yogurt in Fresh Waffle Cone	390	15.5	4.5	350	52	2	32	6
Chocolate Chocolate Frozen Yogurt	190	5	3.5	95	30	1	22	6
Chocolate Chocolate Frozen Yogurt in Cake Cone	210	5	3.5	110	33	1	22	6
Chocolate Chocolate Frozen Yogurt in Premade Waffle Cone	260	6	3.5	185	45	1	28	7
Chocolate Chocolate Frozen Yogurt in Fresh Waffle Cone	340	8.5	4.5	325	54	2	35	6
Chocolate Chocolate Swirl Frozen Yogurt in Cake Cone	150	0.5	0.5	120	35	8	8	6
Chocolate Chocolate Swirl Frozen Yogurt in Premade Waffle Cone	200	1.5	0.5	195	47	8	14	7
Chocolate Chocolate Swirl Frozen Yogurt in Fresh Waffle Cone	280	4	1.5	335	56	9	21	6
Chocolate Chocolate Swirl Frozen Yogurt (NSA)	130	0.5	0.5	105	32	8	8	6
Chocolate Chocolate Swirl Frozen Yogurt (NSA) in Cake Cone	150	0.5	0.5	120	35	8	8	6
Chocolate Chocolate Swirl Frozen Yogurt (NSA) in Premade Waffle Cone	200	1.5	0.5	195	47	8	14	7

Description & Serving	Cal	Fat	Sfat	Sod	Carb	Fiber	Sugar	Prot
Chocolate Chocolate Swirl Frozen Yogurt (NSA) in Fresh Waffle Cone	280	4	1.5	335	56	9	21	6
Chocolate Chunk Cookie Dough Frozen Yogurt	240	9	5	125	37	0	26	4
Chocolate Chunk Cookie Dough Frozen Yogurt in Cake Cone	260	9	5	140	40	0	26	4
Chocolate Chunk Cookie Dough Frozen Yogurt in Premade Waffle Cone	310.	10.	5	215	52	0	32	5
Chocolate Chunk Cookie Dough Frozen Yogurt in Fresh Waffle Cone	390	12.5	6	355	61	1	39	4
Cookies & Cream Frozen Yogurt	210	7	3.5	80	33	0	22	5
Cookies & Cream Frozen Yogurt in Cake Cone	230	7	3.5	95	36	0	22	5
Cookies & Cream Frozen Yogurt in Premade Waffle Cone	280	8	3.5	170	48	0	28	6
Cookies & Cream Frozen Yogurt in Fresh Waffle Cone	360	10.5	4.5	310	57	1	35	5
Cotton Candy Frozen Yogurt	180	5	3.5	90	29	0	20	5
Cotton Candy Frozen Yogurt in Cake Cone	200	5	3.5	105	32	0	20	5
Cotton Candy Frozen Yogurt in Premade Waffle Cone	250	6	3.5	180	44	0	26	6
Cotton Candy Frozen Yogurt in Fresh Waffle Cone	330	8.5	4.5	320	52	1	33	5
Mint Chocolate Chunk Frozen Yogurt	220	8	6	95	33	1	26	4
Mint Chocolate Chunk Frozen Yogurt in Cake Cone	240	8	6	110	36	1	26	4
Mint Chocolate Chunk Frozen Yogurt in Premade Waffle Cone	290	9	6	185	48	1	32	5
Mint Chocolate Chunk Frozen Yogurt in Fresh Waffle Cone	370	11.5	7	325	57	2	39	4
Mocha Almond Frozen Yogurt	230	8	3	170	33	1	24	6
Mocha Almond Frozen Yogurt in Cake Cone	250	8	3	185	36	1	24	6
Mocha Almond Frozen Yogurt in Premade Waffle Cone	300	9	3	260	48	1	30	7
Mocha Almond Frozen Yogurt in Fresh Waffle Cone	380	11.5	4	400	57	2	37	6
Peaches & Cream Frozen Yogurt	170	4.5	3	75	30	0	22	4
Peaches & Cream Frozen Yogurt in Cake Cone	190	4.5	3	90	33	0	22	4
Peaches & Cream Frozen Yogurt in Premade Waffle Cone	240	5.5	3	165	45	0	28	5
Peaches & Cream Frozen Yogurt in Fresh Waffle Cone	320	8	4	305	54	1	35	4
Peanut Butter Delight Frozen Yogurt	270	12	5	160	34	2	24	7
Peanut Butter Delight Frozen Yogurt in Cake Cone	290	12	5	175	37	2	24	7
Peanut Butter Delight Frozen Yogurt in Premade Waffle Cone	340	13	5	250	49	2	30	8
Peanut Butter Delight Frozen Yogurt in Fresh Waffle Cone	420	15.5	6	390	58	3	37	7
Pralines & Cream Frozen Yogurt	220	7	3.5	140	35	0	25	5
Pralines & Cream Frozen Yogurt in Cake Cone	240	7	3.5	155	38	0	25	5
Pralines & Cream Frozen Yogurt in Premade Waffle Cone	290	8	3.5	230	50	0	31	6
Pralines & Cream Frozen Yogurt in Fresh Waffle Cone	370	10.5	4.5	370	59	1	38	5

Description & Serving	Cal	Fat	Sfat	Sod	Carb	Fiber	Sugar	Prot
Rainbow Cream Frozen Yogurt	180	5	3.5	90	29	0	20	5
Rainbow Cream Frozen Yogurt in Cake Cone	200	5	3.5	105	32	0	20	5
Rainbow Cream Frozen Yogurt in Premade Waffle Cone	250	6	3.5	180	44	0	26	6
Rainbow Cream Frozen Yogurt in Fresh Waffle Cone	330	8.5	4.5	320	53	1	33	5
Rocky Road Frozen Yogurt	270	12	6	105	36	2	22	6
Rocky Road Frozen Yogurt in Cake Cone	290	12	6	120	39	2	22	6
Rocky Road Frozen Yogurt in Premade Waffle Cone	340	13	6	195	51	2	28	7
Rocky Road Frozen Yogurt in Fresh Waffle Cone	420	15.5	7	335	60	3	35	6
Strawberries & Cream Frozen Yogurt	170	4	2.5	70	30	0	23	4
Strawberries & Cream Frozen Yogurt in Cake Cone	190	4	2.5	85	33	0	23	4
Strawberries & Cream Frozen Yogurt in Premade Waffle Cone	240	5	2.5	160	45	0	29	5
Strawberries & Cream Frozen Yogurt in Fresh Waffle Cone	320	7.5	3.5	300	54	1	36	4
Vanilla Bean Frozen Yogurt	180	5	3.5	90	29	0	20	5
Vanilla Bean Frozen Yogurt in Cake Cone	130	45	5	35	93	29	0	20
Vanilla Bean Frozen Yogurt in Premade Waffle Cone	180	46	5	110	105	29	6	21
Vanilla Bean Frozen Yogurt in Fresh Waffle Cone	260	48.5	6	250	114	30	13	20
Vanilla Chocolate Chip Frozen Yogurt	220	8	6	85	32	1	24	5
Vanilla Chocolate Chip Frozen Yogurt in Cake Cone	130	70	8	35	88	32	1	24
Vanilla Chocolate Chip Frozen Yogurt in Premade Waffle Cone	180	71	8	110	100	32	7	25
Vanilla Chocolate Chip Frozen Yogurt in Fresh Waffle Cone	260	73.5	9	250	109	33	14	24
Vanilla Fudge Brownie Frozen Yogurt (NSA)	160	3	2	120	34	7	8	6
Vanilla Fudge Brownie Frozen Yogurt (NSA) in Cake Cone	180	3	2	135	37	7	8	6
Vanilla Fudge Brownie Frozen Yogurt (NSA) in Premade Waffle Cone	230	4	2	210	49	7	14	7
Vanilla Fudge Brownie Frozen Yogurt (NSA) in Fresh Waffle Cone	310	6.5	3	350	58	8	21	6
White Chocolate Mousse Frozen Yogurt	290	4	2.5	70	47	0	16	3
White Chocolate Mousse Frozen Yogurt in Cake Cone	310	4	2.5	85	50	0	16	3
White Chocolate Mousse Frozen Yogurt in Premade Waffle Cone	360	5	2.5	160	62	0	22	4
White Chocolate Mousse Frozen Yogurt in Fresh Waffle Cone	440	7.5	3.5	300	71	1	29	3

No Sugar Added/Fat Free, small

Description & Serving	Cal	Fat	Sfat	Sod	Carb	Fiber	Sugar	Prot
Chocolate Frozen Yogurt	160	0	0	180	46	8	12	8
Chocolate Frozen Yogurt in Cake Cone	130	0	0	150	37	6	9	6
Chocolate Frozen Yogurt in Premade Waffle Cone	190	1	0	225	49	6	15	7
Chocolate Frozen Yogurt in Fresh Waffle Cone	270	3.5	1	365	58	7	22	6
Mountain Blackberry Frozen Yogurt	180	0	0	180	48	8	14	8
Mountain Blackberry Frozen Yogurt in Cake Cone	150	0	0	150	39	6	10	6
Mountain Blackberry Frozen Yogurt in Premade Waffle Cone	200	1	0	225	51	6	16	7

Description & Serving	Cal	Fat	Sfat	Sod	Carb	Fiber	Sugar	Prot
Mountain Blackberry Frozen Yogurt in Fresh Waffle Cone	280	3.5	1	365	60	7	23	6
Peach Frozen Yogurt	180	0	0	180	48	8	14	8
Peach Frozen Yogurt in Cake Cone	150	0	0	150	39	6	10	6
Peach Frozen Yogurt in Premade Waffle Cone	200	1	0	225	51	6	16	7
Peach Frozen Yogurt in Fresh Waffle Cone	280	3.5	1	365	60	7	23	6
Strawberry Frozen Yogurt	180	0	0	180	48	8	14	8
Strawberry Frozen Yogurt in Cake Cone	150	0	0	150	39	6	10	6
Strawberry Frozen Yogurt in Premade Waffle Cone	200	1	0	225	51	6	16	7
Strawberry Frozen Yogurt in Fresh Waffle Cone	280	3.5	1	365	60	7	23	6
Vanilla Frozen Yogurt	180	0	0	180	50	10	16	8
Vanilla Frozen Yogurt in Cake Cone	150	0	0	150	40	7	12	6
Vanilla Frozen Yogurt in Premade Waffle Cone	200	1	0	225	52	7	18	7
Vanilla Frozen Yogurt in Fresh Waffle Cone	280	3.5	1	365	61	8	25	6
White Chocolate Macadamia Frozen Yogurt	180	0	0	170	48	8	14	8
White Chocolate Macadamia Frozen Yogurt in Cake Cone	150	0	0	140	39	6	10	6
White Chocolate Macadamia Frozen Yogurt in Premade Waffle Cone	200	1	0	215	51	6	16	7
White Chocolate Macadamia Frozen Yogurt in Fresh Waffle Cone	280	3.5	1	355	60	7	23	6

Sorbet, small

Psychedelic Sorbet	130	0	0	20	34	0	21	0
Psychedelic Sorbet in Cake Cone	150	0	0	35	37	0	21	0
Psychedelic Sorbet in Premade Waffle Cone	200	1	0	110	49	0	27	1
Psychedelic Sorbet in Fresh Waffle Cone	280	3.5	1	250	58	1	34	0
Mango Sorbet	220	0	0	30	52	0	38	0
Mango Sorbet in Cake Cone	180	0	0	35	42	0	28	0
Mango Sorbet in Premade Waffle Cone	230	1	0	110	54	0	34	1
Mango Sorbet in Fresh Waffle Cone	310	3.5	1	250	63	1	41	0
Orange Sorbet	200	0	0	60	48	0	32	0
Orange Sorbet in Cake Cone	160	0	0	60	39	0	24	0
Orange Sorbet in Premade Waffle Cone	220	1	0	135	51	0	30	1
Orange Sorbet in Fresh Waffle Cone	300	3.5	1	275	60	1	37	0
Raspberry Sorbet	200	0	0	20	50	0	32	0
Raspberry Sorbet in Cake Cone	160	0	0	30	40	0	24	0
Raspberry Sorbet in Premade Waffle Cone	220	1	0	105	52	0	30	1
Raspberry Sorbet in Fresh Waffle Cone	300	3.5	1	245	61	1	37	0
Strawberry Kiwi Sorbet	200	0	0	40	48	0	32	0
Strawberry Kiwi Sorbet in Cake Cone	160	0	0	45	39	0	24	0
Strawberry Kiwi Sorbet in Premade Waffle Cone	220	1	0	120	51	0	30	1
Strawberry Kiwi Sorbet in Fresh Waffle Cone	300	3.5	1	260	60	1	37	0

Kids Frozen Yogurt

98% Fat Free

Cake Batter Frozen Yogurt	90	2	1	70	18	2	13	3
Cake Batter Frozen Yogurt in Cake Cone	110	1.5	1	90	22	2	13	3
Cake Batter Frozen Yogurt in Premade Waffle Cone	160	2.5	1	165	34	2	19	4

Description & Serving	Cal	Fat	Sfat	Sod	Carb	Fiber	Sugar	Prot
Cake Batter Frozen Yogurt in Fresh Waffle Cone	240	5	2	305	43	3	26	3
Cheesecake Frozen Yogurt	100	2	1	50	18	2	12	3
Cheesecake Frozen Yogurt in Cake Cone	110	1.5	1	70	22	2	12	3
Cheesecake Frozen Yogurt in Premade Waffle Cone	170	2.5	1	145	34	2	18	4
Cheesecake Frozen Yogurt in Fresh Waffle Cone	250	5	2	285	43	3	25	3
Chocolate Frozen Yogurt	90	2	1	75	18	2	14	3
Chocolate Frozen Yogurt in Cake Cone	110	1.5	1	95	22	2	14	3
Chocolate Frozen Yogurt in Premade Waffle Cone	160	2.5	1	170	34	2	20	4
Chocolate Frozen Yogurt in Fresh Waffle Cone	240	5	2	310	43	3	27	3
Classic Tart Frozen Yogurt	70	0	0	15	17	2	12	2
Classic Tart Frozen Yogurt in Cake Cone	90	0	0	30	20	2	12	2
Classic Tart Frozen Yogurt in Premade Waffle Cone	140	1	0	105	32	2	18	3
Classic Tart Frozen Yogurt in Fresh Waffle Cone	220	3.5	1	245	41	3	25	2
Coffee Frozen Yogurt	100	1	1	65	18	2	13	3
Coffee Frozen Yogurt in Cake Cone	110	1	1	80	22	2	13	3
Coffee Frozen Yogurt in Premade Waffle Cone	170	2	1	155	34	2	19	4
Coffee Frozen Yogurt in Fresh Waffle Cone	250	4.5	2	295	43	3	26	3
Golden Vanilla Frozen Yogurt	100	2	1	75	20	2	14	3
Golden Vanilla Frozen Yogurt in Cake Cone	110	1.5	1	95	24	2	14	3
Golden Vanilla Frozen Yogurt in Premade Waffle Cone	170	2.5	1	170	36	2	20	4
Golden Vanilla Frozen Yogurt in Fresh Waffle Cone	250	5	2	310	45	3	27	3
Peanut Butter Frozen Yogurt	100	2	1	75	21	2	15	4
Peanut Butter Frozen Yogurt in Cake Cone	120	1.5	0.5	95	24	2	16	4
Peanut Butter Frozen Yogurt in Premade Waffle Cone	180	2.5	0.5	170	36	2	22	5
Peanut Butter Frozen Yogurt in Fresh Waffle Cone	260	5	1.5	310	45	3	29	4
Strawberry Frozen Yogurt	90	2	1	70	18	2	13	3
Strawberry Frozen Yogurt in Cake Cone	110	1.5	1	90	22	2	13	3
Strawberry Frozen Yogurt in Premade Waffle Cone	160	2.5	1	165	34	2	19	4
Strawberry Frozen Yogurt in Fresh Waffle Cone	240	5	2	305	43	3	26	3
White Chocolate Mousse Frozen Yogurt	100	2	1	50	18	2	12	3
White Chocolate Mousse Frozen Yogurt in Cake Cone	110	1.5	1	70	22	2	12	3
White Chocolate Mousse Frozen Yogurt in Premade Waffle Cone	170	2.5	1	145	34	2	18	4
White Chocolate Mousse Frozen Yogurt in Fresh Waffle Cone	250	5	2	285	43	3	25	3
Fat Free								
Dutch Chocolate Frozen Yogurt	90	0	0	80	19	2	14	3
Dutch Chocolate Frozen Yogurt in Cake Cone	110	0	0	95	23	2	15	3
Dutch Chocolate Frozen Yogurt in Premade Waffle Cone	160	1	0	170	35	2	21	4
Dutch Chocolate Frozen Yogurt in Fresh Waffle Cone	240	3.5	1	310	44	3	28	3
Old Fashioned Vanilla Frozen Yogurt	90	0	0	50	18	2	12	3
Old Fashioned Vanilla Frozen Yogurt in Cake Cone	110	0	0	70	22	2	12	3

Description & Serving	Cal	Fat	Sfat	Sod	Carb	Fiber	Sugar	Prot
Old Fashioned Vanilla Frozen Yogurt in Premade Waffle Cone	160	1	0	145	34	2	18	4
Old Fashioned Vanilla Frozen Yogurt in Fresh Waffle Cone	240	3.5	1	285	43	3	25	3
Hand-Scooped								
Blueberries & Cream Frozen Yogurt	100	2	1.5	45	16	0	10	2
Blueberries & Cream Frozen Yogurt in Cake Cone	120	2	1.5	60	19	0	10	2
Blueberries & Cream Frozen Yogurt in Premade Waffle Cone	170	3	1.5	120	31	0	16	3
Blueberries & Cream Frozen Yogurt in Fresh Waffle Cone	250	5.5	2.5	275	40	1	23	2
Butter Pecan Frozen Yogurt	120	6	2	6	14	0	9	3
Butter Pecan Frozen Yogurt in Cake Cone	140	6	2	20	17	0	9	3
Butter Pecan Frozen Yogurt in Premade Waffle Cone	190	7	2	95	29	0	15	4
Butter Pecan Frozen Yogurt in Fresh Waffle Cone	270	9.5	3	235	38	1	22	3
Chocolate Chocolate Frozen Yogurt	90	2.5	1.5	45	15	1	11	3
Chocolate Chocolate Frozen Yogurt in Cake Cone	110	2.5	1.5	60	18	1	11	3
Chocolate Chocolate Frozen Yogurt in Premade Waffle Cone	160	3.5	1.5	120	30	1	17	4
Chocolate Chocolate Frozen Yogurt in Fresh Waffle Cone	240	6	2.5	275	39	2	24	3
Chocolate Chocolate Swirl Frozen Yogurt in Cake Cone	90	0	0	70	19	4	4	3
Chocolate Chocolate Swirl Frozen Yogurt in Premade Waffle Cone	140	1	0	125	31	4	10	4
Chocolate Chocolate Swirl Frozen Yogurt in Fresh Waffle Cone	220	3.5	1	285	40	5	17	3
Chocolate Chocolate Swirl Frozen Yogurt (NSA)	70	0	0	55	16	4	4	3
Chocolate Chocolate Swirl Frozen Yogurt (NSA) in Cake Cone	90	0	0	70	19	4	4	3
Chocolate Chocolate Swirl Frozen Yogurt (NSA) in Premade Waffle Cone	140	1	0	125	31	4	10	4
Chocolate Chocolate Swirl Frozen Yogurt (NSA) in Fresh Waffle Cone	220	3.5	1	285	40	5	17	3
Chocolate Chunk Cookie Dough Frozen Yogurt	120	4.5	2.5	60	18	0	13	2
Chocolate Chunk Cookie Dough Frozen Yogurt in Cake Cone	110	3.5	2	40	17	0	11	3
Chocolate Chunk Cookie Dough Frozen Yogurt in Premade Waffle Cone	190	5.5	2.5	130	33	0	19	3
Chocolate Chunk Cookie Dough Frozen Yogurt in Fresh Waffle Cone	270	8	3.5	290	42	1	26	2
Cookies & Cream Frozen Yogurt	90	2.5	1.5	45	15	0	10	3
Cookies & Cream Frozen Yogurt in Cake Cone	130	3.5	2	55	20	0	11	3
Cookies & Cream Frozen Yogurt in Premade Waffle Cone	180	4.5	2	115	32	0	17	4
Cookies & Cream Frozen Yogurt in Fresh Waffle Cone	260	7	3	270	41	1	24	3
Cotton Candy Frozen Yogurt	110	4	3	50	16	0	13	2

Description & Serving	Cal	Fat	Sfat	Sod	Carb	Fiber	Sugar	Prot
Cotton Candy Frozen Yogurt in Cake Cone	110	2.5	1.5	60	18	0	10	3
Cotton Candy Frozen Yogurt in Premade Waffle Cone	160	3.5	1.5	120	30	0	16	4
Cotton Candy Frozen Yogurt in Fresh Waffle Cone	240	6	2.5	275	39	1	23	3
Mint Chocolate Chunk Frozen Yogurt	110	4	1.5	85	17	1	12	3
Mint Chocolate Chunk Frozen Yogurt in Cake Cone	130	4	3	65	19	0	13	2
Mint Chocolate Chunk Frozen Yogurt in Premade Waffle Cone	180	5	3	120	31	0	19	3
Mint Chocolate Chunk Frozen Yogurt in Fresh Waffle Cone	260	7.5	4	280	40	1	26	2
Mocha Almond Frozen Yogurt	90	2	1.5	35	15	0	11	2
Mocha Almond Frozen Yogurt in Cake Cone	130	4	1.5	100	20	1	12	3
Mocha Almond Frozen Yogurt in Premade Waffle Cone	180	5	1.5	145	32	1	18	4
Mocha Almond Frozen Yogurt in Fresh Waffle Cone	260	7.5	2.5	315	41	2	25	3
Peaches & Cream Frozen Yogurt	130	6	1.5	80	17	1	12	3
Peaches & Cream Frozen Yogurt in Cake Cone	110	2	1.5	50	18	0	11	2
Peaches & Cream Frozen Yogurt in Premade Waffle Cone	160	3	1.5	110	30	0	17	3
Peaches & Cream Frozen Yogurt in Fresh Waffle Cone	240	5.5	2.5	265	39	1	24	2
Peanut Butter Delight Frozen Yogurt	110	3.5	2	70	17	0	13	2
Peanut Butter Delight Frozen Yogurt in Cake Cone	150	6	2.5	95	20	1	12	4
Peanut Butter Delight Frozen Yogurt in Premade Waffle Cone	200	7	2.5	140	32	1	18	5
Peanut Butter Delight Frozen Yogurt in Fresh Waffle Cone	280	9.5	3.5	310	41	2	25	4
Pralines & Cream Frozen Yogurt	90	2.5	1.5	45	14	0	10	3
Pralines & Cream Frozen Yogurt in Cake Cone	130	3.5	2	85	20	0	13	2
Pralines & Cream Frozen Yogurt in Premade Waffle Cone	180	4.5	2	135	32	0	19	3
Pralines & Cream Frozen Yogurt in Fresh Waffle Cone	260	7	3	300	41	1	26	2
Rainbow Cream Frozen Yogurt	130	6	3	55	18	1	11	3
Rainbow Cream Frozen Yogurt in Cake Cone	110	2.5	1.5	60	17	0	10	3
Rainbow Cream Frozen Yogurt in Premade Waffle Cone	160	3.5	1.5	120	29	0	16	4
Rainbow Cream Frozen Yogurt in Fresh Waffle Cone	240	6	2.5	275	38	1	23	3
Rocky Road Frozen Yogurt	90	2	1.5	35	15	0	11	2
Rocky Road Frozen Yogurt in Cake Cone	150	6	3	70	21	1	11	3
Rocky Road Frozen Yogurt in Premade Waffle Cone	200	7	3	125	33	1	17	4
Rocky Road Frozen Yogurt in Fresh Waffle Cone	280	9.5	4	285	42	2	24	3
Strawberries & Cream Frozen Yogurt	90	2.5	1.5	45	14	0	10	3
Strawberries & Cream Frozen Yogurt in Cake Cone	110	2	1.5	50	18	0	11	2
Strawberries & Cream Frozen Yogurt in Premade Waffle Cone	160	3	1.5	110	30	0	17	3

Description & Serving	Cal	Fat	Sfat	Sod	Carb	Fiber	Sugar	Prot
Strawberries & Cream Frozen Yogurt in Fresh Waffle Cone	240	5.5	2.5	265	39	1	24	2
Vanilla Bean Frozen Yogurt	110	4	3	40	16	0	12	2
Vanilla Bean Frozen Yogurt in Cake Cone	70	25	2.5	25	48	14	0	10
Vanilla Bean Frozen Yogurt in Premade Waffle Cone	130	26	2.5	95	60	14	6	11
Vanilla Bean Frozen Yogurt in Fresh Waffle Cone	210	28.5	3.5	240	69	15	13	10
Vanilla Chocolate Chip Frozen Yogurt	80	1.5	1	60	17	4	4	3
Vanilla Chocolate Chip Frozen Yogurt in Cake Cone	70	35	4	25	43	16	0	12
Vanilla Chocolate Chip Frozen Yogurt in Premade Waffle Cone	130	36	4	95	55	16	6	13
Vanilla Chocolate Chip Frozen Yogurt in Fresh Waffle Cone	210	38.5	5	240	64	17	13	12
Vanilla Fudge Brownie Frozen Yogurt (NSA)	140	2	1	35	23	0	8	2
Vanilla Fudge Brownie Frozen Yogurt (NSA) in Cake Cone	100	1.5	1	75	20	4	4	3
Vanilla Fudge Brownie Frozen Yogurt (NSA) in Premade Waffle Cone	150	2.5	1	130	32	4	10	4
Vanilla Fudge Brownie Frozen Yogurt (NSA) in Fresh Waffle Cone	230	5	2	290	41	5	17	3
White Chocolate Mousse Frozen Yogurt	70	0	0	10	17	0	11	0
White Chocolate Mousse Frozen Yogurt in Cake Cone	160	2	1	50	26	0	8	2
White Chocolate Mousse Frozen Yogurt in Premade Waffle Cone	210	3	1	110	38	0	14	3
White Chocolate Mousse Frozen Yogurt in Fresh Waffle Cone	290	5.5	2	265	47	1	21	2
No Sugar Added/Fat Free								
Chocolate Frozen Yogurt	60	0	0	70	18	3	5	3
Chocolate Frozen Yogurt in Cake Cone	80	0	0	90	22	3	5	3
Chocolate Frozen Yogurt in Premade Waffle Cone	140	1	0	165	34	3	11	4
Chocolate Frozen Yogurt in Fresh Waffle Cone	220	3.5	1	305	43	4	18	3
Mountain Blackberry Frozen Yogurt	70	0	0	70	19	3	6	3
Mountain Blackberry Frozen Yogurt in Cake Cone	90	0	0	90	23	3	6	3
Mountain Blackberry Frozen Yogurt in Premade Waffle Cone	140	1	0	165	35	3	12	4
Mountain Blackberry Frozen Yogurt in Fresh Waffle Cone	220	3.5	1	305	44	4	19	3
Peach Frozen Yogurt	70	0	0	70	19	3	6	3
Peach Frozen Yogurt in Cake Cone	90	0	0	90	23	3	6	3
Peach Frozen Yogurt in Premade Waffle Cone	140	1	0	165	35	3	12	4
Peach Frozen Yogurt in Fresh Waffle Cone	220	3.5	1	305	44	4	19	3
Strawberry Frozen Yogurt	70	0	0	70	19	3	6	3
Strawberry Frozen Yogurt in Cake Cone	90	0	0	90	23	3	6	3
Strawberry Frozen Yogurt in Premade Waffle Cone	140	1	0	165	35	3	12	4
Strawberry Frozen Yogurt in Fresh Waffle Cone	220	3.5	1	305	44	4	19	3
Vanilla Frozen Yogurt	70	0	0	70	20	4	6	3
Vanilla Frozen Yogurt in Cake Cone	90	0	0	90	24	4	7	3
Vanilla Frozen Yogurt in Premade Waffle Cone	140	1	0	165	36	4	13	4

Description & Serving	Cal	Fat	Sfat	Sod	Carb	Fiber	Sugar	Prot
Vanilla Frozen Yogurt in Fresh Waffle Cone	220	3.5	1	305	45	5	20	3
White Chocolate Macadamia Frozen Yogurt	70	0	0	70	19	3	6	3
White Chocolate Macadamia Frozen Yogurt in Cake Cone	90	0	0	85	23	3	6	3
White Chocolate Macadamia Frozen Yogurt in Premade Waffle Cone	140	1	0	160	35	3	12	4
White Chocolate Macadamia Frozen Yogurt in Fresh Waffle Cone	220	3.5	1	300	44	4	19	3

Kids Sorbet

Description & Serving	Cal	Fat	Sfat	Sod	Carb	Fiber	Sugar	Prot
Psychedelic Sorbet	140	4.5	2.5	75	21	0	13	2
Psychedelic Sorbet in Cake Cone	90	0	0	25	20	0	11	0
Psychedelic Sorbet in Premade Waffle Cone	140	1	0	95	32	0	17	1
Psychedelic Sorbet in Fresh Waffle Cone	220	3.5	1	240	41	1	24	0
Mango Sorbet	90	0	0	10	21	0	15	0
Mango Sorbet in Cake Cone	110	0	0	25	24	0	16	0
Mango Sorbet in Premade Waffle Cone	160	1	0	100	36	0	22	1
Mango Sorbet in Fresh Waffle Cone	240	3.5	1	240	45	1	29	0
Orange Sorbet	80	0	0	25	19	0	13	0
Orange Sorbet in Cake Cone	100	0	0	40	23	0	13	0
Orange Sorbet in Premade Waffle Cone	150	1	0	115	35	0	19	1
Orange Sorbet in Fresh Waffle Cone	230	3.5	1	255	44	1	26	0
Raspberry Sorbet	80	0	0	10	20	0	13	0
Raspberry Sorbet in Cake Cone	100	0	0	25	24	0	13	0
Raspberry Sorbet in Premade Waffle Cone	150	1	0	100	36	0	19	1
Raspberry Sorbet in Fresh Waffle Cone	230	3.5	1	240	45	1	26	0
Strawberry Kiwi Sorbet	80	0	0	15	19	0	13	0
Strawberry Kiwi Sorbet in Cake Cone	100	0	0	30	23	0	13	0
Strawberry Kiwi Sorbet in Premade Waffle Cone	150	1	0	105	35	0	19	1
Strawberry Kiwi Sorbet in Fresh Waffle Cone	230	3.5	1	245	44	1	26	0

Frozen Beverage

Description & Serving	Cal	Fat	Sfat	Sod	Carb	Fiber	Sugar	Prot
Beriyo Smoothie - Berrylicious, 16 oz	290	3	2	65	65	3	5	3
Beriyo Smoothie - Black 'n' Blueberry, 16 oz	280	3	2	65	63	2	54	3
Beriyo Smoothie - Mango Tango, 16 oz	330	3	2	65	76	2	66	3
Beriyo Smoothie - Mangolada, 16 oz	340	6	5	100	70	2	60	3
Beriyo Smoothie - Mondo Mango, 16 oz	310	3	2	65	70	2	63	3
Beriyo Smoothie - Piña Paradise, 16 oz	350	12	9	170	58	1	48	3
Beriyo Smoothie - Pink Pineapple, 16 oz	340	9	7	135	63	2	52	3
Beriyo Smoothie - Straight-Up Strawberry, 16 oz	280	4	2	65	64	1	54	3
Beriyo Smoothie - Strawberry Bananza, 16 oz	320	290	2	65	74	2	61	3
Beriyo Smoothie - Strawberry Fling, 16 oz	340	3	2	65	78	2	67	3
Beriyo Smoothie - Pom Berry Blue, 16 oz	250	3.5	2	60	55	2	46	3
Beriyo Smoothie - Pom Berry Red, 16 oz	250	3	2	60	56	2	45	3
Cappuccino Chiller, 16 oz	410	17	11	190	55	0	55	12
Cappuccino Chiller- Cocoa Berry, 16 oz	480	19	12	250	73	4	35	13
Cappuccino Chiller - Mocha, 16 oz	560	21	13	340	82	1	72	14
Cappuccino Chiller - Oreo Joe, 16 oz	780	29	15	520	115	1	101	19
Cappuccino Chiller - Toffee Coffee, 16 oz	640	28	18	320	86	<1	80	14
Frappe Chiller - Caramel de Leche, 16 oz	240	9	5	190	32	0	28	7

Description & Serving	Cal	Fat	Sfat	Sod	Carb	Fiber	Sugar	Prot
Frappe Chiller - Coffee, 16 oz	190	7	5	150	25	0	22	7
Frappe Chiller - French Vanilla (No Sugar Added), 16 oz	200	9	7	180	23	0	10	7
Frappe Chiller - Hot Chocolate, 16 oz	230	0	8	170	32	<1	27	7
Frappe Chiller - Mocha, 16 oz	240	9	9	170	31	0	25	8
Moo Malt - Chocolate, sml	820	24	10	570	135	0	88	21
Shake - Chocolate, sml	580	19	7	290	92	0	88	15
Shake - Chocolate (w/ Hand-Scooped Frozen Yogurt), 16 oz	690	21	15	310	102	3	85	22
Shake - Cookies & Cream (w/ Hand-Scooped Frozen Yogurt), 16 oz	730	26	16	450	109	1	85	19
Shake - Moussed, sml	720	34	18	330	94	1	82	17
Shake - Oreo, sml	700	23	9	570	111	2	93	18
Shake - Peanut Butter, sml	810	45	13	470	84	2	79	22
Shake - Strawberry, sml	440	11	11	190	75	1	73	15
Shake - Strawberry (w/ Hand-Scooped Frozen Yogurt), 16 oz	680	19	13	300	112	1	98	16
Shake - Vanilla (w/ Hand-Scooped Frozen Yogurt), 16 oz	680	22	15	360	98	<1	82	18
Sorbet Fizz (w/ Soft-Serve Sorbet)	360	0	0	70	90	1	65	0
Sorbet Fizz (w/ Hand-Scooped Sorbet)	410	0	0	65	103	0	70	0

Frozen Treat

Description & Serving	Cal	Fat	Sfat	Sod	Carb	Fiber	Sugar	Prot
Banana Split - Dulce Delight	1120	35	21	530	195	3	138	17
Banana Split - Hand-Scooped Frozen Yogurt - Dulce de Leche	1220	56	34	590	172	4	123	13
Banana Split - Fruit Grove	800	27	20	190	135	4	100	14
Banana Split - Hand-Scooped Frozen Yogurt - Fruit Grove	890	47	33	260	112	5	87	10
Banana Split - Mississippi Mud	750	19	7	400	140	3	112	13
Banana Split - Hand-Scooped Frozen Yogurt - Mississippi Mud	1120	58	36	510	143	5	113	12
Banana Split - Monkey's Uncle	990	45	25	290	139	4	110	17
Banana Split - Hand-Scooped Frozen Yogurt - Monkey's Uncle	1260	74	39	310	138	7	117	16
Banana Split - Hand-Scooped Frozen Yogurt - Traditional	840	52	30	290	86	3	73	10
Parfait - Caramel Crunch	570	15	5	370	103	0	81	11
Parfait - Caramel Crunch (w/ Hand-Scooped Frozen Yogurt)	710	35	17	360	93	<1	69	9
Parfait - Chocolate Dream	560	23	13	220	80	0	76	10
Parfait - Chocolate Dream (w/ Hand-Scooped Frozen Yogurt)	690	43	25	210	69	0	64	8
Parfait - Cookie Dough	660	26	10	470	100	2	58	12
Parfait - Cookie Dough (w/ Hand-Scooped Frozen Yogurt)	790	45	22	460	90	2	45	10
Parfait - Fruity Fudge	610	25	16	180	87	2	83	11
Parfait - Fruity Fudge (w/ Hand-Scooped Frozen Yogurt)	740	45	28	170	77	2	70	9

Description & Serving	Cal	Fat	Sfat	Sod	Carb	Fiber	Sugar	Prot
Parfait - Peanutty Fudge	790	47	17	450	81	2	71	17
Parfait - Peanutty Fudge (w/ Hand-Scooped Frozen Yogurt)	970	70	29	490	72	3	59	16
Parfait - Triple Berry	410	14	12	110	65	3	59	9
Parfait - Triple Berry (w/ Hand-Scooped Frozen Yogurt)	560	34	23	100	58	3	42	7
Shiver - Berry Blend (w/ Hand-Scooped Frozen Yogurt), sml	770	48	30	170	74	1	68	11
Shiver - Cookie Dough, 16 oz	810	29	12	410	129	1	93	17
Shiver - Cookie Dough (w/ Hand-Scooped Frozen Yogurt), sml	1100	69	35	400	115	1	46	14
Shiver - Cookie Dough Monster, 16 oz	710	18	8	410	129	12	77	18
Shiver - DW's Yummy Gummy, 16 oz	510	12	4	120	95	0	71	9
Shiver - Fruit, sml	470	11	7	170	84	<1	83	14
Shiver - Heath, sml	690	26	16	290	104	<1	103	16
Shiver - M&M, sml	750	19	12	320	130	<1	114	22
Shiver - Oreo, sml	660	20	9	460	109	1	97	16
Shiver - Rocky Road, sml	880	40	10	210	116	0	96	26
Shiver - Rocky Road (w/ Hand-Scooped Frozen Yogurt), sml	1140	730	81	180	86	5	73	24
Shiver - Turtle, sml	880	38	13	240	124	0	107	19
Shiver - White Choc Crunch, sml	900	45	24	370	114	2	97	18
Shortcake - Hand-Scooped Frozen Yogurt - Strawberry	550	30	18	310	65	2	47	7
Strawberry Shortcake	450	17	10	310	69	2	53	8
Sundae - Arthur Electric	230	12	8	35	28	0	24	2
Sundae - Buster's Dandy	480	13	6	90	87	0	72	6
Sundae - Butter Cup	1140	68	25	540	116	4	88	22
Sundae - Butter Cup (w/ Hand-Scooped Frozen Yogurt)	1380	90	42	600	119	4	103	24
Sundae - Hot Fudge	720	32	12	360	101	2	90	12
Sundae - Hot Fudge Brownie	840	37	9	510	115	4	94	18
Sundae - Hot Fudge Brownie (Nonfat Frozen Yogurt)	800	33	6	510	115	4	94	18
Sundae - Smart Sundae	280	6	4.5	160	54	11	17	8
Sundae - Specialty	860	29	8	340	142	4	113	17
Sundae - Sundette	360	8	6	140	70	0	52	5
Sundae - Turtle	1000	51	25	320	131	1	101	14
Sundae - Turtle (w/ Hand-Scooped Frozen Yogurt)	1260	77	39	490	135	1	102	13
Sundae - Waffle Berry (w/ Hand-Scooped Frozen Yogurt)	630	37	24	130	69	2	56	8
Yogwich	580	20	7	460	96	1	48	8
Topping								
Almonds	65	6	1	23	2	1	1	2
Blackberries	9	0	0	1	2	1	1	0
Blueberries	7	0	0	0	2	0	1	0
Brownie, 12.3 g	50	2	0	34	7	0	5	0
Butterfinger	66	3	1	33	11	0	7	1
Caramel Fudge	55	0	0	81	13	0	7	0

Description & Serving	Cal	Fat	Sfat	Sod	Carb	Fiber	Sugar	Prot
Cheesecake Topping	48	3	2	44	5	0	3	1
Cherries - Maraschino	7	0	0	0	2	0	2	0
Cherry Topping	28	0	0	4	6	0	5	0
Chocolate Chips	83	5	2	12	9	1	8	1
Chocolate Chips - Mini	92	5	3	13	13	0	12	1
Chocolate Chips - NSA	65	4	3	13	7	1	2	1
Chocolate Cone Coating	119	11	9	1	6	0	5	0
Chocolate Syrup	44	0	0	11	10	0	9	0
Cookie - Chocolate Chip	296	11	3	255	49	1	19	3
Cookie Dough Topping	58	3	1	41	8	0	0	0
Graham Crackers	17	0	0	18	3	0	1	0
Granola	42	2	0	39	6	0	2	1
Gummy Bears	68	0	0	8	17	0	10	0
Heath	68	4	2	32	8	0	8	1
Hot Fudge	91	4	1	50	13	0	11	1
Hot Fudge - NSA/Fat Free	44	0	0	59	10	0	0	0
M&Ms	88	4	2	11	13	0	11	1
Mango Chunks	10	0	0	0	3	0	2	0
Marshmallow Topping	48	0	0	12	12	0	10	0
Oreo	47	2	0	0	7	0	4	0
Peaches (in light syrup)	14	0	0	2	3	0	3	0
Peanut Butter Topping	106	9	2	78	4	0	2	2
Pecans	71	7	1	0	1	1	0	1
Pineapple Chunks	9	0	0	1	2	0	2	0
Rainbow Sprinkles	12	0	0	0	3	0	3	0
Raspberries	9	0	0	0	2	1	1	0
Reese's Peanut Butter Chips	83	4	4	36	7	0	6	3
Reese's Peanut Butter Cups - Mini	78	5	2	47	8	1	7	2
Reese's Pieces	87	4	3	0	11	1	9	2
Reese's Pieces - Mini	85	4	3	33	10	1	9	2
Snickers	54	3	1	28	7	0	6	1
Strawberries	8	0	0	1	2	0	2	0
Walnuts in Syrup	128	7	1	0	15	0	10	2
Whipped Topping	18	2	2	1	1	0	1	0
Yellow Cake	27	1	0	35	4	0	2	0

Yogurt Cake & Pie

Description & Serving	Cal	Fat	Sfat	Sod	Carb	Fiber	Sugar	Prot
Chocolate & Vanilla Yogurt Double Crunch Cake, 1/10 of cake	360	17	10	115	49	<1	36	6
Vanilla Fudge Swirl w/ Chocolate Cake, 1/10 of cake	290	12	8	220	42	<1	31	5
Vanilla Yogurt w/ White Cake, 1/10 of cake	290	13	8	230	39	0	30	5
White Chocolate Mousse Yogurt Cake, 1/10 of cake	300	14	8	210	39	<1	30	5
Yogurt Sheet Cake, 1/24 of cake	270	12	7	140	39	<1	31	5
Chocolate Decadence Deep Dish Pie, 1/10 of cake	340	14	8	140	49	2	36	4
Cookie 'n' Crème Deep Dish Pie, 1/10 of cake	320	14	7	190	45	<1	28	4
Mint 'n' Chips Deep Dish Pie, 1/10 of cake	330	17	10	110	42	<1	32	4

Description & Serving	Cal	Fat	Sfat	Sod	Carb	Fiber	Sugar	Prot
Peanut Buttery Fudge Deep Dish Pie, 1/10 of cake	330	17	8	170	40	<1	29	6
Strawberries 'n' Cream Deep Dish Pie, 1/10 of cake	220	7	4	115	36	0	28	5
Turtle Ripple Deep Dish Pie, 1/10 of cake	310	14	7	130	44	<1	32	4

Tim Hortons

Breakfast

Bagel BELT	440	14	6	940	59	3	10	21
Hashbrown	100	5	0.5	210	12	1	0	1
Sausage, Egg, Cheese Sandwich	510	33	18	950	35	1	3	18
Bacon, Egg, Cheese Sandwich	410	23	14	780	35	1	4	16
Egg, Cheese Sandwich	360	19	13	700	34	1	3	13

Sandwich

Ham & Swiss Sandwich	440	12	5	1690	56	3	7	28
Turkey Bacon Club Sandwich	440	8	2.5	1730	63	2	16	30
Chicken Salad Sandwich	380	9	1.5	980	54	3	6	20
Egg Salad Sandwich	390	13	3	780	52	2	7	17
BLT Sandwich	450	18	5	850	53	2	9	18
Toasted Chicken Club Sandwich	440	7	2.5	1070	70	2	14	25
Whole Wheat Country Bun	230	1	0.3	490	46	4	4	10
White Country Bun	240	1	0.3	510	49	2	5	9

Side/Soup

Chili	300	19	7	1320	17	4	4	26
Baked Beans	270	5	1.5	1140	47	12	14	10
Chicken Noodle Soup	120	2	1	820	18	1	2	5
Hearty Vegetable Soup	70	0.4	0.1	930	14	3	2	4
Vegetable Beef Barley Soup	110	1.5	0.3	930	21	2	2	4
Turkey & Wild Rice Soup	120	1.5	0.2	1000	21	1	2	3
Split Pea w/ Ham Soup	150	2.5	2.5	930	27	5	3	8
Cream of Broccoli Soup	160	9	4	820	16	1	6	6
Hearty Potato Bacon Soup	250	13	6	790	23	1	5	6
Beef Noodle Soup	130	1.5	0.4	930	23	1	3	6
Minestrone Soup	120	3	0.4	750	24	2	4	4
Creamy Field Mushroom Soup	150	3	2	1080	28	1	3	3

Dessert

Apple Fritter Donut	300	11	5	350	49	2	16	4
Blueberry Fritter Donut	330	10	4.5	340	55	2	22	6
Dutchie Donut	250	10	4.5	210	38	1	16	4
Chocolate Dip Donut	210	8	3.5	190	32	1	9	4
Maple Dip Donut	210	8	3.5	190	32	1	9	4
Honey Dip Donut	210	8	3.5	190	33	1	11	4
Old Fashion Plain Donut	260	19	9	230	20	1	7	3
Old Fashion Glazed Donut	320	19	9	230	35	1	22	3
Chocolate Glazed Donut	260	10	4.5	300	39	2	20	4
Sour Cream Plain Donut	270	17	8	230	27	1	10	3
Boston Cream Filled Donut	250	8	3.5	260	40	1	13	4
Strawberry Vanilla Filled Donut	310	8	3.5	220	55	1	28	4

Description & Serving	Cal	Fat	Sfat	Sod	Carb	Fiber	Sugar	Prot
Strawberry Filled Donut	230	8	3.5	220	36	1	12	4
Blueberry Filled Donut	230	8	3.5	210	36	1	11	4
Canadian Maple Filled Donut	260	8	3.5	260	43	1	17	4
Walnut Crunch Donut	360	23	10	320	35	1	19	4
Honey Cruller Donut	320	19	9	220	37	0	23	1
Honey Dip Timbit	60	2	1	50	9	0	4	1
Dutchie Timbit	50	2	1	40	9	0	4	1
Apple Fritter Timbit	50	1.5	1	55	9	0	4	1
Old Fashioned Plain Timbit	70	5	2.5	60	5	0	2	1
Sour Cream Glazed Timbit	90	4.5	2	65	12	0	7	1
Chocolate Glazed Timbit	70	2.5	1	75	10	0	5	1
Raspberry Filled Timbit	60	2	1	50	10	0	4	1
Lemon Filled Timbit	60	2	1	50	9	0	4	1
Strawberry Filled Timbit	60	2	1	55	10	0	4	1
Blueberry Filled Timbit	60	2	1	50	10	0	4	1
Chocolate Chunk Cookie	230	9	6	260	35	1	19	2
Peanut Butter Cookie	280	16	7	260	27	2	16	6
Oatmeal Raisin Spice Cookie	220	8	5	200	35	1	21	3
Triple Chocolate Cookie	250	13	8	220	31	2	20	3
Caramel Chocolate Pecan Cookie	230	11	5	290	32	1	17	3
White Chocolate Macadamia Nut Cookie	240	12	6	270	31	1	17	3

Beverage, 10 oz

	Cal	Fat	Sfat	Sod	Carb	Fiber	Sugar	Prot
Coffee, 1 cream, 1 sugar	75	3.5	2	15	9	0	9	1
Decaffinated Coffee, 1 cream, 1 sugar	75	3.5	2	15	9	0	9	1
Steeped Tea, 1 milk, 1 sugar	50	1	0.5	20	10	0	10	1
Hot Chocolate	240	6	5	360	45	2	38	2
French Vanilla Cappuccino	250	8	7	240	41	1	31	4
English Toffee Cappuccino	240	7	6	220	41	2	30	4
Iced Cappuccino	250	11	6	50	33	0	33	2
Iced Cappuccino, Milk	150	1.5	1	35	32	0	32	3
Café Mocha	180	8	6	170	27	1	24	1
Hot Smoothee	260	10	9	200	39	2	28	5

TOGO'S

Sandwich

	Cal	Fat	Sfat	Sod	Carb	Fiber	Sugar	Prot
Pacific Cobb Sandwich, Regular (6")	710	36	9	2170	68	6	8	34
Pastrami Reuben Sandwich, Regular (6")	990	55	19	2600	67	3	9	52
BBQ Ranch Chicken Sandwich, Regular (6")	750	27	4	2300	88	4	32	42
Chipotle Roast Beef Sandwich, Regular (6")	990	49	12	2450	66	3	7	66
Black Forest Ham & Cheese Sandwich, Regular (6")	670	31	10	2710	67	4	7	35
Turkey & Cheese Sandwich, Regular (6")	670	28	8	2110	68	4	6	42
Turkey, Salami & Cheese Sandwich, Regular (6")	900	40	13	4230	70	4	11	69
Turkey & Cranberry Sandwich, Regular (6")	670	19	3	1860	95	4	33	34
Turkey, Roast Beef & Cheese Sandwich, Regular (6")	770	30	9	2490	69	4	6	59
Roast Beef & Avocado Sandwich, Regular (6")	720	29	5	2120	70	6	6	46
Hummus Sandwich, Regular (6")	650	27	4.5	1770	90	9	6	18
The Italian Sandwich, Regular (6")	860	43	14	3740	71	4	11	51

Description & Serving	Cal	Fat	Sfat	Sod	Carb	Fiber	Sugar	Prot
Capicolla, Dry Salami & Provolone Sandwich, Regular (6")	1080	59	17	4980	69	4	12	73
Mortadella, Salami & Provolone Sandwich, Regular (6")	870	41	14	4180	71	4	11	58
Egg Salad & Cheese Sandwich, Regular (6")	750	39	12	1890	70	4	8	31
Albacore Tuna (Dolphin Safe) Sandwich, Regular (6")	660	28	5	1900	73	4	9	30
Avocado & Cheese Sandwich, Regular (6")	740	40	13	1790	73	9	6	25
Cheese Sandwich, Regular (6")	800	45	20	2260	68	4	6	34
Salami & Cheese Sandwich, Regular (6")	1100	53	17	6230	73	4	15	87
Turkey & Avocado Sandwich, Regular (6")	640	26	4	1800	74	9	7	36
Turkey, Ham & Cheese Sandwich, Regular (6")	690	29	9	2430	68	4	7	42
Avocado & Cucumber Sandwich, Regular (6")	560	25	4	1340	75	9	7	13
Turkey, Ham, Salami & Cheese Sandwich, Regular (6")	920	41	13	4550	71	4	11	70
Chicken Salad Sandwich, Regular (6")	650	29	4.5	2010	74	5	10	26
Turkey Bacon Club Sandwich, Regular (6")	680	32	12	2210	68	4	6	35
Chicken Sandwich, Regular (6")	630	20	3	2070	72	4	8	44
Meatball Sandwich, Regular (6")	690	27	13	2180	78	5	6	33
Roast Beef Sandwich, Regular (6")	730	25	5	2410	67	4	6	58
Pastrami Sandwich, Regular (6")	750	33	12	2280	69	4	6	43
Sicilian Chicken Sandwich, Regular (6")	710	28	9	2010	73	4	8	41
BBQ Beef Sandwich, Regular (6")	670	19	7	2010	85	3	29	40
French Dip Sandwich, Regular (6")	840	33	10	2690	67	3	5	67

Wrap

Description & Serving	Cal	Fat	Sfat	Sod	Carb	Fiber	Sugar	Prot
Cobb Salad Wrap w/ Blue Cheese Dressing, Regular	680	36	9	1330	63	11	6	32
Santa Fe Chicken Salad Wrap w/ Spicy Pepitas Dressing, Regular	800	44	9	1260	75	13	6	34
BBQ Chicken Ranch Salad Wrap w/ Buttermilk Ranch, Regular	630	26	4	1420	77	8	18	27
Asian Chicken Salad Wrap w/ Asian Dressing, Regular	670	32	4.5	1140	74	8	16	28
Chicken Caesar Salad Wrap w/ Caesar Dressing, Regular	550	20	4.5	1310	67	8	6	31
Taco Salad Wrap w/ Taco Sauce, Regular	670	26	10	1580	90	13	13	24
Farmer's Market Salad Wrap w/ Balsamic Vinaigrette, Regular	440	14	3	980	72	9	8	12

Salad

Description & Serving	Cal	Fat	Sfat	Sod	Carb	Fiber	Sugar	Prot
Cobb Salad, Half	180	11	4.5	440	6	4	2	15
Santa Fe Chicken Salad, Half	180	8	2	480	16	5	3	14
BBQ Chicken Ranch Salad, Half	120	2	0	320	16	2	8	10
Asian Chicken Salad, Half	100	4.5	0	210	9	2	3	11
Chicken Caesar Salad, Half	110	3.5	1	340	9	2	2	12
Taco Salad, Half	310	20	10	590	19	5	4	13
Farmer's Market Salad, Half	80	3.5	1.5	220	11	2	3	4

Soup/Chili

Description & Serving	Cal	Fat	Sfat	Sod	Carb	Fiber	Sugar	Prot
Broccoli Cheddar Soup, 8 oz	240	15	8	1110	19	1	4	7
Moroccan Lentil Soup, 8 oz	130	1	0	940	23	8	2	7

Description & Serving	Cal	Fat	Sfat	Sod	Carb	Fiber	Sugar	Prot
Garden Vegetable Soup, 8 oz	80	0.5	0	600	16	3	3	3
Southwestern Chicken & Green Chile Soup, 8 oz	260	18	11	1000	14	1	3	12
Fresh Mushroom & Brie Soup, 8 oz	200	14	8	700	16	2	3	5
Old-Fashioned Chicken Noodle Soup, 8 oz	120	2.5	0.5	1280	18	>1	2	7
Roasted Yukon Baked Potato Soup, 8 oz	300	20	12	880	19	1	3	10
New England Clam Chowder, 8 oz	250	16	8	960	21	>1	5	7
Chili, 8 oz	200	4	1.5	730	30	7	3	11

Kids

	Cal	Fat	Sfat	Sod	Carb	Fiber	Sugar	Prot
Black Forest Ham & Cheese Sandwich	370	19	4.5	1180	33	2	4	16
Turkey & Cheese Sandwich	360	18	4	800	31	2	3	19
Albacore Tuna (Dolphin Safe) Sandwich	330	14	2.5	650	35	2	4	15
Cheese Sandwich	470	31	12	1280	35	2	6	16

Dessert

	Cal	Fat	Sfat	Sod	Carb	Fiber	Sugar	Prot
Chocolate Chunk Brownie	430	22	6	260	57	3	38	6
Dark Chocolate Chunk Cookie	390	19	6	370	51	1	27	4
Peanut Butter Chip Cookie	420	23	10	270	45	2	25	7
Oatmeal Raisin Cookie	360	13	6	230	57	3	32	6

Bread

	Cal	Fat	Sfat	Sod	Carb	Fiber	Sugar	Prot
Classic White Bread, 1"	50	0	0	100	10	0	0	2
Honey Wheat Bread, 1"	50	0.5	0	120	10	>1	1	2
Onion Herb Bread, 1"	50	0	0	100	10	0	1	2
Dutch Crunch Bread, 1"	50	0	0	95	10	0	>1	1
Parmesan Bread, 1"	60	1.5	1	140	9	0	0	3
Spinach Wrap Tortilla, 12"	320	8	1.5	290	53	2	0	7
Sun-Dried Tomato Basil Tortilla Wrap, 12"	320	8	1.5	300	54	2	1	7
Whole Wheat Tortilla Wrap, 12"	300	8	1.5	290	52	6	2	8

Dressing/Condiment

	Cal	Fat	Sfat	Sod	Carb	Fiber	Sugar	Prot
Asian Dressing, 2.5 oz	380	33	4.5	830	10	0	19	0
Low Fat Balsamic Vinaigrette, 2.5 oz	90	3.5	0	780	16	0	6	0
Blue Cheese Dressing, 1.5 oz	260	26	5	780	3	0	3	2
Buttermilk Ranch Dressing, 2.5 oz	250	26	4.5	890	3	0	3	2
Caesar Dressing, 2.5 oz	150	12	2.5	800	8	0	3	2
Fat Free Serano Grape Vinaigrette, 2.5 oz	90	0	0	290	23	0	21	1
Italian Vinaigrette, 2.5 oz	300	32	2.5	420	4	0	0	0
Spicy Pepitas Dressing, 2.5 oz	340	35	6	450	3	0	1	3
Taco Sauce, 1 oz	31	1.8	0	243	7	0	4	0

Tropical Smoothie Café

Smoothie

Low Fat Smoothie

	Cal	Fat	Sfat	Sod	Carb	Fiber	Sugar	Prot
Blimey Limey Smoothie w/ Splenda, 24 oz	211	0.1	NP	2	52.1	1.7	NP	0.5
Blimey Limey Smoothie w/ Turbinado, 24 oz	471	0.1	NP	2	117.1	1.7	NP	0.5
Blue Lagoon Smoothie w/ Splenda, 24 oz	130	0.9	NP	3	29.7	4.7	NP	1.1
Blue Lagoon Smoothie w/ Turbinado, 24 oz	330	0.9	NP	3	79.7	4.7	NP	1.1
Hawaiian Breeze Smoothie w/ Splenda, 24 oz	179	0.1	NP	41	42	1	NP	2.5

Description & Serving	Cal	Fat	Sfat	Sod	Carb	Fiber	Sugar	Prot
Hawaiian Breeze Smoothie w/ Turbinado, 24 oz	379	0.1	NP	41	92	1	NP	2.5
Island Fever Smoothie w/ Splenda, 24 oz	222	0.4	NP	8	53.1	4	NP	1.7
Island Fever Smoothie w/ Turbinado, 24 oz	422	0.4	NP	8	103.1	4	NP	1.7
Jetty Punch Smoothie w/ Splenda, 24 oz	168	0.6	NP	3	38.7	5	NP	1.7
Jetty Punch Smoothie w/ Turbinado, 24 oz	368	0.6	NP	3	88.7	5	NP	1.7
Kiwi Quencher Smoothie w/ Splenda, 24 oz	215	0.1	NP	53	51.1	2.4	NP	2.5
Kiwi Quencher Smoothie w/ Turbinado, 24 oz	415	0.1	NP	53	101.1	2.4	NP	2.5
Mango Magic Smoothie w/ Splenda, 24 oz	199	0.3	NP	43	46	2.5	NP	2.9
Mango Magic Smoothie w/ Turbinado, 24 oz	399	0.3	NP	43	96	2.5	NP	2.9
Paradise Point Smoothie w/ Splenda, 24 oz	249	0.7	NP	4	58.2	6	NP	2.2
Paradise Point Smoothie w/ Turbinado, 24 oz	449	0.7	NP	4	108.2	6	NP	2.2
Peaches 'N Silk Smoothie w/ Splenda, 24 oz	163	0.4	NP	8	38.6	4.2	NP	1.4
Peaches 'N Silk Smoothie w/ Turbinado, 24 oz	363	0.4	NP	8	88.6	4.2	NP	1.4
Pineapple Delight Smoothie w/ Splenda, 24 oz	227	0.4	NP	2	54.8	2.4	NP	1.1
Pineapple Delight Smoothie w/ Turbinado, 24 oz	427	0.4	NP	2	104.8	2.4	NP	1.1
Rockin' Raspberry Smoothie w/ Splenda, 24 oz	201	0.7	NP	2	47	6.8	NP	1.4
Rockin' Raspberry Smoothie w/ Turbinado, 24 oz	425	0.7	NP	2	103.4	6.8	NP	1.4
Strawberry Beach Smoothie w/ Splenda, 24 oz	137	0.2	NP	44	30.7	4.6	NP	3
Strawberry Beach Smoothie w/ Turbinado, 24 oz	449	0.2	NP	44	108.7	4.6	NP	3
Sunny Day Smoothie w/ Splenda, 24 oz	290	0.6	NP	7	69.7	3.4	NP	1.4
Sunny Day Smoothie w/ Turbinado, 24 oz	490	0.6	NP	7	119.7	3.4	NP	1.4
Sunrise Sunset Smoothie w/ Splenda, 24 oz	210	0.3	NP	4	50.2	3.2	NP	0.9
Sunrise Sunset Smoothie w/ Turbinado, 24 oz	410	0.3	NP	4	100.2	3.2	NP	0.9
Power Up Smoothie								
Health Nut Smoothie w/ Splenda, 24 oz	328	6.8	NP	34	42	5.5	NP	24.8
Health Nut Smoothie w/ Turbinado, 24 oz	528	6.8	NP	34	92	5.5	NP	24.8
Immune Blast Smoothie w/ Splenda, 24 oz	241	0.6	NP	61	57.4	3.8	NP	1.6
Immune Blast Smoothie w/ Turbinado, 24 oz	441	0.6	NP	61	107.4	3.8	NP	1.6
Kiwi Citrus Green Tea Smoothie w/ Splenda, 24 oz	276	0.1	NP	51	64.6	3.5	NP	4.1
Kiwi Citrus Green Tea Smoothie w/ Turbinado, 24 oz	476	0.1	NP	51	114.6	3.5	NP	4.1
Lean Machine Smoothie w/ Splenda, 24 oz	161	0.6	NP	3	36.7	5	NP	1.7
Lean Machine Smoothie w/ Turbinado, 24 oz	472	0.6	NP	3	114.7	5	NP	1.7
Muscle Blaster Smoothie w/ Splenda, 24 oz	284	2.8	NP	33	40.7	5	NP	23.7
Muscle Blaster Smoothie w/ Turbinado, 24 oz	484	2.8	NP	33	90.7	5	NP	23.7
Peanut Paradise Smoothie w/ Splenda, 24 oz	490	18.3	NP	221	49.1	2.7	NP	32.2
Peanut Paradise Smoothie w/ Turbinado, 24 oz	690	18.3	NP	221	99.1	2.7	NP	32.2
Stress Defender Smoothie w/ Splenda, 24 oz	264	0.2	NP	43	62.4	3.2	NP	3.3
Stress Defender Smoothie w/ Turbinado, 24 oz	464	0.2	NP	43	112.4	3.2	NP	3.3
Very Berry Green Tea Smoothie w/ Splenda, 24 oz	160	1	NP	4	35.7	3.8	NP	2
Very Berry Green Tea Smoothie w/ Turbinado, 24 oz	360	1	NP	4	85.7	3.8	NP	2
Super Fruit Smoothie								
Acai Berry Boost Smoothie w/ Splenda, 24 oz	231	1.6	NP	9	53.1	5.3	NP	1.4
Acai Berry Boost Smoothie w/ Turbinado, 24 oz	431	1.6	NP	9	103.1	5.3	NP	1.4
Get-Up-and-Goji Smoothie w/ Splenda, 24 oz	232	0.4	NP	30	54.9	4.4	NP	2.6
Get-Up-and-Goji Smoothie w/ Turbinado, 24 oz	432	0.4	NP	30	104.9	4.4	NP	2.6
Pomegranate Plunge Smoothie w/ Splenda, 24 oz	274	0.4	NP	5	67	2.9	NP	0.8
Pomegranate Plunge Smoothie w/ Turbinado, 24 oz	474	0.4	NP	5	117	2.9	NP	0.8

Description & Serving	Cal	Fat	Sfat	Sod	Carb	Fiber	Sugar	Prot
Coffee Smoothie								
Caramel Cream Coffee Smoothie w/ Splenda, 24 oz	591	11.2	NP	351	116.6	0	NP	6.1
Caramel Cream Coffee Smoothie w/ Turbinado, 24 oz	791	11.2	NP	351	166.6	0	NP	6.1
Cinn City Coffee Smoothie w/ Splenda, 24 oz	326	7.6	NP	229	56.3	0.3	NP	8.1
Cinn City Coffee Smoothie w/ Turbinado, 24 oz	526	7.6	NP	229	106.3	0.3	NP	8.1
Coffee Nut Coffee Smoothie w/ Splenda, 24 oz	343	11.2	NP	209	51.8	0.5	NP	8.6
Coffee Nut Coffee Smoothie w/ Turbinado, 24 oz	543	11.2	NP	209	101.8	0.5	NP	8.6
Mocha Madness Coffee Smoothie w/ Splenda, 24 oz	445	12	NP	239	76.1	0	NP	8.1
Mocha Madness Coffee Smoothie w/ Turbinado, 24 oz	645	12	NP	239	126.1	0	NP	8.1
Simply Indulgent Smoothie								
Bahama Mama Smoothie w/ Splenda, 24 oz	345	7.7	NP	60	67.1	3.3	NP	2
Bahama Mama Smoothie w/ Turbinado, 24 oz	545	7.7	NP	60	117.1	3.3	NP	2
Beach Bum Smoothie w/ Splenda, 24 oz	364	5	NP	73	74.7	5	NP	4.7
Beach Bum Smoothie w/ Turbinado, 24 oz	564	5	NP	73	124.7	5	NP	4.7
Chocolate Chiller Smoothie w/ Splenda, 24 oz	354	6.9	NP	152	67	0	NP	6
Chocolate Chiller Smoothie w/ Turbinado, 24 oz	554	6.9	NP	152	117	0	NP	6
Peanut Butter Cup Smoothie w/ Splenda, 24 oz	520	20.5	NP	221	72.6	2.7	NP	11.2
Peanut Butter Cup Smoothie w/ Turbinado, 24 oz	720	20.5	NP	221	122.6	2.7	NP	11.2
Tropi-Colada Smoothie w/ Splenda, 24 oz	312	5.4	NP	17	64.8	2.4	NP	1.1
Tropi-Colada Smoothie w/ Turbinado, 24 oz	512	5.4	NP	17	114.8	2.4	NP	1.1
Breakfast								
All American Breakfast Wrap	558	23.2	7.3	1978	52.6	1.7	NP	35
Early Bird Wrap	617	23.6	7	1545	68.1	2.1	NP	32.9
Salsa Sunrise Wrap	568	23.1	8	1919	53.6	2.2	NP	36.5
Western Wrap	636	27.5	12.1	1811	57.1	2.6	NP	40.2
Sandwich/Wrap								
Cranberry Walnut Chicken Salad Sandwich	737	40.1	4.5	805	70.5	5.8	NP	23.6
Hummus Veggie Sandwich	668	25.5	4.9	1146	84.3	9.3	NP	25.5
The Italian Sandwich	462	15.8	5.3	2259	38.2	3	NP	41.9
Turkey Bacon Ranch Sandwich	429	13	2.7	1590	37	2.8	NP	40.7
Ultimate Club Sandwich	524	19.3	6.3	1687	43.2	2.8	NP	44.3
Wasabi Roast Beef Sandwich	374	10.6	4.7	1358	32.9	2.5	NP	36.7
Baja Chicken Grilled Flatbread Sandwich	455	16.1	5.5	1244	48.3	3.1	NP	29.1
Caribbean Luau Grilled Flatbread Sandwich	452	12	4.7	1243	57.2	2.7	NP	28.7
Chicken Pesto Grilled Flatbread Sandwich	456	17.4	5.7	1227	45.1	2.7	NP	29.8
Honey Ham & Swiss Grilled Flatbread Sandwich	411	11.7	3.5	1200	53	3	NP	23.6
Mediterranean Veggie Grilled Flatbread Sandwich	468	17.1	3.2	1194	61.2	6.5	NP	17.3
Peanut Butter Banana Crunch Grilled Flatbread Sandwich	613	20.9	3.5	713	90.5	4.5	NP	16
Buffalo Chicken Wrap	623	26.2	7.8	2787	60.3	3.1	NP	36.2
Cordon Bleu Wrap	688	32.3	8.6	2391	55	1.7	NP	44.2
Jamaican Jerk Chicken Wrap	624	17.4	6.4	1921	78.8	4.4	NP	38
King Caesar Wrap	604	29.3	6.7	1759	55.7	3.1	NP	29.4
Popeye's Favorite Wrap	623	24.5	11.4	1868	60.1	3.1	NP	40.4
Sesame Chicken Wrap	803	23.3	2.9	2040	112.8	5.9	NP	35.5
Southwest Chicken Wrap	563	20	3.4	1816	69	5.5	NP	27.1

Description & Serving	Cal	Fat	Sfat	Sod	Carb	Fiber	Sugar	Prot
Thai Chicken Wrap	722	15.1	2.1	2267	112.6	5.6	NP	33.6
Totally Turkey Wrap	617	24.6	6	2102	55.2	3.1	NP	43.7
Veggie Veggie Wrap	508	17.1	4.2	1275	72.1	5.8	NP	16.3

Salad

Chicken Caesar Salad	487	38.7	8.1	1151	10.1	3.3	NP	24.3
Cranberry Walnut Chicken Salad	476	37.9	4.5	539	20.1	4.2	NP	13.5
Sesame Chicken Salad	580	19.2	1.2	1519	73.2	5.7	NP	28.4
Southwest Chicken Salad	474	26.8	3.9	1576	33.8	9.4	NP	24.1
Thai Chicken Salad	501	10.5	0.4	1962	73.9	5.3	NP	27.5
TSC Signature Salad	349	12.9	0.9	810	37	6.3	NP	21

Kids

Food

Cheese Pizza	368	12.5	4.7	920	45.3	3	NP	18.4
Cheese Quesadilla	491	22.9	11	1087	51.7	1.7	NP	19.5
Cheese Quesadilla w/ Chicken	542	23.6	11	1420	53	1.7	NP	29.5
Ham & American Flatbread	332	10.1	3	1335	41	2	NP	19.4
Grilled Cheese Flatbread	425	21.9	10	1530	40	2	NP	17
Turkey & Provolone Flatbread	361	10.4	3	1119	41	2	NP	25.8

Smoothie

Awesome Orange Smoothie w/ Splenda, 12 oz	188	2.6	NP	62	39	1.1	NP	2.4
Awesome Orange Smoothie w/ Turbinado, 12 oz	292	2.6	NP	62	65	1.1	NP	2.4
Banana Mania Smoothie w/ Splenda, 12 oz	199	0.8	NP	22	45.2	4.1	NP	2.8
Banana Mania Smoothie w/ Turbinado, 12 oz	303	0.8	NP	22	71.2	4.1	NP	2.8
Chocolate Chimp Smoothie w/ Splenda, 12 oz	156	2.5	NP	36	31.3	1.4	NP	2.1
Chocolate Chimp Smoothie w/ Turbinado, 12 oz	260	2.5	NP	36	57.3	1.4	NP	2.1
Jetty Junior Smoothie w/ Splenda, 12 oz	79	0.4	NP	2	18.3	2.6	NP	0.8
Jetty Junior Smoothie w/ Turbinado, 12 oz	183	0.4	NP	2	44.3	2.6	NP	0.8

Dressing/Condiment

Balsamic Vinaigrette, 1 oz	61	5	0.5	190	4	0	NP	0
Bistro Sauce, 1 oz	121	7.4	1.5	150	13.5	0	NP	0
Buffalo Sauce, 1 oz	8	0	0	940	2	0	NP	0
Caesar Dressing, 1 oz	161	17	3	240	1	0	NP	1
Guacamole, 1 oz	53	4.3	0.5	161	2.8	1.9	NP	0.9
Honey Mustard Dressing, 1 oz	73	0	0	137	18.3	0	NP	0
Jamaican Jerk Sauce, 1 oz	40	0	0	290	9	0	NP	1
Light Ranch Dressing, 1 oz	92	9.5	1.4	274	0.9	0	NP	0.9
Light Southwest Ranch Dressing, 1 oz	88	8.1	1.5	288	3	0	NP	1
Pesto, 1 oz	97	9.4	1.5	174	1	0.5	NP	2
Salsa, 1 oz	4	0	0	100	1	0.5	NP	0
Sesame Dressing, 1 oz	75	4.2	0	284	9.2	0	NP	0
Thai Peanut Dressing, 1 oz	74	3.3	0	500	10	0	NP	1
TSC Signature Dressing, 1 oz	40	2.1	0	142	5.3	0.2	NP	0

Topping

American Cheese, 1 slice	50	4.5	2.5	255	0	0	NP	2.5
Cheddar Cheese, 1/3 cup	177	14.6	9.3	273	0.6	0	NP	10.9

Description & Serving	Cal	Fat	Sfat	Sod	Carb	Fiber	Sugar	Prot
Low Fat Mozzarella Cheese, 1/3 cup	115	7.4	4.7	253	1.3	0	NP	10.7
Pepper Jack Cheese, 1 slice	56	4.4	3.2	96	0	0	NP	4
Swiss Cheese, 1 slice	78	6	3	45	0	0	NP	6
Parmesan Cheese, 1/8 cup	48	3.3	2.1	154	0.4	0	NP	4.2
Provolone Cheese, 1 slice	74	6	3	150	0	0	NP	5

UNO Chicago Grill

Appetizer

Description & Serving	Cal	Fat	Sfat	Sod	Carb	Fiber	Sugar	Prot
Crispy Cheese Dippers, 1/3 of dish	280	16	6	830	27	1	3	12
Buffalo Chicken Quesadillas, 1/3 of dish	350	16	8	890	36	2	4	19
Shrimp & Crab Fondue, 1/5 of dish	220	16	4.5	500	13	0	2	8
Muchos Nachos, 1/3 of dish	460	21	8	810	54	5	4	17
The Chi-Town Tasting Plate, 1/4 of dish	520	36	7	1000	30	3	3	18
Three Way Buffalo Bites, 1/3 of dish	430	21	2.5	1840	39	0	16	31
Steak Quesadillas, 1/3 of dish	390	19	7	900	35	2	4	18
Rhode Island Style Calamari, 1/3 of dish	350	31	3.5	690	28	1	3	13
Onion Strings, 1/3 of dish	600	42	7	630	50	5	6	6
Pizza Skins, 1/5 of dish	480	31	9	720	39	2	2	13
Roasted Vegetable Quesadilla, 1/3 of dish	300	13	5	730	36	2	6	11
Three Way Buffalo Wings, 1/3 of dish	430	35	8	470	3	0	1	21
Buffalo Chicken Quesadilla Lunch, 1/2 of dish	420	17	8	1090	47	3	7	18

Salad

Description & Serving	Cal	Fat	Sfat	Sod	Carb	Fiber	Sugar	Prot
Caesar Side Salad	250	22	5	430	8	2	2	7
House Side Salad	80	5	1	90	9	2	3	2
Gorgonzola Walnut Side Salad	280	23	7	440	16	4	6	9
House Salad w/o dressing, 1/2 of dish	80	5	1	90	9	2	3	2
House Salad w/ Grilled Chicken & no dressing, 1/2 of dish	160	7	1	390	10	2	3	17
Caesar Salad w/ dressing, 1/2 of dish	250	22	5	430	8	2	2	7
Chicken Caesar Salad w/ dressing, 1/2 of dish	290	20	4.5	720	10	2	2	22
Classic Cobb Salad w/ dressing, 1/2 of dish	340	26	8	930	8	3	3	52
Honey Crisp Chicken Salad w/ dressing, 1/2 of dish	410	26	5	790	27	3	9	20
Chicken Milanese Salad w/ dressing, 1/2 of dish	420	28	4.5	1080	20	3	4	25
Spinach, Chicken & Gorgonzola Salad w/ dressing, 1/2 of dish	360	22	5	660	25	4	19	21
Chopped Medium Grilled Shrimp Salad w/ dressing, 1/2 of dish	340	22	4.5	960	20	3	6	17
Asian Chicken Salad	550	28	3	1250	43	7	27	34

Soup/Chili

Description & Serving	Cal	Fat	Sfat	Sod	Carb	Fiber	Sugar	Prot
French Onion Soup	230	14	6	1250	17	1	4	8
New England Clam Chowder	290	18	11	780	20	1	2	11
Veggie Soup	90	1	0	620	18	3	3	4
Broccoli & Cheddar Soup	300	23	13	1450	16	1	4	11
Chipotle Corn Chowder	210	12	10	1100	20	2	2	4
Italian Wedding Soup	120	3.5	1	730	16	2	2	6

Description & Serving	Cal	Fat	Sfat	Sod	Carb	Fiber	Sugar	Prot
Tuscan Pesto Minestrone Soup	100	2	0	930	16	3	2	4
Cuban Black Bean & Lentil Soup	150	3	0	820	23	6	4	8
Beef Barley Soup	90	1.5	0	700	14	2	4	6
Windy City Chili	260	9	3.5	950	33	6	6	14

Sandwich/Burger

Description & Serving	Cal	Fat	Sfat	Sod	Carb	Fiber	Sugar	Prot
Grilled Chicken Sandwich, 2/3 of dish	380	13	3	1010	34	2	3	34
Crispy Chipotle Chicken Sandwich, 2/3 of dish	740	37	5	1260	75	5	3	30
Steak & Cheese Sandwich, 2/3 of dish	730	34	11	1790	56	3	4	37
Turkey Bacon & Swiss Sandwich, 2/3 of dish	550	20	7	1640	55	3	4	61
Crispy Chipotle Chicken Sliders, 2/3 of dish	510	23	3.5	1130	50	3	3	27
Grilled Rosemary Chicken w/ Aged Cheddar Sandwich, 2/3 of dish	620	37	8	1470	39	3	2	57
Firecracker Chicken Sandwich, 2/3 of dish	470	20	5	1270	38	4	2	33
Southwest Steak Panini, 2/3 of dish	740	36	13	1710	63	4	9	31
Buffalo Chicken Panini, 2/3 of dish	650	29	14	1730	64	4	8	33
It's All Greek to Me Panini, 2/3 of dish	520	20	6	1300	60	4	7	24
Calzone, 1/2 of dish	410	18	7	1350	41	2	5	22
The UNO Burger, 1/2 of dish	540	36	14	810	24	2	2	30
Bring Home the Bacon Burger, 1/2 of dish	680	47	18	1220	25	2	2	38
Cabot Aged Cheddar & Mushroom Burger, 1/2 of dish	600	40	16	910	25	2	2	34
BBQ Burger w/ Bacon & Cheddar, 1/2 of dish	700	46	18	1260	32	2	4	41
Philly Burger, 1/2 of dish	590	38	15	890	26	2	2	33
Cheddar Burger, 1/2 of dish	590	39	16	920	25	2	2	33
Gorgonzilla Burger, 1/2 of dish	600	40	17	1010	26	2	2	33
Veggie Burger, 1/2 of dish	310	8	2.5	1170	34	6	3	15
Burger Sliders, 1/2 of dish	600	40	15	790	26	1	2	30

Entrée

Pizza

Description & Serving	Cal	Fat	Sfat	Sod	Carb	Fiber	Sugar	Prot
Cheese & Tomato Deep Dish Pizza, 1/3 of indv pizza OR 1/6 of reg pizza	580	40	12	920	39	2	2	21
Numero UNO Deep Dish Pizza, 1/3 of indv pizza OR 1/6 of reg pizza	640	44	12	1200	41	2	3	21
Spinocolli Deep Dish Pizza, 1/3 of indv pizza OR 1/6 of reg pizza	620	45	11	830	40	3	2	16
Chicken Spinocolli Deep Dish Pizza, 1/3 of indv pizza OR 1/6 of reg pizza	630	45	11	920	40	3	2	20
Buffalo Chicken Deep Dish Pizza, 1/3 of indv pizza OR 1/6 of reg pizza	650	40	10	920	53	2	3	20
Chicken Fajita Deep Dish Pizza, 1/3 of indv pizza OR 1/6 of reg pizza	670	41	11	1090	55	3	4	22
Veggie Deep Dish Pizza, 1/3 of indv pizza OR 1/6 of reg pizza	650	40	11	970	55	3	4	20
Chicago Classic Deep Dish Pizza, 1/3 of indv pizza OR 1/6 of reg pizza	770	55	18	1640	40	2	3	33
Four Cheese Deep Dish Pizza, 1/3 of indv pizza OR 1/6 of reg pizza	640	44	13	920	39	2	2	20

Description & Serving	Cal	Fat	Sfat	Sod	Carb	Fiber	Sugar	Prot
Prima Pepperoni Deep Dish Pizza, 1/3 of indv pizza OR 1/6 of reg pizza	610	42	12	1040	39	2	2	20
Farmer's Market Deep Dish Pizza, 1/3 of indv pizza OR 1/6 of reg pizza	540	35	9	790	42	3	4	15
Bacon, Cheddar & Tomato Deep Dish Pizza, 1/3 of indv pizza OR 1/6 of reg pizza	580	41	12	860	37	1	2	19
Roasted Red Pepper & Chicken Deep Dish Pizza, 1/3 of indv pizza OR 1/6 of reg pizza	680	43	12	970	51	2	2	23
Bianco Deep Dish Pizza, 1/3 of indv pizza OR 1/6 of reg pizza	680	51	13	1040	37	1	2	21
BBQ Chicken Flatbread Pizza, 1/3 of pizza	320	11	4.5	700	36	1	9	22
Cheese & Tomato Flatbread Pizza, 1/3 of pizza	270	11	5	710	31	2	4	16
Mediterranean Flatbread Pizza, 1/3 of pizza	280	15	5	780	29	2	2	13
Pepperoni Flatbread Pizza, 1/3 of pizza	340	17	8	930	30	1	3	20
Gluten Free Veggie Pizza, 1/3 of pizza	320	12	4.5	710	43	2	5	11
Gluten Free Cheese Pizza, 1/3 of pizza	290	11	3.5	660	41	2	4	9
Spinach, Mushroom & Gorgonzola Pizza, 1/3 of pizza	300	14	6	690	30	2	3	16
Roasted Eggplant, Spinach & Feta Flatbread Pizza, 1/3 of pizza	270	10	3.5	570	34	4	6	13
Spicy Chicken Flatbread Pizza, 1/3 of pizza	350	16	7	720	34	2	6	23
Sausage Flatbread Pizza, 1/3 of pizza	330	17	7	960	29	1	3	20
Four Cheese Flatbread Pizza, 1/3 of pizza	340	18	8	740	30	2	3	18
Gluten Free Pepperoni Flatbread Pizza, 1/3 of pizza	340	15	5	830	41	2	4	11
Pasta								
Rattlesnake Pasta, 1/2 of dish	660	38	14	1070	54	3	5	29
Shrimp Scampi, 1/2 of dish	580	32	12	970	53	3	5	22
Chicken Spinoccoli, 1/2 of dish	670	33	15	1510	60	4	7	41
Tuscan Chicken Penne, 1/2 of dish	590	32	4.5	1010	52	9	9	31
Penne Bolognese, 1/2 of dish	380	9	3.5	940	56	3	5	18
Chicken & Broccoli Fettuccine, 1/2 of dish	650	37	14	1010	56	3	5	28
Tuscan Roasted Vegetable Penne, 1/2 of dish	490	29	4.5	590	52	9	9	11
Tortellacci, 1/2 of dish	470	20	10	1280	44	3	4	24
Chicken & Penne w/ Chablis White Wine, 1/2 of dish	600	34	12	1050	54	4	5	24
Chicken								
Grilled Chicken w/ Mango Salsa, 1/2 of dish	110	3	0	520	3	0	1	21
Baked Stuffed Chicken, 1/2 of dish	180	9	3	640	3	1	1	27
Chicken Parmesan, 1/2 of dish	560	21	4	1020	69	4	9	28
Grilled Rosemary Chicken, 1/2 of dish	260	21	2.5	630	1	0	0	20
Chicken Thumb Platter, 1/2 of dish	240	9	1	790	17	1	1	27
Chicken Milanese, 1/2 of dish	420	29	5	1110	20	3	6	27
Seafood								
Fish & Chips, 1/2 of dish	370	32	4	640	29	5	1	13
Baked Haddock, 1/2 of dish	290	17	3	270	6	0	1	27
Lemon Basil Salmon, 1/2 of dish	240	17	2.5	370	0	0	0	21
Grilled BBQ Salmon, 1/2 of dish	290	17	2.5	280	11	0	9	31
Grilled Mahi-Mahi w/ Mango Salsa, 1/2 of dish	120	1	0	490	6	0	4	21

Description & Serving	Cal	Fat	Sfat	Sod	Carb	Fiber	Sugar	Prot
Fisherman's Platter, 1/2 of dish	770	55	7	1450	74	8	5	29
Salmon, Shrimp & Haddock Combo, 1/2 of dish	750	49	6	1640	10	1	1	68
Grilled & Skewered BBQ Shrimp, 1/2 of dish	150	0	0	600	17	0	14	29

Steak/Ribs

6 oz Top Sirloin, 1/2 of dish	150	5	2	290	0	0	0	25
7 oz Filet, 1/2 of dish	290	12	4.5	450	0	0	0	44
Grilled Shrimp & Sirloin, 1/2 of dish	320	14	3.5	750	1	0	0	43
The Chop House Classic, 1/2 of dish	260	9	3.5	320	0	0	0	42
Sirloin Steak Tips, 1/2 of dish	290	14	4	1030	4	1	2	31
Brewmaster's Grill NY Sirloin, 1/2 of dish	260	7	2.5	790	12	0	10	43
Baby Back Ribs, 1/2 of dish	660	45	15	970	34	3	55	34

Side

French Fries	450	33	3.5	1290	36	7	0	5
Skinless Bake	480	31	11	1030	40	3	3	12
Red Bliss Mashed Potatoes	340	19	4	770	39	3	2	4
Steamed Seasonal Vegetables	100	7	1.5	90	10	3	4	2
Brown Rice w/ Cranberries & Mango	180	5	0.5	85	32	2	4	3
Rice Pilaf	220	6	1.5	340	38	1	0	5
Steamed Broccoli	70	6	1	360	5	3	0	3
Roasted Seasonal Vegetables	90	4.5	0	180	12	3	7	2
UNO Breadstick, 1	210	13	4	460	18	1	2	6

Kids

Kid's Cheese Pizza, 1/2 of dish	360	13	6	890	43	2	5	16
Kid's Deep Dish Cheese Pizza, 1/2 of dish	450	32	9	800	29	1	1	15
Kid's Pepperoni Pizza, 1/2 of dish	390	16	7	1030	45	2	5	19
Kid's Deep Dish Pepperoni, 1/2 of dish	490	35	10	930	29	1	1	17
Kid's Kombo, 1/2 of dish	410	23	4	780	36	4	1	17
Tiny Dinos, 1/2 of dish	330	20	2	520	28	4	1	13
Kid's Cheeseburger, 1/2 of dish	360	22	6	1030	26	4	1	14
Kid's Chicken Caesar Salad, 1/2 of dish	160	10	2	420	5	1	1	14
Kid's Grilled Chicken, 1/2 of dish	70	2	0	300	0	0	0	15
Kid's Pasta, 1/2 of dish	150	1.5	0	135	32	2	4	4
Macaroni & Cheese, 1/2 of dish	240	8	2.5	600	34	1	8	9
Kid's Corn	110	5	1	25	17	2	3	2
Kid's Apples & Mandarin Oranges	45	0	0	0	11	1	4	1
Kid's Sundae, 1/2 of dish	430	19	10	260	58	2	47	4
Kid's Slush	70	0	0	10	17	0	16	0

Dressing/Condiment

Fat Free Vinaigrette, 57 g	30	0	0	200	5	1	4	0
Balsamic Vinaigrette, 57 g	220	22	3.5	530	4	0	4	0
Ranch Dressing, 57 g	250	25	4	440	6	0	2	1
Classic Vinaigrette, 57 g	170	16	2.5	190	5	0	4	0
Caesar Dressing, 57 g	290	29	6	440	2	0	1	4
Bleu Cheese Dressing, 57 g	280	29	5	470	2	0	2	2
Avocado Ranch Dressing, 57 g	210	21	3.5	430	5	1	2	1
Honey Mustard Dressing, 57 g	300	28	4	450	12	0	11	1
Low Fat Blueberry Pomegranate Vinaigrette, 28 g	60	3	0	110	8	0	4	0

Description & Serving	Cal	Fat	Sfat	Sod	Carb	Fiber	Sugar	Prot
Asian Sauce, 43 g	110	4.5	0	710	14	0	13	1
Buffalo Wing Sauce, 43 g	20	0.5	0	510	3	0	1	0
Wowza Sauce, 43 g	70	0	0	280	17	0	14	14
Honey BBQ Sauce, 43 g	80	1	0	220	18	0	17	1
Buffalo Garlic Romano Sauce, 43 g	40	3	0	530	3	0	1	2
Sweet & Spicy Sauce, 43 g	40	3	0	530	3	0	1	2
Guacamole, 57 g	90	9	1	240	4	3	1	1

Dessert

	Cal	Fat	Sfat	Sod	Carb	Fiber	Sugar	Prot
The All American, 1/2 of dish	300	14	7	135	42	2	29	3
UNO Deep Dish Sundae, 1/2 of dish	700	34	18	310	95	3	68	7
Chocolate Peanut Butter Cup, 1/2 of dish	800	52	21	420	71	6	55	13
Mega-Sized Deep Dish Sundae, 1/4 of dish	700	34	18	310	95	3	68	7
Brownie Bowl, 1/2 of dish	430	20	12	220	57	2	40	4
Chicago Cheesecake, 1/2 of dish	460	32	20	340	36	1	15	6
Mini Hot Chocolate Brownie Sundae	370	16	8	190	54	2	38	4
Mini White Chocolate Chunk Deep Dish Sundae	660	35	14	390	96	2	63	8
Mini All American Hot Apple Crumble	330	14	7	150	47	2	32	3
Chocolate Cookie Freezer	480	14	4.5	410	83	2	46	9
Strawberry Smoothie	270	6	3	115	52	0	42	5
UNO Raspberry Lime Ricky	170	0	0	0	42	0	35	0
Chocolate Monkey	260	6	0	135	62	1	45	5
Tropical Fruit Freezer	320	4	2	10	71	1	52	1
Wildberry Mango Smoothie	290	6	3	105	47	1	24	3

Vocelli Pizza

Salad

	Cal	Fat	Sfat	Sod	Carb	Fiber	Sugar	Prot
Chicken Caesar Insalata	220	4.5	1.5	120	4	2	2	38
Mediterranean Insalata	270	18	9	1060	20	6	12	13
Garden della Casa Insalata	190	10	4	580	16	5	8	12
Tuscany Chicken Insalata	350	16	6	650	15	5	8	38
Antipasta Insalata	630	50	18	2040	16	5	8	32

Sandwich

	Cal	Fat	Sfat	Sod	Carb	Fiber	Sugar	Prot
Italian Panini	910	42	20	3410	77	4	2	54
Steak Panini	970	46	22	1920	81	5	4	55
Ham Panini	920	43	18	3150	81	5	4	52
Turkey Panini	940	39	16	3560	81	4	5	66
Vegetarian Panini	750	31	15	2110	83	6	5	34
Club Panini	1020	50	20	3550	79	4	4	63
Chicken Panini	900	38	16	2510	81	4	2	54

Pizza, 1 slice

	Cal	Fat	Sfat	Sod	Carb	Fiber	Sugar	Prot
Grande Cheese Pizza	260	6	3	530	38	2	3	13
Grande Pepperoni Pizza	410	20	9	1150	38	2	4	19
Thin Crust Cheese Pizza	210	8	4	390	23	1	2	12
Thin Crust Pepperoni Pizza	350	20	9	1040	23	1	2	20
Spring Veggie Pizza	280	6	3.5	600	41	3	4	13
Garlic Spinaci Pizza	300	10	5	500	40	3	3	15

Description & Serving	Cal	Fat	SFat	Sod	Carb	Fiber	Sugar	Prot
Meat Magnifico Pizza	490	25	10	1440	38	2	3	26
Hawaiian Pizza	360	13	6	890	40	2	5	21
Deluxe Pizza	390	16	7	1100	40	2	4	20
Chicken Spinaci Pizza	330	11	4.5	480	39	3	3	20
Broccoli Chicken Pizza	360	14	7	500	37	2	2	22
Philly Steak Pizza	360	13	6	480	38	2	3	20

Side

Wings - Buffalo	560	39	8	2410	3	0	2	47
Wings - BBQ	610	33	8	2030	26	0	17	47
Wings - Garlic	980	85	17	2550	5	1	2	47
Pepperoni Sticks, 2.5 slices	470	26	9	1090	36	1	2	21
Bread Sticks, 2 slices	230	8	1.5	290	35	1	2	5
Bruschetta, 1 slice	150	8	2.5	315	14	1	0.5	7

Dressing/Topping

Italian Dressing, 43 g	200	32	3	410	4	0	3	0
Fat-Free Italian Dressing, 43 g	20	0	0	700	5	1	3	0
Ranch Dressing, 43 g	260	43	4	240	2	0	2	1
Blue Cheese Dressing, 43 g	230	38	4.5	380	2	0	2	1
Caesar Dressing, 43 g	210	35	3.5	420	2	0	2	1
Greek Dressing, 43 g	220	37	3.5	190	1	0	1	0
Croutons, 7 g	30	1	0	105	5	0	0	1

Wendy's

Burger

Jr. Hamburger	230	8	3	490	26	1	5	13
Jr. Cheeseburger	270	11	5	700	26	1	6	15
Jr. Cheeseburger Deluxe	300	14	6	730	28	2	7	15
Jr. Bacon Cheeseburger	310	16	6	670	25	1	5	17
Double Stack	360	18	8	810	26	1	6	23
Single w/ Everything	430	20	7	870	38	2	9	25
Double w/ Everything & Cheese	700	40	17	1440	38	2	9	47
Triple w/ Everything & Cheese	970	60	27	2010	39	2	10	69
Baconator	830	51	23	1880	35	1	8	56

Sandwich/Wrap

Ultimate Chicken Grill Sandwich	320	7	1.5	950	36	2	8	28
Spicy Chicken Filet Sandwich	440	16	3	1200	49	2	6	26
Homestyle Chicken Filet Sandwich	440	16	3	1050	47	2	6	25
Chicken Club Sandwich	550	26	8	1290	48	2	7	34
Crispy Chicken Sandwich	360	18	3.5	710	36	2	4	15
Grilled Chicken Go Wrap	250	10	3	730	24	1	4	17
Homestyle Chicken Go Wrap	310	15	4.5	800	30	1	2	15
Spicy Chicken Go Wrap	320	15	4	880	30	1	2	16

Nuggets/Wings

Chicken Nuggets, 5 pc	230	16	3.5	480	11	0	0	12
Bold Buffalo Boneless Wings	520	18	3.5	2630	58	2	13	31
Honey BBQ Boneless Wings	580	18	3.5	1990	75	2	34	32
Sweet & Spicy Asian Chicken Boneless Wings	550	18	3.5	2530	67	3	27	31

Description & Serving	Cal	Fat	Sfat	Sod	Carb	Fiber	Sugar	Prot
Salad								
Mandarin Chicken Salad	180	2	0.5	630	16	2	12	24
Chicken Caesar Salad	180	4	2	690	8	3	3	28
Chicken BLT Salad	470	27	10	1210	23	3	5	35
Southwest Taco Salad	400	22	11	1140	26	7	9	27
Kids								
Kids' Meal Hamburger	220	8	3	490	25	1	5	12
Kids' Meal Cheeseburger	260	11	5	700	26	1	5	15
Kids' Meal Crispy Chicken Sandwich	340	15	3	680	35	2	4	15
Kids' Meal Chicken Nuggets, 4 pc	190	13	3	380	9	0	0	9
Kids' Meal French Fries	210	10	2	190	27	3	0	3
Snack/Side								
Side Salad	35	0	0	25	8	2	4	1
Caesar Side Salad	70	4	2	170	4	2	1	6
Mandarin Orange Cup	80	0	0	15	19	1	17	1
Plain Baked Potato	270	0	0	25	61	7	3	7
Sour Cream & Chives Baked Potato	320	3.5	2	50	63	7	4	8
Chili, sml	190	6	2.5	830	19	5	6	14
Chili, lrg	280	9	3.5	1240	29	7	9	21
French Fries, sml	330	16	3	300	44	4	0	4
French Fries, med	420	20	4	380	55	5	0	5
French Fries, lrg	540	26	5	500	71	7	0	7
Topping								
Crispy Noodles	70	2.5	0	190	10	0	0	1
Roasted Almonds	130	11	1	70	4	2	1	5
Homestyle Garlic Croutons	70	2.5	0	125	9	0	0	2
Seasoned Tortilla Strips	110	5	1	160	13	1	0	2
American Cheese Jr.	40	3.5	2	200	0	0	0	2
American Cheese	70	5	3.5	320	1	0	0	3
Swiss Cheese	70	6	3.5	85	0	0	0	5
Bacon, 1 strip	15	1	0	50	0	0	0	1
Dill Pickles, 4 ea	0	0	0	140	0	0	0	0
Tomato, 1 slice	5	0	0	0	1	0	1	0
Onion, 4 rings	5	0	0	0	1	0	1	0
Dressing/Condiment								
Oriental Sesame Dressing	170	10	1.5	360	19	0	18	1
Supreme Caesar Dressing	120	13	2	200	1	0	1	1
Honey Dijon Dressing	250	24	3.5	330	9	0	8	1
Ancho Chipotle Ranch Dressing	90	8	1.5	240	3	0	2	1
Classic Ranch Dressing	200	20	3	340	3	0	2	1
Light Classic Ranch Dressing	90	8	1.5	360	4	0	2	1
Balsamic Vinaigrette Dressing	90	6	1	380	8	0	7	0
Italian Vinaigrette Dressing	130	11	1.5	320	8	0	6	0
Fat Free French Dressing	70	0	0	170	17	1	15	0
Light Honey Dijon Dressing	100	5	1	280	13	1	12	1
Chunky Blue Cheese Dressing	230	24	5	370	2	0	2	2
Thousand Island Dressing	290	28	4.5	530	9	0	7	1

Description & Serving	Cal	Fat	Sfat	Sod	Carb	Fiber	Sugar	Prot
Buttery Best Spread	50	5	1	95	0	0	0	0
Hot Chili Seasoning	5	0	0	270	1	0	1	0
Saltine Crackers	25	0.5	0	80	5	0	0	1
Cheddar Cheese, shredded	70	6	3	105	1	0	0	4
Reduced Fat Acidified Sour Cream	45	3.5	2	25	2	0	1	1
Ketchup, 1 packet	10	0	0	115	3	0	2	0
Coffee Creamer, 1 ea	20	2	1	10	0	0	0	0
Sugar, 1 packet	15	0	0	0	3	0	3	0
Non-Nutritive Sweetener	5	0	0	0	1	0	1	0
Mayonnaise, 1.5 tsp	40	3.5	0.5	55	1	0	0	0
Ketchup, 1 tsp	10	0	0	95	2	0	2	0
Mustard, 3/4 tsp	5	0	0	50	0	0	0	0
Honey Mustard Sauce, 1 tsp	40	3.5	0	60	3	0	2	0
Ranch Sauce	35	3.5	0.5	70	1	0	0	0
Barbecue Nugget Sauce	45	0	0	160	11	0	9	1
Sweet & Sour Nugget Sauce	50	0	0	120	12	0	11	0
Honey Mustard Nugget Sauce	130	12	2	220	6	0	5	0
Heartland Ranch Dipping Sauce	160	17	2.5	220	1	0	1	0

Beverage

Coffee	0	0	0	0	0	0	0	0
Hot Tea	0	0	0	0	0	0	0	0
Sweet Tea, sml	100	0	0	10	26	0	25	0

Dessert

Chocolate Frosty, sml	320	8	5	150	52	0	41	9
Vanilla Frosty, sml	310	8	5	180	52	0	43	8
Vanilla Frosty Float w/ Coca-Cola	380	7	4.5	160	75	0	68	7
Chocolate Fudge Frosty Shake, sml	410	11	7	240	69	1	57	8
Strawberry Frosty Shake, sml	390	11	7	170	65	0	57	7
Vanilla Bean Frosty Shake, sml	380	10	6	170	65	0	56	7
Frosty-cino, sml	390	10	6	170	62	0	52	7
Nestle Toll House Cookie Dough Twisted Frosty, Chocolate	480	16	10	220	77	1	58	10
Nestle Toll House Cookie Dough Twisted Frosty, Vanilla	480	16	10	240	77	1	60	9
M&M's Twisted Frosty, Chocolate	560	19	12	180	86	1	72	10
M&M's Twisted Frosty, Vanilla	550	19	12	210	86	1	74	10
Oreo Twisted Frosty, Chocolate	450	14	7	300	72	1	52	10
Oreo Twisted Frosty, Vanilla	440	14	6	320	72	1	54	9
Coffee Toffee Twisted Frosty, Chocolate	550	21	15	240	83	1	68	9
Coffee Toffee Twisted Frosty, Vanilla	540	20	15	270	83	1	69	9

Whataburger

Breakfast

Biscuit	300	17	8	644	32	1	2	5
Biscuit & Gravy	530	36	14	1823	52	1	7	9

Description & Serving	Cal	Fat	Sfat	Sod	Carb	Fiber	Sugar	Prot
Biscuit Sandwich w/ bacon, egg & cheese	500	32	14	1231	33	1	2	16
Biscuit Sandwich w/ egg & cheese	450	28	13	1028	33	1	2	13
Biscuit Sandwich w/ sausage, egg & cheese	690	49	21	1553	33	1	2	26
Biscuit w/ bacon	350	20	10	847	32	1	2	8
Biscuit w/ sausage	540	37	17	1169	32	1	2	18
Breakfast On A Bun w/ bacon	360	21	6	807	25	1	4	15
Breakfast On A Bun w/ sausage	550	38	14	1129	25	1	4	25
Breakfast Platter w/ bacon	740	45	16	1462	53	2	3	24
Breakfast Platter w/ sausage	930	62	23	1784	53	2	3	34
Cinnamon Roll	390	9	3.5	390	71	3	35	7
Egg Sandwich	310	17	5	604	25	1	4	12
Pancakes w/ bacon	630	12	3	2373	112	5	27	20
Pancakes w/ sausage	820	29	10	2695	112	5	27	30
Pancakes, plain	580	8	2	2170	112	5	27	17
Taquito w/ bacon & egg	380	21	7	932	27	3	2	17
Taquito w/ bacon, egg, & cheese	420	24	9	1157	27	3	2	19
Taquito w/ potato & egg	430	23	7	912	37	3	2	15
Taquito w/ potato, egg & cheese	470	27	9	1137	37	3	2	17
Taquito w/ sausage & egg	410	24	8	909	27	3	2	17
Taquito w/ sausage, egg, & cheese	450	28	11	1134	27	3	2	19

Chicken

Chicken Strip, 1	200	12	2	359	11	0	0	9
Chicken Strips w/ gravy, 4	840	54	9	1858	53	0	2	37

Burger/Sandwich

Justaburger	290	15	4.5	727	26	1	4	13
Whataburger Jr.	300	15	4.5	730	28	1	5	13
Whataburger	620	30	10	1262	58	2	13	26
Whataburger w/ bacon & cheese	780	43	16	1997	59	2	13	36
Whataburger, double meat	870	49	18	1510	58	2	13	43
Whataburger, triple meat	1120	68	26	1759	58	2	13	61
Grilled Chicken Sandwich	470	19	4	1018	49	3	11	27
Whatacatch Sandwich	460	29	5	878	38	2	5	15
Whatachick'n Sandwich	550	20	3.5	1408	65	4	11	26
Whatacatch Dinner, 2 pc	1580	92	19	1661	161	8	88	29

Kids

Kid's Meal Chicken Strips	770	51	10	720	53	2	0	22
Kid's Meal Justaburger	550	28	8	747	56	3	4	17

Side

French Fries, sml	260	13	3.5	26	31	2	0	4
French Fries, med	400	20	5	39	47	4	0	6
French Fries, lrg	530	27	7	52	63	5	0	8
Hash Brown Sticks	200	12	2.5	366	20	1	0	2
Honey Butter Chicken Biscuit	610	38	12	1072	51	1	9	14
Onion Rings, lrg	630	42	19	742	55	4	25	8
Onion Rings, med	420	28	13	494	36	3	17	5
Texas Toast, 1	150	7	1	170	20	1	3	3

Description & Serving	Cal	Fat	Sfat	Sod	Carb	Fiber	Sugar	Prot
Salad								
Chicken Strips Salad	430	25	5	713	33	4	6	19
Garden Salad	50	1	1	13	11	4	6	1
Grilled Chicken Salad	220	8	2.5	633	18	4	6	21
Dressing/Condiment/Topping								
Gravy, White Peppered (for chicken strips)	60	5	1	421	8	0	2	0
Ranch Sauce	480	51	7	731	4	0	3	1
Cheese, American (lrg slice)	90	7	4.5	431	1	0	0	5
Cheese, American (sml slice)	45	4	2.5	225	0	0	0	2
Jalapeno, sliced (for lrg burger)	0	0	0	168	0	1	0	0
Jalapeno, sliced (for sml burger)	0	0	0	126	0	1	0	0
Jalapeno, whole	0	0	0	143	0	1	0	0
Dessert								
Cookie, Chocolate Chunk	230	11	7	150	33	1	21	2
Cookie, White Chocolate Chunk Macadamia Nut	250	14	8	130	30	0	20	3
Hot Apple Pie	230	11	2.5	285	29	2	1	3
Hot Lemon Pie	230	12	2.5	280	35	1	13	3
Malt, chocolate, kids	520	13	9	230	94	2	88	11
Malt, chocolate, lrg	1460	35	24	642	264	5	246	29
Malt, chocolate, med	1050	25	18	460	188	3	175	21
Malt, chocolate, sml	670	15	11	297	123	2	115	13
Malt, strawberry, kids	520	12	9	199	94	0	89	10
Malt, strawberry, lrg	1450	33	23	548	263	0	250	26
Malt, strawberry, med	1040	24	17	397	188	0	178	19
Malt, strawberry, sml	670	15	10	250	123	0	117	12
Malt, vanilla, kids	470	13	9	205	77	0	72	11
Malt, vanilla, lrg	1300	37	26	569	215	0	201	29
Malt, vanilla, med	940	27	19	409	155	0	144	21
Malt, vanilla, sml	600	17	12	259	98	0	92	13
Shake, chocolate, kids	500	13	4	219	86	2	80	11
Shake, chocolate, lrg	1380	36	25	610	241	5	222	31
Shake, chocolate, med	1000	26	18	439	171	3	158	22
Shake, chocolate, sml	630	16	11	281	111	2	103	14
Shake, strawberry, kids	500	13	3.5	188	86	0	81	10
Shake, strawberry, lrg	1370	35	24	516	240	0	226	28
Shake, strawberry, med	990	26	18	376	171	0	161	20
Shake, strawberry, sml	630	16	11	234	111	0	105	13
Shake, vanilla, kids	440	14	10	194	69	0	64	11
Shake, vanilla, lrg	1220	38	27	534	191	0	176	31
Shake, vanilla, med	890	28	19	388	139	0	128	22
Shake, vanilla, sml	560	17	12	243	87	0	80	14

White Castle

Breakfast								
Sausage, Egg, Cheese, Golden Bun	340	25	9	660	14	<1	3	15
Sausage, Cheese, Golden Bun	250	17	7	590	14	<1	2	9

Description & Serving	Cal	Fat	Sfat	Sod	Carb	Fiber	Sugar	Prot
Sausage, Egg, Golden Bun	320	23	8	530	14	<1	3	14
Sausage, Golden Bun	220	15	6	460	13	<1	2	8
Bacon, Egg, Cheese, Golden Bun	230	14	5	540	14	<1	3	13
Bacon, Cheese, Golden Bun	150	7	3	470	14	<1	2	7
Bacon, Egg, Golden Bun	210	12	3.5	410	14	<1	3	12
Bacon, Golden Bun	120	5	2	340	13	<1	2	5
Egg, Cheese, Golden Bun	190	10	4	350	14	<1	3	10
Egg, Golden Bun	160	8	2.5	220	14	<1	3	9
Bologna, Egg, Cheese, Golden Bun	280	18	6	740	16	<1	4	14
Bologna, Cheese, Golden Bun	190	11	4	570	15	<1	3	7
Bologna, Egg, Golden Bun	260	16	5	620	16	<1	4	12
Hamburger, Egg, Cheese, Golden Bun	260	16	6	480	15	<1	3	14
Hamburger, Cheese, Golden Bun	160	8	4	310	14	<1	2	8
Hamburger, Egg, Golden Bun	240	14	5	360	15	<1	3	13
Egg	90	7	2	70	0	0	1	6
Hashbrown	170	11	4	380	16	2	0	2
Hamburger Meat	70	6	2.5	15	0	0	0	4
Sausage	150	14	5	310	0	0	0	5
Bologna	80	8	2.5	300	1	0	1	3
Strip of Bacon	50	4	1.5	190	0	0	0	3

Burger/Sandwich

Single White Castle	140	7	2.5	210	14	<1	2	6
Cheeseburger	170	9	4	330	15	<1	2	7
Jalapeno Cheeseburger	180	10	4.5	380	15	<1	2	8
Bacon Cheeseburger	200	11	5	480	15	<1	2	10
Bacon Jalapeno Cheeseburger	210	12	6	480	15	<1	2	11
Chicken Ring Sandwich on Golden Bun	180	8	2	380	19	<1	2	7
Chicken Ring Sandwich w/ Cheese on Golden Bun	200	10	3	500	19	<1	2	8
Chicken Breast Sandwich on Golden Bun	180	6	1	580	21	1	2	11
Chicken Breast Sandwich w/ Cheese on Golden Bun	210	8	2.5	710	21	1	2	13
Fish Sandwich on Golden Bun	160	6	1	300	18	<1	2	8
Fish w/ Cheese on Golden Bun	190	8	2	430	20	<1	2	10
Traditional Bun w/ Cheese	100	3.5	2	280	13	<1	1	3
Pulled Pork BBQ Sandwich	170	4.5	1.5	490	24	1	12	9
Chicken Supreme on Golden Bun	230	10	3.5	860	21	1	2	14
Surf & Turf w/ Cheese	390	22	9	670	28	1	4	20
Surf & Turf w/o Cheese	340	18	6	420	28	1	4	17
Double White Castle	250	13	5	340	22	1	2	11
Double Cheeseburger	300	17	8	590	23	1	2	14
Double Jalapeno Cheeseburger	320	19	9	680	23	1	2	15
Double Bacon Cheeseburger	370	22	10	880	23	1	2	19
Double Fish w/o Cheese on Golden Bun	290	11	1.5	540	32	1	3	16
Double Fish w/ Cheese on Golden Bun	340	15	4.5	790	32	1	3	18

Side

French Fries, reg	310	15	3	250	39	4	1	4
French Fries, sack	700	34	6	560	89	9	3	9

Description & Serving	Cal	Fat	Sfat	Sod	Carb	Fiber	Sugar	Prot
Onion Chips, reg	480	23	4	670	62	2	9	7
Onion Chips, sack	980	47	8	1350	125	5	18	13
Onion Rings, reg	200	9	1.5	220	28	1	4	2
Onion Rings, sack	390	17	3	400	53	2	8	5
Homestyle Onion Rings, reg	400	21	3.5	460	49	1	7	4
Homestyle Onion Rings, sack	750	39	6	860	91	2	13	8
Chicken Rings, 3	150	10	2	340	8	0	0	8
Clam Strips, reg	250	22	3.5	620	5	0	1	8
Clam Strips, sack	500	44	7	1250	9	0	2	16
Fish Nibblers, reg	280	16	3.5	870	24	5	0	19
Fish Nibblers, sack	1090	56	12	2980	82	17	0	65
Mozzarella Cheese Sticks, 3	250	14	6	750	22	1	2	10
Dressing/Condiment/Topping								
BBQ Sauce, 28 g	35	0.5	0	390	8	0	8	0
Cheese Sauce (Nacho), 47 g	50	4	1	400	3	0	0	0
Cheese Sauce, 43 g	130	10	3.5	560	6	0	3	3
Fat Free Honey Mustard Sauce, 28 g	50	0	0	120	13	0	7	0
Marinara Sauce, 28 g	15	0	0	260	3	0	1	1
Ranch Dressing, 28 g	150	17	2.5	200	1	0	1	0
Seafood Sauce, 28 g	30	0	0	340	7	0	6	0
Tartar Sauce, 28 g	90	8	1	220	5	0	3	0
White Castle Zesty Zing Sauce, 28 g	120	11	1.5	190	4	0	3	0
BBQ Sauce, 9 g	15	0	0	130	3	0	3	0
Fat Free Honey Mustard Sauce, 12 g	20	0	0	50	5	0	3	0
Hot Sauce, 7 g	5	0	0	170	1	<1	0	0
Ketchup, 9 g	10	0	0	100	3	0	2	0
Lemon Juice, 4 g	5	0	0	0	1	0	0	0
Mayonnaise, 9 g	70	7	1	55	0	0	0	0
Mustard, 5.5 g	5	0	0	85	<1	0	0	0
Tartar Sauce, 9 g	25	2.5	0	85	1	0	1	0
Grape Jelly, 14 g	35	0	0	0	9	0	7	0
Maple Syrup, 43 g	120	0	0	25	31	0	21	0
Butter, 5 g	30	3.5	2.5	30	0	0	0	0
Cream Cheese, 28 g	100	10	6	110	0	0	0	2
Strawberry Jam, 14 g	40	0	0	0	10	0	7	0
American Cheese Slice	25	2	1.5	125	0	0	0	1
Jalapeno Cheese Slice	35	3	2	170	0	0	0	2
Bacon	30	2.5	1	140	0	0	0	2
Beverage (shakes vary by region)								
Hot Chocolate, 12 oz	220	6	0.5	300	40	<1	32	1
Hot Chocolate, 16 oz	300	8	1	410	55	<1	43	2
Hot Chocolate, 20 oz	370	10	1	510	68	<1	53	2
Chocolate Shake, 10 oz	190	2	1.5	135	39	0	35	3
Chocolate Shake, 21 oz	390	4.5	3	280	82	0	73	6
Chocolate Shake, 32 oz	600	7	4.5	430	125	0	112	9
Chocolate Shake, 44 oz	820	9	6	590	172	0	154	13
Vanilla Shake, 10 oz	150	2	1.5	130	31	0	27	3
Vanilla Shake, 21 oz	320	4.5	3	280	65	0	56	6

Description & Serving	Cal	Fat	Sfat	Sod	Carb	Fiber	Sugar	Prot
Vanilla Shake, 32 oz	490	7	4.5	430	99	0	86	9
Vanilla Shake, 44 oz	680	9	6	590	136	0	118	13
Strawberry Shake, 10 oz	190	2	1.5	135	40	0	36	3
Strawberry Shake, 21 oz	400	4.5	3	280	83	0	74	6
Strawberry Shake, 32 oz	610	7	4.5	430	127	0	114	9
Strawberry Shake, 44 oz	830	9	6	590	174	0	156	13

Wienerschnitzel

Breakfast

	Cal	Fat	Sfat	Sod	Carb	Fiber	Sugar	Prot
Burrito w/ Egg, Bacon & Cheese	490	25	8	1380	39	1	3	24
Burrito w/ Egg, Sausage & Cheese	590	34	12	1500	43	1	3	25
Chorizo Breakfast Burrito	670	41	14	1640	38	1	1	34
Chili Cheese Burrito	470	21	6	1720	43	2	2	25
Biscuit w/ Bacon	330	17	5	1120	35	1	4	10
Biscuit w/ Sausage	430	26	9	1240	39	1	4	11
Biscuit w/ Egg & Bacon	390	21	6	1270	36	1	4	16
Biscuit w/ Egg & Sausage	490	30	10	1390	40	1	4	17
Biscuit w/ Egg, Bacon & Cheese	440	25	9	1520	36	1	4	18
Biscuit w/ Egg, Sausage & Cheese	540	34	12	1640	40	1	4	19
Croissant w/ Egg, Bacon & Cheese	520	31	17	990	40	1	8	19
Croissant w/ Egg, Sausage & Cheese	620	40	21	1110	44	1	8	20
Sandwich w/ Egg, Bacon & Cheese	300	15	6	830	26	1	1	16
Sandwich w/ Egg, Sausage & Cheese	400	24	10	950	30	1	1	17
Breakfast Platter w/ Bacon	600	40	15	960	40	3	1	20
Breakfast Platter w/ Sausage	700	49	19	1080	44	3	1	21
Country Breakfast	640	40	13	1820	47	1	4	24
Biscuit	260	11	3	890	35	1	4	6
Biscuit w/ Egg	320	15	4	1040	36	1	4	12
Biscuit & Gravy	350	17	5	1180	42	1	4	8
Hash Browns	290	25	10	240	14	2	0	1
French Toast Sticks	490	29	11	460	49	5	11	6

Hot Dog

	Cal	Fat	Sfat	Sod	Carb	Fiber	Sugar	Prot
Original Chili Cheese Dog, standard bun	340	17	6	1260	31	1	4	14
Original Chili Dog, standard bun	290	13	4	1000	31	1	3	11
Original Mustard Dog, standard bun	260	12	4	690	28	1	4	9
Original Relish Dog, standard bun	270	12	4	720	30	1	5	9
Original Kraut Dog, standard bun	260	12	4	890	28	1	4	9
Original Deluxe Dog, standard bun	270	12	4	1080	30	2	5	9
Original BBQ Bacon Dog, standard bun	380	21	8	970	33	1	9	14
Original Plain Hot Dog, standard bun	270	13	4	640	28	1	5	9
Original Stadium Dog, standard dog	370	20	7	1360	32	1	6	14
Original Chicago Dog, standard bun	410	20	7	2510	43	2	13	15
Original Pastrami Dog, standard bun	510	32	12	1960	31	1	5	23
Angus All Beef Chili Cheese Dog, seeded bun	600	37	15	2050	40	2	4	29
Angus All Beef Chili Dog, seeded bun	490	27	9	1870	39	2	3	22
Angus All Beef Mustard Dog, seeded bun	450	26	9	1530	36	1	3	20
Angus All Beef Relish Dog, seeded bun	460	26	9	1590	39	1	5	20

Description & Serving	Cal	Fat	Sfat	Sod	Carb	Fiber	Sugar	Prot
Angus All Beef Kraut Dog, seeded bun	460	26	9	1760	37	1	3	20
Angus All Beef Deluxe Dog, seeded bun	470	26	9	1950	39	2	5	20
Angus All Beef BBQ Bacon Dog, seeded bun	570	34	13	1840	42	1	8	25
Angus All Beef Plain Hot Dog, seeded bun	460	26	9	1510	37	1	4	20
Angus All Beef Stadium Dog, seeded bun	470	26	9	1630	39	1	6	20
Angus All Beef Chicago Dog, seeded bun	520	27	9	2780	50	2	13	21
Angus All Beef Pastrami Dog, seeded bun	600	38	13	2230	38	2	4	29
Big Original Chili Cheese Dog, standard bun	510	32	13	1490	42	1	5	22
Big Original Chili Dog, standard bun	400	23	7	1310	41	1	4	15
Big Original Mustard Dog, standard bun	370	22	7	970	38	1	4	13
Big Original Relish Dog, standard bun	380	22	7	1030	41	1	6	13
Big Original Kraut Dog, standard bun	370	22	7	1190	39	1	4	13
Big Original Deluxe Dog, standard bun	380	22	7	1390	41	2	6	13
Big Original BBQ Bacon Dog, standard bun	480	30	11	1280	44	1	9	18
Big Original Plain Hot Dog, standard bun	370	22	7	940	39	1	5	13
Big Original Stadium Dog, standard bun	380	22	7	1060	41	1	7	13
Big Original Chicago Dog, standard bun	430	22	7	2210	52	2	14	14
Big Original Pastrami Dog, standard bun	520	33	11	1670	40	1	5	22
Chili Cheese Dog on a Pretzel Bun	480	20	7	1330	57	2	8	17
Chili Dog on a Pretzel Bun	430	16	5	1070	57	2	7	14
Mustard Dog on a Pretzel Bun	400	15	5	750	54	1	8	12
Relish Dog on a Pretzel Bun	410	15	5	780	56	1	9	12
Kraut Dog on a Pretzel Bun	400	15	5	950	54	2	8	12
Deluxe Dog on a Pretzel Bun	410	15	5	1150	56	2	9	12
BBQ Bacon Dog on a Pretzel Bun	510	23	9	1040	59	1	12	17
Plain Dog on a Pretzel Bun	400	15	5	700	54	1	8	12
Stadium Dog on a Pretzel Bun	510	23	8	1420	58	1	10	17
Chicago Dog on a Pretzel Bun	550	23	8	2570	69	2	17	18
Pastrami Dog on a Pretzel Bun	640	34	13	2030	57	2	8	26
Angus All Beef Chili Cheese Dog on a Pretzel Bun	680	37	13	2040	59	2	8	28
Angus All Beef Chili Dog on a Pretzel Bun	570	28	9	2860	58	2	7	21
Angus All Beef Mustard Dog on a Pretzel Bun	530	27	9	1520	55	1	7	19
Angus All Beef Relish Dog on a Pretzel Bun	540	27	9	1580	58	1	9	19
Angus All Beef Kraut Dog on a Pretzel Bun	540	27	9	1740	56	1	7	19
Angus All Beef Deluxe Dog on a Pretzel Bun	550	27	9	1940	58	2	9	19
Angus All Beef BBQ Bacon Dog on a Pretzel Bun	650	35	13	1830	61	1	12	24
Angus All Beef Plain Dog on a Pretzel Bun	540	27	9	1490	56	1	8	19
Angus All Beef Stadium Dog on a Pretzel Bun	550	27	9	1610	58	1	10	19
Angus All Beef Chicago Dog on a Pretzel Bun	600	27	9	2760	69	2	17	20
Angus All Beef Pastrami Dog on a Pretzel Bun	680	38	14	2220	57	2	8	28
Big Original Chili Cheese Dog on a Pretzel Bun	640	34	14	1550	68	2	8	25
Big Original Chili Dog on a Pretzel Bun	530	25	8	1370	67	2	7	18
Big Original Mustard Dog on a Pretzel Bun	500	24	8	1030	64	1	7	16
Big Original Relish Dog on a Pretzel Bun	510	24	8	1090	67	1	9	16
Big Original Kraut Dog on a Pretzel Bun	500	24	8	1260	65	1	7	16
Big Original Deluxe Dog on a Pretzel Bun	510	24	8	1450	67	2	9	16
Big Original BBQ Bacon Dog on a Pretzel Bun	610	32	12	1340	70	1	12	21
Big Original Plain Hot Dog on a Pretzel Bun	500	24	8	1010	65	1	8	16
Big Original Stadium Dog on a Pretzel Bun	510	24	8	1130	67	1	10	16

Description & Serving	Cal	Fat	Sfat	Sod	Carb	Fiber	Sugar	Prot
Big Original Chicago Dog on a Pretzel Bun	560	24	8	2280	78	2	17	17
Big Original Pastrami Dog on a Pretzel Bun	650	35	12	1730	66	2	8	25
Sea Dog	350	17	3	640	38	1	5	11
Corn Dog	250	17	6	490	15	1	1	7
Mini Corn Dogs, 6	320	22	7	540	22	1	1	8
1/3 lb Spicy Polish Sausage Dog	650	34	11	1750	62	4	10	23

Burger/Sandwich/Burrito

Original Burger	290	9	3	790	29	1	4	20
Deluxe Hamburger	400	19	4	990	33	2	7	21
Deluxe Cheeseburger	450	23	7	1250	33	2	7	23
Chili Cheeseburger	350	13	5	1270	29	1	2	25
Chili Burger	310	9	3	1000	29	1	2	22
Double Chili Cheeseburger	560	24	10	2270	35	2	4	45
Pastrami Burger	510	26	9	1050	30	1	4	34
Pastrami Sandwich	580	34	11	1680	36	2	2	30
Polish Sausage Sandwich	490	29	11	1870	39	3	4	22
Italian Sausage Sandwich	350	17	4	940	31	2	6	17
Italian Sausage Sandwich - mustard only	350	18	4	950	28	1	6	17
Chicken Deluxe Sandwich	430	21	9	970	37	2	4	23
Chipotle Ranch Pupsters	440	24	7	980	43	2	11	23
Chili Cheese Fries Burrito	470	21	9	1650	53	3	2	14

Side

Fries, reg	300	22	11	400	25	2	0	2
Fries, lrg	430	31	15	630	35	3	0	3
Chili Cheese Fries	540	38	19	1380	39	4	1	12
Jalapeno Poppers, 3	210	11	6	670	21	2	3	6
Side Salad	70	5	3	95	2	1	1	4

Dressing/Condiment

Ranch Dressing, 35 g	160	17	3	320	2	0	1	1
Italian Dressing, 12 g	40	4	1	115	1	0	1	0
Syrup	120	0	0	25	31	0	21	0

Dessert

Old Fashion Sundae, Hot Fudge	400	16	11	250	63	1	50	7
Old Fashion Sundae, Chocolate	390	14	9	250	64	2	51	7
Old Fashion Sundae, Strawberry	370	14	9	220	59	1	48	7
Old Fashion Sundae, Caramel	400	14	9	250	66	1	53	7
Old Fasion Sundae, Pineapple	370	14	9	230	59	1	49	7
Cone, 6 oz Plain	300	11	6	220	49	1	36	6
Cone, 6 oz Chocolate Dipped	490	29	23	240	57	2	42	7
Cone, 4 oz Kids Plain	210	7	4	150	34	1	24	4
Cone, 4 oz Kids Chocolate Dipped	400	25	21	170	43	2	31	5
Banana Split	820	24	12	340	149	8	122	13
Shake, Vanilla	650	23	13	440	110	2	91	13
Shake, Chocolate	650	23	13	480	110	3	91	13
Shake, Strawberry	650	23	13	440	111	2	92	13
Freezee, Oreo	630	25	13	410	99	3	76	13
Freezee, M&M	630	25	15	420	99	2	80	13

Description & Serving	Cal	Fat	SFat	Sod	Carb	Fiber	Sugar	Prot
Freezee, Butterfinger	620	24	14	440	100	3	78	13
Freezee, Reese's Peanut Butter Cup	630	26	14	460	97	3	78	14
Tastee Float, Mountain Dew	440	12	7	290	85	1	75	7
Tastee Float, Mug Root Beer	440	12	7	290	83	1	73	7
Tastee Float, Tropicana Strawberry Lemonade	450	12	7	350	82	1	72	7
Mini Sundae, Hot Fudge	250	9	6	160	40	1	32	4
Mini Sundae, Chocolate	230	7	4	170	42	1	34	4
Mini Sundae, Strawberry	210	7	4	140	37	1	31	4
Mini Sundae, Caramel	140	7	4	170	44	1	36	4
Mini Sundae, Pineapple	210	7	4	140	37	1	31	4

Winchell's

Donut

	Cal	Fat	SFat	Sod	Carb	Fiber	Sugar	Prot
Apple Fritters-Glazed, 1	600	23	3	690	93	5	39	8
Bars-Chocolate Iced, 1	380	19	4.5	490	44	2	14	6
Bars-Maple Iced, 1	380	19	5	480	44	2	14	6
Bear Claw, 1	700	33	8	980	89	4	27	12
Blueberry Fritters-Glazed, 1	540	23	6	490	75	2	38	6
Butterfly-Glazed, 1	530	23	6	620	74	4	30	8
Buttermilk Bar-Chocolate Iced, 1	420	19	4.5	370	61	4	35	4
Buttermilk Bar-Glazed, 1	420	18	4.5	330	61	3	35	3
Buttermilk Bar-Maple Iced, 1	420	19	5	340	62	3	35	3
Buttermilk Bar-Plain, 1	300	18	4.5	330	32	3	10	3
Chocolate Cake-Choc Iced w/ Choc Sprinkles, 1	260	11	2.5	340	42	3	24	4
Chocolate Cake-Choc Iced w/ Rainbow Sprinkles, 1	260	11	2.5	340	42	3	24	4
Chocolate Cake-Chocolate Iced, 1	240	10	2.5	340	36	3	19	4
Chocolate Cake-Chocolate Iced w/ Coconut, 1	290	14	6	340	41	3	19	4
Chocolate Cake-Chocolate Iced w/ Peanuts, 1	280	13	3	340	38	4	19	5
Chocolate Cake-Plain, 1	190	10	2.5	320	25	3	9	3
Donut Holes w/ Cinnamon Crumb Topping, 1	340	17	4	320	46	3	27	3
Donut Holes w/ Cinnamon Sugar Topping, 1	350	13	3	230	59	4	45	3
Donut Holes w/ Coconut Topping, 1	370	21	11	240	44	2	24	3
Donut Holes w/ Donut Sugar, 1	370	16	4	250	54	1	30	2
Donut Holes w/ Sprinkles, 1	360	15	3.5	240	55	2	41	2
Donut Holes-Glaze, 1	270	13	3	230	36	2	22	2
Filled Donut-Vanilla Cream w/ Chocolate Icing, 1	410	16	4	680	59	2	13	8
Filled Jelly Donut-Apple w/ Cinnamon Crumb, 1	450	18	4.5	730	65	3	15	8
Filled Jelly Donut-Lemon w/ Donut Sugar, 1	430	16	4	670	62	2	18	7
Filled Jelly Donut-Raspberry w/ Glaze, 1	480	15	3.5	620	78	3	34	7
Filled Jelly Donut-Raspberry w/ Peanut Butter, 1	480	18	4	620	70	3	29	9
Filled Jelly Donut-Strawberry w/ Peanut Butter, 1	480	18	4.5	620	69	3	28	9
Filled Jelly Donut-Strawberry w/ Sugar, 1	460	15	4	630	74	3	32	7
French Donut-Cherry Iced, 1	270	14	4	340	32	1	16	3
French Donut-Chocolate Iced, 1	270	15	4	350	31	1	15	3
French Donut-Glazed, 1	270	14	4	330	32	1	15	3
French Donut-Maple Iced, 1	270	14	4	340	32	1	16	3
French Donut-Plain, 1	150	12	3	200	8	1	0	2
French Donut-Vanilla Iced, 1	270	14	4	340	32	1	16	3

Description & Serving	Cal	Fat	Sfat	Sod	Carb	Fiber	Sugar	Prot
Old Fashioned-Chocolate Glazed, 1	420	18	4.5	400	59	2	37	5
Old Fashioned-Glazed, 1	410	17	4	360	60	2	37	4
Old Fashioned-Maple Iced, 1	410	18	4.5	370	60	2	37	4
Old Fashioned-Plain, 1	300	17	4	360	31	2	12	4
Pineapple Fritters-Glazed, 1	680	34	8	660	81	2	36	8
Raised Round-Glazed, 1	220	9	2	290	31	1	12	4
Raised Round-Sugared, 1	230	9	2	290	34	1	17	4
Raised Round-Chocolate Iced, 1	220	9	2	310	31	1	12	4
Twist-Chocolate Iced, 1	400	19	4.5	560	48	2	14	7
Twist-Glazed, 1	390	19	4.5	540	48	2	14	7
Twist-Sugared, 1	430	19	4.5	540	58	2	26	7
Wheat & Spice-Cinnamon Crumb Topping, 1	390	19	4.5	390	52	4	26	5
Wheat & Spice-Glazed, 1	310	15	3.5	300	42	3	21	4
White Cake-Cherry Iced, 1	310	14	3.5	350	46	2	26	4
White Cake-Cherry Iced w/ Rainbow Sprinkles, 1	340	14	3.5	360	51	2	31	4
White Cake-Chocolate Iced, 1	320	14	3.5	370	45	3	25	4
White Cake-Donut Sugar, 1	300	14	3.5	350	40	2	19	4
White Cake-Lemon Iced, 1	310	14	3.5	350	46	2	26	4
White Cake-Maple Iced, 1	320	14	3.5	350	46	2	26	4
White Cake-Orange Iced, 1	310	14	3.5	350	46	2	26	4
White Cake-Plain, 1	240	13	3	350	28	2	11	4
White Cake-Vanilla Iced, 1	320	14	3.5	350	46	2	26	4
White Cake-Vanilla Iced w/ Chocolate Sprinkles, 1	340	14	3.5	360	51	2	32	4
White Cake-Vanilla Iced w/ Coconut, 1	370	18	8	360	50	3	27	4
White Cake-Vanilla Iced w/ Peanuts, 1	360	17	4	350	47	3	26	5
White Cake-Vanilla Iced w/ Rainbow Sugar, 1	340	14	3.5	360	51	2	32	4
White Cake-w/ Cinnamon Crumb, 1	340	16	4	410	46	3	24	4

Muffin/Pastry

Description & Serving	Cal	Fat	Sfat	Sod	Carb	Fiber	Sugar	Prot
Apple Spice Muffin, 1	490	19	4	710	77	3	41	6
Banana Nut Muffin, 1	610	33	4.5	640	67	3	39	12
Blueberry Muffin, 1	430	18	4	640	63	1	37	6
Bran Muffin, 1	450	16	3	990	74	8	45	7
Cranberry Orange Muffin w/o Crystal Sugar, 1	470	18	3.5	640	73	4	44	6
Chocolate Chip Muffin, 1	580	27	10	640	82	2	53	7
Cranberry Nut Muffin, 1	670	37	5	640	74	5	43	14
Cream Cheese Muffin, 1	610	27	10	840	81	1	56	9
Double Chocolate Muffin, 1	640	29	9	830	91	3	59	8
Lemon Poppy Seed Muffin, 1	470	20	4	660	68	2	40	7
Pineapple Coconut Muffin, 1	600	27	13	720	83	2	47	7
Pineapple Cream Cheese Muffin, 1	620	27	10	840	83	1	58	9
Pineapple Upsidedown Muffin, 1	470	17	3.5	640	75	1	49	6
Puffies w/ Vanilla Cream Filling, 1	150	8	2.5	250	16	1	3	2
Pumpkin Nut Muffins, 1	580	31	4.5	640	66	4	37	12
Carrot Cake, 1 slice	670	29	9	790	98	4	62	10
Cinnamon Buns, 1	460	18	9	600	68	3	30	8
Cinnamon Rolls-Glazed, 1	630	31	8	710	80	5	30	9
Croissant, 1	510	26	15	940	58	3	14	10
Sticky Buns, 1	400	20	10	560	47	3	13	8

Description & Serving	Cal	Fat	Sfat	Sod	Carb	Fiber	Sugar	Prot
Bread/Bagel								
Banana Nut Bread, 1 slice	430	25	3.5	430	45	2	26	9
Blueberry Bread, 1 slice	430	18	4	640	63	1	37	6
Chocolate Chip Bread, 1 slice	540	25	8	640	77	2	50	7
Cranberry Orange Bread, 1 slice	310	12	2.5	430	49	2	29	4
Cranberry Nut Bread, 1 slice	430	23	3	430	49	3	29	9
Cream Cheese Bread, 1 slice	410	18	7	560	54	0	37	6
Lemon Poppy Seed Bread, 1 slice	330	13	2.5	450	48	1	28	4
Pineapple Coconut Bread, 1 slice	390	17	8	480	54	1	31	5
Pumpkin Nut Bread, 1 slice	370	19	3	430	44	3	24	7
Quesadilla Bread, 1 slice	610	33	9	830	69	2	41	9
Blueberry Bagel-Plain, 1	280	1	0	390	60	2	11	9
Blueberry Bagel -w/ Cream Cheese, 1	380	11	6	480	61	2	11	11
Blueberry Bagel w/ Butter, 1	380	12	8	390	60	2	11	9
Blueberry Bagel w/ Margarine, 1	380	12	2	490	60	2	11	9
Cinnamon Raisin Bagel-Plain, 1	280	1	0	390	59	2	9	9
Cinnamon Raisin Bagel w/ Cream Cheese, 1	380	11	6	480	60	2	10	11
Cinnamon Raisin Bagel w/ Butter, 1	380	12	8	390	59	2	9	9
Cinnamon Raisin Bagel w Margarine, 1	380	12	2	490	59	2	9	9
Egg Bagel-Plain, 1	280	1	0	420	57	1	4	10
Egg Bagel w/ Cream Cheese, 1	370	11	6	510	58	1	5	12
Egg Bagel w/ Butter, 1	380	12	8	420	57	1	4	10
Egg Bagel w/ Margarine, 1	380	12	2	520	57	1	4	10
Jalapeno Bagel-Plain, 1	250	1	0	410	51	1	4	9
Jalapeno Bagel w/ Cream Cheese, 1	350	11	6	500	52	1	5	11
Jalapeno Bagel w/ Butter, 1	350	12	8	410	51	1	4	9
Jalapeno Bagel w/ Margarine, 1	350	12	2	510	51	1	4	9
Onion Bagel-Plain, 1	270	1.5	0	410	55	1	4	10
Onion Bagel w/ Cream Cheese, 1	370	11	6	500	56	1	5	11
Onion Bagel w/ Butter, 1	370	12	8	410	55	1	4	10
Onion Bagel w/ Margarine, 1	370	12	2	510	55	1	4	10
Plain Bagel-Plain, 1	280	1	0	420	57	1	4	10
Plain Bagel w/ Cream Cheese, 1	380	11	6	510	58	1	5	12
Plain Bagel w/ Butter, 1	380	12	8	420	57	1	4	10
Plain Bagel w/ Margarine, 1	380	12	2	520	57	1	4	10
Whole Wheat Bagel-Plain, 1	260	1	0	390	55	4	5	10
Whole Wheat Bagel w/ Cream Cheese, 1	360	11	6	480	56	4	6	11
Whole Wheat Bagel w/ Butter, 1	360	12	8	390	55	4	5	10
Whole Wheat Bagel w/ Margarine, 1	360	12	2	500	55	4	5	10
Sandwich								
Bacon & Cheddar on Plain Bagel	440	14	7	800	57	1	4	21
Bacon & Cheddar on Croissant	670	39	22	1320	58	3	14	21
Chipotle Sandwich on Plain Bagel	660	31	15	840	63	3	8	31
Chipotle Sandwich on Croissant	900	57	30	1360	63	5	18	32
Chorizo Sandwich on Plain Bagel	1040	67	35	1940	67	1	10	44
Chorizo Sandwich on Croissant	1270	92	49	2450	67	3	20	45
Egg & Cheese on Plain Bagel	780	43	23	1360	64	1	10	34
Egg & Cheese on Croissant	1010	68	37	1870	64	3	20	35

Description & Serving	Cal	Fat	Sfat	Sod	Carb	Fiber	Sugar	Prot
Ham & Cheese on Plain Bagel	610	28	17	1130	62	1	9	27
Ham & Cheese on Croissant	750	43	24	1650	63	3	19	28
Ham, Egg, Cheese on Plain Bagel	830	45	24	1360	65	1	11	41
Ham, Egg, Cheese on Croissant	1060	70	38	1870	65	3	20	42
Ranchero on Plain Bagel	850	45	24	1620	66	1	13	41
Ranchero on Croissant	1080	70	38	2140	67	3	22	42
Beverage								
Hot Chai Tea, 12 oz	280	9	9	130	49	1	38	4
Hot Cocoa, 12 oz	270	9	7	240	46	1	40	4
Hot French Vanilla Cappuccino, 12 oz	290	10	10	290	48	0	38	3
Hot Mocha Cappuccino, 12 oz	280	9	9	280	47	0	36	4
Chai Chilla, 16 oz	630	24	19	270	92	2	71	8
French Vanilla Cappuccino Chilla, 16 oz	650	30	19	430	85	0	63	5
French Vanilla Caramel Cappuccino Chilla, 16 oz	760	30	19	440	111	0	88	5
Mocha Cappuccino Chilla, 16 oz	610	21	20	570	95	1	75	11
Mocha Caramel Cappuccino Chilla, 16 oz	670	19	18	510	115	1	96	9
Strawberry Banana Chilla, 16 oz	400	9	4	10	79	4	62	1

Zaxby's

Description & Serving	Cal	Fat	Sfat	Sod	Carb	Fiber	Sugar	Prot
Appetizer								
Tater Chips	799	53	9	1316	76	8	0	8
Spicy Fried Mushrooms w/o sauce	432	28	6	954	37	3	3	7
Onion Rings	625	41	7	1534	55	4	4	7
Chicken								
Buffalo Wings Meal Deal w/ Fries & w/o drink or sauce	738	39	9	397	53	4	0	46
Chicken Finger Sandwich Meal Deal w/ Fries & w/o drink	1266	69	12	2376	116	9	17	46
Grilled Chicken Sandwich Meal Deal w/ Fries & w/o drink	1071	48.8	8.7	1748	107	7	15	49
Kickin' Chicken Sandwich Meal Deal w/ Fries & w/o drink	1204	67.1	12.1	2630	107.3	8	9	44
Boneless Wings Meal Deal w/ Fries & Sweet & Spicy Glaze, no drink	1098	57.7	10.1	1929	114.5	7	28	32
Big Zax Snack Meal Deal w/ Fries & w/o drink or sauce	766	34	7	1260	78	7	2	39
Niddler Meal Deal w/ Fries & w/o drink	1293	66	11.9	2105	125.6	8.3	19	49
Chicken Parmesan Sandwich Meal w/ Texas Toast & w/o drink	1100	56.5	10.5	2090	105	9	10	45
Chicken Finger Plate w/ Fries, Coleslaw, & Texas Toast	1053	49.9	10.8	1920	91.1	10.9	10	60
Large Chicken Finger Plate w/ Fries, Coleslaw, & Texas Toast	1592	73	16	2701	147	16	13	86
Wings & Thighs w/ Fries & Texas Toast	1138	57	13	1963	80	7	2	79
Large Wings & Thighs w/ Fries & Texas Toast	1676	80	17	2261	134	12	5	106
5 Buffalo Wings	368	23	6	192	0	0	0	40

Description & Serving	Cal	Fat	Sfat	Sod	Carb	Fiber	Sugar	Prot
5 Chicken Fingerz	422	20	3	1317	8	3	0	51
5 Buffalo Chicken Fingerz	424	20	3	1336	8	3	0	51
5 Boneless Wings w/o sauce	390	20	4	1060	29	3	0	24
Sandwich								
Zaxby's Club Sandwich Basket w/ Fries & Texas Toast	1221	69	15	2138	102	8	7	49
Cajun Club Sandwich Basket w/ Fries	1186	56.8	13	2709	107.6	7	14	58
Salad								
The House Zalad, No Chicken, w/ Texas Toast	419	25	12	667	36	5	7	16
The House Zalad, Fried, w/ Texas Toast	757	41	15	1719	43	8	7	56
The House Zalad, Grilled, w/ Texas Toast	607	30	13	1515	36	5	7	50
The Caesar Zalad, No Chicken	327	18	7	712	24	5	3	17
The Caesar Zalad, Fried	665	34	10	1764	31	8	3	57
The Caesar Zalad, Grilled	515	23	8	1560	24	5	3	51
The Blue Zalad, No Chicken, w/ Texas Toast	400	23	11	740	36	6	6	14
The Blue Zalad, Fried & Buffaloed, w/ Texas Toast	753	39	14	2095	46	9	7	54
The Blue Zalad, Blackened, w/ Texas Toast	588	27	12	1712	37	6	6	49
Zensation Zalad w/ Vegetable Egg Roll	836	39	8	2509	77	10	31	49
Kids								
Kiddie Finger Meal w/ Fries	390	17	3	711	34	4	0	23
Kiddie Cheese Meal w/ Fries & Texas Toast	437	20	7	732	55	4	3	9
Bug Bites	140	5	2	125	23	0	9	2
Chocolate Chip Cookie	174	7	4	125	24	1	16	2
White Chocolate Macadamia Nut Cookie	158	8	4	114	20	2	13	2
Unsweet Tea, kids (170 g)	14	0	0	0	0	0	0	0
Sweet Tea, kids (170 g)	76	0	0	0	20	0	20	0
Side								
Nibbler Bun w/o garlic margarine	130	3	1	180	22	1	5	4
Nibbler Bun w/ garlic margarine	160	7	1	210	21	1	5	4
Crinkle Fries	592	25	5	394	84	7	0	9
Basket of Celery	7	0	0	92	2	0	1	0
Texas Toast w/ garlic margarine	144	6	2	268	20	1	2	3
Texas Toast, Dry	99	1	0	226	19	1	2	3
Texas Toast Basket w/ garlic margarine	432	18	5	803	60	4	6	10
Coleslaw	117	8	3	130	10	2	8	0
Chicken Nibbler A La Carte w/o sauce	85	4.1	0.7	265	1.7	0.7	0	10
Onion Rings	312	21	4	767	28	2	2	4
Side Salad	17	0	0	0	4	1	3	1
Dressing/Condiment								
Blue Cheese Dressing, 35 g	180	19	3.5	350	2	0	2	1
Caesar Dressing, 35 g	160	17	2.5	260	2	0	1	0
Citrus Vinaigrette, 29 g	116	10	1	162	7	0	6	0
Honey French Dressing, 35 g	150	12	2	260	9	0	8	0
Honey Mustard Dressing, 35 g	150	13	2	230	6	0	5	0
Lite Ranch Dressing, 35 g	90	8	1.5	390	3	0	1	1

Description & Serving	Cal	Fat	Sfat	Sod	Carb	Fiber	Sugar	Prot
Lite Vinaigrette Dressing, 35 g	50	2	0	290	7	0	6	0
Mediterranean Dressing, 35 g	140	14	2	530	4	1	3	0
Ranch Dressing, 35 g	160	16	2.5	260	2	0	1	1
Thousand Island Dressing, 35 g	230	24	3.5	180	3	0	3	0
BBQ Sauce, 70 g	90	0	0	710	23	1	19	0
Hot Honey Mustard Sauce, 60 g	160	17	3	780	10	1	8	1
Insane Sauce, 65 g	40	2	0	280	6	2	2	1
Ketchup, 9 g	10	0	0	108	2	0	2	0
Nuclear Sauce, 65 g	30	1	0	1650	5	1	2	1
Original Sauce, 62 g	56	5	1	1060	2	1	0	0
Sweet & Spicy Glaze, 70 g	140	2	0	490	30	0	27	1
Teriyaki Sauce, 73 g	110	0	0	1180	25	0	24	2
Tongue Torch Sauce, 65 g	33	1	0	680	6	0	3	0
Wimpy Sauce, 65 g	50	0	0	1340	10	0	7	0
Zax Sauce, 43 g	180	17	3	620	6	0	4	1
Zestable Dip, 36 g	160	15	2	290	5	1	3	1

Beverage

Description & Serving	Cal	Fat	Sfat	Sod	Carb	Fiber	Sugar	Prot
Unsweet Tea, reg (340 g)	28	0	0	0	0	0	0	0
Sweet Tea, reg (340 g)	153	0	0	0	41	0	41	0

Part III
Common Food Guide

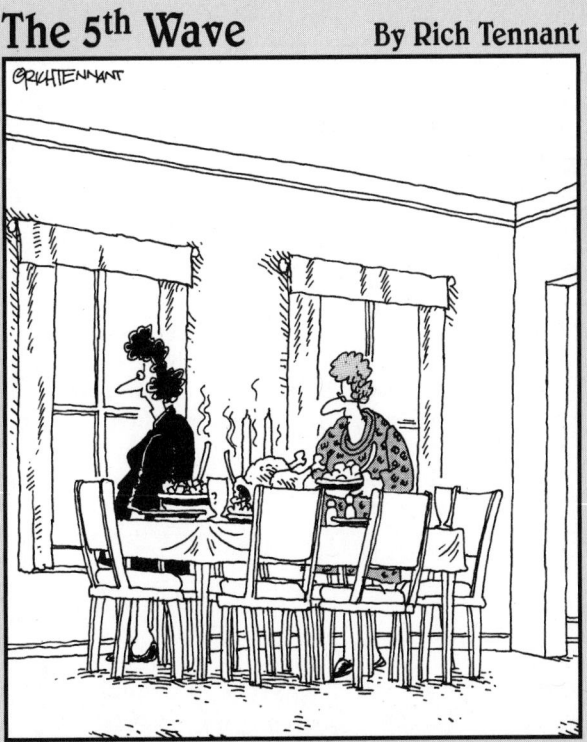

The 5th Wave   By Rich Tennant

"I guess I can't complain about them being late for dinner. I'm the one who insisted everyone take a walk before meals."

In this part . . .

*E*ating nutritious home-cooked meals is an important part of a balanced diet, but unless you're a walking encyclopedia of nutrition information, you probably don't know the nutrition stats for an artichoke versus a carrot. Never fear. This part is your easy-to-digest reference for the nutrient values of common foods. The information is arranged by category (such as dairy, fruits, vegetables, and so on), and the foods themselves are listed alphabetically so you can easily access what you're looking for.

Description & Serving	Cal	Fat	Sfat	Sod	Carb	Fiber	Sugar	Prot

Beans & Bean Products

Beans, 1 cup

Description & Serving	Cal	Fat	Sfat	Sod	Carb	Fiber	Sugar	Prot
Black beans, cooked, boiled, w/o salt	227	1	0	2	41	15	NP	15
Broadbeans, cooked, boiled, w/o salt	187	1	0	8	33	9	3	13
Chickpeas, canned	286	3	0	718	54	11	NP	12
Great northern beans, cooked, boiled, w/o salt	209	1	0	4	37	12	NP	15
Kidney beans, all types, cooked, boiled, w/o salt	225	1	0	2	40	11	1	15
Lentils, cooked, boiled, w/o salt	230	1	0	4	40	16	4	18
Lima beans, lrg, cooked, boiled, w/o salt	216	1	0	4	39	13	5	15
Navy beans, cooked, boiled, w/o salt	255	1	0	0	47	19	1	15
Peas, split, cooked, boiled, w/o salt	231	1	0	4	41	16	6	16
Pigeon peas, cooked, boiled, w/o salt	203	1	0	8	39	11	NP	11
Pink beans, cooked, boiled, w/o salt	252	1	0	3	47	9	1	15
Pinto beans, cooked, boiled, w/o salt	245	1	0	2	45	15	1	15
White beans, small, cooked, boiled, w/o salt	254	1	0	4	46	19	NP	16

Peanut Products

Description & Serving	Cal	Fat	Sfat	Sod	Carb	Fiber	Sugar	Prot
Peanuts, all types, dry-roasted, w/ salt, 1 oz	166	14	2	230	6	2	1	7
Peanut butter, chunk style, w/ salt, 2 tbsp	188	16	3	156	7	3	3	8
Peanut butter, smooth style, w/ salt, 2 tbsp	188	16	4	147	6	2	3	8

Soy Products

Description & Serving	Cal	Fat	Sfat	Sod	Carb	Fiber	Sugar	Prot
Soybeans, cooked, boiled, w/o salt, 1 cup	298	15	2	2	17	10	5	29
Soy milk, fluid, 1 cup	131	4	1	124	15	2	10	8
Soy sauce made from soy & wheat (shoyu), 1 tbsp	8	0	0	902	1	0	0	1
Soy sauce made from soy (tamari), 1 tbsp	11	0	0	1005	1	0	0	2
Tempeh, 1 cup	320	18	4	15	16	NP	NP	31
Tofu, raw, regular, 1 cup	151	9	1	20	4	1	2	16

Breads, Flours, Grains, Pasta

Breads

Description & Serving	Cal	Fat	Sfat	Sod	Carb	Fiber	Sugar	Prot
Bagels, plain, 1	146	1	0	255	29	1	3	6
Bagel, cinnamon-raisin, 1	156	1	0	184	31	1	3	6
Bagels, oat bran, 1	145	1	0	289	30	2	1	6
Bread crumbs, dry, grated, plain, 1 cup	427	6	1	791	78	5	7	14
Breadsticks, plain, 1 small	21	0	0	33	3	0	0	1
Dinner rolls, wheat, 1 roll (1 oz)	76	2	0	95	13	1	0	2
Egg bread, 1 slice	113	2	1	197	19	1	1	4
English muffins, plain, 1	129	1	0	242	25	2	2	5
English muffins, whole-wheat, 1	134	1	0	312	27	4	5	6
French rolls, 1	105	2	0	231	19	1	0	3
French or Vienna bread, 1 slice	277	2	0	624	54	2	2	11
Hamburger or hot dog, 1	120	2	0	206	21	1	3	4
Hard rolls, 1	167	2	0	310	30	1	1	6
Italian bread, 1 slice	81	1	0	175	15	1	0	3
Mixed-grain bread, 1 slice	109	2	0	172	18	3	3	5
Oatmeal bread, 1 slice	73	1	0	162	13	1	2	2
Phyllo dough, 1 sheet	57	1	0	92	10	0	0	1
Pita, white, enriched bread, 1	165	1	0	322	33	1	1	5

Description & Serving	Cal	Fat	Sfat	Sod	Carb	Fiber	Sugar	Prot
Pita, whole-wheat bread, 1	170	2	0	340	35	5	1	6
Pumpernickel bread, 1 slice	65	1	0	174	12	2	0	2
Raisin, enriched bread, 1 slice	88	1	0	125	17	1	2	3
Rye bread, 1 slice	83	1	0	211	15	2	1	3
Wheat (incl wheat berry) bread, 1 slice	66	1	0	130	12	1	1	3
White bread crumbs, 1 cup	120	1	0	306	23	1	2	3
Taco shells, baked, 1	98	4	1	82	13	1	0	1
Tortillas, corn, 1	52	1	0	11	10	2	0	1
Tortillas, flour, 1	94	1	1	191	15	1	1	2
Crispbread, rye, 1	37	0	0	26	8	2	0	1
Matzoh, plain, 1	111	1	0	1	23	1	0	3
Melba toast, plain, 1 cup	117	1	0	249	23	2	0	4
Rye, wafers, plain, 1 cracker	37	0	0	87	9	3	0	1
Saltine oyster crackers, 1 cup	189	4	1	502	33	1	1	4
Wheat cracker, 1	9	0	0	16	1	0	0	0

Flours, 1 cup

Description & Serving	Cal	Fat	Sfat	Sod	Carb	Fiber	Sugar	Prot
Buckwheat flour, whole-groat	402	4	1	13	85	12	3	15
Cornmeal, degermed, enriched, white	587	3	0	11	126	6	3	12
Cornmeal, degermed, enriched, yellow	587	3	0	11	126	6	3	12
Cornmeal, whole-grain, white	442	4	1	43	94	9	1	10
Cornmeal, whole-grain, yellow	442	4	1	43	94	9	1	10
Cracker meal	440	2	0	32	93	3	0	11
Rice flour, brown	574	4	1	13	121	7	1	11
Rice flour, white	578	2	1	0	127	4	0	9
Rye flour, dark	415	3	0	1	88	29	1	18
Rye flour, medium	361	2	0	3	79	15	1	10
Rye flour, light	374	1	0	2	82	15	1	9
Wheat flour, durum	651	5	1	4	137	0	NP	26
Wheat flour, whole-grain	651	5	0	4	137	NP	NP	26
Wheat flour, white, all-purpose, enriched, bleached	455	1	0	2	95	3	0	13
Wheat flour, white, all-purpose, enriched, unbleached	455	1	0	2	95	3	0	13

Grains, 1 cup

Description & Serving	Cal	Fat	Sfat	Sod	Carb	Fiber	Sugar	Prot
Barley, pearled, cooked	193	1	0	5	44	6	0	4
Buckwheat groats, roasted, cooked	155	1	0	7	34	5	2	6
Bulgur, cooked	151	0	0	9	34	8	0	6
Corn grits, white, reg & quick, enriched, cooked w/ water, w/ salt	143	0	0	540	31	1	0	3
Corn grits, yellow, reg & quick, enriched, cooked w/ water, w/o salt (corn)	143	0	0	5	31	1	0	3
Couscous, cooked	176	0	0	8	36	2	0	6
Farina, unenr, dry	649	1	0	5	137	3	NP	19
Hominy, canned, white	119	1	0	346	24	4	3	2
Hominy, canned, yellow	115	1	0	336	23	4	NP	2
Millet, cooked	207	2	0	3	41	2	0	6
Oat bran, cooked	88	2	0	2	25	6	NP	7
Oats, reg & quick & instant, w/o fort, cooked w/ water, w/o salt (oats)	166	4	1	9	28	4	1	6
Oats, instant, fort, plain, prep w/ water (oats), cooked	159	3	0	115	27	4	1	6
Quinoa, cooked	222	4	NP	13	39	5	NP	8
Rice, brown, long-grain, cooked	216	2	0	10	45	4	1	5
Rice, brown, medium-grain, cooked	218	2	0	2	46	4	NP	5

Description & Serving	Cal	Fat	Sfat	Sod	Carb	Fiber	Sugar	Prot
Rice, white, long-grain, reg, cooked, enriched, w/ salt	205	0	0	604	45	1	0	4
Rice, white, glutinous, cooked	169	0	0	9	37	2	0	4
Semolina, enriched	601	2	0	2	122	7	NP	21
Sorghum	651	6	1	12	143	12	NP	22
Wheat germ, toasted, plain	432	12	2	5	56	17	9	33
Whole wheat hot nat crl, cooked w/water, w/o salt, (wheat)	150	1	0	0	33	4	0	5
Wild rice, cooked	166	1	0	5	35	3	1	7

Pasta, 1 cup

Description & Serving	Cal	Fat	Sfat	Sod	Carb	Fiber	Sugar	Prot
Macaroni, cooked, enriched elbow shaped	221	1	0	1	43	3	1	8
Macaroni, whole-wheat, cooked elbow shaped	174	1	0	4	37	4	1	7
Noodles, egg, cooked, enriched	221	3	1	8	40	2	1	7
Noodles, egg, spinach, cooked, enriched	211	3	1	19	39	4	1	8
Noodles, Chinese, chow mein	237	14	2	198	26	2	0	4
Noodles, Japanese, soba, cooked	113	0	0	68	24	NP	NP	6
Spaghetti, cooked, enriched, w/o salt	221	1	0	1	43	3	1	8
Spaghetti, spinach, cooked	182	1	0	20	37	NP	NP	6
Spaghetti, whole-wheat, cooked	174	1	0	4	37	6	1	7

Dairy

Butter, 1 tbsp

Description & Serving	Cal	Fat	Sfat	Sod	Carb	Fiber	Sugar	Prot
Butter, w/o salt	102	12	7	2	0	0	0	0
Butter, w/ salt	102	12	7	82	0	0	0	0
Butter, whipped, w/ salt	67	8	5	78	0	0	0	0

Cheese

Description & Serving	Cal	Fat	Sfat	Sod	Carb	Fiber	Sugar	Prot
Blue, 1 oz	100	8	5	395	1	0	0	6
Camembert, 1 wedge	114	9	6	320	0	0	0	8
Cheddar, 1 cup, diced	532	44	28	820	2	0	1	33
Colby, 1 cup, diced	520	42	27	797	3	0	1	31
Cottage cheese, creamed, lrg curd, 1 cup unpacked	206	9	4	764	7	0	6	23
Cottage cheese, uncreamed, dry, lrg or sml curd, 1 cup unpacked	104	0	0	478	10	0	3	15
Cottage cheese, 2% fat, 1 cup unpacked	194	6	2	746	8	0	8	27
Cottage cheese, 1% fat, 1 cup unpacked	163	2	1	918	6	0	6	28
Cream cheese, 1 tbsp	50	5	3	47	1	0	0	1
Cream cheese, fat free, 100 g	105	1	1	702	8	0	5	16
Edam, 1 oz	101	8	5	274	0	0	0	7
Feta, 1 oz	75	6	4	316	1	0	1	4
Goat cheese, semisoft type, 1 oz	103	8	6	146	1	0	1	6
Goat cheese, soft type, 1 oz	76	6	4	104	0	0	0	5
Goat cheese, hard type, 1 oz	128	10	7	98	1	0	1	9
Gouda, 1 oz	101	8	5	232	1	0	1	7
Gruyere, 1 cup, diced	545	43	25	444	0	0	0	39
Limburger, 1 oz	93	8	5	227	0	0	0	6
Monterey, 1 cup, diced	492	40	25	708	1	0	1	32
Mozzarella, whole milk, 1 oz	85	6	4	178	1	0	0	6
Mozzarella, part skim milk, 1 oz	72	5	3	131	1	0	0	7
Muenster, 1 cup, diced	486	40	25	829	1	0	1	31
Neufchatel, 1 oz	72	6	4	95	1	0	1	3

Description & Serving	Cal	Fat	Sfat	Sod	Carb	Fiber	Sugar	Prot
Parmesan, grated, 1 tbsp	22	1	1	76	0	0	0	2
Port de salut, 1 cup, diced	465	37	22	705	1	0	1	31
Provolone, 1 oz	100	8	5	248	1	0	0	7
Queso Anejo, 1 cup, crumbled	492	40	25	1493	6	0	6	28
Queso Asadero, 1 cup, diced	470	37	24	865	4	0	4	30
Queso Chihuahua, 1 cup, diced	494	39	25	814	7	0	7	28
Ricotta, whole milk, 1 cup	428	32	20	207	7	0	1	28
Ricotta, part skim milk, 1 cup	339	19	12	308	13	0	1	28
Romano, 1 oz	110	8	5	340	1	0	0	9
Roquefort, 1 oz	105	9	5	513	1	0	NP	6
Swiss, 1 cup, diced	502	37	23	253	7	0	2	36

Egg

Description & Serving	Cal	Fat	Sfat	Sod	Carb	Fiber	Sugar	Prot
Whole, raw, fresh, 1 ex lrg	80	6	2	78	0	0	0	7
White, raw, fresh, 1 lrg	16	0	0	55	0	0	0	4
Yolk, raw, fresh, 1 lrg	54	5	2	8	1	0	0	3

Milk

Description & Serving	Cal	Fat	Sfat	Sod	Carb	Fiber	Sugar	Prot
Whole, 3.25% fat, 1 cup	146	8	5	98	11	0	13	8
Lowfat, 2% fat, w/ vit A, 1 cup	122	5	3	100	11	0	12	8
Lowfat, 1% fat, w/ vit A, 1 cup	102	2	2	107	12	0	13	8
Skim, w/ vit A, 1 cup	83	0	0	103	12	0	12	8
Buttermilk, cultured, from skim milk, 1 cup	98	2	1	257	12	0	12	8
Canned, condensed, sweetened, 1 cup	982	27	17	389	166	0	166	24
Canned, evaporated, whole, w/ vit A, 1 fl oz	42	2	1	33	3	0	NP	2
Canned, evaporated, skim, 1 cup	200	1	0	294	29	0	29	19
Dry, skim, nonfat sol, reg, w/ vit A, 1 cup	434	1	1	642	62	0	62	43
Dry, whole, 1 cup	635	34	21	475	49	0	49	34
Goat, 1 cup	168	10	7	122	11	0	11	9

Cream

Description & Serving	Cal	Fat	Sfat	Sod	Carb	Fiber	Sugar	Prot
Half and half, 1 tbsp	20	2	1	6	1	0	0	0
Sour cream, cultured, 1 cup	444	45	30	184	7	0	8	5
Sour cream, cultured, 1 tbsp	23	2	1	10	0	0	0	0
Sour cream, imitation, cultured, 1 cup	478	45	41	235	15	0	15	6
Whipping cream, light, 1 cup, fluid (yields 2 cups whipped)	698	74	46	81	7	0	0	5
Whipping cream, heavy, 1 cup, fluid (yields 2 cups whipped)	821	88	55	90	7	0	0	5
Whipping cream, heavy, 1 tbsp	52	6	3	6	0	0	0	0

Ice Cream, 1/2 cup

Description & Serving	Cal	Fat	Sfat	Sod	Carb	Fiber	Sugar	Prot
Ice cream, chocolate	143	7	4	50	19	1	17	3
Ice cream, strawberry	127	6	3	40	18	1	NP	2
Ice cream, vanilla	137	7	4	53	16	1	14	2
Ice cream, vanilla, light	125	4	2	56	20	0	17	4

Yogurt, 1 cup

Description & Serving	Cal	Fat	Sfat	Sod	Carb	Fiber	Sugar	Prot
Plain, whole milk	149	8	5	113	11	0	11	9
Plain, lowfat	154	4	2	172	17	0	17	13
Plain, skim milk	137	0	0	189	19	0	19	14

Description & Serving	Cal	Fat	Sfat	Sod	Carb	Fiber	Sugar	Prot

Fats & Oils

Fats

Description & Serving	Cal	Fat	Sfat	Sod	Carb	Fiber	Sugar	Prot
Chicken fat, 1 tbsp	115	13	4	0	0	0	0	0
Lard, 1 tbsp	115	13	5	0	0	0	0	0
Margarine, reg, hard, corn (hydr), 1 tsp	34	4	1	44	0	0	0	0
Margarine, soft, corn (hydr & reg), 1 tsp	34	4	1	51	0	0	0	0
Margarine blend, 60% corn oil & 40% butter, 1 tbsp	102	11	4	127	0	0	0	0

Oils, 1 tbsp

Description & Serving	Cal	Fat	Sfat	Sod	Carb	Fiber	Sugar	Prot
Almond oil	120	14	1	0	0	0	0	0
Canola oil	124	14	1	0	0	0	0	0
Corn, salad or cooking oil	120	14	2	0	0	0	0	0
Grapeseed	120	14	1	0	0	0	0	0
Olive, salad or cooking oil	119	14	2	0	0	0	0	0
Peanut, salad or cooking oil	119	14	2	0	0	0	0	0
Sesame, salad or cooking oil	120	14	2	0	0	0	0	0
Soybean, salad or cooking oil (hydrognated)	120	14	2	0	0	0	0	0
Wheat germ oil	120	14	3	0	0	0	0	0

Fruits

Description & Serving	Cal	Fat	Sfat	Sod	Carb	Fiber	Sugar	Prot
Apples, raw, w/ skin, 3.25" diam	116	0	0	2	31	5	23	1
Apples, dried, sulfured, uncooked, 1 cup	209	0	0	75	57	7	49	1
Apple juice, canned or bottled, unsweetened, w/ vit C, 1 cup	114	0	0	10	28	1	24	0
Apple sauce, unsweetened, 1 cup	102	0	0	5	28	3	23	0
Apricots, raw, 1 cup, halves	74	1	0	2	17	4	14	2
Apricots, canned, juice pk, w/ skin, sol & liquids, 1 cup, halves	117	0	0	10	30	4	26	2
Apricots, dried, sulfured, uncooked, 1 half	8	0	0	0	2	0	2	0
Apricot nectar, canned, w/ vit C, 1 cup	141	0	0	8	36	2	NP	1
Avocados, raw, California, 1 fruit, w/o skin & seeds	227	21	3	11	12	9	0	3
Avocados, raw, Florida, 1 fruit, w/o skin & seeds	365	31	6	6	24	17	7	7
Bananas, raw, 1 cup, sliced	134	0	0	2	34	4	18	2
Blackberries, raw, 1 cup	62	1	0	1	14	8	7	2
Blueberries, raw, 1 cup	84	0	0	1	21	4	15	1
Cherries, sour, red, raw, 1 cup w/ pits	52	0	0	3	13	2	9	1
Cherries, sweet, raw, 1 cup, w/ pits	87	0	0	0	22	3	18	1
Clementine, raw, 1 fruit	35	0	NP	1	9	1	7	1
Cranberries, dried, sweetened, 1 cup	383	2	0	4	102	7	81	0
Cranberry sauce, canned, sweetened, 1 cup	418	0	0	80	108	3	105	1
Currants, European black, raw, 1 cup	71	0	0	2	17	NP	NP	2
Currants, zante, dried, 1 cup	408	0	0	12	107	10	97	6
Dates, domestic, nat & dry, 1 cup, chopped	415	1	0	3	110	12	93	4
Elderberries, raw, 1 cup	106	1	0	9	27	10	NP	1
Figs, dried, uncooked, 1 fig	21	0	0	1	5	1	4	0
Gooseberries, canned, light syrup pk, sol & liquids, 1 cup	184	1	0	5	47	6	NP	2
Grapefruit, raw, pink & red & white, all areas, 1 cup sections w/ juice	74	0	0	0	19	3	16	1

Description & Serving	Cal	Fat	Sfat	Sod	Carb	Fiber	Sugar	Prot
Grapefruit juice, white, canned, unsweetened, 1 cup	94	0	0	2	22	0	22	1
Grapes, American type (slip skin), raw, 1 cup	62	0	0	2	16	1	15	1
Grapes, red or green European type (adherent skin), raw, 1 cup, seedless	104	0	0	3	27	1	23	1
Grape juice, canned or bottled, unsweetened, w/o vit C, 1 cup	152	0	0	13	37	1	36	1
Guavas, common, raw, 1 cup	112	2	0	3	24	9	15	4
Kiwifruit, fresh, raw, 1 lrg fruit, w/o skin	56	0	0	3	13	3	8	1
Kumquats, raw, 1 fruit, w/o refuse	13	0	0	2	3	1	2	0
Lemon juice, raw, 1 fl oz	8	0	0	0	3	0	1	0
Lichis, raw, 1 fruit, w/o refuse	6	0	0	0	2	0	1	0
Lime juice, raw, 1 fl oz	8	0	0	1	3	0	1	0
Mangos, raw, 1 fruit, w/o refuse	135	1	0	4	35	4	31	1
Melons, cantaloupe, raw, 1 cup, balls	60	0	0	28	14	2	14	1
Melons, honeydew, raw, 1 cup, diced (approx 20 pc per cup)	61	0	0	31	15	1	14	1
Nectarines, raw, 1 fruit (2.5" diam)	62	0	0	0	15	2	11	2
Olives, ripe, canned (small-extra lrg), 1 lrg	5	0	0	38	0	0	0	0
Olives, ripe, canned (jumbo-super colossal), 1 jumbo	7	1	0	75	0	0	0	0
Oranges, raw, California, Valencias, 1 fruit (2.625" diam, sphere)	59	0	0	0	14	3	NP	1
Oranges, raw, navels, 1 fruit (2.875" diam)	69	0	0	1	18	3	12	1
Oranges, raw, Florida, 1 fruit (2.675" diam, sphere)	65	0	0	0	16	3	13	1
Orange juice, raw, 1 cup	112	1	0	2	26	1	21	2
Tangerines (mandarin oranges), raw, 1 med (2.5" diam)	47	0	0	2	12	2	9	1
Tangerines (mandarin oranges), canned, juice pk, 1 cup	92	0	0	12	24	2	22	2
Papayas, raw, 1 cup, cubes	55	0	0	4	14	3	8	1
Papaya nectar, canned, 1 cup	142	0	0	12	36	2	35	0
Passion fruit, purple, raw, 1 fruit, w/o refuse	17	0	0	5	4	2	2	0
Peaches, raw, 1 lrg (2.75" diam) (approx 2.5 per lb)	68	0	0	0	17	3	15	2
Peaches, dried, sulfured, uncooked, 1 half	31	0	0	1	8	1	5	0
Peach nectar, canned, w/o vit C, 1 cup	134	0	0	17	35	2	33	1
Pears, raw, 1 med (approx 2.5 per lb)	103	0	0	2	28	6	17	1
Pears, dried, sulfured, uncooked, 1 half	197	0	0	1	13	1	11	0
Persimmons, native, raw, 1 fruit, w/o refuse	32	0	NP	0	8	NP	NP	0
Pineapple, raw, 1 cup, chunks	82	0	0	2	22	2	16	1
Pineapple juice, canned, unsweetened, w/o vit C, 1 cup	132	0	0	5	32	1	25	1
Plantains, cooked, 1 cup, slices	179	0	0	8	48	4	22	1
Plums, raw, 1 fruit (2.125" diam)	30	0	0	0	8	1	7	0
Pomegranates, raw, 1 pomegranate (4" diam)	234	3	0	8	53	11	39	5
Pomegranate, juice, bottled, 1 cup	134	1	0	22	33	0	32	0
Prickly pears, raw, 1 fruit, w/o refuse	42	1	0	5	10	4	NP	1
Prunes, dried, uncooked, 1 prune, pitted	23	0	0	0	6	1	4	0
Prune juice, canned, 1 cup	182	0	0	10	45	3	42	2
Quinces, raw, 1 fruit, w/o refuse	52	0	0	4	14	2	NP	0
Raisins, seedless, 1 cup, packed	493	1	0	18	131	6	98	5
Raspberries, raw, 1 cup	64	1	0	1	15	8	5	1
Rhubarb, frozen, uncooked, 1 cup, diced	29	0	0	3	7	3	2	1
Strawberries, raw, 1 cup, halves	49	0	0	2	12	3	7	1
Watermelon, raw, 1 cup, balls	46	0	0	2	12	1	10	1

Description & Serving	Cal	Fat	Sfat	Sod	Carb	Fiber	Sugar	Prot
Herbs, Spices, & Condiments								
Allspice, ground, 1 tsp	5	0	0	1	1	0	NP	0
Anise seed, 1 tsp	7	0	0	0	1	0	NP	0
Basil, ground, 1 tsp	4	0	0	0	1	1	0	0
Bay leaf, crumbled, 1 tsp	2	0	0	0	0	0	NP	0
Capers, canned, 1 tbsp	2	0	0	255	0	0	0	0
Caraway seed, 1 tsp	7	0	0	0	1	1	0	0
Cardamom, ground, 1 tsp	6	0	0	0	1	1	NP	0
Catsup, 1 tbsp	15	0	0	167	4	0	3	0
Celery seed, 1 tsp	8	1	0	3	1	0	0	0
Chervil, dried, 1 tsp	1	0	0	0	0	0	NP	0
Chili powder, 1 tsp	8	0	0	26	1	1	0	0
Chives, freeze-dried, 1 tbsp	1	0	0	0	0	0	NP	0
Chives, raw, 1 tsp chopped	1	0	0	0	0	0	0	0
Cinnamon, ground, 1 tsp	6	0	0	0	2	1	0	0
Cloves, ground, 1 tsp	7	0	0	5	1	1	0	0
Coriander leaf, dried, 1 tsp	2	0	0	1	0	0	0	0
Coriander seed, 1 tsp	5	0	0	1	1	1	NP	0
Cumin seed, 1 tsp	8	0	0	4	1	0	0	0
Curry powder, 1 tsp	6	0	0	1	1	1	0	0
Dill seed, 1 tsp	6	0	0	0	1	0	NP	0
Dill weed, dried, 1 tsp	3	0	0	2	1	0	NP	0
Dill weed, fresh, 5 sprigs	0	0	0	1	0	0	NP	0
Fennel, bulb, raw, 1 cup, sliced	27	0	0	45	6	3	NP	1
Fennel seed, 1 tsp	7	0	0	2	1	1	NP	0
Fenugreek seed, 1 tsp	12	0	0	2	2	1	NP	1
Garlic, raw, 1 tsp	4	0	0	0	1	0	0	0
Ginger, ground, 1 tsp	6	0	0	1	1	0	0	0
Horseradish, prepared, 1 tsp	2	0	0	16	1	0	0	0
Mace, ground, 1 tsp	8	1	0	1	1	0	NP	0
Marjoram, dried, 1 tsp	2	0	0	0	0	0	0	0
Mustard, prepared yellow, 1 tsp or 1 packet	3	0	0	57	0	0	0	0
Mustard seed, yellow, 1 tsp	15	1	0	0	1	1	0	1
Nutmeg, ground, 1 tsp	12	1	1	0	1	1	1	0
Onion powder, 1 tsp	8	0	0	1	2	0	1	0
Oregano, ground, 1 tsp	6	0	0	0	1	1	0	0
Paprika, 1 tsp	6	0	0	1	1	1	0	0
Parsley, dried, 1 tsp	1	0	0	2	0	0	0	0
Parsley, raw, 1 tbsp	1	0	0	2	0	0	0	0
Pepper, black, 1 tsp	5	0	0	1	1	1	0	0
Pepper, red or cayenne, 1 tsp	6	0	0	1	1	1	0	0
Pepper, white, 1 tsp	7	0	0	0	2	1	NP	0
Pickles, cucumber, dill, 1 cup (about 23 slices)	19	0	0	1356	4	2	2	1
Pickle, cucumber, sweet, 1 cup	139	1	0	699	32	2	28	1
Pickle, cucumber, sour, 1 lrg (4" long)	15	0	0	1631	3	2	1	0
Pickle relish, sweet, 1 tbsp	20	0	0	122	5	0	4	0
Pimento, canned, 1 tbsp	3	0	0	2	1	0	0	0
Poppy seed, 1 tsp	15	1	0	1	1	1	0	1
Poultry seasoning, 1 tsp	5	0	0	0	1	0	0	0
Pumpkin pie spice, 1 tsp	6	0	0	1	1	0	0	0
Rosemary, dried, 1 tsp	4	0	0	1	1	1	NP	0
Rosemary, fresh, 1 tsp	1	0	0	0	0	0	NP	0

Description & Serving	Cal	Fat	Sfat	Sod	Carb	Fiber	Sugar	Prot
Saffron, 1 tsp	2	0	0	1	0	0	NP	0
Sage, ground, 1 tsp	2	0	0	0	0	0	0	0
Salt, table, 1 tbsp	0	0	0	6976	0	0	0	0
Savory, ground, 1 tsp	4	0	0	0	1	1	NP	0
Spearmint, dried, 1 tsp	1	0	0	2	0	0	NP	0
Tarragon, ground, 1 tsp	5	0	0	1	1	0	NP	0
Thyme, fresh, 1 tsp	1	0	0	0	0	0	NP	0
Thyme, ground, 1 tsp	4	0	0	1	1	1	0	0
Turmeric, ground, 1 tsp	8	0	0	1	1	1	0	0
Vanilla extract, 1 tbsp	37	0	0	1	2	0	2	0
Vinegar, balsamic, 1 tbsp	14	0	0	4	3	NP	2	0
Vinegar, cider, 1 tbsp	3	0	0	1	0	0	0	0
Vinegar, distilled, 1 tbsp	3	0	0	0	0	0	0	0

Meats

Beef, 3 oz

Description & Serving	Cal	Fat	Sfat	Sod	Carb	Fiber	Sugar	Prot
Brisket	575	22	9	146	0	0	0	89
Chuck roast	257	16	6	42	0	0	0	26
Rib, roasted	298	24	10	54	0	0	NP	19
Shortribs	400	36	15	42	0	0	0	18
Bottom round	210	10	4	37	0	0	0	28
Eye of round	177	8	3	31	0	0	0	24
Tenderloin	223	14	6	48	0	0	0	23
Ground, 95% lean	145	6	3	55	0	0	0	22
Ground, 70% lean	191	13	5	57	0	0	0	18
Ground, reg	251	19	7	65	0	0	0	20
Corned beef brisket	213	16	5	964	0	0	0	15

Lamb, 3 oz

Description & Serving	Cal	Fat	Sfat	Sod	Carb	Fiber	Sugar	Prot
Leg	162	7	2	58	0	0	0	24
Loin	263	20	9	54	0	0	0	19
Leg & shoulder, cubed for stew	190	7	3	60	0	0	0	29

Veal, 3 oz

Description & Serving	Cal	Fat	Sfat	Sod	Carb	Fiber	Sugar	Prot
Leg	128	3	1	58	0	0	NP	24
Loin	149	6	2	82	0	0	0	22
Rib	150	6	2	82	0	0	NP	22
Ground	146	6	3	71	0	0	0	21

Pork, 3 oz

Description & Serving	Cal	Fat	Sfat	Sod	Carb	Fiber	Sugar	Prot
Ham	179	8	3	54	0	0	0	25
Ham, cured	151	8	3	1275	0	0	0	19
Loin	178	8	3	49	0	0	0	24
Center loin chops, bone-in	153	6	2	48	0	0	0	23
Center rib chops, bone-in	158	7	2	48	0	0	0	22
Sirloin roast, bone-in	173	8	2	50	0	0	0	24
Shoulder	194	11	4	68	0	0	NP	23
Spareribs	337	26	9	79	0	0	0	25

Bacon

Description & Serving	Cal	Fat	Sfat	Sod	Carb	Fiber	Sugar	Prot
Bacon, cured, 1 slice	43	3	1	185	0	0	0	3
Canadian-style bacon, 2 slices	87	4	1	727	1	0	0	11

Description & Serving	Cal	Fat	Sfat	Sod	Carb	Fiber	Sugar	Prot
Chicken, 1/2 chicken, boneless								
Light meat, meat & skin, fried, batter	521	29	8	540	18	0	NP	44
Light meat, meat & skin, fried, flour	320	16	4	100	2	0	0	40
Light meat, meat & skin, roasted	293	14	4	99	0	0	NP	38
Light meat, meat & skin, stewed	302	15	4	94	0	0	NP	39
Dark meat, meat & skin, fried, batter	828	52	14	820	26	0	NP	61
Dark meat, meat & skin, roasted	423	26	7	145	0	0	NP	43
Dark meat, meat & skin, stewed	429	27	7	129	0	0	NP	43
Duck								
Meat & skin, roasted, 1 cup	472	40	14	83	0	0	0	27
Meat only, roasted, 1 cup	281	16	6	91	0	0	0	33
Goose								
Meat & skin, roasted, 1 cup	427	31	10	98	0	0	0	35
Meat only, roasted, 1/2 goose	1407	75	27	449	0	0	NP	171
Turkey								
Breast, meat & skin, roasted, 1/2 breast	1633	64	18	544	0	0	NP	248
Leg, meat & skin, roasted, 1 leg	1136	54	17	420	0	0	0	152
Luncheon meat								
Bologna, beef, 1 slice	87	8	3	302	1	0	0	3
Bologna, turkey, 1 serving	59	4	1	351	1	0	1	3
Chicken roll, light meat, 2 slices	63	2	0	604	3	0	0	9
Frankfurter, beef, 1	148	13	5	513	2	0	2	5
Frankfurter, chicken, 1	100	7	2	380	1	0	0	7
Frankfurter, turkey, 1	100	8	2	485	2	0	1	6
Ham, sliced, extra lean (approx. 5% fat), 1 slice	26	1	0	254	0	0	0	5
Ham, sliced, reg (approx. 11% fat), 1 slice	46	2	1	365	1	0	0	5
Salami, beef & pork, 1 slice	41	3	1	178	0	0	0	3
Salami, turkey, 1 serving	47	3	1	281	0	0	0	5
Salami, pork, 1 slice	41	3	1	226	0	0	NP	2
Turkey breast, 1 slice	22	0	0	213	1	0	1	4
Turkey roll, light meat, 1 slice	28	0	0	302	1	0	0	4
Turkey roll, light & dark meat, 2 slices	85	4	1	334	1	0	0	10

Nuts & Seeds

Nuts & Nut Products

Description & Serving	Cal	Fat	Sfat	Sod	Carb	Fiber	Sugar	Prot
Almonds, 1 cup	529	45	3	1	20	11	4	20
Almonds, dry roasted, w/o salt, 1 cup	824	73	6	1	27	16	7	30
Almonds, oil roasted, w/o salt, 1 cup	953	87	7	2	28	17	7	33
Almond paste, 1 oz	130	8	1	3	14	1	10	3
Brazil nuts, dried, unblanched, 1 cup, whole	872	88	20	4	16	10	3	19
Cashew nuts, dry roasted, w/o salt, 1 cup	786	64	13	22	45	4	7	21
Cashew nuts, oil roasted, w/o salt, 1 cup	748	62	11	17	39	4	6	22
Chestnuts, Chinese, boiled and steamed, 1 oz	43	0	0	1	10	NP	NP	1
Coconut meat, raw, 1 cup	283	27	24	16	12	7	5	3
Coconut meat, dried, not swtnd, 1 oz	187	18	16	10	7	5	2	2
Coconut cream, raw, 1 tbsp	50	5	5	1	1	0	NP	1
Filberts or hazelnuts, blanched, 1 oz	178	17	1	0	5	3	1	4

Description & Serving	Cal	Fat	Sfat	Sod	Carb	Fiber	Sugar	Prot
Filberts or hazelnuts, dry roasted, w/o salt, 1 oz	183	18	1	0	5	3	1	4
Filberts or hazelnuts, oil roasted, unblanched, w/o salt, 1 oz	187	18	1	1	5	2	NP	4
Macadamia nuts, raw, 1 oz	204	21	3	1	4	2	1	2
Macadamia nuts, oil roasted, w/o salt, 1 cup	962	103	15	9	17	12		10
Pecans, dry roasted, w/o salt, 1 oz	201	21	1	0	4	3	1	3
Pecans, oil roasted, w/o salt, 1 oz	203	21	2	0	4	3	1	3
Pine nuts, dry roasted, w/o salt, 1 cup	702	57	7	12	34	13	10	26
Pistachio nuts, dry roasted, w/o salt, 1 cup	702	57	7	12	34	13	10	26

Seeds

Description & Serving	Cal	Fat	Sfat	Sod	Carb	Fiber	Sugar	Prot
Sesame butter, tahini, 1 tbsp	89	8	1	17	3	1	0	3
Sunflower seed kernels, dry roasted, w/ salt, 1 cup	745	64	7	525	31	12	3	25
Sesame seeds, whole, dried, 1 tbsp	52	4	1	1	2	1	0	2
Sunflower seed kernels, dried, 1 cup, w/ hulls	269	24	2	4	9	4	1	10
Walnuts, black, dried, 1 cup	772	74	4	2	12	9	1	30

Seafood

Fish, cooked

Description & Serving	Cal	Fat	Sfat	Sod	Carb	Fiber	Sugar	Prot
Bass, freshwater, dry heat, 3 oz	124	4	1	76	0	0	NP	21
Bass, striped, dry heat, 3 oz	105	3	1	75	0	0	NP	19
Bluefish, dry heat, 3 oz	135	5	1	65	0	0	NP	22
Carp, dry heat, 3 oz	138	6	1	54	0	0	NP	19
Catfish, channel, farmed, dry heat, 3 oz	129	7	2	68	0	0	NP	16
Caviar, black & red, granular, 1 tbsp	40	3	1	240	1	0	0	4
Cod, Atlantic, dry heat, 3 oz	89	1	0	66	0	0	0	19
Cod, Pacific, dry heat, 3 oz	89	1	0	77	0	0	NP	20
Cuttlefish, moist heat, 3 oz	134	1	0	632	1	0	NP	28
Dolphinfish, dry heat, 3 oz	93	1	0	96	0	0	NP	20
Drum, freshwater, dry heat, 3 oz	130	5	1	82	0	0	NP	19
Eel, dry heat, 1 oz, boneless	67	4	1	18	0	0	NP	7
Flatfish, dry heat, 3 oz	99	1	0	89	0	0	0	21
Grouper, dry heat, 3 oz	100	1	0	45	0	0	NP	21
Haddock, dry heat, 3 oz	95	1	0	74	0	0	NP	21
Haddock, smoked, 1 oz, boneless	33	0	0	216	0	0	0	7
Halibut, Atlantic & Pacific, dry heat, 3 oz	119	3	0	59	0	0	NP	23
Herring, Atlantic, pickled, 1 oz, boneless	74	5	1	247	3	0	2	4
Herring, Atlantic, kippered, 1 oz, boneless	62	4	1	260	0	0	0	7
Mackerel, Atlantic, dry heat, 3 oz	223	15	4	71	0	0	NP	20
Monkfish, dry heat, 3 oz	82	2	0	20	0	0	NP	16
Mullet, striped, dry heat, 3 oz	128	4	1	60	0	0	NP	21
Perch, dry heat, 3 oz	99	1	0	67	0	0	NP	21
Pike, northern, dry heat, 3 oz	96	1	0	42	0	0	NP	21
Pike, walleye, dry heat, 3 oz	101	1	0	55	0	0	NP	21
Pollock, Atlantic, dry heat, 3 oz	100	1	0	94	0	0	NP	21
Pollock, walleye, dry heat, 3 oz	96	1	0	99	0	0	0	20
Pompano, Florida, dry heat, 3 oz	179	10	4	65	0	0	NP	20
Roe, dry heat, 1 oz	58	2	1	33	1	0	NP	8
Roughy, orange, dry heat, 3 oz	89	1	0	59	0	0	0	19
Sablefish, smoked, 3 oz	218	17	4	626	0	0	NP	15
Salmon, chinook, smoked (lox), reg, 3 oz	99	4	1	1700	0	0	NP	16

Description & Serving	Cal	Fat	Sfat	Sod	Carb	Fiber	Sugar	Prot
Salmon, Atlantic, wild, dry heat, 3 oz	155	7	1	48	0	0	NP	22
Salmon, chinook, dry heat, 3 oz	196	11	3	51	0	0	NP	22
Salmon, chum, dry heat, 3 oz	131	4	1	54	0	0	NP	22
Salmon, pink, dry heat, 3 oz	127	4	1	73	0	0	NP	22
Salmon, sockeye, dry heat, 3 oz	184	9	2	56	0	0	NP	23
Sardine, Atlantic, canned in oil, drained sol w/ bone, 1 oz	59	3	0	143	0	0	0	7
Sea bass, dry heat, 3 oz	105	2	1	74	0	0	NP	20
Shad, American, dry heat, 3 oz	214	15	0	55	0	0	NP	18
Smelt, rainbow, dry heat, 3 oz	105	3	0	65	0	0	NP	19
Snapper, dry heat, 3 oz	109	1	0	48	0	0	NP	22
Sturgeon, smoked, 3 oz	147	4	1	628	0	0	0	27
Surimi, 3 oz	84	1	0	122	6	0	0	13
Swordfish, dry heat, 3 oz	132	4	1	98	0	0	NP	22
Trout, rainbow, wild, dry heat, 3 oz	128	5	1	48	0	0	NP	19
Tuna, fresh, bluefin, dry heat, 3 oz	156	5	1	42	0	0	NP	25
Tuna, yellowfin, fresh, dry heat, 3 oz	118	1	0	40	0	0	NP	25
Turbot, European, dry heat, 3 oz	104	3	0	163	0	0	NP	17
Whitefish, smoked, 1 oz, boneless	31	0	0	289	0	0	0	7

Shellfish, cooked

Description & Serving	Cal	Fat	Sfat	Sod	Carb	Fiber	Sugar	Prot
Abalone, fried, 3 oz	161	6	1	502	9	0	NP	17
Clam, moist heat, 20 small clams	281	4	0	213	10	0	NP	49
Crab, Alaska king, moist heat, 1 leg	130	2	0	1436	0	0	NP	26
Crab, blue, moist heat, 1 cup (not packed)	138	2	0	377	0	0	0	27
Crab, dungeness, moist heat, 1 crab	140	2	0	480	1	0	NP	28
Crab, queen, moist heat, 3 oz	98	1	0	587	0	0	NP	20
Crayfish, farmed, moist heat, 3 oz	74	1	0	82	0	0	NP	15
Lobster, northern, moist heat, 3 oz	83	1	0	323	1	0	0	17
Mussel, blue, moist heat, 3 oz	146	4	1	314	6	0	NP	20
Oyster, eastern, wild, raw, 6 med	57	2	1	177	3	0	0	6
Oyster, eastern, wild, moist heat, 6 med	58	2	1	177	3	0	NP	6
Oyster, eastern, wild, dry heat, 6 med	42	1	0	144	3	0	NP	5
Oyster, Pacific, raw, 3 oz	69	2	0	90	4	0	NP	8
Oyster, Pacific, moist heat, 3 oz	139	4	1	180	8	0	0	16
Scallop, breaded & fried, 2 lrg scallops	67	3	1	144	3	NP	NP	6
Shrimp, moist heat, 4 lrg	22	0	0	49	0	0	0	5
Squid, fried, 3 oz	149	6	2	260	7	0	NP	15

Vegetables

Description & Serving	Cal	Fat	Sfat	Sod	Carb	Fiber	Sugar	Prot
Artichokes (globe or French), cooked, boiled, drained, w/o salt, 1 med	64	0	0	72	14	10	1	3
Arugula, raw, 1 cup	5	0	0	5	1	0	0	1
Asparagus, raw, 1 small spear (5" long or less)	2	0	0	0	0	0	0	0
Bamboo shoots, cooked, boiled, drained, w/o salt, 1 cup (.5" slices)	14	0	0	5	2	1	NP	2
Beans, snap, green, cooked, boiled, drained, w/o salt, 1 cup	44	0	0	1	10	4	2	2
Beets, cooked, boiled, drained, 1/2 cup slices	37	0	0	65	8	2	7	1
Broccoli, raw, 1 cup, chopped	31	0	0	30	6	2	2	3
Brussels sprouts, cooked, boiled, drained, w/o salt, 1/2 cup	28	0	0	16	6	2	1	2

Description & Serving	Cal	Fat	Sfat	Sod	Carb	Fiber	Sugar	Prot
Cabbage, raw, 1 cup, shredded	18	0	0	13	4	2	2	1
Cabbage, cooked, boiled, drained, w/o salt, 1/2 cup shredded	17	0	0	6	4	1	2	1
Cabbage, red, raw, 1 cup, shredded	22	0	0	19	5	2	3	1
Cabbage, red, cooked, boiled, drained, w/o salt, 1/2 cup shredded	22	0	0	21	5	2	2	1
Cabbage, savoy, cooked, boiled, drained, w/o salt, 1 cup, shredded	35	0	0	35	8	4	NP	3
Cabbage, Chinese (pak-choi), cooked, boiled, drained, w/o salt, 1 cup, shredded	20	0	0	58	3	2	1	3
Carrots, raw, 1 cup, grated	45	0	0	76	11	3	5	1
Carrots, baby, raw, 1 med	4	0	0	8	1	0	0	0
Carrots, cooked, boiled, drained, w/o salt, 1/2 cup slices	27	0	0	45	6	2	3	1
Carrot juice, canned, 1 cup	94	0	0	68	22	2	9	2
Cauliflower, raw, 1 cup	25	0	0	30	5	3	2	2
Cauliflower, cooked, boiled, drained, w/o salt, 1/2 cup (1" pieces)	14	0	0	9	3	1	1	1
Cauliflower, green, raw, 0.2 head	29	0	0	21	6	3	NP	3
Cauliflower, green, cooked, no salt, 0.2 head	29	0	0	21	6	3	NP	3
Celery, raw, 1 cup, chopped	16	0	0	81	3	2	2	1
Chard, Swiss, cooked, boiled, drained, w/o salt, 1 cup, chopped	35	0	0	313	7	4	2	3
Chicory, witloof, raw, 1/2 cup	8	0	0	1	2	1	NP	0
Collards, cooked, boiled, drained, w/o salt, 1 cup, chopped	49	1	0	30	9	5	1	4
Corn, sweet, yellow, cooked, boiled, drained, w/o salt, 1 baby ear	9	0	0	0	2	0	0	0
Cress, garden, raw, 1 cup	16	0	0	7	3	1	2	1
Cucumber, w/ peel, raw, 1/2 cup slices	8	0	0	1	2	0	1	0
Eggplant, cooked, boiled, drained, w/o salt, 1 cup (1" cubes)	35	0	0	1	9	3	3	1
Endive, raw, 1/2 cup, chopped	4	0	0	6	1	1	0	0
Hearts of palm, canned, 1 cup	41	1	0	622	7	4	NP	4
Kale, cooked, boiled, drained, w/o salt, 1 cup, chopped	36	1	0	30	7	3	2	2
Kohlrabi, cooked, boiled, drained, w/o salt, 1 cup, sliced	48	0	0	35	11	2	5	3
Leeks (bulb & lower leaf portion), cooked, boiled, drained, w/o salt, 1/4 cup chopped or diced	8	0	0	3	2	0	1	0
Lettuce, butterhead (incl Boston & bibb types), raw, 1 cup, shredded or chopped	7	0	0	3	1	1	1	1
Lettuce, cos or romaine, raw, 1/2 cup shredded	4	0	0	2	1	1	0	0
Lettuce, iceberg (incl crisphead types), raw, 1 cup, shredded or chopped	10	0	0	7	2	1	1	1
Lettuce, looseleaf, raw, 1/2 cup shredded	3	0	0	5	1	0	0	0
Mushrooms, raw, 1 cup, whole	21	0	0	4	3	1	2	3
Mushrooms, enoki, raw, 1 lrg	2	0	NP	0	0	0	0	0
Mushrooms, oyster, raw, 1 lrg	64	1	0	27	10	3	2	5
Mushrooms, shiitake, dried, 1	11	0	0	0	3	0	0	0

Description & Serving	Cal	Fat	Sfat	Sod	Carb	Fiber	Sugar	Prot
Mushrooms, shiitake, cooked, w/o salt, 1 cup (pieces)	81	0	0	6	21	3	5	2
Okra, cooked, boiled, drained, w/o salt, 8 pods (3" long)	19	0	0	5	4	2	2	2
Onions, raw, 1 cup, chopped	64	0	0	6	15	3	7	2
Onions, cooked, boiled, drained, w/o salt, 1 cup	92	0	0	6	21	3	10	3
Onions, spring (incl tops & bulb), raw, 1 tbsp chopped	2	0	0	1	0	0	0	0
Parsley, raw, 1 cup	22	0	0	34	4	2	1	2
Parsnips, cooked, boiled, drained, w/o salt, 1/2 cup slices	55	0	0	8	13	3	4	1
Peas, green, cooked, boiled, drained, w/o salt, 1 cup	134	0	0	5	25	9	9	9
Peppers, sweet, green, raw, 1 cup, chopped	30	0	0	4	7	3	4	1
Peppers, sweet, yellow, raw, 10 strips	14	0	0	1	3	1	NP	1
Potatoes, baked, flesh, w/o salt, 1 potato (2.33" × 4.75")	145	0	0	8	34	2	3	3
Potatoes, baked, skin, w/o salt, 1 potato skin	115	0	0	12	27	5	1	2
Potatoes, boiled, cooked in skin, flesh, w/o salt, 1 potato (2.5" diam, sphere)	118	0	0	5	27	2	1	3
Pumpkin, cooked, boiled, drained, w/o salt, 1 cup, mashed	49	0	0	2	12	3	3	2
Radicchio, raw, 1 cup, shredded	9	0	0	9	2	0	0	1
Radishes, raw, 1 cup, slices	19	0	0	45	4	2	2	1
Rutabagas, cooked, boiled, drained, w/o salt, 1 cup, mashed	94	1	0	48	21	4	14	3
Spinach, cooked, boiled, drained, w/o salt, 1 cup	41	0	0	126	7	4	1	5
Squash, summer, zucchini, incl skin, raw, 1 cup, sliced	18	0	0	11	4	1	2	1
Squash, summer, zucchini, incl skin, frz, cooked, boiled, drained, w/o salt, 1 cup	38	0	0	4	8	3	4	3
Squash, winter, acorn, cooked, baked, w/o salt, 1 cup, cubes	115	0	0	8	30	9	NP	2
Squash, winter, butternut, cooked, baked, w/o salt, 1 cup, cubes	82	0	0	8	22	NP	4	2
Squash, winter, hubbard, cooked, baked, w/o salt, 1 cup, cubes	102	1	0	16	22	NP	NP	5
Squash, winter, spaghetti, cooked, boiled, drained, or baked, w/o salt, 1 cup	42	0	0	28	10	2	4	1
Succotash (corn & limas), cooked, boiled, drained, w/o salt, 1 cup	221	2	0	33	47	9	NP	10
Sweet potato, cooked, baked in skin, w/o salt, 1 lrg	162	0	0	65	37	6	12	4
Sweet potato, cooked, boiled, w/o skin & salt, 1 med	115	0	0	41	27	4	9	2
Tomatoes, red, ripe, raw, year round avg 1 cup, chopped or sliced	32	0	0	9	7	2	5	2
Tomatoes, red, ripe, cooked, boiled, w/o salt, 2 med	44	0	0	27	10	2	6	2
Turnips, cooked, boiled, drained, w/o salt, 1 cup, mashed	51	0	0	37	12	5	7	2
Watercress, raw, 1 cup, chopped	4	0	0	14	0	0	0	1

Description & Serving	Cal	Fat	Sfat	Sod	Carb	Fiber	Sugar	Prot

Beverages

Coffee & Tea

	Cal	Fat	Sfat	Sod	Carb	Fiber	Sugar	Prot
Coffee, brewed, 1 cup (8 fl oz)	5	0	0	5	1	0	0	0
Coffee, instant, 6 fl oz	4	0	0	5	1	0	0	0
Coffee, instant, decaffeinated, 1 cup (8 fl oz)	4	0	0	5	1	0	0	0
Tea, brewed, 1 cup (8 fl oz)	2	0	0	7	1	0	0	0
Tea, herbal, chamomile, brewed, 1 cup (8 fl oz)	2	0	0	2	0	0	0	0

Alcoholic Beverages

	Cal	Fat	Sfat	Sod	Carb	Fiber	Sugar	Prot
Alcoholic beverage, distilled (gin, rum, vodka, whiskey) 80 proof, 1 fl oz	64	0	0	0	0	0	0	0
Alcoholic beverage, distilled (gin, rum, vodka, whiskey) 86 proof, 1 fl oz	70	0	0	0	0	0	0	0
Alcoholic beverage, distilled, all 100 proof, 1 fl oz	82	0	0	0	0	0	0	0
Beer, 1 can (12 fl oz)	153	0	0	14	13	0	0	1
Beer, light, 1 can (12 fl oz)	103	0	0	14	6	0	0	1
Wine, red, 1 glass (3.5 fl oz)	74	0	0	5	2	0	1	0
Wine, white , 1 glass (3.5 fl oz)	70	0	0	5	1	0	1	0

Carbonated Beverages

	Cal	Fat	Sfat	Sod	Carb	Fiber	Sugar	Prot
Club soda, 1 can (16 fl oz)	0	0	0	100	0	0	0	0
Cola, 1 can (16 fl oz)	202	0	0	20	51	0	44	0
Cola, low calorie, w/ aspartame, 1 can (16 fl oz)	5	0	0	28	0	0	0	0
Cola, low calorie, or pepper-types, w/saccharin, 1 can (16 fl oz)	0	0	0	76	0	0	0	0
Ginger ale, 1 can (16 fl oz)	166	0	0	34	42	0	42	0
Tonic water, 1 bottle (11 fl oz)	114	0	0	13	30	0	30	0

Business/Accounting & Bookkeeping

Bookkeeping For Dummies
978-0-7645-9848-7

eBay Business
All-in-One For Dummies,
2nd Edition
978-0-470-38536-4

Job Interviews
For Dummies,
3rd Edition
978-0-470-17748-8

Resumes For Dummies,
5th Edition
978-0-470-08037-5

Stock Investing
For Dummies,
3rd Edition
978-0-470-40114-9

Successful Time
Management
For Dummies
978-0-470-29034-7

Computer Hardware

BlackBerry For Dummies,
3rd Edition
978-0-470-45762-7

Computers For Seniors
For Dummies
978-0-470-24055-7

iPhone For Dummies,
2nd Edition
978-0-470-42342-4

Laptops For Dummies,
3rd Edition
978-0-470-27759-1

Macs For Dummies,
10th Edition
978-0-470-27817-8

Cooking & Entertaining

Cooking Basics
For Dummies,
3rd Edition
978-0-7645-7206-7

Wine For Dummies,
4th Edition
978-0-470-04579-4

Diet & Nutrition

Dieting For Dummies,
2nd Edition
978-0-7645-4149-0

Nutrition For Dummies,
4th Edition
978-0-471-79868-2

Weight Training
For Dummies,
3rd Edition
978-0-471-76845-6

Digital Photography

Digital Photography
For Dummies,
6th Edition
978-0-470-25074-7

Photoshop Elements 7
For Dummies
978-0-470-39700-8

Gardening

Gardening Basics
For Dummies
978-0-470-03749-2

Organic Gardening
For Dummies,
2nd Edition
978-0-470-43067-5

Green/Sustainable

Green Building
& Remodeling
For Dummies
978-0-470-17559-0

Green Cleaning
For Dummies
978-0-470-39106-8

Green IT For Dummies
978-0-470-38688-0

Health

Diabetes For Dummies,
3rd Edition
978-0-470-27086-8

Food Allergies
For Dummies
978-0-470-09584-3

Living Gluten-Free
For Dummies
978-0-471-77383-2

Hobbies/General

Chess For Dummies,
2nd Edition
978-0-7645-8404-6

Drawing For Dummies
978-0-7645-5476-6

Knitting For Dummies,
2nd Edition
978-0-470-28747-7

Organizing For Dummies
978-0-7645-5300-4

SuDoku For Dummies
978-0-470-01892-7

Home Improvement

Energy Efficient Homes
For Dummies
978-0-470-37602-7

Home Theater
For Dummies,
3rd Edition
978-0-470-41189-6

Living the Country Lifestyle
All-in-One For Dummies
978-0-470-43061-3

Solar Power Your Home
For Dummies
978-0-470-17569-9

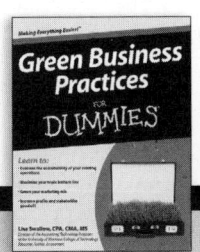
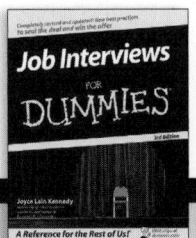
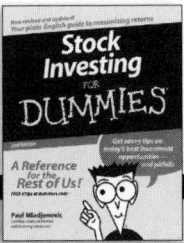
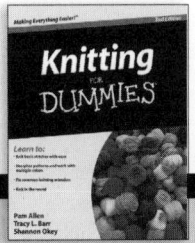

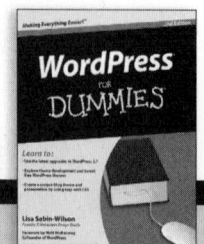 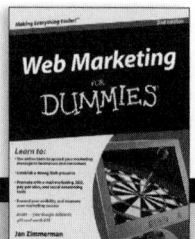 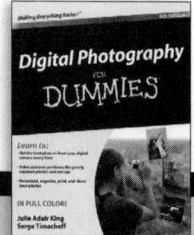 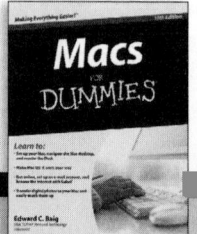